Current Progress in Experimental Pharmacology

Current Progress in Experimental Pharmacology

Edited by **Mark Avis**

SYRAWOOD
PUBLISHING HOUSE
New York

Published by Syrawood Publishing House,
750 Third Avenue, 9th Floor,
New York, NY 10017, USA
www.syrawoodpublishinghouse.com

Current Progress in Experimental Pharmacology
Edited by Mark Avis

International Standard Book Number: 978-1-68286-355-8 (Hardback)

Printed in China.

Contents

Preface

This book aims to highlight the current researches and provides a platform to further the scope of innovations in this area. This book is a product of the combined efforts of many researchers and scientists from different parts of the world. The objective of this book is to provide the readers with the latest information in the field.

Pharmacology is a branch of medical science which has undergone much advancement over time. The recent scientific and technological progresses aided the growth of this discipline. This book is meant for students who are looking for an elaborate reference text on experimental pharmacology and has lucid descriptions of significant topics such as drug-target interactions, pharmacokinetics, drug synthesis, etc. This book contains many latest researches which will be extremely beneficial for students and scholars pursuing pharmacology and allied disciplines.

I would like to express my sincere thanks to the authors for their dedicated efforts in the completion of this book. I acknowledge the efforts of the publisher for providing constant support. Lastly, I would like to thank my family for their support in all academic endeavors.

Editor

The effects of polyunsaturated fatty acids in alcohol dependence treatment - a double-blind, placebo-controlled pilot study

Marina N Fogaça[1], Ruth F Santos-Galduróz[2], Jaqueline K Eserian[1] and José Carlos F Galduróz[3*]

Abstract

Background: The lipid fraction of cell membranes consists of polyunsaturated fatty acids (PUFAS), and chronic alcohol use alters it, modifying its permeability, what might contribute for the dysfunctional metabolism observed in the central nervous system of alcohol dependent patients. Therefore, the supplementation of PUFAS can be an important adjuvant in alcoholism treatment.

Methods: This was a placebo controlled, double blind, randomized study where, 80 alcohol dependent patients, according to DSM-IV, were allocated in four groups with 20 patient each: 'PUFAS', 'Naltrexone', 'Naltrexone + PUFAS' and 'Placebo'. Those substances were administered for 90 days and scales were applied to assess patients craving (OCDS) and alcohol dependence severity (SADD) at baseline and after 90 days. PUFAS serum levels were assessed before and after treatment by high performance liquid chromatography assay.

Results: Forty-three patients completed the trial. There was a significant improvement over time on drinking days, SADD and OCDS scores in all groups ($p < 0.001$). The drinking days comparison between groups did not show statistical significant difference. The same effect was observed for compulsion (OCDS) and severity of dependence scale (SADD). The serum levels of PUFAS increased in all the supplemented groups after treatment, although not significantly.

Conclusions: The oral supplementation of 2 g PUFAS for 3 months did not significantly differ from placebo in reducing the amount of alcohol ingestion, or OCDS and SADD scores in a group of alcohol dependent patient.

Trial registration: NCT01211769

Background

Polyunsaturated fatty acids (PUFAS) are unsaturated fatty acids whose carbon chain has more than one double bond per molecule. Of those, omega-3 (n-3) and omega-6 (n-6) are known as "essential" fatty acids, as humans are unable to synthesize them.

The n-3 series are derived from alpha-linolenic acid (ALA) and the n-6 series, from linoleic acid (LA). The main ALA derivates are eicosapentaenoic acid (EPA) and docosahexaenoic acid (DHA). Gamma linolenic acid (GLA), dihomogamma linolenic acid (DGLA) and arachidonic acid (AA) are the main LA products. GLA is produced from LA by the enzyme delta-6-desaturase and is further metabolized to DGLA. A small amount of DGLA can also be converted to AA by the enzyme delta-5-desaturase. Human conversion of ALA and LA to their derivates is limited, and the existence of them depends on the ingestion of certain food sources.

PUFAS are key components to the brain and count up to 15-20% of its dry mass [1]. Other relevant roles of PUFAS are the influence over fluidity of neuronal membranes and acting as second messengers in neurotransmitter systems [2]. According to Naliwaiko, et al. [3], changes in cell membrane fatty acid composition occurs in the central nervous system (CNS) depending on PUFAS dietary intake [4,5]. Therefore it has been postulated that adequate supplementation of omega-3 and omega-6 would have beneficial effects on brain

* Correspondence: galduroz@psicobio.epm.br
[3]Psychobiology Department, Federal University of São Paulo, Edifício de Ciências Biomédicas, Rua Botucatu 862 - 1° Andar, São Paulo, Brasil
Full list of author information is available at the end of the article

functions, although the ratio between them has not yet been established [6].

Omega-3 fatty acids have been associated with several benefits. This is particularly true for two essential fatty acids of the omega-3 family; docosahexaenoic acid (DHA) and eicosapentaenoic acid (EPA). As an example, it has been used as an adjuvant treatment of systemic hypertension, Crohn's disease, rheumatoid arthritis, age-related macular disease and asthma with favorable outcomes. There are also reports of effectiveness in reducing risk of primary cardiac and promising data on the prevention of breast and lung cancer [7,8].

In psychiatry, the strongest evidence of the beneficial effects of omega-3 is in mood disorders. A meta-analysis involving patients with major depressive disorder and bipolar disorder provided evidence that 1 to 2 grams daily of omega-3 PUFA supplementation can reduce symptoms of depression [9]. Furthermore, it has been suggested that supplementation with eicosapentaenoic acid may be more beneficial than that of docosahexaenoic acid in these disorders [10-12]. Although several factors do not allow definitive conclusions about what kind of omega-3 would bring better results. Other studies also support the action of PUFAS in reducing the number of relapses of cocaine addicts, minimizing the aggressiveness [13,14], improving bipolar disorders [15] and borderline personality disorder symptoms [16,17].

In 1987, Glen et al. summarized alcohol effects in PUFAS metabolism. He stated that ethanol consumption leads to an increase in the ratio of linoleic to arachidonic acid in the phospholipids of tissues. Some of the main contributors for this PUFAS altered ratio would be a reduced intake, absorption, and alteration in fatty acid metabolism [18]. Alcohol also inhibits ∂-6 and ∂-5-desaturases, enzymes associated with the conversion of linoleic acid to gamma linolenic (GLA), and dihomogamma linolenic acids to arachidonic acid [19]. Moreover alcohol has a direct effect on cell membranes composition. A relative increase in n-6 PUFAS in the membranes increases the fluidity resulting in cell damage. Interestingly, it has been reported that this pathological effect could be reduced, at least partially by fatty acid supplementation, especially n-3 PUFAS [18].

Previous studies have evaluated the role of PUFAS in alcoholism. They are linked to the action of neurotransmitters [20], liver damage produced by alcohol [21,22], their effects on tolerance [23] and even as attenuators of the negative effects of chronic alcohol use [24]. Treatment with omega-3 looks promising, but few studies have been published so far. Further studies are needed to identify individuals likely to be benefited by this type of treatment, assess the durability of these effects and to determine dosage and treatment time recommended [25].

There is no literature to date, associating PUFAS as a potential treatment to prevent compulsion for alcohol. This association seems plausible, since the lipid fraction of cell membranes consists of PUFAS, and chronic alcohol use alter the absorption of these acids, modifying its permeability. The aim of this study was to investigate the effects of PUFAS in alcohol-dependent patients, and to evaluate the possible reduction in craving for alcohol.

Methods

The present study is a placebo controlled, double blind, randomized trial. It was approved by the Institutional Board Review (IRB) at Federal University of Sao Paulo - UNIFESP (CEP 0185/06).

Patients Selection

The research was announced in the media (radio and Metro newspaper) and Federal University of Sao Paulo internal network, and followed by an initial selection of volunteers (initial telephone contact). For this initial screening, the inclusion criteria were: male subjects, aged between 30 and 50, dependent of alcohol according to DSM-IV [26], with no history of known clinical disease, Axis I psychiatric comorbidities, or other substance misuse in the past month (except for tobacco).

After the screening, patients were invited to a clinical interview. The interview included medical and psychiatric history and physical examination. Following the interview, volunteers underwent laboratorial workup which consisted of: uric acid, albumin, amylase, bilirubin and fractions, calcium, phosphorus, total cholesterol, HDL, LDL, creatinine, alkaline phosphatase, fasting glucose, complete blood count, lipid profile T3, T4 and TSH, SGOT, SGPT, triglycerides, urea, urinalysis, VDRL, Serologic tests for (Hepatitis A, Hepatitis B, Hepatitis C, Chagas disease and Elisa for HIV), Screening for drugs of abuse (cocaine, THC, methamphetamine, barbiturates, phencyclidine, amphetamine, morphine and benzodiazepines).

The volunteers eligible to participate in the study received written information pertinent to the research, including the safety aspects and risks of the administered substances, and signed the informed consent.

Treatment arms

After selection patients were randomized into four groups: 'Placebo', 'Naltrexone', 'PUFAS' and 'Naltrexone + PUFAS'. The composition of PUFAS capsules was of 1 g *Borago officinalis* oil (rich in omega 6) and another of 1 g of fish oil (rich in omega 3). The capsules were provided from Herbarium Laboratório Botânico (Colombo, PR, Brazil) and contained respectively 120 mg of GLA and 400 mg EPA + DHA, which corresponds to a ratio of approximately (3, 5: 1) between omega-3 and omega-6, similar to the previous ratio suggested benefic [6]. The fish oil capsule composition was 160 mg of EPA and 240 mg of DHA. Capsules of liquid paraffin composed the placebo version of PUFAS. Cristália Produtos Químicos Farmacêuticos LTDA (Itapira, SP, Brazil) provided Naltrexone 50 mg and also identical placebo-Naltrexone pills.

The medications were administered daily, after an initial period of seven days of detoxification. Patients were then followed monthly for 90 days, allowing observation of possible side effects that might implicate in volunteers exclusion from the study. Patient returned the empty bottles of medication on each visit (end of first, second and third month), as well as a calendar with the marked days in which they took the medication.

Follow-up measurements

The serum level of PUFAS (EPA, DHA, AA and Linoleic acid) was dosed at the baseline and last day of follow-up. The quantification protocol of PUFAS dosage was conducted as described by Naliwako et al [3] using the high performance liquid chromatography technique (HPLC). Briefly, total lipids were extracted from plasma, using chloroform-methanol (2:1 vol/vol). Fatty acids were derivatized with 4-bromomethyl-7-coumarin and then separated on a Shimadzu LC-10A high performance liquid chromatograph using an octa- decylsilica column (25 cm £ 4:6 mm i.d.; particle size 5 mm). Fatty acids were resolved isocratically using a mobile phase of acetonitrile-water (gradient from 77:23 to 90:10 vol/vol) at a flow rate of 1 ml/min. Fatty acid derivatives were detected by fluorescence (325-nm excitation; 395-nm emission).

During the study, two scales were applied to assess patients craving and alcohol dependence severity, at the baseline visit and three months after the initiation of treatment. The SADD questionnaire (Short Alcohol Dependence Data), a self-completion questionnaire designed to evaluate the presence and the degree of severity of alcohol dependence, adapted and validated for use in Brazil by Jorge & Masur [27]; and the OCDS Scale (Obsessive-Compulsive Drinking Scale), also a self rating scale, looking at obsessive thinking and compulsive desire to use alcohol.

Statistical Analysis

Continuous variables were tested by means of tests of normality, to verify pre-requisites for the implementation of parametric tests. Shapiro Wilk tests were performed for normality and variables without normal distribution were tested with non-parametric tests. To assess whether in baseline, the groups had similar results in relation to the "drinking days" and measures of the scales SADD and OCDS, we used the non-parametric test Kruskal-Wallis, which showed no statistical difference between groups. To compare if there were differences on Drinking Days or SADD and OCDS scales between the groups and over the time of follow-up, repeated measures ANOVA were performed.

To assess if there was any difference between the analyzed groups, scores of SADD and OCDS were ranked, and chi-square tests were performed. SADD questionnaire was ranked in "low dependence" (1 - 9), "medium dependence" (10 - 19) and "high dependence" (20 - 45), as previously reported by Raistrick *et al* [28]. The OCDS scores were separated in "insignificant" (0 - 5), "low craving" (6 - 14), "medium craving" (15 - 25) and "severe craving" (26 and above), as in previous publication [29].

The statistical software Statistica for Windows (version 9.0) was used to perform the above-mentioned analysis.

Results

A total of 80 patients, 20 per group were enrolled. The groups did not differ at the baseline from demographic characteristics, such as: marital status, educational level or employment status. At the end of three moth follow-up period, 43 patients were still in the study: PUFAS (n = 12), naltrexone (n = 11), naltrexone + PUFAS (n = 9) and Placebo (n = 11). Thirty-seven patients were excluded: 30 due to incomplete follow-up, 2 for clinical complications and 5 were referred to inpatient unit care.

All groups improved at the end of 3 months. The repeated measures ANOVA showed significant effect of time in relation to "drinking days", SADD and OCDS in all groups ($p < 0.001$). At the beginning of the study, patient referred to have drunk in 20.49 (± 9.78) of the 30 days previous to the scheduled appointment. In the final visit it was reduced to 7.95 days (± 10.80).

As for SADD questionnaire, the baseline score was 33.17 (± 10.39) and the final measure was 10.86 (± 13.49). Dependence severity was ranked as: severe dependents 90% of the patients (n = 72), moderate dependents 9% (n = 7) and only one patient was considered to have a low severity. Remarkably, in the final appointment, of the 43 patients that remained in the study, 23% were still severe dependents (n = 10), 14% had a moderate classification (n = 6), 28% were ranked as low dependents (n = 12) and 35% did not point at all in the questionnaire (n = 15). A Chi-square test performed did not show any difference between the groups according to the SADD analysis.

Regarding the OCDS scale, in the baseline assessment, patient had a mean score of 40.81 (± 13.07) and 14, 67 (± 16.33) in the final visit. When ranked, 72 of the 80 patients were considered to have a strong craving, 5 patient a moderate and 3 were classified as low in the baseline moment. When OCDS was last performed, the 43 patients had their craving ranked respectively as strong 21% (n = 9), moderate 16% (n = 7), low 19% (n = 8) and insignificant 64% (n = 19). Again, the Chi-square test was performed, and no difference was observed between the studied groups.

There was no statistical significant difference in the drop-out rate between the studied groups (PUFAS, Placebo, Naltrexone and Naltrexone + PUFAS). There was a statistical significant difference of treatment completion in "drinking days" (p = 0.03). The mean "drinking days" in the last month of patient that completed the trial was 18.46 (± 1.46), while in the "drop-out" group, it was of 23.08 (± 1.57). There was no statistical difference of SADD (p = 0.50) or OCDS (p = 0.69) scores in the baseline moment, between patients who dropped out.

The accumulated data suggest that OCDS scores increases in relationship to the severity of the alcohol dependence syndrome [30]. In our study it was observed a highly significant correlation between the two instruments (+ 0.94). The initial and final mean values obtained for drinking days, SADD and OCDS in each group are demonstrated in Figure 1.

Regarding the laboratory work-up, there was no difference between the groups or over time for total cholesterol, HDL, LDL, alkaline phosphate, SGOT, SGPT, GGT and all other general exams performed. As for PUFAS dosage, the repeated measures ANOVA did not show a significant difference between groups and from the baseline to final visit dosages for EPA, DHA, AA or Linoleic acid. Figure 2 illustrates the results in each group.

No patients had any serious adverse event. Some of them (16, 21%, n = 80) complained of minor gastrointestinal disturbance.

Discussion

In this study, the daily administration of PUFAS and Naltrexone, for a period of 3 months did not significantly differ from placebo in reducing the amount of alcohol ingestion, or OCDS and SADD scores in a group of severe alcohol dependent patient.

Overall all the four groups reduced significantly the amount of alcohol ingestion, dependence severity and compulsion for alcohol, when compared the baseline and the last visit values. This could be possibly explained by the severity of patient's dependence in the present trial. As patients had extremely severe dependence, high scores on SADD scale (mean SADD 33.55; ± 10.09), they might have benefited from the simple fact of been followed for a three-month period, received medical consultation, as well as "pharmacological treatment" (studied drugs or placebo). This could be an explanation of why the placebo group had similar improvement as the other treatment groups.

Several clinical studies have investigated the time and dose-dependent incorporation and successive washout of n-3 PUFAS in different biological tissues following dietary supplementation [31]. The evidence to date indicates that modest amounts of n-3 PUFAS can rapidly change the composition of fatty acids in blood cell membranes. A low-dose approach (1 g/day) appears justified by the concordance of biological and clinical findings. The International Society for the Study of Fatty Acids and Lipids (ISSFAL) for cardiovascular health, recommends a daily intake of EPA and DHA of 500 mg. Hibbeln et al. have proposed that the amount which would protect against major psychiatric diseases should be as high as 3.5 g per day [32]. The present trial supplemented 400 mg of EPA+DHA and 120 mg of GLA, which could not be an optimal dose for patients that are

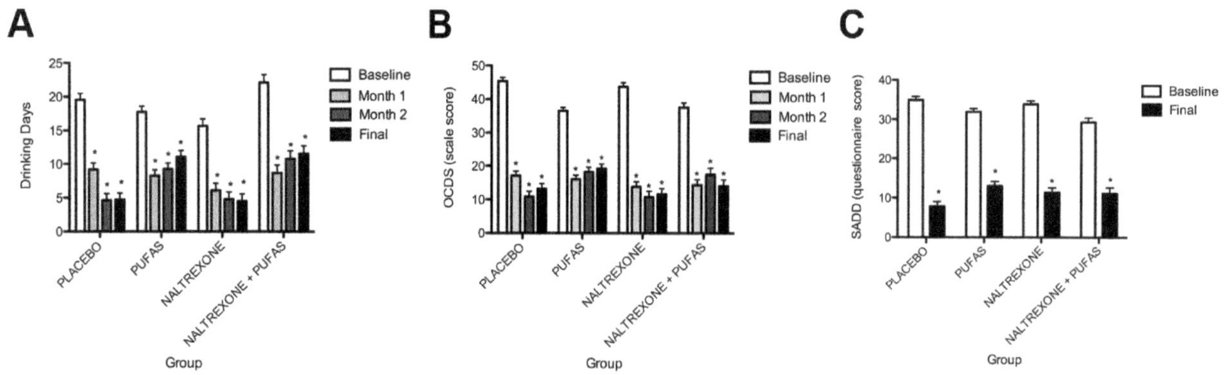

Figure 1 Repeated Measures ANOVA of "Drinking Days", OCDS scale and SADD questionnaire. (A) This graph represents the repeated measures ANOVA comparing the mean values of "drinking days" from baseline over time between the studied groups. (B) This graph represents the repeated measures ANOVA comparing the mean values of OCDS scale from baseline over time between the studied groups. (C) This graph represents the repeated measures ANOVA comparing the mean values of SADD questionnaire from baseline over time between the studied groups. * p values ≤ 0.001.

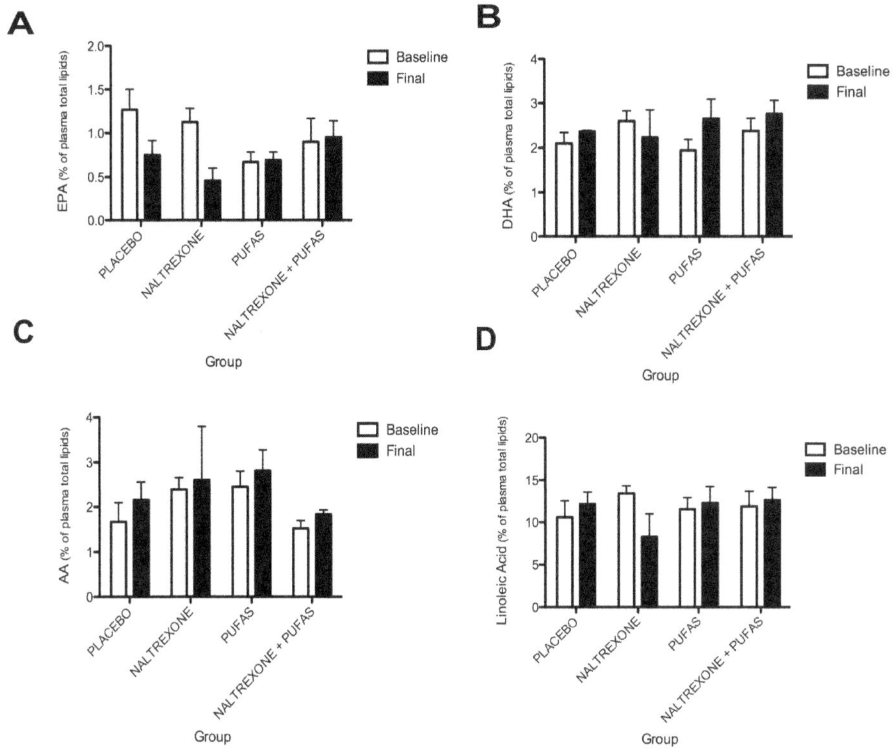

Figure 2 Repeated Measures ANOVA of PUFAS serum measures. (A) This graph represents the repeated measures ANOVA comparing the mean values of the percentage of EPA obtained from plasma total lipids, from baseline over time between the studied groups. (B) This graph represents the repeated measures ANOVA comparing the mean values of the percentage of DHA obtained from plasma total lipids, from baseline over time between the studied groups. (C) This graph represents the repeated measures ANOVA comparing the mean values of the percentage of AA obtained from plasma total lipids, from baseline over time between the studied groups. (D) This graph represents the repeated measures ANOVA comparing the mean values of the percentage of Linoleic Acid obtained from plasma total lipids, from baseline over time between the studied groups.

already depleted from those substances, as alcohol dependents. Therefore, it is possible that the amount of PUFAS administrated was not high enough to benefit the studied population, what could justify the lack of an expected positive effect.

It is important to remark that even though no statistical differences were found between the groups, all PUFAS measurements increased in the groups to whom it was supplemented (Figure 2). Apparently, this increase was less intense in the group that also received naltrexone. Also, in the group that was given naltrexone alone, EPA, DHA and Linoleic acid dosages decreased. This effect could be related to the hipolipaemic effect cased by naltrexone, previously reported in both animal and human studies. Naltrexone prevented the stress-induced increase in total and LDL cholesterol in rats during stress caused by immobilization and a decrease in HDL-C levels [33]. Also, in patients treated with naltrexone, there was a significant decrease in total cholesterol (TC) concentration after 16 weeks of pharmacotherapy. Patients treated with naltrexone had lower mean TC ($P < 0.03$) and LDL-C ($P < 0.01$) than patients of the remaining pharmacotherapy groups [33]. In our study, even with only 12 weeks of treatment, a trend in naltrexone effects over PUFAS, TC and LDL-C could be observed (Figures 2 and 3).

It would have been interesting to obtain a dietary daily report of PUFAS ingestion by those patients. As they were treated on an outpatient basis and many kept drinking during the study, this could have helped to differentiate an inadequate diet from the deleterious effect of alcohol, in incorporating PUFAS to the cell membrane [34].

Another point to consider is the interaction between n-3 and n-6 series. Most of the studied conducted until now, administered only one PUFAS series, usually n-3. The patients enrolled in our study could be extremely depleted in the n-3 series, even more than from n-6 series. If that was true, they could benefit more from n-3 administration as monotherapy. It would be interesting, in future trials, to assess which would be a reference mean rate of PUFAS serum dosages in alcohol dependent patients, what would help to define which PUFAS

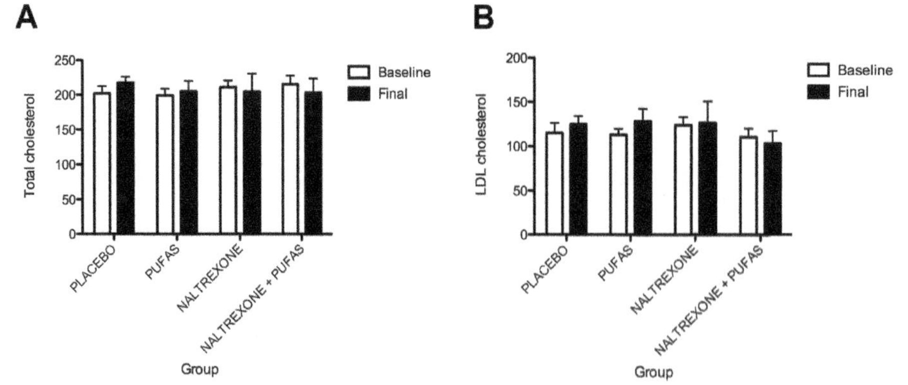

Figure 3 Repeated Measures ANOVA of LDL and total cholesterol. (A) This graph represents the repeated measures ANOVA comparing the mean values of Total cholesterol from baseline over time between the studied groups. (B) This graph represents the repeated measures ANOVA comparing the mean values of LDL cholesterol from baseline over time between the studied groups.

series and dosage of supplementation might bring better outcomes.

An important consideration to be made is that, even though there was an increase on PUFAS serum dosages on the supplemented groups, the lack of adherence to the medications administered is still a concern. Despite being given calendar with dates and times (to check individually) and guided of its correct usage, some patients reported having completed the calendar at the day of consultation, because they forgot to check it in advance.

Comparisons also might have failed to reach statistical significance because the relatively small number of patients failed to lend enough power to the statistical analyses. As in other clinical trials for substance dependence, specially in an outpatient basis, most of the patients who start treatment do not accomplish to complete it [35]. Subsequent studies with more participants are needed to assess the possible benefit of the administration of polyunsaturated fatty acids to alcohol-dependent patients, either as monotherapy or in combination with naltrexone.

Our interpretation of the data should be taken in the context of our study's possible limitations. It should be pointed out that, to date, there is no data on the efficacy of PUFAS in alcohol dependence treatment. There are some studies aiming substance abuse population, but most of them have patient in use of more than one substance or medication such as methadone and antidepressants [6,36,37]. We aimed a very specific population of severe dependent patient that had no clinical comorbidities and in no use of other drugs of abuse as cocaine, heroin, cannabis or even benzodiazepines and other prescribed psychotropic medications.

Study Limitations

Studies aiming substance abuse or dependence and PUFAS supplementation are very limited and to our knowledge, there is no combination proven to have positive effects on alcohol consumption or alcohol dependence severity.

In this study patient were given, 160 mg of EPA, 240 mg of DHA and 120 mg of GLA. The administration of both omega-3 and omega-6 aimed an increase of polyunsaturated and consequent decrease of saturated fatty acids membrane content. A low dosage was chosen because previous studies had demonstrated positive effects in other population. Another major concern in an outpatient trial is compliance, as patient would have to take a greater number of capsules in order to enlarge PUFAS supplementation.

EPA, DHA and GLA are major PUFAS components of cell membrane and have shown several benefits to human health. EPA and DHA are the two types of omega-3 fatty acids that serve as important precursors for lipid-derived modulators of cell signaling, gene expression and inflammatory processes [38]. GLA, a n-6 fatty acid have gained importance in the last four decades for its anti-inflammatory and anti-cancer actions. GLA and its metabolites also affect expression of various genes and play a significant role in immune functions and apoptosis [39]. Omega-6 fatty acids possibly also play a role as second messengers in the process of signal transduction across cell membranes [40].

Several clinical trials have supplemented PUFAS to the most diverse population. There is a wide range of dosage administered and combination of fatty acids. Some examples are a 6-month trial supplementing 80 mg EPA and 120 mg DHA that significantly protected an elderly population from a rise in serum triglycerides [41]; 80 mg AA daily for 3 weeks which increased the composition of AA, but did not decrease the composition of n-3 in young woman [42]; 324 mg EPA + 216 mg DHA + 480 mg LA and 258 mg GLA daily improved pulmonary status, inflammatory and anthropometric parameters in adults with cystic fibrosis [43]; and supplementation with only 200 mg DHA for 2 weeks induced an antioxidant effect, not achieved with 1600 mg [44].

There was an important drop-out from the start of the study until its completion 3 months later (from 80 patients to 43). A drop-out rate was expected, as the study was designed in an outpatient basis, but this loss overcame our expectations. Perhaps if they had additional visits, or associated psychotherapy, we could have had better results. As in majority of trials, patient who do not complete, tend to be the most severe ones. However, there was no statistical significant difference in the drop-out rate between the studied groups (PUFAS, Placebo, Naltrexone and Naltrexone + PUFAS) as previously discussed.

Another curious question is why there were no significant differences from baseline to final visit in EPA, DHA, AA and LA. It is possible that the given dosages were small and as the difference in PUFAS blood dosage was not statistical significant. We also have to consider that patient might not have taken their medication properly. They filled a calendar, as well as returned their empty medication container, but this does not necessary mean that they took the capsules as recommended. It is also important to take in account a possible hypolipaemic effect of Naltrexone as previously mentioned in the text.

Conclusions

The administration of 120 mg of GLA and 400 mg EPA + DHA (160 mg EPA and 240 mg DHA), for 3 months did not significantly differ from placebo in reducing the amount of alcohol ingestion, or OCDS and SADD scores in a group of alcohol dependent patient. Subsequent studies with more participants are needed to assess the possible benefit of the administration of polyunsaturated fatty acids to alcohol-dependent patients, either as monotherapy or in combination with naltrexone.

List of abbreviations

AA: Arachidonic acid; ALA: Alpha-linolenic acid; CNS: Central Nervous System; DHA: Docosahexaenoic acid; DPA: Docosapentaenoic acid; DSM-IV: Diagnostic and Statistical Manual of Mental Disorders; EPA: Eicosapentaenoic acid; GGT: Gamma-glutamyl transpeptidase; GLA: Gamma linolenic acid; HDL: High Density Lipoprotein; HIV: Human immunodeficiency virus; LA: Linoleic acid; LDL: Low Density Lipoprotein; n-3: Omega-3; n-6: Omega-6; OCDS: Obsessive compulsive drinking scale; PUFAS: Polyunsaturated fatty acids; SADD: Short Alcohol dependence data questionnaire; SGOT: Serum glutamic-oxaloacetic transaminase; SGPT: Serum glutamic-pyruvic transaminase; T3: Triiodothyronine; T4: Tetraiodothyronine or thyroxine; THC: Thetrahydrocannabinol; TSH: Thyroid-stimulating hormone; UNIFESP: Universidade Federal de São Paulo; VDRL: Venereal Disease Research Laboratory.

Acknowledgements

Funding for this study was provided by: "Fundação de Amparo a Pesquisa do Estado de São Paulo" - FAPESP, Grant 06/01641-6. The study was also supported by "Coordenação de Aperfeiçoamento de Pessoal de Nível Superior" - CAPES and "Associação Fundo de Incentivo a Psicofarmacologia" - AFIP. FAPESP, CAPES and AFIP had no further role in study design; in the collection, analysis and interpretation of data; in writing the report; or in the decision to submit the paper for publication. RFSG and JCFG receive a CNPQ grant for studying alcohol dependence.

Author details

[1]Psychobiology Department, Federal University of São Paulo, Edifício de Ciências Biomédicas, Rua Botucatu 862 - 1° Andar, São Paulo, Brasil. [2]Laboratory of Physical Activity and Aging of Rio Claro Biosciences Institute - Universidade Paulista Júlio de Mesquita Filho, Rio Claro, São Paulo, Brasil and Centro de Matemática, Computação e Cognição da UFABC, Santo André, São Paulo, Brasil. [3]Psychobiology Department, Federal University of São Paulo, Edifício de Ciências Biomédicas, Rua Botucatu 862 - 1° Andar, São Paulo, Brasil.

Authors' contributions

The study was designed by RFSG and JCFG and JCFG wrote the protocol. Authors MNF and JCFG performed the clinical appointments and JKE was responsible for PUFAS quantification. The statistical analysis was made by MNF and RFSG, and MNF wrote the first draft of the manuscript. All authors contributed to and have approved the final manuscript.

Competing interests

The authors declare that they have no competing interests.

References

1. Yehuda S, Rabinovitz S, Mostofsky DI: **Essential fatty acids are mediators of brain biochemistry and cognitive functions.** *J Neurosci Res* 1999, **56(6)**:565-570.
2. Borsonelo EC, Galduroz JC: **The role of polyunsaturated fatty acids (PUFAs) in development, aging and substance abuse disorders: review and propositions.** *Prostaglandins Leukot Essent Fatty Acids* 2008, **78(4-5)**:237-245.
3. Naliwaiko K, Araujo RL, da Fonseca RV, Castilho JC, Andreatini R, Bellissimo MI, Oliveira BH, Martins EF, Curi R, Fernandes LC, *et al*: **Effects of fish oil on the central nervous system: a new potential antidepressant?** *Nutritional neuroscience* 2004, **7(2)**:91-99.
4. Carlson SE: **Docosahexaenoic acid and arachidonic acid in infant development.** *Semin Neonatol* 2001, **6(5)**:437-449.
5. Fernstrom JD: **Effects of dietary polyunsaturated fatty acids on neuronal function.** *Lipids* 1999, **34(2)**:161-169.
6. Buydens-Branchey L, Branchey M: **n-3 polyunsaturated fatty acids decrease anxiety feelings in a population of substance abusers.** *J Clin Psychopharmacol* 2006, **26(6)**:661-665.
7. Freeman MP: **Omega-3 fatty acids in psychiatry: a review.** *Ann Clin Psychiatry* 2000, **12(3)**:159-165.
8. Mazza M, Pomponi M, Janiri L, Bria P, Mazza S: **Omega-3 fatty acids and antioxidants in neurological and psychiatric diseases: an overview.** *Progress in neuro-psychopharmacology & biological psychiatry* 2007, **31(1)**:12-26.
9. Ross BM, Seguin J, Sieswerda LE: **Omega-3 fatty acids as treatments for mental illness: which disorder and which fatty acid?** *Lipids in health and disease* 2007, **6**:21.
10. Adams PB, Lawson S, Sanigorski A, Sinclair AJ: **Arachidonic acid to eicosapentaenoic acid ratio in blood correlates positively with clinical symptoms of depression.** *Lipids* 1996, **31(Suppl)**:S157-161.
11. Edwards R, Peet M, Shay J, Horrobin D: **Omega-3 polyunsaturated fatty acid levels in the diet and in red blood cell membranes of depressed patients.** *Journal of affective disorders* 1998, **48(2-3)**:149-155.
12. Su KP, Huang SY, Chiu CC, Shen WW: **Omega-3 fatty acids in major depressive disorder. A preliminary double-blind, placebo-controlled trial.** *Eur Neuropsychopharmacol* 2003, **13(4)**:267-271.

13. Buydens-Branchey L, Branchey M, McMakin DL, Hibbeln JR: **Polyunsaturated fatty acid status and aggression in cocaine addicts.** *Drug Alcohol Depend* 2003, **71(3)**:319-323.
14. Buydens-Branchey L, Branchey M, McMakin DL, Hibbeln JR: **Polyunsaturated fatty acid status and relapse vulnerability in cocaine addicts.** *Psychiatry Res* 2003, **120(1)**:29-35.
15. Chiu CC, Huang SY, Su KP, Lu ML, Huang MC, Chen CC, Shen WW: **Polyunsaturated fatty acid deficit in patients with bipolar mania.** *Eur Neuropsychopharmacol* 2003, **13(2)**:99-103.
16. Hallahan B, Hibbeln JR, Davis JM, Garland MR: **Omega-3 fatty acid supplementation in patients with recurrent self-harm. Single-centre double-blind randomised controlled trial.** *Br J Psychiatry* 2007, **190**:118-122.
17. Zanarini MC, Frankenburg FR: **omega-3 Fatty acid treatment of women with borderline personality disorder: a double-blind, placebo-controlled pilot study.** *The American journal of psychiatry* 2003, **160(1)**:167-169.
18. Glen I, Skinner F, Glen E, MacDonell L: **The role of essential fatty acids in alcohol dependence and tissue damage.** *Alcohol Clin Exp Res* 1987, **11(1)**:37-41.
19. Nervi AM, Peluffo RO, Brenner RR, Leikin AI: **Effect of ethanol administration on fatty acid desaturation.** *Lipids* 1980, **15(4)**:263-268.
20. Hibbeln JR, Linnoila M, Umhau JC, Rawlings R, George DT, Salem N Jr: **Essential fatty acids predict metabolites of serotonin and dopamine in cerebrospinal fluid among healthy control subjects, and early- and late-onset alcoholics.** *Biol Psychiatry* 1998, **44(4)**:235-242.
21. Pita ML, Rubio JM, Murillo ML, Carreras O, Delgado MJ: **Chronic alcoholism decreases polyunsaturated fatty acid levels in human plasma, erythrocytes, and platelets–influence of chronic liver disease.** *Thrombosis and haemostasis* 1997, **78(2)**:808-812.
22. Shiraishi K, Matsuzaki S, Itakura M, Ishida H: **Abnormality in membrane fatty acid compositions of cells measured on erythrocyte in alcoholic liver disease.** *Alcohol Clin Exp Res* 1996, **20(1 Suppl)**:56A-59A.
23. Meehan E, Beauge F, Choquart D, Leonard BE: **Influence of an n-6 polyunsaturated fatty acid-enriched diet on the development of tolerance during chronic ethanol administration in rats.** *Alcohol Clin Exp Res* 1995, **19(6)**:1441-1446.
24. Duffy O, Menez JF, Leonard BE: **Attenuation of the effects of chronic ethanol administration in the brain lipid content of the developing rat by an oil enriched in gamma linolenic acid.** *Drug Alcohol Depend* 1992, **31(1)**:85-89.
25. Haag M: **Essential fatty acids and the brain.** *Canadian journal of psychiatry* 2003, **48(3)**:195-203.
26. Association AP: *Diagnostic and Statistical Manual of Mental Disorders.* 4 edition. Washington, DC; 1994.
27. Jorge MR, De Padua FC, Masur J: **Lack of agreement between two questionnaires that evaluate the severity of the alcohol dependence syndrome.** *Drug Alcohol Depend* 1986, **18(4)**:355-360.
28. Raistrick D, Dunbar G, Davidson R: **Development of a questionnaire to measure alcohol dependence.** *British journal of addiction* 1983, **78(1)**:89-95.
29. Araujo RB, Oliveira MS, Nunes MLT, Piccoloto LB, Melo WV: **A avaliac ão do craving em alcoolistas na siíndrome de abstine ncia.** *Psico-USF* 2004, **9(1)**:71-76.
30. Anton RF: **Obsessive-compulsive aspects of craving: development of the Obsessive Compulsive Drinking Scale.** *Addiction* 2000, **95(Suppl 2)**: S211-217.
31. Masson S, Latini R, Tacconi M, Bernasconi R: **Incorporation and washout of n-3 polyunsaturated fatty acids after diet supplementation in clinical studies.** *J Cardiovasc Med (Hagerstown)* 2007, **8(Suppl 1)**:S4-10.
32. Hibbeln JR, Nieminen LR, Blasbalg TL, Riggs JA, Lands WE: **Healthy intakes of n-3 and n-6 fatty acids: estimations considering worldwide diversity.** *The American journal of clinical nutrition* 2006, **83(6 Suppl)**:1483S-1493S.
33. Budzynski J, Rybakowski J, Swiatkowski M, Torlinski L, Klopocka M, Kosmowski W, Ziolkowski M: **Naltrexone exerts a favourable effect on plasma lipids in abstinent patients with alcohol dependence.** *Alcohol Alcohol* 2000, **35(1)**:91-97.
34. Hibbeln JR, Umhau JC, Linnoila M, George DT, Ragan PW, Shoaf SE, Vaughan MR, Rawlings R, Salem N Jr: **A replication study of violent and nonviolent subjects: cerebrospinal fluid metabolites of serotonin and dopamine are predicted by plasma essential fatty acids.** *Biol Psychiatry* 1998, **44(4)**:243-249.
35. Schmitz JM, Mooney ME, Moeller FG, Stotts AL, Green C, Grabowski J: **Levodopa pharmacotherapy for cocaine dependence: choosing the optimal behavioral therapy platform.** *Drug Alcohol Depend* 2008, **94(1-3)**:142-150.
36. Buydens-Branchey L, Branchey M: **Long-chain n-3 polyunsaturated fatty acids decrease feelings of anger in substance abusers.** *Psychiatry Res* 2008, **157(1-3)**:95-104.
37. Buydens-Branchey L, Branchey M, Hibbeln JR: **Low plasma levels of docosahexaenoic acid are associated with an increased relapse vulnerability in substance abusers.** *Am J Addict* 2009, **18(1)**:73-80.
38. Riediger ND, Othman RA, Suh M, Moghadasian MH: **A systemic review of the roles of n-3 fatty acids in health and disease.** *Journal of the American Dietetic Association* 2009, **109(4)**:668-679.
39. Kapoor R, Huang YS: **Gamma linolenic acid: an antiinflammatory omega-6 fatty acid.** *Current pharmaceutical biotechnology* 2006, **7(6)**:531-534.
40. Benatti P, Peluso G, Nicolai R, Calvani M: **Polyunsaturated fatty acids: biochemical, nutritional and epigenetic properties.** *Journal of the American College of Nutrition* 2004, **23(4)**:281-302.
41. Fakhrzadeh H, Ghaderpanahi M, Sharifi F, Mirarefin M, Badamchizade Z, Kamrani AA, Larijani B: **The effects of low dose n-3 fatty acids on serum lipid profiles and insulin resistance of the elderly: a randomized controlled clinical trial.** *International journal for vitamin and nutrition research Internationale Zeitschrift fur Vitamin- und Ernahrungsforschung* **80(2)**:107-116.
42. Hirota S, Adachi N, Gomyo T, Kawashima H, Kiso Y, Kawabata T: **Low-dose arachidonic acid intake increases erythrocytes and plasma arachidonic acid in young women.** *Prostaglandins Leukot Essent Fatty Acids* **83(2)**:83-88.
43. Olveira G, Olveira C, Acosta E, Espildora F, Garrido-Sanchez L, Garcia-Escobar E, Rojo-Martinez G, Gonzalo M, Soriguer F: **Fatty acid supplements improve respiratory, inflammatory and nutritional parameters in adults with cystic fibrosis.** *Archivos de bronconeumologia* **46(2)**:70-77.
44. Guillot N, Caillet E, Laville M, Calzada C, Lagarde M, Vericel E: **Increasing intakes of the long-chain omega-3 docosahexaenoic acid: effects on platelet functions and redox status in healthy men.** *Faseb J* 2009, **23(9)**:2909-2916.

2

In utero exposure to low dose arsenic via drinking water impairs early life lung mechanics in mice

Kathryn A Ramsey[1,2*], Alexander N Larcombe[1,2], Peter D Sly[3] and Graeme R Zosky[1,2]

Abstract

Background: Exposure to arsenic via drinking water is a significant environmental issue affecting millions of people around the world. Exposure to arsenic during foetal development has been shown to impair somatic growth and increase the risk of developing chronic respiratory diseases. The aim of this study was to determine if *in utero* exposure to low dose arsenic via drinking water is capable of altering lung growth and postnatal lung mechanics.

Methods: Pregnant C57BL/6 mice were given drinking water containing 0, 10 (current World Health Organisation (WHO) maximum contaminant level) or 100μg/L arsenic from gestational day 8 to birth. Birth outcomes and somatic growth were monitored. Plethysmography and the forced oscillation technique were used to collect measurements of lung volume, lung mechanics, pressure-volume curves and the volume dependence of lung mechanics in male and female offspring at two, four, six and eight weeks of age.

Results: *In utero* exposure to low dose arsenic via drinking water resulted in low birth weight and impaired parenchymal lung mechanics during infancy. Male offspring were more susceptible to the effects of arsenic on growth and lung mechanics than females. All alterations to lung mechanics following *in utero* arsenic exposure were recovered by adulthood.

Conclusions: Exposure to arsenic at the current WHO maximum contaminant level *in utero* impaired somatic growth and the development of the lungs resulting in alterations to lung mechanics during infancy. Deficits in growth and lung development in early life may contribute to the increased susceptibility of developing chronic respiratory disease in arsenic exposed human populations.

Keywords: Animal model, Arsenic, Environmental exposure, Growth & development, Lung function

Background

Arsenic is a toxic metalloid that contaminates drinking water through both natural and anthropogenic sources [1]. Millions of people around the world are exposed to arsenic in drinking water at levels above the current World Health Organisation (WHO) maximum contaminant level (MCL) of 10μg/L [2,3]. Several studies have established the link between arsenic exposure and increased lung cancer risk; however, emerging data suggest an important role for arsenic in non-malignant lung disease. Epidemiological data have linked arsenic exposure via drinking water to chronic cough [4], chronic bronchitis [5], bronchiectasis [6] and obstructive lung diseases [7]. Ingestion of arsenic in drinking water has also been associated with respiratory symptoms such as shortness of breath and morning cough [8], and decrements in lung function, including reduced FEV_1 (forced expiratory volume in 1 s) and reduced forced vital capacity [8-10].

Of particular concern, is the mounting evidence that exposure to arsenic in foetal or early postnatal life has the greatest effect on respiratory health. Exposure to arsenic *in utero*, through maternal drinking water, has been shown to alter the expression of genes in the lungs at birth in rats [11], and result in the development of pulmonary tumours in adult mice [12]. Following a discrete exposure event in Antofagasta, Chile in the 1950-1970s, it was found that exposure to arsenic *in utero* and early postnatal life resulted in a standardised mortality ratios for bronchiectasis in young adults of

* Correspondence: kramsey@ichr.uwa.edu.au
[1]Division of Clinical Sciences, Telethon Institute for Child Health Research, 100 Roberts Road, Subiaco, WA 6008, Australia
[2]Centre for Child Health Research, University of Western Australia, 100 Roberts Road, Subiaco, WA 6008, Australia
Full list of author information is available at the end of the article

46.2 (95% CI, 21.1–87.7) compared to 12.4 (95% CI, 3.3–31.7) if the exposure only occurred postnatally [13]. These data suggest that early life exposure to arsenic can have profound effects on lung health decades after the exposure event.

Exposure to environmental toxins *in utero* may have significant effects on growth and organ development, and have long term implications for disease risk [14]. Arsenic is a known transplacental toxin which is able to cross the placenta and enter foetal circulation at levels equivalent to maternal circulation [15]. In contrast, low levels of arsenic are excreted in the breast milk and breastfeeding is thought to be protective in arsenic exposed areas [16]. In arsenic exposed areas of Bangladesh and West Bengal, exposure to arsenic during pregnancy is associated with infants being born small for gestational age [17] and at a greater risk of developing lower respiratory tract infections in infancy [18]. A mouse study investigating the effects of *in utero* and postnatal exposure to arsenic, at the current WHO MCL of 10μg/L, found that exposed offspring had significant deficits in growth after birth compared with unexposed offspring [19], highlighting the potency of arsenic as an early life toxicant.

Exposure to arsenic during the critical window of development in foetal life may not just restrict growth, but also impair development of the lungs [20]. Foetal growth restriction is associated with worse lung function and greater respiratory morbidity in early childhood [21-23] and adulthood [24,25]. In this study, we determined the effects of *in utero* exposure to low dose arsenic on somatic growth, lung growth and lung mechanics using a mouse model. We hypothesised that *in utero* arsenic exposure would alter the growth and development of the lungs resulting in impairments to postnatal lung mechanics.

Methods

Animals and exposure protocol

Time-mated C57BL/6 dams (Animal Resource Centre; Murdoch, Western Australia) were housed at the Telethon Institute for Child Health Research with a 12 h: 12 h light/dark cycle. All experiments were conducted with the approval of the Telethon Institute for Child Health Research Animal Ethics Committee and conformed to the guidelines of the National Health and Medical Research Council of Australia. Dams were given drinking water containing 0 (control), 10 or 100μg/L arsenic in the form of soluble sodium arsenite ($NaAs_2O_3$). This water was provided *ad libitum* from day 8 gestation to delivery (~ day 20 gestation) which ensured that the foetus was exposed to arsenic prior to the development of the lung buds (e9) [26]. Concentrations of arsenic in drinking water were confirmed by inductively coupled plasma-mass spectrometry (ICP-MS; Geotechnical Services, Western Australia). Maternal water consumption, gestation period and litter size were recorded along with somatic growth (body weight and snout-vent length) at birth and the day lung function measurements were taken. Lung function was assessed in male and female offspring at two, four, six and eight weeks of age.

Animal preparation

Mice were anaesthetised by intraperitoneal injection of a mixture containing xylazine (2mg/mL; Troy Laboratories, New South Wales, Australia) and ketamine (40mg/mL; Troy Laboratories, New South Wales, Australia) at a dose 0.1mL/10g body weight. Mice were tracheotomised and a tracheal cannula inserted (23G stainless steel for two and four week old mice; 1.26 mm outer diameter polyethylene tube for six and eight week old mice) and secured with suture. Mice were ventilated (MiniVent, Harvard Apparatus, Germany) at a tidal volume of 8mL/kg, respiratory rate of 400 breaths per minute and positive end expiratory pressure of 2 cmH_2O. This elevated respiratory rate was used to suppress spontaneous breathing thus allowing the apnoeic periods required for measurement of lung function without the need for paralysis.

Thoracic gas volume

Plethysmography was used to measure thoracic gas volume (TGV) as described previously [27]. Briefly, the trachea was occluded at end expiration (transrespiratory pressure, P_{rs} = 0 cmH_2O) and the intercostal muscles were stimulated with intramuscular electrodes to induce inspiratory efforts. Six 20V pulses of 2-3ms in duration were delivered over a 6s period while recording changes in tracheal pressure and plethysmograph box pressure. TGV was calculated using Boyle's law after correcting for the impedance and thermal properties of the plethysmograph [27].

Baseline lung mechanics

Lung mechanics were measured using the forced-oscillation technique as described previously [28]. The forcing function (9 frequencies from 4 – 38 Hz) was generated by a loudspeaker and delivered to the animal via a wave tube during pauses in ventilation. The respiratory system impedance spectrum (Z_{rs}) was measured and a 4-parameter model with constant phase tissue impedance was fitted to the data to partition Z_{rs} into components representing the mechanical properties of the airways and parenchyma [29]. This model allowed the calculation of airway resistance (R_{aw}) and inertance (I_{aw}) and coefficients of tissue damping (G) and elastance (H). The resistance and inertance of the tracheal cannula were subtracted from R_{aw} and I_{aw} respectively. As most of the inertance is contained in the tracheal cannula, values of I_{aw} were insignificant and are not reported.

Volume dependence of lung mechanics

The volume dependence of lung mechanics was assessed during a slow inflation-deflation (ID) manoeuvre from 0 to 20 cmH_2O P_{rs}. Inspiration was induced by applying a controlled negative pressure to the plethysmograph and expiration was achieved by the slow equilibration of the plethysmograph to atmospheric pressure through a resistor. During the manoeuvre, an oscillatory signal was applied to the lung as described above. The 4-parameter model was fitted to the Z_{rs} using 0.5s data epochs extracted from the signal during the recording period. By monitoring plethysmograph pressure, integrating flow and calculating starting TGV we were also able to construct absolute pressure-volume curves.

Experimental protocol

To establish a volume history two ID manoeuvres were performed separated with 5 min of regular ventilation. Two measurements of TGV were recorded followed by 6 measurements of baseline lung mechanics at 0 cmH_2O P_{rs}. TGV was recorded again before a final ID manoeuvre (used for analyses).

Statistical analysis

Maternal and birth outcome means were compared by one-way ANOVA using GraphPad Prism (Version 5.02, GraphPad Software, San Diego, CA USA). Somatic growth, TGV and lung mechanics within each sex were analysed by two-way ANOVA using Sigma Plot with Holm-Sidak post-hoc analysis (Version 11.0, Systat Software, Chicago, IL USA). A p value of less than 0.05 was considered significant.

Results

Effects of exposure to arsenic on maternal, birth and growth outcomes

There was no difference in the amount of water consumed per day between dams exposed to either concentration of arsenic or control water ($p = 0.57$), nor were there any differences in litter size ($p = 0.45$) or gestational period ($p = 0.32$) between arsenic and control water exposed mice (Table 1). At birth, offspring exposed *in utero* to 100μg/L arsenic were significantly smaller in weight ($p < 0.001$) and length ($p < 0.001$) than controls, but there were no differences in birth weight or length between offspring exposed to 10μg/L arsenic and controls ($p > 0.47$) (Table 1). The number of offspring tested from each exposure group at each age is shown in Table 2. There was no effect of *in utero* arsenic exposure on body weight in male ($p > 0.58$) or female ($p > 0.22$) offspring at two, four, six or eight weeks of age. Likewise, there was no effect of arsenic on TGV in males ($p > 0.30$) or females ($p > 0.57$) at any age (Figure 1).

Effects of *in utero* exposure to arsenic on early life lung mechanics

Two week old male offspring exposed to 10μg/L and 100μg/L arsenic had higher tissue damping ($p < 0.001$) and tissue elastance ($p < 0.001$) compared to male controls (Figure 2). Two week old male offspring exposed to 10μg/L arsenic had lower airway resistance ($p = 0.03$) compared to male controls (Figure 2). There were no differences in airway resistance between two week old male mice exposed to 100μg/L arsenic and male controls ($p > 0.42$). Although female mice showed similar trends in the data as males, there were no significant effects of arsenic on parenchymal lung mechanics (G, $p = 0.31$; H, $p = 0.64$) or airway resistance ($R_{aw,}$ $p = 0.14$) in two week old female offspring exposed *in utero* to 10 or 100μg/L arsenic via drinking water (Figure 2).

The maximum TGV reached during inflation to P_{rs} = 20 cmH_20 was significantly lower in two week old male offspring exposed to 100μg/L arsenic ($p = 0.02$) compared to male controls (Figure 3). Exposure to arsenic at 10μg/L *in utero* had no effect on maximum TGV during inflation in two week old males ($p > 0.95$ in all cases). There were no significant effects of arsenic, at either dose, on maximum TGV at P_{rs} = 20 cmH_20 in two week old female offspring ($p > 0.41$ in both cases) (Figure 3).

Two week old male offspring exposed to 100μg/L arsenic had significantly higher tissue elastance and tissue damping at P_{rs} = 20 cmH_20 compared to male controls (H $p = 0.02$; G $p = 0.03$, Figure 4). Exposure to arsenic at 10μg/L *in utero* had no effect on tissue elastance or

Table 1 Maternal and birth outcomes for C57BL/6J dams exposed to 0 (control), 10 or 100μg/L arsenic via drinking water (mean ± SD)

	Control	10μg/L As	100μg/L As
Maternal water consumption (mL/day)	5.11 ± 1.41	4.97 ± 1.36	4.91 ± 1.33
Gestation period (days)	20.1 ± 0.92	20.4 ± 0.88	20.0 ± 0.81
Litter size (pups/dam)	5.63 ± 1.98	4.79 ± 1.87	5.54 ± 2.23
Birth weight (g)	1.34 ± 0.16	1.35 ± 0.19	1.27 ± 0.18 *
Birth length (mm)	29.1 ± 1.74	28.8 ± 1.94	28.4 ± 1.90 *

There were no differences in maternal water consumption, gestation period or litter size between control and arsenic exposed mice. Offspring exposed to 100μg/L arsenic were born significantly smaller than control mice in both weight and length (* indicates significantly different to controls).

Table 2 Numbers of offspring tested at each age from each exposure group.

Numbers of offspring tested	Control	10μg/L As	100μg/L As
2 weeks - males	24	11	23
2 weeks - females	25	13	15
4 weeks - males	22	9	7
4 weeks - females	13	9	9
6 weeks - males	14	7	24
6 weeks - females	14	4	11
8 weeks - males	17	5	12
8 weeks - females	17	9	12

tissue damping at P_{rs} = 20 cmH_20 in two week old males (G and H, $p > 0.33$). There were no differences in airway resistance at P_{rs} = 20 cmH_20 between two week old male offspring exposed to arsenic and control water ($p > 0.21$ in all cases, Figure 3). Exposure to arsenic at 10 or 100μg/L *in utero* had no effect on parenchymal mechanics (G or H, $p > 0.54$) or airway resistance (R_{aw} $p > 0.30$, in all cases) at P_{rs} = 20 cmH_20 in females at two weeks (Figure 4).

Effects of *in utero* exposure to on lung mechanics throughout life

There were no significant effects of arsenic on tissue damping ($p > 0.31$) or tissue elastance ($p > 0.61$, Figure 5) in male or female offspring at 4, 6 or 8 weeks of age. There were also no effects of arsenic on airway resistance ($p > 0.34$) in either male or female offspring at 4, 6 or 8 weeks of age (data not shown). There were no effects of arsenic maximum TGV at P_{rs} = 20 cmH_20 in male or female offspring at 4, 6 or 8 weeks of age compared to controls ($p > 0.47$ in all cases, data not shown). There were also no effects of arsenic on airway or parenchymal mechanics at P_{rs} = 20 cmH_20 in male or female offspring at 4, 6 and 8 weeks of age ($p > 0.21$ in all cases, data not shown).

Discussion

In this study a brief exposure of pregnant mice to environmentally low doses of arsenic altered *in utero* growth and lung development of their offspring resulting in deficits in postnatal lung mechanics. This is the first study to show that *in utero* exposure alone to low doses of arsenic via drinking water is capable of impairing postnatal lung function. Exposure to the current WHO MCL of 10μg/L arsenic significantly impaired lung function suggesting that the current MCL may fail to protect against the non-malignant effects of arsenic on the lung. The lung mechanics of male mice were impaired more than those of female mice indicating that males may be more susceptible to the adverse effects of arsenic on the lungs. These deficits in lung mechanics were evident in early life but resolved with age.

Arsenic exposure had a direct effect on *in utero* growth in male offspring exposed to 100μg/L resulting in lower birth weight and length in males compared with

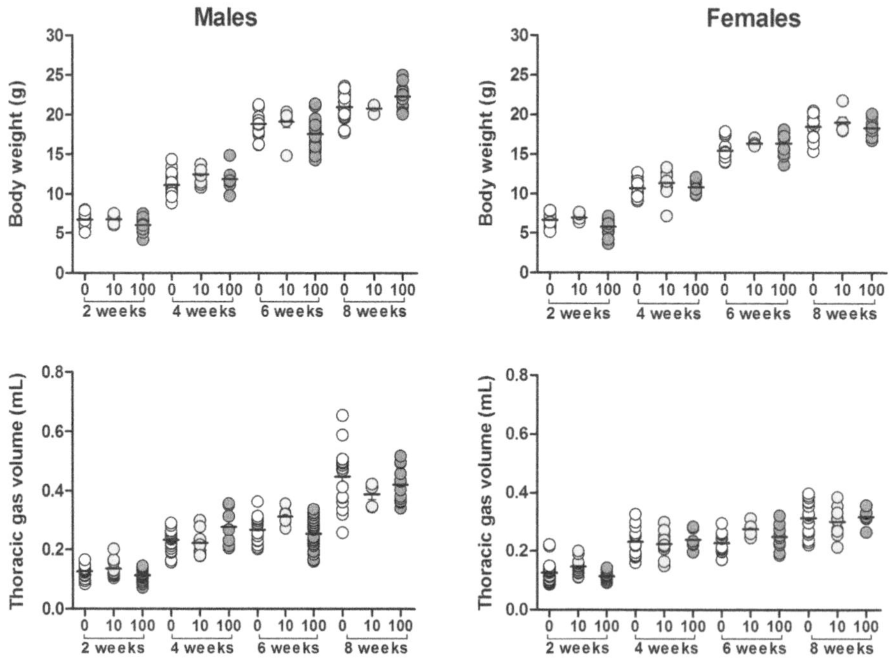

Figure 1 Body weight and thoracic gas volume in two, four, six and eight week old male and female C57BL/6 offspring exposed *in utero* to drinking water containing 0 (control), 10 or 100μg/L arsenic (mean). There were no differences in body weight or thoracic gas volume between offspring exposed to arsenic and controls at two, four, six or eight weeks of age.

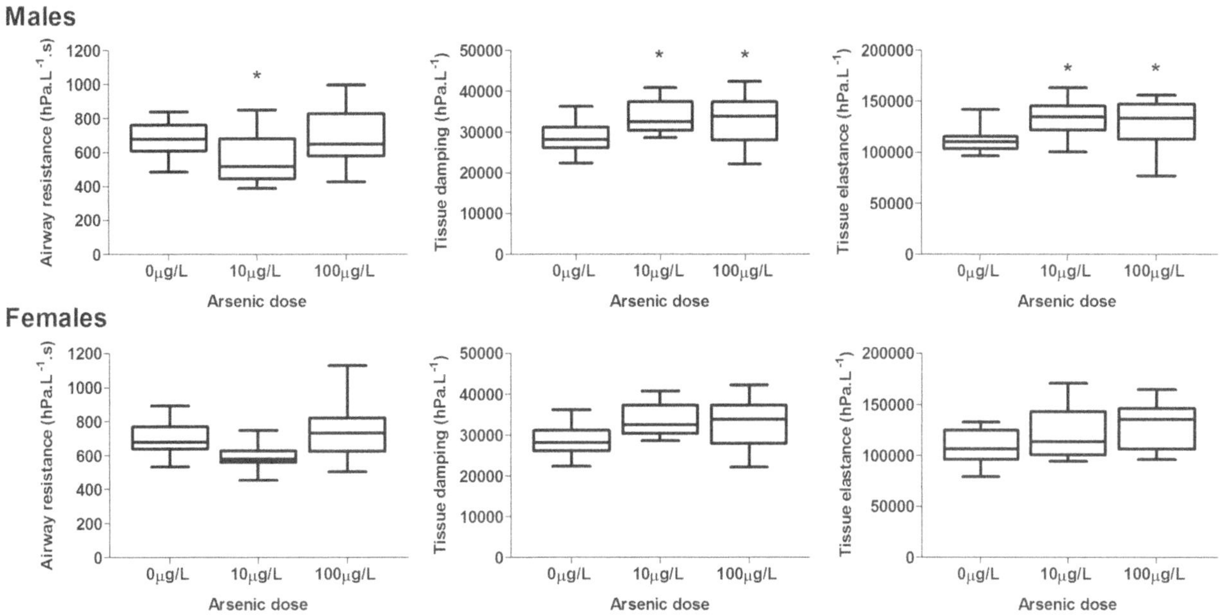

Figure 2 Airway resistance, tissue damping and tissue elastance at P_{rs} = 0 cmH_20 in two week old male and female C57BL/6 offspring exposed *in utero* to drinking water containing 0 (control), 10 or 100μg/L arsenic (mean ± SD). Tissue damping and tissue elastance were higher in two week old male offspring exposed to 10 or 100μg/L arsenic compared with controls. There was no effect of arsenic, at either dose, on lung mechanics in two week female offspring (* indicates significantly different to controls).

controls. There were no differences in the gestational age at birth between offspring exposed to arsenic compared with controls. These mice were therefore small for gestational age, indicating that arsenic exposure *in utero* caused intrauterine growth restriction. Similarly in epidemiological studies, exposure to low dose (<100μg/L) arsenic during pregnancy was linked to low birth weight and size but not to gestational age [17,30]. The mechanism for this is not fully understood but may be a result of arsenic-induced oxidative stress resulting in placental insufficiency [31] or disruption of the endocrine control of glucose homeostasis and cellular growth [32,33]. Being small for gestational age can induce alterations in metabolism, hormonal output and distribution of cardiac output, and have a lifelong impact on the potential for development and survival [34,35]. Foetal growth restriction is associated with increased respiratory morbidity during early childhood [21,22,36] and children who are small for gestational age are more likely to be hospitalised for respiratory tract infections [37,38]. Low birth weight is significantly associated with worse lung function in adulthood and increased mortality from obstructive lung disease [20,24]. There are clear associations between maternal smoking during pregnancy

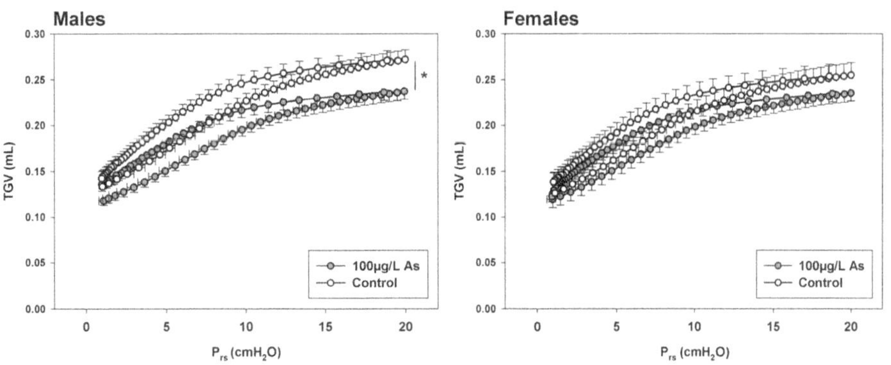

Figure 3 Pressure-volume curve during inflation to P_{rs} = 20 cmH_2O and exhalation to functional residual capacity plotted against TGV in male and female two week old C57BL/6 offspring exposed *in utero* to drinking water containing 0 (control) or 100μg/L arsenic (mean ± SD). The maximum TGV reached during inflation was lower in male offspring exposed to 100μg/L arsenic compared to male controls. There was no effect of 100μg/L arsenic on maximum TGV in two week female offspring (* indicates significantly different to controls).

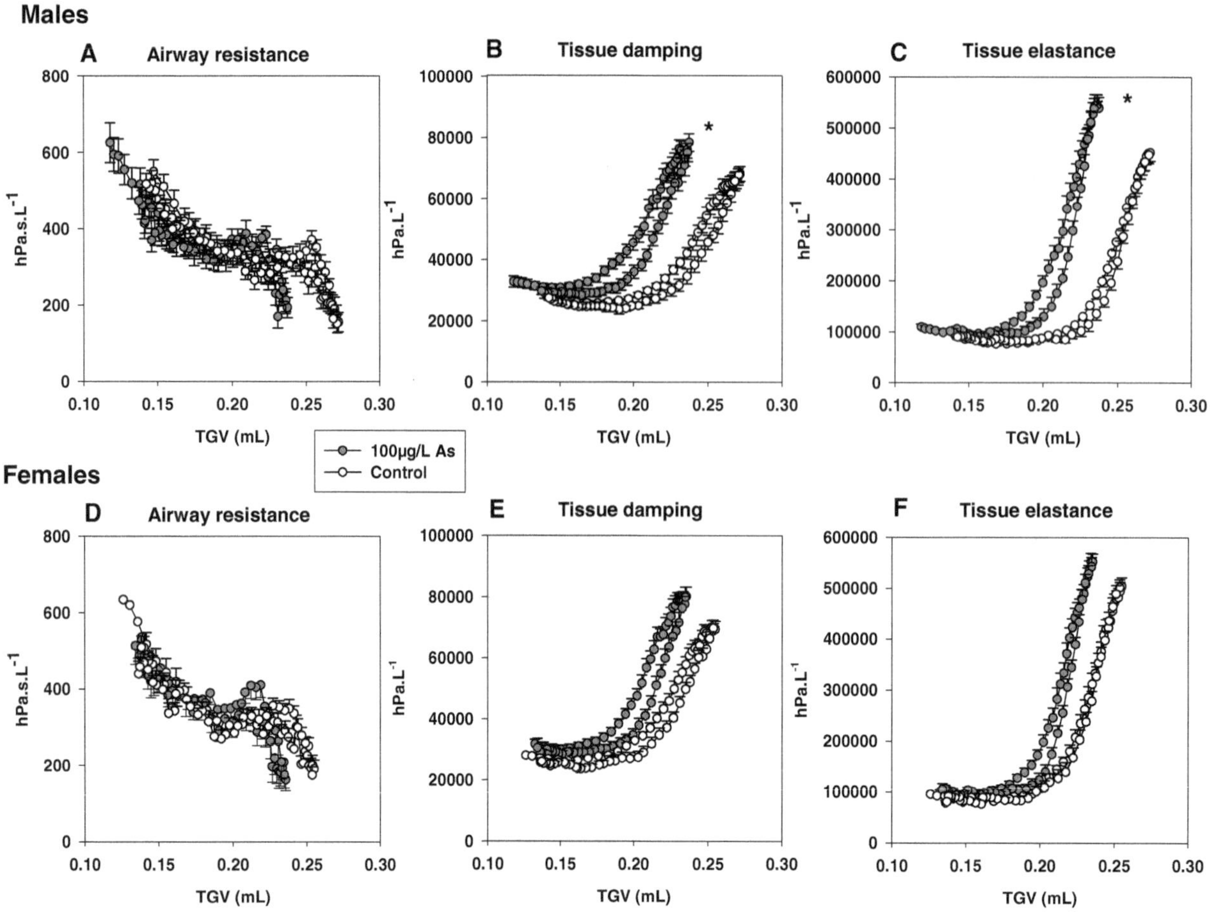

Figure 4 Volume dependence of airway resistance, tissue damping and tissue elastance during inflation to P_{rs} = 20 cmH_2O and exhalation to functional residual capacity in two week old male (A, B, C) and female (D, E, F) offspring exposed *in utero* to drinking water containing 0 (control) or 100µg/L arsenic (mean). Tissue damping and tissue elastance at P_{rs} = 20 cmH_2O were significantly higher in male offspring exposed to 100µg/L arsenic compared to male controls. There was no effect of arsenic exposure on tissue mechanics in females and no effect of arsenic on airway resistance in either sex (* indicates significantly different to controls).

and small for gestational age infants [39], reduced lung function [40] and increased respiratory infections in early childhood [41]. Therefore, arsenic-induced intrauterine growth restriction resulting in low birth weight infants may play a significant role in the childhood morbidity and increased the susceptibility to obstructive lung disease seen in arsenic exposed populations.

Despite the offspring exposed to 100µg/L arsenic being smaller at birth, these mice were not smaller in weight or length at two, four, six and eight weeks of age compared

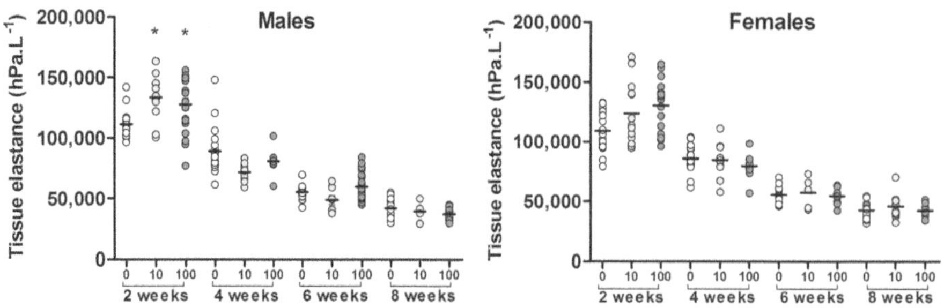

Figure 5 Tissue elastance at P_{rs} = 0 cmH_2O in two, four, six and eight week old male and female C57BL/6 offspring exposed *in utero* to drinking water containing 0 (control), 10 or 100µg/L arsenic (mean). Arsenic-induced impairments to lung mechanics in male two week old offspring were resolved at four, six and eight weeks of age (* indicates significantly different to controls).

with age-matched controls. In a similar study by Kozul *et al.* mice exposed to 10μg/L arsenic *in utero* had normal birth weight, but did have deficits in body weight during infancy compared with controls [19]. The low birth weight offspring in our study displayed catch-up growth during the first two weeks of life. There is evidence that infants who demonstrate catch-up growth and show early and complete recovery from intrauterine growth restriction are at greatest risk for developing metabolic diseases [42]. Similarly, in low birth weight infants, weight gain during infancy has been shown to be inversely related to lung function in infancy [43], with one study finding that the lowest lung function outcomes were seen in infants of below average birth weight with above average postnatal weight gain [44]. Therefore, despite showing no deficits in body weight later in life, the catch-up growth shown in the first two weeks of life may be related to intrauterine stress and poorer outcomes later in life.

As well as altering the pattern of somatic growth, we have shown that *in utero* exposure to low doses of arsenic (10 and 100μg/L) had direct effects on lung development in males resulting in deficits in lung function two weeks after birth. The abnormalities that we detected were mostly in the parenchymal tissue of the lungs in arsenic exposed offspring. Both tissue elastance and tissue damping were significantly higher in male mice exposed to arsenic compared with male controls, indicative of increased stiffness of the parenchymal lung tissue. When inflated to P_{rs} = 20 cmH_2O, male offspring exposed to 100μg/L arsenic reached a lower maximum TGV than controls signifying a loss of lung compliance. These data suggest that intrauterine stress caused by arsenic exposure is hindering the development of the distal airways and alveolar tissue in the lungs. Animal models of early life arsenic exposure, that included exposure post-natally, have shown both increased smooth muscle actin in small airways [45], which would increase the resistance of the small peripheral airways (tissue damping), and increased expression of collagen and elastin in the lung parenchyma [46], which would increase tissue stiffness (tissue elastance). As it is well established that sufficient nutrition *in utero* is essential for the healthy development of the lungs [47,48], it is unclear from this study whether the changes in lung mechanics in arsenic exposed mice are a result of suboptimal nutrition during development or a direct effect of arsenic itself.

In our study, male offspring were more susceptible to the harmful effects of *in utero* arsenic exposure on the lung than female offspring. While female mice showed similar trends in deficits in lung mechanics as males, the deficits were not statistically significant. Epidemiological studies also indicate that males may be more susceptible to the health effects of arsenic than females [8,49] which has been attributed to the differences in the way females metabolise arsenic [50]. When inorganic arsenic is ingested, it is absorbed into the blood and transported to the liver where it is reduced and sequentially methylated to monomethylarsonate (MMA) and dimethylarsinate (DMA) [51]. MMA is a highly toxic intermediate product and levels of MMA in the urine correlate strongly with levels of MMA found in the body [52]. DMA is a less toxic end product of arsenic methylation and can also be identified in urine [50]. Females have been shown to metabolise arsenic more efficiently than males, resulting in less MMA and more DMA in the urine [50]. While it is still largely unknown how the effects of arsenic manifest differently in males and females, sex dependent differences in the metabolism of arsenic may have contributed to the difference in susceptibility seen in our study.

We found that *in utero* arsenic exposure alone did not produce a lasting effect on respiratory mechanics, rather the early life deficits recovered with age. This data has two implications from a public health point perspective. Firstly, early life alterations in lung development induced by arsenic exposure may be recovered provided there is access to uncontaminated water. Secondly, we postulate that arsenic-induced impairments lung development may increase the susceptibility to respiratory infections in early life by inhibiting effective clearance of pathogens. This is consistent with the observation that there are increased respiratory infections in children exposed to arsenic-contaminated drinking water *in utero* [18]. Infancy represents a period of high susceptibility to respiratory infections and other harmful environmental exposures. The incidence of respiratory infections leading to bronchitis, pneumonia, or whooping cough in infancy has been shown to reduce adult lung function and increase the risk of mortality from obstructive lung disease [20]. Additionally, animal studies have shown that arsenic compromises the lung's immune response to viral infections resulting in greater viral load and higher mortality [53]. In humans, early life exposure to arsenic (before age 10) had long term effects on lung function outcomes in adults, with an 11.5% decrease in FEV_1 and 12.2% decrease in forced vital capacity (FVC) compared to unexposed adults [9]. It is unclear, however, whether the deficits in long term lung function were a result of the direct effects of arsenic on the lung, or an effect of arsenic exacerbating the effects of other respiratory infections or environmental exposures in early life. Arsenic-induced alterations to somatic growth and lung development *in utero* may result in individuals being more susceptible to postnatal insults, and contribute to long term alterations in lung function and disease risk.

Conclusions

We have shown that the lung is highly susceptible to the adverse effects of arsenic during the *in utero* period of lung development. Exposure to arsenic for a brief period during gestation impaired *in utero* somatic growth and lung development resulting in impaired lung function two weeks after birth (infancy). Alterations to lung function during infancy, a period of high susceptibility to respiratory system insults, may contribute to the increased susceptibility to respiratory infections and diseases in arsenic exposed populations. The deficits following exposure to the current WHO 'safe' dose of arsenic highlights the potency of arsenic toxicity and draws attention to the need for ongoing review of regulations regarding safe contaminant levels in community drinking supplies and the particular susceptibility of children to arsenic.

Abbreviations

WHO: World Health Organisation; MCL: Maximum contaminant level; $NaAs_2O_3$: Sodium arsenite; ICP-MS: Inductively coupled plasma-mass spectroscopy; TGV: Thoracic gas volume; P_{rs}: Transrespiratory pressure; Z_{rs}: Respiratory system impedance; R_{aw}: Airway resistance; I_{aw}: Airway intertance; G: Tissue damping; H: Tissue elastance; ID: Inflation-deflation.

Competing interests

The authors declare that they do not have any competing interests.

Authors' contributions

KR was involved in the conception and design of the research question, acquisition, analysis and interpretation of data, drafting and revising the manuscript and approving the final version for publication. AL and PS were involved in the conception and design of the research question, analysis and interpretation of data, revising the manuscript and approving the final version for publication. GZ was involved in the conception and design of the research question, acquisition, analysis and interpretation of data, revising the manuscript and approving the final version for publication.

Author details

[1]Division of Clinical Sciences, Telethon Institute for Child Health Research, 100 Roberts Road, Subiaco, WA 6008, Australia. [2]Centre for Child Health Research, University of Western Australia, 100 Roberts Road, Subiaco, WA 6008, Australia. [3]Queensland Children's Medical Research Institute, University of Queensland, Level 4, Foundation Building, Herston Road, Herston, QLD 4029, Australia.

References

1. Mukherjee A, Sengupta MK, Hossain MA, Ahamed S, Das B, Nayak B, Lodh D, Muhmudur Rahman M, Chakraborti D: **Arsenic contamination in ground water: a global perspective with emphasis on the Asian scenario.** *J Health Popul Nutr* 2006, **24**(2):142–163.
2. Chakraborti D, Sengupta MK, Rahman MM, Ahamed S, Chowdhury UK, Hossain MA, Mukherjee SC, Pati S, Saha KC, Dutta RN, *et al*: **Groundwater arsenic contamination and its health effects in the Ganga-Meghna -Brahmaputra plain.** *J Environ Monit* 2004, **6**(6):74N–83N.
3. World Health Organization: *Arsenic in drinking-water*, WHO guidelines for drinking water. Geneva, Switzerland: World Health Organization; 2003.
4. von Ehrenstein OS, Mazumder DNG, Yuan Y, Samanta S, Balmes J, Sil A, Ghosh N, Hira-Smith M, Haque R, Purushothamam R, *et al*: **Decrements in lung function related to arsenic in drinking water in West Bengal, India.** *Am J Epidemiol* 2005, **162**(6):533–541.
5. Milton AH, Rahman M: **Respiratory effects and arsenic contaminated well water in Bangladesh.** *Int J Environ Health Res* 2002, **12**(2):175–179.
6. Guha Mazumder D, Steinmaus C, Bhattacharya P, von Ehrenstein O, Ghosh N, Gotway M, Sil A, Balmes J, Haque R, Hira-Smith M, *et al*: **Bronchiectasis in persons with skin lesions resulting from arsenic in drinking water.** *Epidemiology* 2005, **16**(6):760–765.
7. De B, Majumdar D, Sen S, Guru S, Kunda S: **Pulmonary involvement in chronic arsenic poisoning from drinking contaminated ground-water.** *J Assoc Physicians India* 2004, **52**:395–400.
8. Guha Mazumder DN: **Chronic arsenic toxicity: clinical features, epidemiology, and treatment: experience in West Bengal.** *J Environ Sci Health A Tox Hazard Subst Environ Eng* 2003, **38**(1):141.
9. Dauphiné D, Ferreccio C, Guntur S, Yuan Y, Hammond S, Balmes J, Smith A, Steinmaus C: **Lung function in adults following in utero and childhood exposure to arsenic in drinking water: preliminary findings.** *Int Arch Occup Environ Health* 2011, **84**(6):591–600.
10. Parvez F, Chen Y, Brandt-Rauf PW, Bernard A, Dumont X, Slavkovich V, Argos M, D'Armiento J, Foronjy R, Hasan MR, *et al*: **Nonmalignant respiratory effects of chronic arsenic exposure from drinking water among never-smokers in Bangladesh.** *Environ Health Perspect* 2007, **116**(2):190–195.
11. Petrick J, Blachere F, Selmin O, Lantz R: **Inorganic arsenic as a developmental toxicant: *In utero* exposure and alterations in the developing rat lungs.** *Mol Nutr Food Res* 2009, **53**(5):583–591.
12. Waalkes MP, Ward JM, Liu J, Diwan BA: **Transplacental carcinogenicity of inorganic arsenic in the drinking water: induction of hepatic, ovarian, pulmonary, and adrenal tumors in mice.** *Toxicol Appl Pharmacol* 2003, **186**(1):7–17.
13. Smith AH, Marshall G, Yan Y, Ferreccio C, Liaw J, von Ehrenstein O, Steinmaus C, Bates MN, Selvin S: **Increased mortality from lung cancer and bronchiectasis in young adults after exposure to arsenic in utero and in early childhood.** *Environ Health Perspect* 2006, **114**(8):1293–1296.
14. Merkus PJFM: **Effects of childhood respiratory diseases on the anatomical and functional development of the respiratory system.** *Paediatr Respir Rev* 2003, **4**(1):28–39.
15. Concha G, Vogler G, Lezcano D, Nermell B, Vahter M: **Exposure to inorganic arsenic metabolites during early human development.** *Toxicol Sci* 1998, **44**(2):185–190.
16. Concha G, Vogler G, Nermell B, Vahter M: **Low-level arsenic excretion in breast milk of native andean women exposed to high levels of arsenic in the drinking water.** *Int Arch Occup Environ Health* 1998, **71**(1):42–46.
17. Huyck KL, Kile ML, Mahiuddin G, Quamruzzaman Q, Rahman M, Breton CV, Dobson CB, Frelich J, Hoffman E, Yousuf J, *et al*: **Maternal arsenic exposure associated with low birth weight in Bangladesh.** *J Occup Environ Med* 2007, **49**(10):1097–1104.
18. Rahman A, Vahter M, EkstrÃm E-C, Persson L-Ãk: **Arsenic exposure in pregnancy increases the risk of lower respiratory tract infection and diarrhea during infancy in Bangladesh.** *Environ Health Perspect* 2011, **119**(5):719–724.
19. Kozul-Horvath CD, Zandbergen F, Jackson BP, Enelow RI, Hamilton JW: **Effects of low-dose drinking water arsenic on mouse fetal and postnatal growth and development.** *PLoS One* 2012, **7**(5):e38249.
20. Barker DJ, Godfrey KM, Fall C, Osmond C, Winter PD, Shaheen SO: **Relation of birth weight and childhood respiratory infection to adult lung function and death from chronic obstructive airways disease.** *BMJ* 1991, **303**(6804):671–675.
21. Chan KN, Noble-Jamieson CM, Elliman A, Bryan EM, Silverman M: **Lung function in children of low birth weight.** *Arch Dis Child* 1989, **64**(9):1284–1293.
22. Rona RJ, Gulliford MC, Chinn S: **Effects of prematurity and intrauterine growth on respiratory health and lung function in childhood.** *BMJ* 1993, **306**(6881):817–820.
23. Shaheen S, Barker DJ: **Early lung growth and chronic airflow obstruction.** *Thorax* 1994, **49**(6):533–536.
24. Stein CE, Kumaran K, Fall CH, Shaheen SO, Osmond C, Barker DJ: **Relation of fetal growth to adult lung function in south India.** *Thorax* 1997, **52**(10): 895–899.
25. Stick S: **Pediatric origins of adult lung disease. 1. The contribution of airway development to paediatric and adult lung disease.** *Thorax* 2000, **55**(7):587–594.
26. Burri PH: **Fetal and postnatal development of the lung.** *Ann Rev Physiol* 1984, **46**:617–628.
27. Janosi TZ, Adamicza A, Zosky GR, Asztalos T, Sly PD, Hantos Z: **Plethysmographic estimation of thoracic gas volume in apneic mice.** *J Appl Physiol* 2006, **101**(2):454–459.
28. Sly P, Collins R, Thamrin C, Turner D, Hantos Z: **Volume dependence of airway and tissue impedance in mice.** *J Appl Physiol* 2003, **94**:1460–1466.
29. Hantos Z, Adamicza A, Govaerts E, Daroczy B: **Mechanical impedances of lungs and chest wall in the cat.** *J Appl Physiol* 1992, **73**(2):427–433.
30. Rahman A, Vahter M, Smith AH, Nermell B, Yunus M, El Arifeen S, Persson L-A, Ekstrom E-C: **Arsenic exposure during pregnancy and size at birth:**

a prospective cohort study in Bangladesh. *Am J Epidemiol* 2009, **169**(3):304–312.
31. Vahter ME: **Interactions between arsenic-induced toxicity and nutrition in early life.** *J Nutr* 2007, **137**(12):2798–2804.
32. Bodwell JE, Kingsley LA, Hamilton JW: **Arsenic at very Low concentrations alters glucocorticoid receptor (GR)-mediated gene activation but Not GR-mediated gene repression: complex doseâ˘'Response effects Are closely correlated with levels of activated GR and require a functional GR DNA binding domain.** *Chem Res Toxicol* 2004, **17**(8):1064–1076.
33. Davey JC, Nomikos AP, Wungjiranirun M, Sherman JR, Ingram L, Batki C, Lariviere J, Hamilton JW: **Arsenic as an endocrine disruptor: arsenic disrupts retinoic acid receptor– and thyroid hormone receptor–mediated gene regulation and thyroid hormone–mediated amphibian tail metamorphosis.** *Environ Health Perspect* 2008, **116**:165–172.
34. Barker DJ: **The fetal and infant origins of adult disease.** *BMJ* 1990, **301**(6761):1111.
35. McCormick MC: **The contribution of low birth weight to infant mortality and childhood morbidity.** *N Engl J Med* 1985, **312**(2):82–90.
36. Hulskamp G, Lum S, Stocks J, Wade A, Hoo AF, Costeloe K, Hawdon J, Deeptha K, Pillow JJ: **Association of prematurity, lung disease and body size with lung volume and ventilation inhomogeneity in unsedated neonates: a multicentre study.** *Thorax* 2009, **64**(3):240–245.
37. Taylor B, Wadsworth J: **Maternal smoking during pregnancy and lower respiratory tract illness in early life.** *Arch Dis Child* 1987, **62**(8):786–791.
38. Vik T, Vatten L, Markestad T, Ahlsten G, Jacobsen G, Bakketeig LS: **Morbidity during the first year of life in small for gestational age infants.** *Arch Dis Child Fetal Neonatal Ed* 1996, **75**(1):F33–37.
39. Haddow JE, Knight GJ, Palomaki GE, Kloza EM, Wald NJ: **Cigarette consumption and serum cotinine in relation to birthweight.** *Br J Obstet Gynaecol* 1987, **94**(7):678–681.
40. Stick SM, Burton PR, Gurrin L, Sly PD, LeSouef PN: **Effects of maternal smoking during pregnancy and a family history of asthma on respiratory function in newborn infants.** *Lancet* 1996, **348**(9034):1060–1064.
41. Strachan DP, Cook DG: **Health effects of passive smoking. 1. Parental smoking and lower respiratory illness in infancy and early childhood.** *Thorax* 1997, **52**(10):905–914.
42. Cianfarani S, Germani D, Branca F: **Low birthweight and adult insulin resistance: the "catch-up growth" hypothesis.** *Arch Dis Child Fetal Neonatal Ed* 1999, **81**(1):F71–73.
43. Turner S, Zhang G, Young S, Cox M, Goldblatt J, Landau L, Le Souëf P: **Associations between postnatal weight gain, change in postnatal pulmonary function, formula feeding and early asthma.** *Thorax* 2008, **63**(3):234–239.
44. Lucas JS, Inskip HM, Godfrey KM, Foreman CT, Warner JO, Gregson RK, Clough JB: **Small size at birth and greater postnatal weight gain.** *Am J Respir Crit Care Med* 2004, **170**(5):534–540.
45. Lantz RC, Chau B, Sarihan P, Witten ML, Pivniouk VI, Chen GJ: **In utero and postnatal exposure to arsenic alters pulmonary structure and function.** *Toxicol Appl Pharmacol* 2009, **235**(1):105–113.
46. Lantz RC, Hays AM: **Role of oxidative stress in arsenic-induced toxicity.** *Drug Metab Rev* 2006, **38**(4):791–804.
47. Romieu I: **Nutrition and lung health state of the Art.** *Int J Tuberc Lung Dis* 2005, **9**(4):362–374.
48. Sahebjami H: **Nutrition and lung structure and function.** *Exp Lung Res* 1993, **19**(2):105–124.
49. Guha Mazumder DN, Haque R, Ghosh N, De BK, Santra A, Chakraborti D, Smith AH: **Arsenic in drinking water and the prevalence of respiratory effects in West Bengal, India.** *Int J Epidemiol* 2000, **29**(6):1047–1052.
50. Lindberg A-L, Rahman M, Persson L, Vahter M: **The risk of arsenic induced skin lesions in Bangladeshi men and women is affected by arsenic metabolism and the age at first exposure.** *Toxicol Appl Pharmacol* 2008, **230**:9–16.
51. Lindberg A-L, Ekström E-C, Nermell B, Rahman M, Lönnerdal B, Persson L-Å, Vahter M: **Gender and age differences in the metabolism of inorganic arsenic in a highly exposed population in Bangladesh.** *Environ Res* 2008, **106**(1):110–120.
52. Huang Y-K, Huang Y-L, Hsueh Y-M, Yang M-H, Wu M-M, Chen S-Y, Hsu L-I, Chen C-J: **Arsenic exposure, urinary arsenic speciation, and the incidence of urothelial carcinoma: a twelve-year follow-up study.** *Cancer Causes Control* 2008, **19**:829–839.
53. Kozul CD, Ely KH, Enelow RI, Hamilton JW: **Low-dose arsenic compromises the immune response to influenza A infection *in vivo*.** *Environ Health Perspect* 2009, **117**(9):1441–1447.

Tocopheryl acetate 20% spray for elimination of head louse infestation: a randomised controlled trial comparing with 1% permethrin creme rinse

Ian F Burgess*, Nazma A Burgess and Elizabeth R Brunton

Abstract

Background: Tocopheryl acetate is viscous oily fluid used in a range of preparations for skin and scalp care in Italy. Observational and *in vitro* data have suggested a high level of efficacy against head louse infestation. The purpose of this investigation was to confirm the activity of tocopheryl acetate in a clinical setting in comparison with a standard widely used preparation.

Methods: A spray formulation containing tocopheryl acetate 20% in cyclomethicone was compared with permethrin 1% creme rinse for treatment of head louse infestation in a randomised, assessor blind, trial. Forty-five people were treated on two occasions 7 days apart. The spray was applied to dry hair for 20 minutes then washed. Participants treated with permethrin washed their hair and towel dried it before treatment for 10 minutes. Assessments were made by dry detection combing 1, 6, 9, and 14 days after first treatment.

Results: The tocopheryl acetate 20% spray was significantly ($p = 0.033$) more effective than permethrin 1%, using intention to treat worst case analysis, in which there were 13/23 (56.5%) successful treatments for tocopheryl acetate compared with 5/22 (22.7%) for permethrin. After unprecedented issues of re-infestation within households had been taken into account the underlying cure rate was 17/23 (73.9%) for tocopheryl acetate compared with 5/22 (22.7%), Odds Ratio 9.63 (95% CI, 2.46 to 37.68) ($p < 0.001$).

Conclusions: The tocopheryl acetate spray was significantly more effective than the permethrin product, was cosmetically acceptable, and not affected by current problems with resistance.

Trial registration: Current Controlled Trials ISRCTN45553737.

Keywords: Head lice, Pediculosis, Medical device, Medicinal product, Permethrin, Tocopheryl acetate, Vitamin-E

Background

Tocopheryl acetate, a vitamin-E ester, has long been used as a skin emollient and anti-oxidant in a variety of cosmetic and cosmeceutical preparations. Tocopheryl acetate has limited applications on its own because it is a high viscosity (>700 centistokes (cSt)), high surface tension (0.0337 newtons/metre (N/m)) oil, and is therefore normally formulated in more fluid materials such as decamethylcyclopentasiloxane, a low surface tension (0.018 N/m), low viscosity (2.4 cSt) silicone solvent. This type of mixture is capable of delivering small quantities of the active substance to target sites that would otherwise be inaccessible to the viscous fluid.

Fluid medical devices based on synthetic oils are widely used in Europe, Australia, and South America to control head lice and are generally claimed to block the respiratory structures of the insects [1-4]. However, increasing numbers of consumers express an interest to use naturally derived materials rather than mineral oils. Relatively few fixed plant oils have been shown to have activity and some are relatively unstable or have only been tested in developing countries [5,6], which may explain why, in several European countries, the use of neurotoxic insecticides against head lice persists despite evidence that many of the products are no longer effective.

* Correspondence: ian@insectresearch.com
Medical Entomology Centre, Insect Research & Development Limited, Cambridge, UK

Tocopheryl acetate in various formulations is used for a variety of protective or preventive barrier applications on inflamed or dry skin and in the spray dosage form was also designed to be suitable for application to the hair and scalp as a general conditioning agent. This use was incidentally seen to have novel potential as an anti-head louse agent. As a preliminary to investigating clinical control of head lice using the 20% tocopheryl acetate spray, we ran a series of *ex vivo* tests against head lice, which confirmed that 20% tocopheryl acetate completely immobilises lice and inhibits the hatching of louse eggs in a similar way to dimeticone based products [7]. As a result a class I medical device based on this activity was registered in Italy in 2010.

Here we report a clinical investigation conducted using the methodologies underpinning the recently published guidelines for trials of pediculicides [8]. The study compared a patented tocopheryl acetate 20% spray with an insecticide product based on 1% permethrin, the most potent of the pyrethroid insecticides used against lice.

Methods

Objective and participants

Participants were recruited to the study in essentially the same way as used for previous trials by advertising on local radio and by direct contact with previous study participants who had expressed an interest in taking part in further research. Potential participants were supplied with an information booklet prior to recruitment, and an enrolment visit arranged a minimum of 24 hours later.

We screened all assenting members of each household for presence of live lice by using a plastic detection comb ("PDC" comb, KSL Consulting, Helsinge, Denmark) on dry hair. Each infested member could be enrolled if: older than 6 months; had not been treated with head louse products during the previous 2 weeks; or treated with trimethoprim containing products during the previous 4 weeks. We also excluded those who had used permanent waves or hair colours during the previous 4 weeks because some products in these categories still use thiol-based ingredients that may exert an insecticidal effect, particularly against louse eggs, and some prospective participants had used them for this purpose in the past. We asked all prospective participants to confirm that they were unaware of allergy or sensitivity to pyrethroid insecticides or any other ingredient of the test products. Adult females also confirmed they were not breast feeding or pregnant, and using adequate contraception. We excluded people with long-term scalp conditions other than head louse infestation, earlier participants in this trial, and anyone who had participated in another clinical study within 1 month before screening.

At the first visit we also collected baseline demographic data on gender, age, hair characteristics, and previous pediculicide use. All treatments and assessment visits were domiciliary and no payment was offered for participation. Any ineligible people infested with lice were offered a standard of care treatment (4% dimeticone liquid gel) to minimise the risk of reinfestation of study participants.

Ethics

Ethical approval for the study was granted by NRES Committee South Central - Berkshire B (EudraCT 2011-001892-38).

The study was conducted in conformity with the principles of the Declaration of Helsinki, of European Union Directive 2001/20/EC, and of the ICH Topic E11 guideline. All participants stated before giving consent that they had read the participation information booklet (PIB) and understood the purpose and requirements of the study. Parents or guardians gave written consent for children younger than 16 years. Children also provided written or verbal assent, according to age, witnessed by the parent or guardian.

Treatment

The products were different both physically and in the method of application, so this study was single blinded with post-treatment assessments performed by investigators unaware of which treatment products had been used (assessor blinded). The products were applied following the instructions for use given by the manufacturers.

Tocopheryl acetate 20% spray (LiceKO®, Panin S.r.l, Rovigo, Italy) is made from allergen free, nature identical, tocopheryl acetate dissolved in decamethylcyclopentasiloxane (cyclomethicone) in a 20:80 ratio [7]. It was supplied in 100 mL bag-in-can sprays, i.e. the pressurised air propellant gas is not mixed with the product so pH stabilisation is not an issue. We applied the spray directly to dry hair, massaging it in with fingers, working systematically around the scalp to ensure even coverage. The treatment time was 20 minutes followed by washing with shampoo and rinsing out.

Permethrin 1% creme rinse (Lyclear® creme rinse, Omega Pharma UK, London, UK) is made from 1% 25:75 cis:trans permethrin in a conditioning base containing 20% propan-2-ol as a co-solvent. It was supplied in 59 mL plastic bottles with a flip cap dispenser. It was applied after washing the hair with a non-medicated shampoo followed by towel drying. We applied the rinse a few millilitres at a time and massaged in to thoroughly coat the hair and scalp. It was left in place for 10 minutes followed by rinsing out with water. Parents/care givers performed the hair washing and rinsing.

The first treatment day was designated Day 0. We repeated the treatments 7 days later. We asked participants not to use nit combs or other louse treatments during the course of the study.

Outcome measures

The primary outcome measure for the study was elimination of lice after two applications of product. We assessed efficacy by dry detection combing on Days 1 and 6, before the second treatment, then on Days 9 and 14. Any lice found were collected, fixed into the case record, and examined by microscope to determine the development stage. A successful treatment was defined as no lice found on Days 9 and 14.

Outcomes of treatment were classified as cure, reinfestation following cure, or treatment failure.

Sample size

We designed the study so we could detect superior activity of either product. We assumed that all participants were independent. Although there is ample evidence of widespread resistance to permethrin it is still used as a benchmark for comparison with novel treatments. Consequently, we expected a considerable difference in outcome between the two treatments and, using previously reported outcomes for permethrin [9-11], we estimated a success rate of about 30%. *Ex vivo* data for tocopheryl acetate indicated a potential for complete success [7], but such outcomes are rarely encountered in practice so our estimate for clinical success was likely to be of the order of 90%.

We estimated a sample size of 44 participants (22 per group) had more than 95% confidence and 90% power to detect a difference in the success rates of 60% between the two products, following the second treatment. The sample size made allowance for dropout. This sample size was also able to detect a difference of 42% with 90% confidence and 80% power.

Randomisation and blinding

The randomised treatment allocation sequence was derived using an online computer generated list from http://www.randomization.com (seed 10028, 23rd September 2011). We used instruction sheets enclosed in opaque, sealed, sequentially numbered envelopes, distributed to investigators in balanced blocks of 8, to hide the allocation until the point of delivery. A copy of the listing was prepared in case an emergency code break was required. Investigators allocated the numbered envelopes in sequence. Randomisation was by individual so different family members could receive different treatments.

Statistics and outcome measures

Statistical analyses were performed blind of treatment allocation. Fisher exact tests were used for presence/absence variables. Differences in success rates were measured by the 95% confidence interval calculated using a normal approximation to the binomial distribution. Quantitative variables were compared by using the Mann–Whitney U test. We conducted analyses using Oxstat II, version 1.1, EpiInfo, version 6, and purpose built calculators for normal approximation and Kruskal-Wallis/Mann–Whitney tests.

Results

Participants

We performed this study in Cambridgeshire, UK. Between 10th October 2011 and 2nd February 2012, we screened 75 people for head lice and enrolled 45 participants in the study from 28 households. A further 60 household members either declined screening, were ineligible, or were unavailable. Enrolled people comprised 39 children and 6 adults aged between 2 and 45 years, median 9 years. Demographic characters of this study population showed no significant differences from populations enrolled in recent previous studies [9-12]. The proportion of participants with heavier infestations at enrolment was also similar to previous studies.

We enrolled 10 households with more than one participating family member: 7 families having two, and one family each for three, four, and six participants. The most common household sizes were five (8 houses), four (7 houses), three and six (6 houses) each. We planned for equal numbers of people receiving each treatment (22 per group) with a final enrolment of 23 receiving tocopheryl acetate 20% spray and 22 receiving permethrin 1% creme rinse. All 45 participants completed all study assessments and there were no instances of non-compliance. Consequently, all participants were included in both the intention to treat (ITT) and per-protocol (PP) analyses (Figure 1).

The main endpoint analysis was the comparison of rate of cure in the 45 participants in the ITT population. According to this criterion, using worst case analysis, tocopheryl acetate 20% spray performed significantly better ($p = 0.033$, 95% confidence interval (CI), 0.05 to 0.62) with success achieved for 13/23 (56.5%) of the participants compared with 5/22 (22.7%) of those treated with permethrin 1% creme rinse, a difference of 33.8% (Odds Ratio (OR) 4.42, 95% CI, 1.21 to 16.12).

The reason we performed a worst case analysis is because randomisation in this study produced an unusually high proportion of households in which at least two members received different treatments. The result was that tocopheryl acetate eliminated lice from several people who were then reinfested from family members receiving the much less effective permethrin. When we analysed the lice collected during post-treatment assessments it indicated a higher actual treatment success rate for tocopheryl acetate of 17/23 (73.9%), without a similar change in the outcome for permethrin, a difference of 51.2% (OR 9.63, 95% CI, 2.46 to 37.68). This analysis also revealed that the 20% tocopheryl acetate spray was not able to prevent all

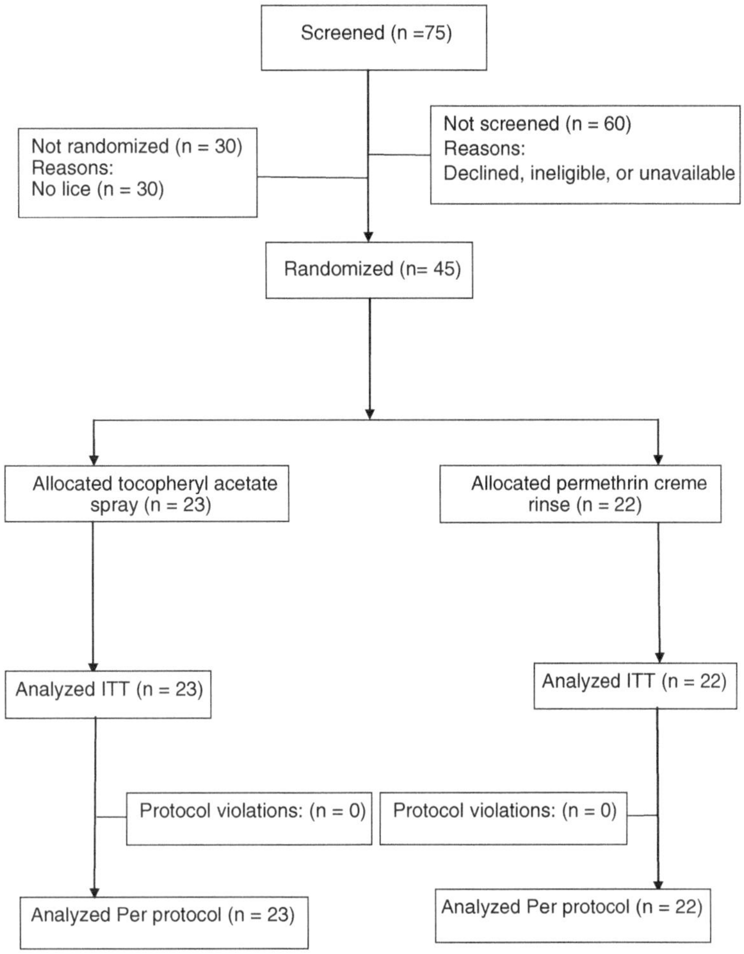

Figure 1 Flowchart of participants enrolled in the study.

louse eggs from hatching because small numbers of newly emerged nymphs were found on 14 participants between the first and second treatments. Six participants (26.1%) also had newly emerged nymphs following the second application of spray, showing that some eggs may take longer than 7 days to hatch.

Although we found lice in both groups before the second treatment on Day 7, applying the spray a second time eliminated the majority of infestation. After the second treatment, people in the tocopheryl acetate 20% group had significantly ($p < 0.05$) fewer lice of any development stage except adult females at Day 9, and adults and third stage nymphs at Day 14. These adult lice and older nymphs, which had migrated from infested family members treated with permethrin, reduced the overall efficacy outcome for tocopheryl acetate from 73.9% to 56.5%. We also analysed the distribution of outcome and success rates for subsets of the population by various factors: sex, age, level of initial infestation, hair length, hair thickness, hair curl, and hair type. Additional tests were made for the significance of variations in the rates of cure or re-infestation by levels of these factors and the results are summarised in Table 1.

Given the small sample size, it was not surprising that few differences or trends were significant at $p < 0.05$. However, we did find significant trend differences ($p < 0.05$) between the treatment groups for females, and those with a "light" infestation at enrolment, and in the populations overall. The most highly significant difference of outcome was in those with "wavy" hair ($p < 0.01$), possibly due to the quantity of preparation that could be held by the hair, which would have influenced the level of contact between the product and the lice and louse eggs. Nearly all (20/23) people treated with tocopheryl acetate and their carers expressed a preference for using the spray compared with the permethrin creme rinse with respect to comfort and convenience, as well as success of outcome.

We weighed the containers of product before and after use to measure product usage. Slightly more treatment was applied on the first occasion than the second, with a mean application of 39.5 g of spray. In contrast the mean quantity of creme rinse used was nearly double for

Table 1 Rates of cure overall and by data subgroup - ITT population

		Success rate				p value
		Tocopheryl acetate 20%		Permethrin 1%		
		n/N	%	n/N	%	
Whole population						
Elimination of initial infestation		17/23	73.9	5/22	22.7	<0.001
Worst case analysis		13/23	56.5	5/22	22.7	0.033
Data subgroup						
Sex	- males	1/2	50.0	1/3	33.3	NS
	- females	12/21	57.1	4/19	21.1	0.027
Age	- 2 to 9	10/13	76.9	4/11	36.4	NS
	- 10 to 15	1/7	14.3	0/8	0.0	NS
	- 16+	2/4	50.0	1/3	33.3	NS
Infestation	- light	9/12	75.0	3/11	27.3	0.039
	- moderate	2/4	50.0	2/5	40.0	NS
	- heavy	2/7	28.6	0/5	0.0	NS
Hair length	- above ears	1/2	50.0	1/3	33.3	NS
	- ears to shoulders	5/9	55.6	1/7	14.3	NS
	- below shoulders	7/12	58.3	3/12	25.0	NS
Hair thickness	- fine	3/4	75.0	2/4	50.0	NS
	- medium	4/6	66.7	1/6	16.7	NS
	- thick	6/13	46.2	2/12	16.7	NS
Hair curl	- straight	4/11	36.4	4/14	28.6	NS
	- wavy	6/8	75.0	0/6	0.0	<0.01
	- curly	3/4	75.0	1/2	50.0	NS
Hair type	- dry	1/2	50.0	1/2	50.0	NS
	- normal	11/19	57.9	5/18	27.8	NS
	- greasy	1/2	50.0	0/2	0.0	NS

each treatment at 76.3 g, from which the cost of a single treatment application proved to be similar for each product at approximately €6.50 to €6.85.

Adverse events

There were 13 adverse events in 13 participants, of which 11 were simple accidents or childhood infections not related to treatment. One adverse event in each group was an application site event of stinging or itching considered to have some relationship to treatment or the washing process involved in removing the treatment. In the case of permethrin creme rinse, stinging occurred during the treatment application process, indicating irritation of existing excoriations by the treatment. In the case of tocopheryl acetate spray, itching occurred during the washing off process that was possibly associated with the shampoo used.

Discussion

We have found that tocopheryl acetate, applied as a 20% spray, was significantly more effective to eliminate head lice than the insecticide permethrin. We have also found evidence that resistance to pyrethroid insecticides like permethrin has not diminished in the study area despite reduced use of the insecticide during the past few years. However, the presentation of resistance in the UK is largely different from that in some other countries where susceptibility to pyrethroids may be reduced, but not eliminated, and resistance to alternative insecticides like malathion is either not found or is of limited impact [13,14]. Although knockdown resistance (*kdr*) is present in the country it appears to play only a minor role in treatment failure compared with a double resistance to permethrin and malathion mediated by elevated levels of non-specific esterases [Burgess IF, unpublished] [15]. As a result, the impact of resistance has continued to reduce efficacy of insecticide based products to the point that they are now effectively useless for many consumers [9-12,16].

The mode of action of tocopheryl acetate to kill head lice is currently unconfirmed but, as it is hydrophobic and has a high viscosity (>700 cSt), we believe it has an occlusive effect on the louse surface and blocks the spiracular structures in a similar manner to the high molecular weight dimeticone used in some of the most widely used products in Europe [3].

Since 2005, physically acting medical device products for control of head louse infestation have increased in number, availability, and variety of dosage form and have largely replaced insecticides in several countries in Europe, and have a large market share in Australia and New Zealand. However, clinical data are only available in the public domain for a limited number of these products. This treatment concept is generally popular with consumers because the products do not contain insecticides and most do not contain irritating solvents or preservatives. But comments from consumers indicate that some are not effective and others are difficult to use.

In recent times an additional problem for all families attempting to eliminate head louse infestation has been reinfestation. Irrespective of the effectiveness of the product they are using there is no protection after washing the treatment off so the children could potentially be reinfested from the next contact with their friends. Fortunately in most households everyone is normally treated using the same product so that everyone is usually either cured or not at the same time. In clinical studies randomised by individual it is often the case that some households have different members receiving different treatments. For most medications this does not constitute an issue but for head louse studies, if there is a disparity of efficacy, those receiving the more effective product are at continual risk of reinfestation from those on the less effective one. This is an issue we have addressed in the past by development of an algorithm to identify where the few cases of reinfestation occur [9-12,16]. However, in this study a high proportion of households had people in receipt of different treatments, and most people receiving permethrin still had lice after treatment. As a result it was inevitable that any siblings who had been treated with tocopheryl acetate would be at risk of reinfestation, which was identified by being found to be free from lice after treatment but infested again by adult lice and third stage nymphs by the end of the study. Of course, it is impossible to confirm absolutely that the reinfestation arose from such contacts, which is why we conducted a worst case analysis also. Perhaps for this reason it would be wiser to consider randomisation by household in future studies but this has drawbacks because it requires larger numbers of participants, which could make the cost of investigations prohibitive for small companies, and has hitherto not been favoured by some regulatory agencies who have preferred randomisation by individual because each person is seen as being independent [12].

Fixed vegetable oils, such as olive and coconut oils, have been used as hair grooming agents for centuries in several cultures while others such as neem have been used to treat infections and infestations. Whether they have any real activity against head lice is unknown but modern folklore from the USA, and other western cultures where these oils are not routinely used, suggests they occlude the louse respiratory tract, similar to the activity of synthetic oils. However, with a low viscosity of the order of 80–90 cSt combined with a low surface tension, these oils would form a thin film on lice and hairs that could only act slowly and may not deliver sufficient material to the respiratory structures of the lice. Certainly, in geographic areas where these vegetable oils are routinely used on hair, lice are common and appear to survive unhindered by the oils. Neem seed oil, which is marketed as a shampoo formulated material, is reported to demonstrate a rapid activity, killing lice within a few minutes [5,6]. Such speed of effect is unlikely to occur by occlusion alone because neem oil is chemically similar to extra virgin olive oil but with the addition of small quantities of a number of complex terpenoids. The reported rapid activity of neem shampoo either suggests a pharmacological activity, which would place the preparations into the sphere of medicinal products rather than devices, or else the activity must be due to formulation components other than neem such as powerful surfactants stripping the lipid from the louse surface. Similarly, eucalyptus and tea tree oils, as well as other monoterpene based products, are reported to show good efficacy [4,9,17-19] but these oils have a recognised activity to inhibit acetylcholine esterase and other enzymes [20], which would make them pharmacologically active also.

Tocopheryl acetate is different from other products based on natural materials because it has a high viscosity causing it to adhere to lice or hair without absorption across the insect cuticle. As a 20% spray in a low viscosity carrier, tocopheryl acetate becomes an effective physical occlusive agent that is not easily removed from the hydrophobic louse cuticle by shampoo. Consequently, even a short application time of 20 minutes proved effective because the immobilised lice remain coated with the active material. As a preparation we have found it to be of similar efficacy to other widely accepted physically acting preparations but with the added appeal for consumers that it is "naturally" based. Like the original cosmetic tocopheryl acetate spray upon which this product was based (Vea® Spray, Hulka S.r.l., Rovigo, Italy), it has the added effect to reduce inflammation of the scalp resulting from previous louse bites, thus reducing irritation and dryness. Future investigations will look at ways to limit flow of the sprayed fluid along the hair shafts, which should reduce the quantity of product required for an adequate treatment and improve the performance of the product overall, particularly against louse eggs.

Conclusion

In this randomized, controlled, assessor-blinded, clinical investigation we have shown that a 20% tocopheryl acetate based spray (LiceKO® spray) was significantly more effective than a 1% permethrin creme rinse. The product was both better tolerated and more cosmetically acceptable.

Competing interests

IFB is a consultant to several major and minor manufacturers of pediculicides, medical devices, and combs for use against head lice and their eggs. The other authors declare they have no competing interests in this work.

Author contributions

All three authors contributed towards the design of the study. Participant enrolment was performed by IFB and ERB and the majority of outcome data were acquired by NAB. ERB managed the study documentation and IFB conducted the analyses and drafted the manuscript. All three authors agreed the manuscript.

Acknowledgments

This study was sponsored and financed by Panin S.r.l., Rovigo, Italy, who played no role in design, interpretation of results, or writing of the manuscript. Thanks to Dr.ssa Franca Maria Astolfi and Ms Jules West Erhabor who arranged for supply of investigational clinical materials. Investigator members of the study team not listed as authors were Audrey Pepperman and Rebecca French. Thanks also to Dr.ssa Francesca Brazzo for monitoring of study documents. Dr Paul Silverston was the study consultant physician who reviewed all adverse events.

References

1. Burgess IF, Brown CM, Lee PN: **Treatment of head louse infestation with 4% dimeticone lotion: randomised controlled equivalence trial.** *Br Med J* 2005, **330**(7505):1423–1425.
2. Heukelbach J, Pilger D, Oliveira FA, Khakban A, Ariza L, Feldmeier H: **A highly efficacious pediculicide based on dimeticone: randomized observer blinded comparative trial.** *BMC Infect Dis* 2008, **8**:115.
3. Burgess IF: **The mode of action of dimeticone 4% lotion against head lice.** *Pediculus capitis. BMC Pharmacol* 2009, **9**:3.
4. Barker SC, Altman PM: **A randomised, assessor blind, parallel group comparative efficacy trial of three products for the treatment of head lice in children - melaleuca oil and lavender oil, pyrethrins and piperonyl butoxide, and a "suffocation" product.** *BMC Dermatol* 2010, **10**:6.
5. Abdel-Ghaffar F, Semmler M: **Efficacy of neem seed extract shampoo on head lice of naturally infected humans in Egypt.** *Parasitol Res* 2007, **100**:329–332.
6. Abdel-Ghaffar F, Al-Quraishy S, Al-Rasheid KA, Mehlhorn H: **Efficacy of a single treatment of head lice with a neem seed extract: an in vivo and in vitro study on nits and motile stages.** *Parasitol Res* 2012, **110**:277–280.
7. Panin G: **Use of vitamin E or its esters for the control of ectoparasites.** *European Patent, EP* 2008, **2334186**:B1.
8. Barker SC, Burgess I, Meinking TL, Mumcuoglu KY: **International guidelines for clinical trials with pediculicides.** *Int J Dermatol* 2012, **51**:853–858.
9. Burgess IF, Brunton ER, Burgess NA: **Clinical trial showing superiority of a coconut and anise spray over permethrin 0.43% lotion for head louse infestation, ISRCTN964697.** *Eur J Pediatr* 2010, **169**:55–62.
10. Burgess IF, Lee PN, Brown CM: **Randomised, controlled, parallel group clinical trials to evaluate the efficacy of isopropyl myristate/ cyclomethicone solution against head lice.** *Pharm J* 2008, **280**:371–375.
11. Burgess IF, Burgess NA, Brunton ER: **Soya oil based shampoo superior to 0.5% permethrin lotion against head louse infestation: randomized clinical trial.** *Medical Devices: Evidence and Research* 2011, **4**:35–42.
12. Burgess IF, Lee PN, Kay K, Jones R, Brunton ER: **1,2-octanediol, a novel surfactant, for treating head louse infestation: identification of activity, formulation, and randomised, controlled trials.** *PLoS ONE* 2012, **7**(4):e35419.
13. Bouvresse S, Berdjane Z, Durand R, Bouscaillou J, Izri A, Chosidow O: **Permethrin and malathion resistance in head lice: Results of ex vivo and molecular assays.** *J Am Acad Dermatol* 2012, **67**:1143–1150.
14. Clark JM: **Permethrin resistance due to knockdown gene mutations is prevalent in human head louse populations.** *Open Dermatol J* 2010, **4**:63–68.
15. Downs AMR, Stafford KA, Harvey I, Coles GC: **Evidence for double resistance to permethrin and malathion in head lice.** *Br J Dermatol* 1999, **141**:508–511.
16. Burgess IF, Brunton ER, Burgess NA: **Single application of 4% dimeticone liquid gel versus two applications of 1% permethrin creme rinse for treatment of head louse infestation: a randomised controlled trial.** *BMC Dermatol* 2013, **13**:5.
17. Barker SC, Altman PM: **An ex vivo, assessor blind, randomised, parallel group, comparative efficacy trial of the ovicidal activity of three pediculicides after a single application–melaleuca oil and lavender oil, eucalyptus oil and lemon tea tree oil, and a "suffocation" pediculicide.** *BMC Dermatol* 2011, **11**:14.
18. Grieve KA, Altman PM, Rowe SJ, Staton JA, Oppenheim VMJ: **A randomised, double-blind, comparative efficacy trial of three head lice treatment options: malathion, pyrethrins with piperonyl butoxide and MOOV Head Lice Solution.** *Aust Pharmacist* 2007, **26**:738–743.
19. McCage CM, Ward SM, Paling CA, Fisher DA, Flynn PJ, McLaughlin JL: **Development of a paw paw herbal shampoo for the removal of head lice.** *Phytomedicine* 2002, **9**:743–748.
20. Mills C, Cleary BJ, Gilmer JF, Walsh JJ: **Inhibition of acetylcholinesterase by Tea Tree oil.** *J Pharm Pharmacol* 2004, **56**:375–379.

4

Influence of Vitamin C and Vitamin E on testicular zinc content and testicular toxicity in lead exposed albino rats

Oluseyi C Ayinde*, Sunday Ogunnowo† and Rita A Ogedegbe†

Abstract

Background: Occupational and environmental exposures to lead remain a public health problem as lead alters physiological processes by inducing oxidative stress and mimicking divalent cations. This study was designed to investigate the effects of Vitamin C (VC) and Vitamin E (VE) on the reproductive function of lead exposed male rats. Experimental animals were exposed to oral doses of lead, VC and VE at 60 mg/kg body weight, 40 mg/kg body weight, and 150 mg/kg body weight respectively, while control animals received 0.9% saline solution. Oral administration spanned for six weeks after which changes in testicular redox status, lead deposition, testicular zinc content, serum androgen content, semen quality and testis histology were examined.

Results: There were significant ($p < 0.05$) increases in oxidative stress indices and testicular lead content. A significant ($p < 0.05$) depletion of zinc in the testis of lead exposed animals was also observed. Fluctuations were observed in androgen levels of lead treated animals with a significant increase ($p < 0.05$) in Serum follicle stimulating hormone (FSH) and testosterone (TT) content, while there was no significant change in luteinizing hormone (LH) content. Testicular tissue showed an alteration in its normal histology with degeneration of the seminiferous epithelium accompanied by a significant reduction ($p < 0.05$) in the number of luminal spermatozoa. A downgrade in the semen appearance and semen quality –sperm motility, morphology, and count was also observed after lead exposure. VC and VE treatment showed a significant ($p < 0.05$) reversal of the physiological alteration induced by lead.

Conclusions: Lead exposure resulted in a decline in the reproductive function of male rats by inducing oxidative stress, inhibiting enzymes and depleting testicular zinc contents. However, results clearly showed that VC and VE attenuated the deleterious impact of lead on the reproductive system.

Keywords: Lead, Zinc, Vitamin C, Vitamin E, Oxidative stress, Testicular toxicity

Background

Lead poisoning is an age long environmental hazard [1]. Industries account for an annual production of about 2.5 million tons of lead globally [2]. Lead is present in batteries, leaded gasoline [3], paints, water pipes, insecticides, and some cosmetics. Air, water, soil, food and consumer products are the major routes of human exposure to lead [4]. The accumulation of lead in various tissues and its interference with bioelements accounts for its pathophysiology [5]. The toxic effect of lead on reproduction is pervasive affecting basically all aspects of the reproductive system [6]. One mechanism by which lead exerts its adverse effect is by inducing oxidative stress (OS). Oxidative stress represents an imbalance between the production of reactive oxygen species (ROS) and a biological system's antioxidant defence mechanism [7]. Because of a high content of polyunsaturated membrane lipids testicular tissue becomes one of the targets for OS [8].

Zinc (Zn) plays an important role in the reproductive system [9]. It is the only metal found in almost all classes of enzymes. High concentrations of zinc found in the testes and accessory sex glands show its pivotal role in the reproductive system [10]. Zn deficiency has been

* Correspondence: oluseyiayinde@yahoo.com
†Equal contributors
Department of Biochemistry, College of Medicine, University of Lagos, Idi-Araba, Lagos, Nigeria

linked to hypogonadism [11] and impaired sperm function [12].

Studies have shown that antioxidants have a far-reaching effect in andrology [13]. Vitamins A, E, D and C were reported to possess antioxidant functions, and their inhibitory effects on ROS accumulation vary from one vitamin to the other [14]. L-Ascorbic acid (Vitamin C) is a water soluble vitamin derived from dietary sources such as fruits and vegetables [15]. Vitamin C (VC) plays an efficient protective role directly or indirectly in a systemic detoxification of Pb [16]. Vitamin E (VE) a term that encompasses a group of potent, lipid-soluble, chain breaking antioxidants [11] which acts as a naturally occurring antioxidant. VE locates itself in biological membranes where it functions to inhibit oxidation and oxidative damage to membrane polyunsaturated fatty acid (PUFA) [17].

Since the environment remains an integral portion of human existence coupled with lead's pervasiveness within the environment, it has become imperative to find out inexpensive and simple ways by which the body can be made to maintain homeostasis after lead exposure. This work, therefore, aims at finding out whether or not oral administration of VC and VE either individually or in combination would proffer any form of ameliorative effect on testicular toxicity, zinc concentration and testicular lead burden in lead exposed rats.

Results

Data in Table 1 show that rats exposed to lead exhibited a significant decrease in the glutathione content, superoxide dismutase and catalase enzyme activity in the testis when compared with the control group. More so, lead treatment increased significantly the amount of lipid peroxidation products (MDA), total protein and nitric oxide content in the testis. However vitamin C and/or vitamin E treatment significantly increased glutathione content, superoxide dismutase and catalase enzyme activity, while also decreasing lipid peroxidation products, total protein and nitric oxide contents when compared to the lead only group.

Data in Table 2 reveal that lead treatment resulted in a significant increase in lead accumulation in the testis of lead exposed animals, with a concomitant decrease in zinc content when compared to the control. Nevertheless, vitamin C and/or E treatment reduced lead content and increased zinc content in the testes of lead treated animals when compared with lead only group.

Table 3 shows that lead treatment accounted for a significant decrease in serum follicle stimulating hormone and testosterone of lead treated rats. However, no significant decrease was observed in the luteinising hormone content when compared to the control. Vitamin C and/or vitamin E treatment increased significantly the contents of follicle stimulating hormone, and testosterone content in the serum of lead treated rats when compared to the lead alone group.

Table 4 shows that lead exposed animals had a significant decrease in the percentage of sperm motility and sperm count when compared with the control group. They also had an increase in abnormal sperm morphology. However vitamin C and/or vitamin E treatment significantly increased sperm motility and count in lead treated animals, and also reduced the percentage of abnormal sperm morphology in lead exposed animals, when compared to the lead alone group

Figure 1 presents the histological changes in lead exposed animals, lead exposed animals had a reduction in the seminiferous epithelium accompanied with a reduction in the lumina spermatozoa when compared to control group. However improvements were observed with vitamin C and/or E treatment.

Discussion

Occupational and environmental exposures to heavy metals are known to have deleterious effects on human reproduction. In rats lead (Pb) has been implicated in male reproductive dysfunction [18]. In this study our

Table 1 Oxidative stress markers of albino rats

Parameter	Control	Pb	Pb + VC	Pb + VE	Pb + VC + VE
GSH (U/mg Protein)	0.69 ± 0.04	0.10 ± 0.02 ^{a}	0.51 ± 0.03 ^{ab}	0.52 ± 0.03 ^{ab}	0.57 ± 0.02 ^{ab}
SOD (U/mg Protein)	9.19 ± 0.69	1.20 ± 0.17 ^{a}	5.40 ± 0.43 ^{ab}	6.04 ± 0.55 ^{ab}	6.17 ± 0.07 ^{ab}
CAT (U/mg Protein)	42.48 ± 2.37	9.48 ± 0.36 ^{a}	28.90 ± 0.78 ^{ab}	26.44 ± 1.33 ^{ab}	31.30 ± 0.69 ^{ab}
MDA (Mmol/g tissue)	0.35 ± 0.02	0.94 ± 0.03 ^{a}	0.44 ± 0.02 ^{ab}	0.47 ± 0.02 ^{ab}	0.43 ± 0.01 ^{ab}
PRT (mg/g tissue)	20.36 ± 0.71	30.29 ± 1.75 ^{a}	21.54 ± 1.55 ^{b}	18.69 ± 1.71 ^{b}	21.00 ± 1.04 ^{b}
NO (mg/dL)	15.84 ± .86	42.12 ± 1.70 ^{a}	25.42 ± 1.65 ^{ab}	26.98 ± 1.60 ^{ab}	22.96 ± 1.24 ^{ab}

Values are expressed as Mean ± S. E. M.
a: Significant with control.
b: Significant with lead only group.
c: Significant with Vitamin C group.
d:Significant with Vitamin E group.
Significant at $p < 0.05$.
The number of animals in each experimental group was 5.

Table 2 Metal contents in the testes of albino rats

Metals	Control	Pb	Pb + VC	Pb + VE	Pb + VE + VC
LEAD (mg/g tissue)	0.0245 ± 0.002	1.256 ± 0.008 [a]	0.586 ± 0.048 [ab]	0.840 ± 0.041 [abc]	0.521 ± 0.011 [abd]
ZINC (mg/g tissue)	0.541 ± 0.014	0.107 ± 0.012 [a]	0.233 ± 0.009 [ab]	0.1401 ± 0.007 [ac]	0.281 ± 0.007 [abcd]

Values are expressed as Mean ± S. E. M.
a: Significant with control.
b: Significant with lead only group.
c: Significant with Vitamin C group.
d:Significant with Vitamin E group.
Significant at $p < 0.05$.
The number of animals in each experimental group was 5.

results clearly demonstrates that lead acetate exposure can seriously alter the testes and reproductive function of adult male rats. Oxidative stress parameters were examined in testicular homogenate, and lipid peroxidation as measured by the amount of MDA was significantly ($p < 0.05$) elevated in the testes of lead treated rats (Table 1). Lipid peroxidation has been implicated in the aetiology of damage to subcellular membranes by inactivating cell constituents through oxidation or causing oxidative stress by undergoing radical chain reaction [19]. The stimulation of lipid peroxidation, seemingly caused by lead treatment is related to the formation of free radicals after depletion of antioxidants. Table 1, shows a significant ($p < 0.05$) decline in the production of glutathione in the testes of lead exposed animals, as well as lead alteration in the function of some antioxidant enzymes markers. Lead exposure resulted in a significant ($p < 0.05$) decrease in superoxide dismutase and catalase enzyme activities in the testes of the rats. This observations are similar to those made by Salawu *et al.,* [20]. Our study also showed that there was a significant ($p < 0.05$) increase in the levels of nitric oxide content in the testes of the animals similar to observations made by Moniem *et al.,* [6]. All these culminate to a depletion of total antioxidant content and an increase in reactive oxidant specie. Vigeh *et al.,* [21] describes lead's ability to elevate ROS in biological systems as correlated to its active inhibition of sulfhydryl antioxidants synthesis, inhibition of enzyme reactions, damage to nucleic acids and inhibition of DNA repair. As such our results indicate that lead acetate induced an embellished inhibitory effect on GSH, SOD and CAT.

Testicular protein content was significantly ($p < 0.05$) increased in lead treated animals. Afaf *et al.,* [22], hypothesised that these changes in protein content could result from reduction in the synthetic activity in testes, since testicular fluid contains both stimulatory factors and inhibitory factors that alter protein secretions [23]. Furthermore, Afaf *et al.,* [24] suggested that protein accumulation in the testes could be due to androgen deprivation.

Zinc is essential in spermatogenesis, a cofactor of metalloenzymes, involved in DNA transcription, involved in steroid receptor expression, and protein synthesis [25]. Results in Table 2 showed that lead treated animals showed a significant ($p < 0.05$) decrease in testicular zinc content. Victery *et al.,* [26] reported a similar reduction in zinc content in the plasma and testes of lead exposed male rats. They further revealed that lead's ability to significantly increase urinary excretion of zinc was a possible mechanism for loss of testicular zinc. More so, another mechanism in which Pb exerts its toxicity is by substituting Zn in zinc-mediated processes [27]. This trend could also explain the lead induced SOD-enzyme inhibitory effect as lead replaces Zn in its sites. Such interaction has been demonstrated where lead replaces Zn to form Cu-Pb-SOD [14]. Our studies revealed that lead treated animals also showed an elevation in testicular tissue lead content. Therefore a possible relationship could be drawn between lead exposure and zinc depletion in the testes of albino rats.

Table 3 Hormone profile in the blood sera of albino rats

Hormone	Control	Pb	Pb + VC	Pb + VE	Pb + VE + VC
LH(mIU/L)	1.02 ± 0.05	0.46 ± 0.10	0.86 ± 0.08	1.1 ± 0.26 [b]	1.04 ± 0.10
FSH(mIU/L)	1.68 ± 0.12	0.68 ± 0.11 [a]	1.46 ± 0.05 [b]	1.16 ± 0.05 [ab]	1.44 ± 0.08 [b]
TT(nmol/L)	39.00 ± 1.18	9.64 ± 0.52 [a]	35.60 ± 1.03 [b]	21.80 ± 1.16 [abc]	36.40 ± 0.93 [bd]

Values are expressed as Mean ± S. E. M.
a: Significant with control.
b: Significant with lead only group.
c: Significant with Vitamin C group.
d:Significant with Vitamin E group.
Significant at $p < 0.05$.
The number of animals in each experimental group was 5.

Table 4 Status of spermatozoa in albino rats

Parameter	Control	Pb	Pb + VC	Pb + VE	Pb + VE + VC
MOTILITY(%)	46.40 ± 1.21	28.20 ± 1.28 ^{a}	35.20 ± 0.86 ^{ab}	37.60 ± 0.93 ^{ab}	43.60 ± 1.03 ^{bcd}
COUNT(sperm x10 ^{6}/ml)	53.75 ± 2.24	36.00 ± 1.28 ^{a}	44.25 ± 2.04 ^{ab}	41.25 ± 1.63 ^{a}	45.55 ± 2.18^{ab}
MORPHOLOGY CHANGE (%)	6.00 ± 0.95	21.00 ± 1.38 ^{a}	8.80 ± 0.37 ^{ab}	11.60 ± 0.75 ^{ab}	7.80 ± 0.5 ^{bd}

Values are expressed as Mean ± S. E. M.
a: Significant with control.
b: Significant with lead only group.
c: Significant with Vitamin C group.
d:Significant with Vitamin E group.
Significant at $p < 0.05$.
The number of animals in each experimental group was 5.

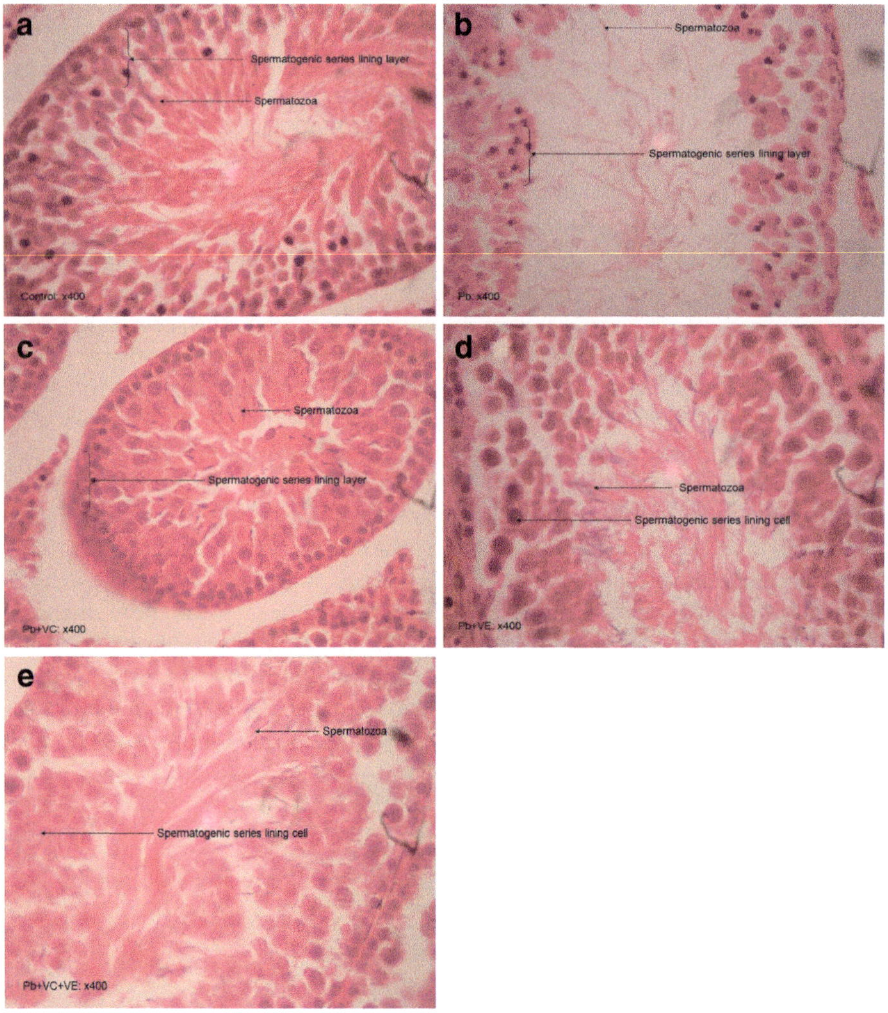

Figure 1 Histological changes in testes of rats (magnification x400) (spermatogenic series and spermatozoa illustrated). (**a**). Control testes showing normal* cell histology. (**b**). Pb only group- testes showing Mild reduction in seminiferous epithelium, empty lumen and reduction in number luminal spermatozoa in areas. (**c**). Pb + VC group-testes showing normal* cell histology. (**d**). Pb + VE group-testes showing an increase in luminal spermatozoa. (**e**). Pb + VC + VE group- Increase in luminal spermatozoa. *Normal: Seminiferous tubules contain 3–5 cell layered spermatogenic epithelium, with moderate amount of luminal spermatozoa.

Results in Table 2 also show that vitamin C and vitamin E treatment either individually, or in combination ameliorated the inhibitory action of lead by removing ROS once formed. Interestingly, Vitamin C treatment significantly ($p < 0.05$) reduced the testicular lead content and increased the Zinc contents in the lead treated rats when compared to vitamin E treatment. The biochemical parameters considered in this study showed a significant increase in total antioxidant content, and a reduction in lipid peroxidation products in vitamin C and/or vitamin E treatment (Tables 1 and 2).

Table 3 showed that serum FSH and TT levels in the animals were altered in the lead exposed animals, this was similar to the study of Ait *et al.,* [28]. LH results showed no significant alteration in lead exposed animals when compared to the control group. This is in agreement with El-tohamy [29] who observed that lead suppressed TT production with no significant alteration to LH content. However, studies carried out by Salawu *et al.,* [20] showed no significant decrease in serum TT level in lead treated rats. Nevertheless, reduction of LH and TT levels in animals exposed to lead indicates enzyme inhibition in the steroidogenetic pathway [30]. More so, increased blood lead content has been associated with disruption of hypothalamic secretion of hormones and spermatogenesis [28].

The testicular sperm counts and daily sperm production are important indicators of spermatogenesis [31]. In this study (Table 4), administration of lead acetate resulted in an obvious decline in sperm density, significantly ($p < 0.05$) reducing sperm counts, sperm motility, and increasing the amount of anomalous spermatozoa, [32]. OS is associated with sperm function impairment and plays a major role in the aetiology of defective sperm function [14]. Lead's direct toxicity on testicular histology or its action on the hypothalamic-pituitary axis or a combined defect involving the gonad and hypothalamic-pituitary sites could inhibit spermatogenesis [33]. Zinc deficiency has also been reported to affect sperm membrane integrity, and to reduce sperm motility. A possible correlation could also be drawn from lead induced zinc deficiency and sperm quality in rats.

Nonetheless vitamin C and/or vitamin E treatment on lead intoxicated animals showed a significant increase in reproductive hormones and an ameliorative effect on the semen quality assessed. Vitamin C treatment showed a higher ameliorative effect on testosterone, follicle stimulating hormone levels, and sperm motility and morphology when compared to vitamin E treatment.

Histological examination in Figure 1 shows deformities in the testicular tissue architecture of lead treated animals, with serious damages within the semniferous tubules. Lead treated animals showed reduction in seminiferous epithelium, an empty lumen with concomitant reduction in the number luminal spermatozoa. These findings are in agreement with Moniem *et al.,* [6] whose work showed that lead exposure caused progressive vascular, tubular and interstitial testicular damage. One possible mechanism for this impairment could be attributed to zinc reduction, as zinc deficiency in rats have been suggested to result in atrophy of seminiferous tubules [10]. More so lead induced OS could also cause oxidative damage to cellular materials.

Treatment of lead exposed animals with vitamin C and/or vitamin E showed an increase in luminal spermatozoa and seminiferous epithelium, with VC treatment potentiating better effects as viewed in the tissue histology. Zhu *et al.,* [34] reported a similar increase in the density of semineferous cells and luminal spermatozoa in Boer goats supplemented with vitamin E.

The ability for Vitamin C to exhibit ameliorative effect stems from its antioxidant, and chelating properties. In previous studies administration of ascorbic acid decreased significantly but not completely Pb circulation in the blood. Some other studies in rats demonstrated that ascorbic acid decreased the intestinal absorption of lead [35] and increased the renal clearance of lead [36]. VC has also been reported to protect the cells and sperm from oxidative stress and loss of motility, respectively [37]. VC inhibits lipid peroxidation, regenerate spent VE and protects against hydrogen peroxide induced DNA damage [15].

More so, VE was found to exhibit a protective effect on the testis of rats. It is a major chain-breaking antioxidant in the sperm membranes. It acts as a free radical scavenger, scavenging superoxide, hydrogen peroxide, and hydroxyl radicals [13]. Adding VE in diet increased the activity of some antioxidant enzymes, decreased nitric oxide content and lipid peroxidation products in the testis of Boer goat [34].

Vitamin C and E have both been implicated in protecting sperm DNA from oxidative stress of free radicals and improving fertility [38]. The differential in the ameliorative effect of Vitamin C and Vitamin E on the Pb-exposed animals could be related to the ability of vitamin C to chelate lead, thereby reducing leads capacity to substitute zinc in zinc mediated processes, recycling vitamin E and also directly participating in antioxidant activity by helping to replenish glutathione.

Conclusions

In conclusion, the present study showed that oral administration of lead was responsible for histological damage and disturbances in the metabolism of male reproductive organs. Nonetheless ameliorative effects where observed with vitamin C and/or Vitamin E treatment, with vitamin C potentiating a better ameliorative effect than vitamin E. Vitamin C and E proved to be ameliorative by improving the redox status, replenishing testes zinc content, reducing lead burden, reverting androgen levels, semen quality and testicular histology towards normal physiology.

Methods

Animals

Twenty five sexually matured, 12 weeks old albino Sprague Dawley Male rats (120-160 g) were obtained from the animal house of the College of Medicine, University of Lagos, Idi-araba Lagos state, Nigeria. This research was conducted in accordance with the internationally accepted principles for laboratory animal use and care as found in the US guidelines (NIH publication # 85–23, 1985) and approved by the committee on ethics in animal experimentation of the college of medicine, university of Lagos, Lagos Nigeria. The animals were kept in plastic cages and maintained under standard animal house conditions of illumination (illuminated for 12 h per day 0700-1900 h), and ventilation (kept in a room with a temperature of 28 ± 2°C). They had access to standard rat chow and water *ad libitum*.

Experimental Design

The animals were randomly and equally divided into five (5) groups. The rats were housed 5 in a plastic cage, and acclimatized for 14 days. After 14 days of acclimatization, a sub chronic study of six weeks was conducted. Lead was administered at 60 mg/kg body weight as lead acetate; Ascorbic acid was administered at 40 mg/Kg body weight as L ascorbic acid (VC), and α-tocopherol (VE) at 150 mg/Kg body weight as α-tocopheryl acetate. The first group served as control and received normal saline (0.9% w/v NaCl), the second group served as the lead (Pb) only group and received lead only, the third group served as the lead and L ascorbic acid (Pb + VC) group and received Pb and twenty minutes later VC. The fourth group served as the lead and α- tocopheryl acetate (Pb + VE) group and received Pb and twenty minutes later VE. The fifth group served as the lead and L ascorbic acid and α-tocopheryl acetate (Pb + VC + VE) group and received Pb and twenty minutes later L ascorbic acid and α-tocopheryl acetate.

The administration, of saline, lead, L ascorbic acid, and α-tocopheryl acetate was done three (3) times a week, every other day. All administrations were done via oral route.

Laboratory procedures and sample collection

At the end of the six weeks exposure and consequently after 24 h of the last oral administration, blood samples were collected via the orbital plexus into a standard test tubes from all animals and the animals were sacrificed by cervical dislocation. Blood samples stood for half an hour and then centrifuged at 500x g for 15 mins at 4°C to separate serum and stored at −70°C.Also the testes were quickly excised suspended in cold normal saline to rinse, weighed and kept cold for homogenisation.

Histological examination

After sacrificing rats in each group, the testis was quickly removed. The tissue was immersed in 10% formal saline for 16 hr for tissue fixation. Afterwards it was rinsed with distilled water, dehydrated in graded alcohol, cleared in xylene, and embedded in paraffin. Finally, they were cut into 5 µm section with a rotary microtome and stained with haematoxylin and eosin and examined under a microscope [39].

Biochemical indices

Determination of serum hormones

Serum testosterone (TT), follicle stimulating hormone (FSH) and luteinizing hormones (LH) where quantitatively measured by adopting enzyme-linked immunosorbent assay (ELISA) technique using kits purchased from Rapid Labs Ltd., (Essex, U.K).

Determination of lipid peroxidation products (MDA)

Malondialdehyde, formed from the breakdown of polyunsaturated fatty acids, serve as a convenient index for determining the extent of lipid peroxidation that reacts with thiobarbituric acid to give a red specie absorbing at 535 nm [40].

Determination of reduced gluthatione content (GSH)

Determination of reduced glutathione is based on the formation of a yellow colour after reacting with 5,5'dithiobis-2-nitrobenzoic acid (DTNB) which is then read at 412 nm [41].

Determination of super oxide dismutase (SOD) activity

SOD activity was determined according to the method by Sum and Zigma, [42]. Here the SOD enzyme assay is determined by the difference between superoxide anion decomposition and production i.e. its ability to inhibit the autoxidation of epinephrine, determined by the increase in absorbance at 320 nm.

Determination of catalase enzyme activity (CAT)

The activity of the enzyme catalase was analysed according to Cohen *et al.,* [43], which measures the initial rate of hydrogen peroxide (50 mM) decomposition. Where one unit is the amount of enzyme that hydrolyses 1 mol of H2O2 per minute and per milligram of protein at 25°C and pH 8.0.

Determination of total protein content (PRT) This method is based on the reaction between the tryptophan and tyrosine residues of the protein and the phosphomolybdic - phosphotungestic acid reagent (Folin Ciocalteu's reagent) in alkaline copper solution. The developed blue colour was then measured colouremetrically at a wave-length of 690 nm [44].

Sperm analysis and evaluation

Sperm samples obtained from the distal region of the vas deferens of the rats were used. This involved excision of a small piece of the vas deferens just distal to the cauda epididymis. The excised pieces were placed in a Petri dish containing 4 ml of normal saline (0.9% sodium chloride) at 37°C and homogenized. Sperm motility, count and morphology were determined through microscopic examination [45].

Metal analysis

Testes were digested with concentrated nitric acid and digests were diluted to a constant volume with deionised water. Lead and zinc concentration where then determined from the resultant solution by atomic absorption spectrophotometry (AAS).

Statistical analysis

Results were presented as Mean± S.E.M. Statistical analysis was conducted using one way ANOVA to compare the means and Tukey's test for post hoc. P-value <0.05 was considered significant. Statistical analysis was done using SPSS® 16 statistical software for windows.

Abbreviations

Pb: Lead; VC: Vitamin C; VE: Vitamin E; ROS: Reactive Oxygen Species; OS: Oxidative Stress; GSH: Glutathine; SOD: Superoxide Dismutase; CAT: Catalase; MDA: Malondialdehyde; NO: Nitric Oxide; TT: Testosterone; LH: Luteinising hormone; FSH: Follicle stimulating hormone; PRT: Total protein content; Zn: Zinc.

Competing interests

The authors declare that they have no competing interests.

Authors' contributions

RAO was involved in the histological examination, and participated in animal care. SO carried out the immunoassays. OCA conceived of the study, and participated in its design and coordination, OCA participated in animal care, participated in enzyme assay and metal analysis and drafted the manuscript. All authors read and approved the final manuscript.

Acknowledgements

Many thanks to Miss. Esther Abraham, and Mr. Oyesola Ojewunmi for their inputs to this study.

References

1. Flora SJ, Mittal M, Mehta A: **Heavy metal induced oxidative stress & its possible reversal by chelation therapy.** *Indian J Med Res* 2008, **128**(4):501–523.
2. Mostafa MH, Hoda SI, Yousria AM, Seham MA, Amal SA, Amany MH: **Effect of Alpha Lipoic Acid and Vitamin E on Heavy Metals Intoxication in Male Albino Rats.** *J Am Sci* 2010, **8**:56–63.
3. Chowdhury RA: **Recent Advances in Heavy Metals Induced Effect on Male Reproductive Function—A Retrospective.** *Al Ameen J Med Sci* 2009, **2**(2):37–42.
4. Hammond PB: **Exposure of humans to lead.** *Annu Rev Pharmacol Toxicol* 1977, **17**:197–214.
5. Berrahal AA, Lasram M, El Elj N, Kerkeni A, Gharbi N, El-Fazaa S: **Effect of age-dependent exposure to Lead on hepatotoxicity and nephrotoxocity in male rats.** *Environ Toxicol* 2011, **26**:68–78.
6. Moniem A, Dkhil M, Al-Quraishy S: **Protective role of flaxseed oil against lead acetate induced oxidative stress in testes of adult rats.** *Afr J Biotechnol* 2010, **9**(42):7216–7223.
7. Singh RP, Shashwat S, Suman K: **Free Radicals and Oxidative Stress in Neurodegenerative Diseases: Relevance of Dietary Antioxidants.** *Journal of Indian Academy of Clinical Medicine JIACM* 2004, **5**(3):218–225.
8. Mishra M, Acharya UR: **Protective action of vitamins on the spermatogenesis in lead-treated Swiss mice.** *J Trace Elem Med Biol* 2004, **18**(2):173–178.
9. Bedwal RS, Bahugana A: **Zinc, Copper and Selenium in reproduction.** *Experientaia* 1994, **50**:626–640.
10. Tuncer I, Sunar F, Toy H, Baltaci AK, Mogulkoc R: **Histological effect of zinc and melatonin on rat testes.** *Bratisl Lek Listy* 2011, **112**(8):425–427.
11. Krause MV, Mahan KL: *Food, Nutition, and Diet Therapy*, Volume 4-6. 7th edition.: W.B. Sanders company; 1984:71–133.
12. Lewis-Jones DI, Aird IA, Biljan MM, Kingsland CR: **Effects of sperm activity on zinc and fructose concentrations in seminal plasma.** *Hum Reprod* 1996, **11**(1):2465–2467.
13. Kartikeya M, Ashok A, Rakesh S: **Oxidative stress & male infertility.** *Indian J Med Res* 2009, **129**:357–367.
14. El-Tohamy MM, El-Nattat WS: **Effect of Antioxidant on Lead-Induced Oxidative Damage and Reproductive Dysfunction in Male Rabbits.** *J Am Sci* 2010, **6**(11):613–622.
15. Adeniyi TT, Ajayi GO, Akinloye OA: **Effect of Ascobic acid and *Allium sativum* on Tissue lead level in female *Rattus navigicus*.** *Niger J Health Biomed Sci* 2008, **7**(2):38–41.
16. Calabrese EJ, Stoddard A, Leonard DA, Dinardi SE: **The effects of vitamin C supplementation on blood and hair levels of cadmium, lead, and mercury.** *Ann NY Acad Sci* 1987, **498**:347–358.
17. Sugiyama M: **Role of physiological antioxidants in chromium (VI)-induced cellular injury.** *Free Radical Biol Med* 1992, **12**:397–407.
18. Nathan E, Huang HF, Pogach L, Giglio W, Bogden JD, Seebode J: **Lead acetate does not impair secretion of Sertoli cell function marker proteins in the adult Sprague Dawley rat.** *Arch Environ Health* 1992, **47**:370–375.
19. Abdel-Wahhab MA, Omara EA, Abdel-Galil MM, Hassan NS, Nada SA, Saeed A, Elsayed MM: **Zizyphus spina-christi extract protects against aflatoxin b (1)-intitiated hepatic carcinogenicity.** *Afr J Tradit Complement Altern Med* 2007, **4**(3):248–256.
20. Salawu O, Adeeyo OA, Falokun OP, Yusuf UA, Oyerinde A, Adeleke AA: **Tomato (Lycoperscion esculentum) prevents lead-induced testicular toxicity.** *J Hum Reprod Sci* 2009, **2**(1):30–34.
21. Vigeh M, Derek R, Ping-Chi H: **How does lead induce male infertility.** *IJRM* 2011, **9**(1):1–8.
22. Afaf AE: **Influence of Subchronic Exposure of Profenofos onBiochemical Markers and Microelements in Testicular Tissue of Rats.** *J Am* 2009, **5**(1):19–28.
23. Brooks DE: **Effect of androgen on protein synthesis and secretion in various regions of the rat epididymis, as analysed by two dimensional gel electrophoresis.** *Mol Cell Endocrinol* 1983, **29**:255–270.
24. Afaf AE, Hanan AT: **Chlorpyrifos (from different sources): Effect on Testicular Biochemistry of Male Albino Rats.** *J Am Sci* 2010, **6**(7):251–261.
25. Hamdi SA, Nassif OI, Ardawi MS: **Effect of marginal or severe dietary zinc deflciency on testlcular development and functions of the rat.** *Arch Androl* 1997, **38**:243–253.
26. Victery M, Thomas D, Schoeps P, Vander AJ: **Lead imcreases urinary excretion in rats.** *Biological trace elements research* 1982, **4**:211–219.
27. Lidsky TI, Schneider JS: **Lead neurotoxicity in children: basic mechanisms and clinical correlates.** *Brain* 2003, **126**:5–19.
28. Ait HN, Slimani M, Merad-Boudia B, Zaoui C: **Reproductive toxicity of lead acetate in adult male rats.** *Am J Scientific Res* 2009, **1**(3):38–50.
29. El-tohamy MM: *Reproductive potential in female and male domestic fowl exposed to lead acetate*, XIII Congress of the World Veterinary poultry association, 19–23. 17th edition. Denver: Co-sponsored by the American

Association of avian pathologist and the American veterinary Medicine Association; 2003:113.
30. Imran A, Muhammad S, Khalid FY: **Study of the effects of lead poisoning on the testes in albinos rats.** *Pakistan J Med Res* 2003, **42**(3):1–9.
31. Wang XJ, Zhang YM, Cui JS: **Study of effects of lead acetate on reproductive function in male mice.** *Chin J Ind Med* 2004, **17**(4):237–239.
32. Jensen TK, Bonde JP, Joffe M: **The influence of occupational exposure on male reproductive function.** *Occup Med* 2006, **56**(8):544–553.
33. Thoreux-Manlay A, de la Calle JFV, Olivier MF, Soufir JC, Masse R, Pinon-Lataillade G: **Impairment of testicular endocrine function after lead intoxication in the adult rat.** *Toxicology* 1995, **26:**101–109.
34. Zhu H, Luo HL, Meng H, Zhang GJ: **Effect of Vitamin E supplementation on development of reproductive organs in Boer goat.** *Anim Reprod Sci* 2009, **113:**93–101.
35. Morton AP, Partridge S, Blair JA: **The intestinal uptake of lead.** *Chem Br* 1985, **15:**923–927.
36. Niazi S, Lim J, Bederka JP: **Effect of ascorbic acid on the renal excretion of lead in rats.** *J Pharm* 1982, **71:**1189–1190.
37. Patra RC, Swarup D, Dwivedi SK: **Antioxidant effects of alpha tocopherol, ascorbic acid and L-methionine on lead induced oxidative stress to the liver, kidney and brain in rats.** *Toxicology* 2001, **162**(2):81–88.
38. Tarin JJ, Brines J, Cano A: **Antioxidants may protect against infertility.** *Hum Reprod* 1998, **13:**1415–1416.
39. Luna LG: *Manual Histological staining methods of the armed forces institute of pathology.* New York, USA: McGraw Hill Book Co; 1968:58–62.
40. Buege JA, Aust SD: **Microsomal lipid peroxidation methods.** *Enzymol* 1978, **52:**302–310.
41. Ellman GL: **Tissue sulfhudryl groups.** *Arch Biochem Biophys* 1959, **82**(1):70–77.
42. Sum M, Zigman S: **An improved spectrophotometric assay for superoxide dismutase based on epinephrine autoxidation.** *Anal Biochem* 1978, **90:**81–89.
43. Cohen G, Kim M, Ogwa V: *A modified catalase assay suitable for a plate reader.* 1996:56. Order article via Infotrieve.
44. Lowry OH, Rosenbrough NJ, Parr AL, Fandall RJ: **Protein measurement with Folin phenolreagent.** *J Biol Chem* 1951, **1951**(193):265–275.
45. Seed J, Chapin RE, Clegg ED, Dostal LA, Foote RH, Hurtt ME, *et al*: **Methods for assessing sperm motility, morphology, and counts in the rat, rabbit, and dog: a consensus report. ILSI Risk Science Institute Expert Working Group on Sperm Evaluation.** *Reprod Toxicol* 1996, **10:**237–244.

5

Unplanned medication discontinuation as a potential pharmacovigilance signal: a nested young person cohort study

Angela Peichen Sun[1], Bradley Kirby[1], Corri Black[1], Peter John Helms[1], Marion Bennie[2] and James Stuart McLay[1,3*]

Abstract

Background: Because of relatively small treatment numbers together with low adverse drug reaction (ADR) reporting rates the timely identification of ADRs affecting children and young people is problematic. The primary objective of this study was to assess the utility of unplanned medication discontinuation as a signal for possible ADRs in children and young people.

Methods: Using orlistat as an exemplar, all orlistat prescriptions issued to patients up to 18 years of age together with patient characteristics, prescription duration, co-prescribed medicines and recorded clinical (Read) codes were identified from the Primary Care Informatics Unit database between 1st Jan 2006-30th Nov 2009. Binary logistic regression was used to assess association between characteristics and discontinuation.

Results: During the study period, 79 patients were prescribed orlistat (81% female, median age 17 years). Unplanned medication discontinuation rates for orlistat were 52% and 77% at 1 and 3-months. Almost 20% of patients were co-prescribed an anti-depressant. One month unplanned medication discontinuation was significantly lower in the least deprived group (SIMD 1–2 compared to SIMD 9–10 OR 0.09 (95% CI0.01 – 0.83)) and those co-prescribed at least one other medication. At 3 months, discontinuation was higher in young people (≥17 yr versus, OR 3.07 (95% CI1.03 – 9.14)). Read codes were recorded for digestive, respiratory and urinary symptoms around the time of discontinuation for 24% of patients. Urinary retention was reported for 7.6% of patients.

Conclusions: Identification of unplanned medication discontinuation using large primary care datasets may be a useful tool for pharmacovigilance signal generation and detection of potential ADRs in children and young people.

Keywords: Pharmacovigilance, Pharmacoepidemiology, Obesity, Child, Orlistat, Adverse drug reaction, Medical records systems, Computerized, Young people

Background

Although adverse drug reactions (ADR) represent a major source of morbidity and mortality in adults, the nature and frequency of ADRs affecting children and young people remains poorly defined. Published data suggest that ADRs account for 1.5-2.1% of paediatric hospital admissions and affect 2.6-9.3% of paediatric in-patients and 1.5-11.1% of paediatric outpatients [1-10].

* Correspondence: j.mclay@abdn.ac.uk
[1]Division of Applied Health Sciences, University of Aberdeen, King's College, Aberdeen AB24 3FX, UK
[3]Department of Child Health, Royal Aberdeen Children's Hospital, Westburn Road, Aberdeen, Scotland AB25 2ZG, UK
Full list of author information is available at the end of the article

In the past children and young people have frequently been excluded from clinical trials and where trials are undertaken, they are often insufficiently powered to detect even relatively common ADRs. This means that children and young people are often prescribed medication with limited information about a treatment's ADR profile, at doses which are not evidence based, and "off–label"; a practice which itself is associated with increased risk of ADRs [2].

Post marketing surveillance is an essential tool in enabling the detection of potentially serious ADRs; however, to detect an ADR with a frequency of 1:10,000, at least 30,000 individuals need to be treated with the drug for at least 1 case to be identified. Therefore, post-marketing surveillance requires the monitoring of large patient cohorts exposed to a medication to detect ADRs. Currently, pharmacovigilance systems rely primarily on spontaneous reporting of ADRs. However under-reporting of ADRs is a significant issue affecting all European ADR monitoring systems. It is widely accepted that only 10% of UK and European healthcare professionals take part in the process of ADR reporting and that only 6-9% of ADRs affecting adults, which should be reported, are actually reported to the regulatory authorities [11-15]. Despite extending spontaneous ADR reporting in the UK to the public, and a wider group of healthcare professionals, public reporting rates still remain low, and significantly lower for children and young people than adults [16].

A growing area of medical concern and drug treatment is that of obesity [17,18]. Obese adolescents tend to be become obese adults, and it is well recognised that obesity in adults is associated with increased morbidity and mortality [19,20].

In the UK, orlistat, is currently the only anti-obesity drug licensed for use in severely obese (Body Mass Index, BMI ≥30 kg/m^2) adult patients or obese patients with comorbidities. Use in adults is associated with a 30% discontinuation within 3 months due to intolerable ADRs [21-24]. In pediatric/adolescent clinical trials, orlistat use has also been associated with a high level of ADRs (97-100%) and medication discontinuation (3.4-30%). However the majority of these orlistat studies have included less than 30 subjects so the ADR profile in children and young people is poorly understood [25-27].

In the UK, the majority of children and young people who require medical intervention for obesity, even when assessed in secondary care, are routinely reviewed and prescribed their medication in primary care. Primary Care electronic administrative data provide a record of relevant clinical information, service contacts and prescribing information and can, therefore, be used to assess the effectiveness of medications and potentially to generate pharmacovigilance signals. Such datasets which have been previously used for pharmacoepidemiology t have not been widely used for pharmacovigilance and have the potential to offer a complementary approach to routine pharmacovigilance methodologies.

Unplanned medication discontinuation (UMD), as a signal for the identification of possible ADRs, has been previously assessed in the adult population using Primary Care electronic administrative data. This approach is based on the recognition of an early, unplanned discontinuation of the prescription for a medication, possibly accompanied by switching to alternative medication. A close agreement has been previously reported between the UMD rate and ADR rates reported in the literature for a variety of adult medications [28].

The primary objective of this study was to assess the utility of UMD as a signal for possible ADRs in children and young people. Using a large Primary Care electronic administrative dataset and orlistat as an exemplar, we assessed prescribing pattern, medicine use and the potential to generate pharmacovigilance signals for medicines prescribed with low frequency to special populations such as children and young people.

Methods

Data source

The Primary Care Clinical Informatics Unit (PCCIU) research database is a large administrative dataset covering, in 2006, 179 Primary Care practices across Scotland [29]; representing approximately 20% of the Scottish population (1 million patients).

The PCCIU database, contains demographic data including gender, date of birth and socioeconomic status based on the practice post code (the Scottish Index of Multiple Deprivation (SIMD) 2006 quintiles) [30]: clinical information including diagnoses, procedures and practice encounter data, all recorded as Read codes, and prescribing data. Read codes are a national coding system used in primary care to code and record relevant information arising from a patient encounter in a standardised format. Read codes permit codification of a patient's history, symptoms, examination findings, physical signs, diagnostic procedures, therapeutic and administrative procedures, drugs, appliances, occupation and social information [31]. PCCIU contains validated clinical data on a large representative proportion of the Scottish population [30,32,33].

Study population

The study population included a closed cohort, all children and young people aged 0–16 years of age registered with a General Practice on the 1st January 2006. This cohort was then followed until they reached their 19th birthday or 30th November 2009.

Exposure

All children and young people newly prescribed orlistat (British National Formulary code 4.5) were identified and tracked through the study period.

For this study, a "new prescription" was defined as the first prescription for orlistat during the study period with no previous prescription in the preceding 3 months.

Primary outcome

The primary outcome of interest was identification of a potential pharmacovigilance signal, defined as the discontinuation of orlistat for at least 3 months without a subsequent prescription. Unplanned medication discontinuations were categorised based on duration of treatment as: <1 month, 1–3 months, 4–6 months or >6 months. Duration was calculated from the date of the first prescription to the date of the last prescription. If prescriptions were ongoing at the end of the study, the child was categorised as continuing treatment.

Because the majority of patient records identified in the PCCIU dataset did not contain a specific reason for drug discontinuation, clinical symptoms, diagnoses, investigations and procedures recorded as Read codes around the time of medication discontinuation were examined. All Read codes occurring after starting orlistat were identified. Potential signal associations were limited to codes recorded during the 3 months before and 3 months after the last prescription. Read codes were reported and summarised according to the International Classification of Diseases (ICD)-10 top level categories.

Other covariates

All co-prescriptions were extracted from the date of the first orlistat prescription up to 3 months after the last orlistat prescription date and classified into their respective British National Formulary (BNF) therapeutic drug classes [33]. The number of therapeutic drug classes prescribed for each patient was then determined and classified into 3 groups: no co-prescriptions issued, 1–4 therapeutic drug classes prescribed and >4 drug classes prescribed.

As national guidelines recommend that the BMI be calculated for the purposes of diagnosis, monitoring and initiation of pharmacological treatment, the date of the last recorded weight and height was also noted, and if assessed more than 1 year before start of orlistat was treated as missing.

To allow comparison between gender and developmental stages, the BMI standard deviation score (BMI SDS) was calculated based on Cole's LMS method [34].

Individuals with a BMI SDS between 2.5 – 3.49 were classified as overweight to obese, those with a BMI SDS over 3.5 classified as severely obese and those over 4 as very severely obese.

Statistical analysis

Descriptive statistics (percentages, mean (SD), median (IQR)) were used to report the characteristics of the cohort. The incidence rate for orlistat prescription was calculated for 2006.

Discontinuations were summarised as percentages and reported graphically.

To explore factors that might influence the discontinuation of orlistat treatment, we compared those who discontinued orlistat treatment at one and three months with those continuing treatment. We used binary logistic regression to calculate unadjusted odds ratios (OR) and 95% confidence intervals (CI). The factors considered included: gender, age, socioeconomic status, co-prescribing of antidepressants, and number of co-prescriptions. Analysis was performed using SPSS for windows 19.0 (SPSS Inc, Chicago, Illinois, USA).

Ethics and approvals

Data were anonymised and no personally identifiable information was sought. Approval for the study was granted by the Primary Care Clinical Informatics Unit research steering committee in accordance with their research governance process.

Results

From the study population of 166,726 children and young people (49% female) aged 0–16 years and registered with a participating primary care practice in Jan 2006, a cohort of 79 young people newly prescribed orlistat during the study period were identified. In 2006, at cohort inception, the incidence of orlistat was 0.06/1000/year for children aged 0–16 years.

Characteristics of the individuals prescribed orlisat

The median age at first orlistat prescription was 17 years (IQR 16 – 18), 81% were female and 55% were from General Practices situated in the most deprived socioeconomic areas (SIMD deciles 7–10) (Table 1). Of the 79 children and young people prescribed orlistat, only 54 (68.3%) had a BMI recorded, of which 42 (53.2%) had a BMI measured within 1 year, and 28 (35.4%) within one month of orlistat initiation. For the 42 individuals in whom BMI was measured within a year of orlistat initiation, the median time between BMI measurement and the index orlistat prescription was 0.3 months (IQR 0.0 – 2.2 months). The mean BMI SDS was 3.31 (SD0.9) with only 16 (20.3%) of all patients prescribed orlistat having a recorded BMI SDS greater than 3.5. The demographic characteristics of individuals prescribed orlistat is described in Table 1.

Two thirds (65.8%) of patients were co-prescribed between 1–4 drug classes/items. The medicines most commonly co-prescribed were antibiotics (17.4% of all prescriptions), topical skin treatments (12.4%), analgesics (10.7%), oral contraceptives (9.9%), asthma medications (7.4%) and antidepressants (4.1%). Four (5%) patients prescribed orlistat were also prescribed metformin. For three of these, metformin was initiated immediately following cessation of the orlistat prescription.

Orlistat discontinuation

Fifty-two percent of patients (41) discontinued orlistat medication within 1 month of the index prescription and 77% (61) within 3 months.

Discontinuation within 1 month was not affected by age or gender but was significantly less likely if the patient had received any co-prescription (OR 0.12 (95% CI

Table 1 Patient characteristics at time of first orlistat prescription during the follow up period (1st Jan 2006 -30th Nov 2009)

	Orlistat population (N = 79)	Male (N = 15) (19% of total)	Female (N = 64) (81% of total)
Age n (%)			
Children (under 17 years)	24 (30.5%)	4 (26.7%)	20 (31.3%)
Young people (17 – 18 years)	55 (69.6%)	11 (73.3%)	44 (68.7%)
Median (IQR)	*17 (16–18)*		
BMI SDS n (%)			
<2.5	12 (15.2%)	0	12 (18.8%)
2.5 – 3.49	24 (30.4%)	6 (40%)	18 (28.1%)
>3.5	18 (22.8%)	6 (40%)	12 (18.8%)
Missing	25 (31.6%)	3 (20%)	22 (34.4%)
Mean (SD)	*3.13 (1.0)*		
Deprivation SIMD (2006) n (%)			
1-2 (least deprived)	8 (10.1%)	1 (6.7%)	7 (10.9%)
3-4	7 (8.9%)	2 (13.3%)	5 (7.8%)
5-6	20 (25.3%)	3 (20.0%)	17 (26.6%)
7-8	18 (22.8%)	7 (46.7%)	11 (17.2%)
9-10 (most deprived)	26 (32.9%)*	2 (13.3%)	24 (37.5%)
Co-prescribed drug classes n (%)			
0	24 (30.4%)	7 (46.7%)	17 (26.6%)
1-4	52 (65.8%)	8 (53.3%)	44 (68.8%)
>4	3 (3.8%)	0 (0.0%)	3 (4.7%)
Median (IQR)	*1 (0–2)*		

*All percentage calculated from column total. *Chi squared test for trend p = 0.03.*
SIMD: Scottish Index of Multiple Deprivation, IQR: Inter-quartile range, BMI SDS: Body mass index standard deviation score.

0.03 – 0.41) or was in the least deprived group (OR 0.09 (95% CI 0.01 – 0.84) (SIMD 1–2) though there was no obvious trend by deprivation category.

Gender, co-prescription and socio-economic status, were not significantly related to 3-month discontinuation, however young people over 17 years of age were three times more likely to discontinue their prescription at 3-months when compared with those under 17 years of age (OR 3.07; 95%Cl 1.03 – 9.14) (Table 2).

Read codes and possible adverse events

In total, 404 Read codes were recorded from the start of orlistat treatment to 3 months after the last orlistat prescription for 77.2% (61) of the study population. The median number of Read codes per individual was 5; IQR 1–6 (range 0–51), and 20.3% (82) of these Read codes related specifically to symptoms or treatments. Eight (10.1%) patients had a Read Code recorded for: the respiratory, seven (8.9%) for the genitourinary, six (7.6%) for skin, six (7.6%) for endocrine, four (5.1%) for obstetric and gynaecological, four (5.1%) for gastrointestinal, four (5.1%) for musculoskeletal, 3 (3.8%) for mental health and behavioural and 3 (3.8%) for the CNS systems. (Symptoms and diagnoses are listed in Table 3).

Of note 8.9% (7, all female) of all patients prescribed orlistat had a Read code recorded within three months of orlistat discontinuation for the genitourinary system, of whom five were recorded as having urinary catheterisation and one urinary retention. None of these individuals were prescribed any medication or items during the three year study period to suggest neurological, bowel, bladder or malignant disease, which might explain the need for urinary catheterisation.

Discussion

We demonstrate that using UMD as a surrogate for possible adverse events, routinely collected primary care datasets may be used for pharmacovigilance signal generation, although validation of generated signals and confirmation of potential ADRs will require appropriately designed prospective studies. We believe that this approach will be complementary to the spontaneous reporting systems currently in use and enhance the capability of these systems to widen the breadth of ADRs detected while reducing

Table 2 Crude odds ratios for 1 month and 3 month discontinuation for factors such as: gender, age, deprivation score, prescription of anti-depressants and co-prescription of other therapeutic drug classes

	Duration of treatment				Duration of treatment			
	<1 month	≥1 month	OR	95% CI	<3 month	≥3 month	OR	95% CI
	N = 41	N = 38			N = 61	N = 18		
Gender *n (%)*								
Female	33 (80.5%)	31 (81.6%)	Ref		48 (78.7%)	16 (88.9%)	Ref	
Male	8 (19.5%)	7 (18.4%)	1.07	0.35–3.31	13 (21.3%)	2 (11.1%)	2.17	0.44– 10.65
Age bands *n (%)*								
Children (under 17 years)	9 (22.0%)	15 (39.5%)	Ref		15 (24.6%)	9 (50.0%)	Ref	
Young people (17-18 years)	32 (78.0%)	23 (60.5%)	2.32	0.87–6.21	46 (75.4%)	9 (50.0%)	3.07	1.03– 9.14
Deprivation SIMD 2006 *n (%)*								
1-2	1 (2.4%)	7 (18.4%)	0.09	0.01–0.84	5 (8.2%)	3 (16.7%)	0.23	0.03-1.41
3-4	3 (7.3%)	4 (10.5%)	0.47	0.09–2.55	6 (9.8%)	1 (0.6%)	0.78	0.07– 8.93
5-6	12 (29.3%)	8 (21.1%)	0.94	0.28–3.09	15 (24.6%)	5 (27.8%)	0.39	0.08– 1.89
7-8	9 (22.0%)	9 (23.7%)	0.63	0.19–2.11	12 (19.7%)	6 (33.3%)	0.26	0.06– 1.23
9-10	16 (39.0%)	10 (26.3%)	Ref		23 (37.7%)	3 (16.7%)	Ref	
Antidepressants *n (%)*								
Yes	37 (90.2%)	28 (73.7%)	Ref		51 (83.6%)	14 (77.8%)	Ref	
No	4 (9.8%)	10 (26.3%)	0.30	0.09–1.07	10 (16.4%)	4 (22.2%)	0.69	0.19– 2.52
Co-prescriptions issued *n (%)*								
Yes	20 (48.8%)	4 (10.5%)	Ref		22 (36.1%)	2 (11.1%)	Ref	
No	21 (51.2%)	34 (89.5%)	0.12	0.03–0.41	39 (63.9%)	16 (88.9%)	0.22	0.05– 1.06

CI; Confidence Interval. OR; Odds Ratio.
All percentage calculated from column total. SIMD: Scottish Index of Multiple Deprivation.

cost and time to ADR detection. Furthermore such an approach permits assessment of prescribing appropriateness together with real life prescribing patterns. In this study, one in every two patients prescribed orlistat discontinued within a month, and more than three quarters discontinued within three months, of starting treatment.

For medicines such as orlistat, continued use is likely to reflect patient acceptability and perceived effectiveness. In this context it is likely that early discontinuation reflects the appearance of unwanted poorly tolerated ADRs, while later discontinuation represents a perceived lack of response [35]. The levels of UMD in this study are similar to those reported by Viner at al, who noted orlistat discontinuations of 45% at one month, 75% at 3 months and 90% at 6 months [36].

Discontinuation at three months was significantly more frequent in the young people aged 17 years and over, possibly reflecting the effects of emerging autonomy and loss of parental influence [37-39]. One month discontinuation was significantly associated with social class and the presence of other co-prescribed medication, with patients from the most affluent social groups and those co-prescribed other medications less likely to discontinue orlistat therapy. While the association between social deprivation and poor adherence is well recognised the observation that medication discontinuation was less likely in those co-prescribed other medications runs counter to the perceived wisdom that higher levels of non-adherence are observed among adolescents and young adults prescribed multiple medicines [40,41].

In this study orlistat was prescribed predominantly to adolescents females, and those from the most socially deprived areas. Although the relationship between obesity and social deprivation is well recognised, this is the first study to report a link between social deprivation and orlistat prescribing [42-46].

Seventy percent of the cohort prescribed orlistat was co-prescribed medications including antibiotics, topical treatments for skin conditions and analgesia. Five percent of patients were also prescribed metformin, licensed for use in individuals aged 10 years and older for type II diabetes mellitus, but which is being increasingly used for the treatment of obesity and insulin resistance [46-51].

In the present study, one fifth of all patients (predominantly female) prescribed orlistat were also prescribed antidepressants at some point during the study period. In the general adolescent population antidepressants are reportedly prescribed to 1-5/1000 individuals per year [52-54], therefore the high level of use observed in our study suggests a significantly greater prevalence of depression in the

Table 3 Actual Symptoms and diagnoses recorded as Read codes by the treating primary care physician within 3 months of orlistat discontinuation (n = 79)

System	Number of patients (%)	Symptoms	Frequency
Respiratory	8 (10.1%)	Influenza	3
		Acute tonsillitis	3
		Acute bronchitis and bronchiolitis	2
		Asthma	1
		Chest infection	1
		Acute laryngitis and tracheitis	1
		Upper respiratory infection	1
		Cough	1
		Respiratory symptom	1
Genitourinary	7 (8.9%)	Treatment via bladder catheter	5
		Retention of urine	1
		Urinary tract infection (UTI)	1
		Suspected UTI	2
		Cystitis	1
Dermatology	6 (7.6%)	Rash and other non-specific skin eruption	1
		Dermatitis	1
		Skin cyst	1
		Chalazion (meibomian cyst)	1
		Acne vulgaris	1
		Unilateral mastalgia	1
		Lump in breast	1
		Psoriasis and similar disorders	1
Endocrine	6 (7.6%)	Obesity	4
		Acquired hypothyroidism	2
		Gynaecomastia	3
Obstetrics & Gynaecology	4 (5.1%)	Menorrhagia	1
		Dysmenorrhoea	1
		Spontaneous abortion	1
		Codes related to spontaneous abortion	6
		Polycystic ovarian syndrome	1
Gastrointestinal	4 (5.1%)	Non-infective gastritis	1
		Gastritis	1
		Abdominal pain	3
		Abdominal discomfort	1
		Irritable bowel syndrome	1
Musculoskeletal	4 (5.1%)	Backache	1
		Pain in lumbar spine	1
		Closed fracture of radius	1
		Temporomandibular joint disorder	1
		Arthralgia of knee	1
Mental health and behavioural	3 (3.8%)	Social phobias	4
		Loss of confidence	1
		Anxiety state	1
		Depressed mood	4
		At risk of deliberate self harm	1
Central nervous system	3 (3.8%)	In-coordination	1
		Tiredness	1
		Migraine	1
		Headache	1
		Infantile autism	1
Infection	3 (3.8%)	Viral infection	3

obese t population a finding consistent with studies in both young people and adults [54-56].

Read code, describing clinical symptoms and treatments, were recorded by a primary care physician for approximately a fifth of patients around the time of orlistat discontinuation. Respiratory, genitourinary, endocrine, skin, gynaecological and gastrointestinal symptoms were reported to occur in 10%, 8.9%, 7.6%, 7.6%, 5.1% and 5.1% of patients respectively. Data from pediatric/young person orlistat trials suggest that adverse effects, primarily diarrhoea, affect 97-100% of individuals, leading to a discontinuation rate of 2% - 30% [26,27,57]. In this study a Read code for gastrointestinal symptoms (all of which were abdominal pain) was only recorded for 5.1% of patients. The reasons for this apparent difference between our data and that from clinical trials may be that patients were pre-warned about possible gastrointestinal symptoms and therefore did not report the ADR, or that gastrointestinal side effects were so common that primary care physicians did not record them as a reason for discontinuation.

An unexpected finding was the number of individuals for whom urological system Read codes, urinary catheterisation and urinary retention, were recorded. The reasons for this finding are not clear. While urinary retention is frequently associated with neurological disorders and or constipation, assessment of co-prescribed medicines and items for these individuals, identified only one subject prescribed laxatives and none prescribed medicines or items commonly used for the treatment of neurological, bowel, bladder, malignant or infective conditions during the study period. Although orlistat use has been associated with nephrolithiasis and acute renal injury [58,59], there are currently no data in the literature linking orlistat with urinary retention. However as of November 2013 (current reporting period), the Medicines and Healthcare products Regulatory Agency, the UK government medicine regulatory agency, had received two "Yellow Card" reports for urinary retention possibly associated with orlistat use [60], raising the possibility that the association between orlistat use and urological symptoms observed in this study may be real. Although the approach used in this study doesn't allow us to attribute causality, it is reassuring to observe that the symptoms and diagnoses recorded by primary care physicians around the time of orlistat discontinuation, such as influenza infection, upper respiratory infection, headache and menstrual irregularities are in close agreement with those reported for adults in the real world [61].

Current clinical guidelines make it clear that prior to the initiation of orlistat therapy, height and weight should be recorded. In our study, 70% of the study cohort had this information recorded, and of these only a third had measurements recorded within a month of their initial prescription. The failure to undertake appropriate BMI assessment prior to orlistat initiation means that it is not possible to determine for the majority of patients whether orlistat was prescribed appropriately, according to the UK guidelines.

We have previously reported that electronic prescribing databases can be used to identify UMD in adult patients, and that such UMD rates can be used as a surrogate for ADR/AE rates [28,35]. However, the use of UMD does not identify the reasons for discontinuation or the nature of possible ADRs/AEs. The UMD and ADR results we obtained for orlistat are in close agreement with previously published UMD and ADR rates obtained using more traditional methods of ascertainment, indicating that UMD obtained from routinely collected data may represent a surrogate marker for ADR/ADE occurrence. Using this approach together with more traditional spontaneous reporting systems [62], may reveal potential pharmacovigilance signals at an earlier stage following introduction of a medicine and permit a more accurate assessment of ADR incidence than is currently possible.

The use of large primary care electronic datasets enables the linkage of whole population prescription information with recorded clinical symptoms, diagnoses and encounters. As we have demonstrated, this approach permits the assessment of prescribing trends and identification of individuals who discontinue their medication at an early stage before clinical effectiveness might be expected. Assessment of clinical symptoms and diagnosis recorded around the time of orlistat discontinuation identified unexpected findings which might indicate, although not prove, the occurrence of an ADR to the study medication.

There were several limitations to our study. It is possible that the small number of patients prescribed orlistat in this study may reduce the generalisability of the orlistat specific findings; however it does not alter the overall conclusion that the linkage of UMD with medical Read codes identifies possible pharmacovigilance signals of interest. Moreover, the PCCIU-R database, like most other prescribing/dispensing databases, only reflects primary care prescribing and does not provide information on secondary care prescribing or over the counter purchase of orlistat. It is therefore possible that patients for whom an initial prescription was issued in secondary care or who purchased their medication OTC may have been missed. However this is unlikely to be a major issue in the Western world, where primary care remains the major source of medication prescriptions. A further limitation is the lack of a specific recorded reason for orlistat discontinuation in the PCCIU-R database, and this is the reason why all Read codes at or about the time of discontinuation were identified and examined.

Conclusions

Using orlistat as the exemplar, we have demonstrated that when unplanned medication discontinuation are linked to clinical codes for events occurring at the time of discontinuation, it is possible to generate both predictable and unpredicted pharmacovigilance signals. These findings support the use of this approach together with traditional pharmacovigilance methodologies to identify possible signals and plan more specific and focused pharmacovigilance studies with the aim of validating suspected ADRs.

Patient consent

As all data analyzed was fully anonymised and non attributable the approval for the study was granted by the Primary Care Clinical Informatics Unit research steering committee in accordance with their research governance process and individual patient consent was not necessary.

Abbreviations

ADR: Adverse drug reaction; BMI: Body mass index; BMISDS: Body mass index standard deviation score; BNF: British National Formulary; ICD: International Classification of Diseases; MHRA: Medicines and healthcare products regulatory agency; PCCIUR: Primary care clinical informatics unit research; NICE: National institute for health and clinical excellence; SIMD: Scottish index of multiple deprivation; SIGN: Scottish intercollegiate guidelines network.

Competing interests

The authors declare that they have no competing interests.

Authors' contributions

AS: assisted in conceptualization, design and analysis of the study, drafted the initial manuscript, and approved the final manuscript as submitted. BK: assisted in conceptualization, design and analysis of the study and approved the final manuscript as submitted. PH: assisted in conceptualization, design and analysis of the study and approved the final manuscript as submitted. CB: assisted in conceptualization, design and analysis of the study and approved final manuscript as submitted. MB: assisted in conceptualization, design and analysis of the study and approved the final manuscript as submitted. JM: conceptualized and designed the study, assisted with analysis and interpretation of results, and approved the final manuscript as submitted. JM acts as study guarantor. All authors read and approved the final manuscript.

Acknowledgement
The authors wish to acknowledge that the data contained herein were provided by the Primary Care Clinical Informatics Unit (PCCIU) at the University of Aberdeen. The views in this publication are not necessarily the views of the University of Aberdeen, it's agents, or employees. The authors also wish to acknowledge the Chief Scientists Office, Scotland who funded this study and the Scottish Children's Research Network (ScotCRN).

Funding source
All phases of this study were supported by a Scottish Government, Chief Scientist Office project grant. Grant Number: ARPG/07/4.

Financial disclosure
The authors have no financial relationships relevant to this article to disclose.

Author details
[1]Division of Applied Health Sciences, University of Aberdeen, King's College, Aberdeen AB24 3FX, UK. [2]National Medicines Utilisation Unit, Information Services Division, NHS National Services Scotland, Edinburgh, Scotland. [3]Department of Child Health, Royal Aberdeen Children's Hospital, Westburn Road, Aberdeen, Scotland AB25 2ZG, UK.

References

1. Turner S, Nunn AJ, Fielding K, Choonara I: **Adverse drug reactions to unlicensed and off-label drugs on paediatric wards.** *Acta Paediatr* 1999, **88**(9):965–968.
2. Horen B, Montastruc JL, Lapeyre-Mestre M: **Adverse drug reactions and off label drug use in paediatric outpatients.** *Br J Clin Pharmacol* 2002, **54**:665–670.
3. Impicciatore P, Choonara I, Clarkson A, Provasi D, Pandolfini C, Bonati M: **Incidence of adverse drug reactions in paediatric in/out patients: a systematic review and meta-analysis of prospective studies.** *Br J Clin Pharmacol* 2001, **52**(1):77–83.
4. Gargon E, Kirkham J, Cresswell L, Golder S, Smyth R, Williamson P: **Adverse drug reactions in children—a systematic review.** *PLOS One* 2012.
5. Jonville-Bera AP, Giraudeau B, Blanc P, Beau-Salinas F, Autret-Leca E: **Frequency of adverse drug reactions in children: a prospective study.** *Br J Clin Pharmacol* 2002, **53**(2):207–210.
6. Whyte J, Greenan E: **Drug usage and adverse drug reactions in paediatric populations.** *Acta Paediatr Scand* 1977, **66**(6):767–775.
7. Martinez-Mir I, Garcia-Lopez M, Palop V, Ferrer JM, Rubio E, Morales-Olivas FJ: **A prospective study of adverse drug reactions in hospitalised children.** *Br J Clin Pharmacol* 1999, **47**(6):681–688.
8. Weiss J, Krebs S, Hoffman C, Werner U, Neubert A, Brune K, Rascher W: **Survey of adverse drug reactions on a paediatric ward: a strategy for early and detailed detection.** *Pediatrics* 2002, **110**(2 Pt 1):254–257.
9. Kramer MS, Hutchinson TA, Flegel KM, Naimark L, Contardi R, Leduc DG: **Adverse drug reactions in general paediatric outpatients.** *J Paediatr* 1985, **106**(2):305–310.
10. Davies EC, Green CF, Mottram DR, Pirmohamed M: **Adverse drug reactions in hospital in-patients: a pilot study.** *J Clin Pharmacol Ther* 2006, **31**:335–341.
11. Martin RM, Kapoor KV, Wilton LV, Mann RD: **Underreporting of suspected adverse drug reactions to newly marketed ("black triangle") drugs in general practice: observational study.** *BMJ* 1998, **317**:119–120.
12. **Reporting adverse drug reactions. A guide for healthcare professionals.** 2006. BMA Board of Science. British Medical Association, BMA House, Tavistock Square,London, WC1H 9JP. http://www.isoponline.org/documents/news/BMAreport.pdf. © British Medical Association.
13. Smith CC, Bennet PM, Pearce HM, Harrison HI, Reynolds DJM, Aronson JK, Graeme-Smith DG: **Adverse drug reactions in a hospital general medical unit meriting notification to the Committee on the Safety of Medicines.** *Brit J Clin Pharmacol* 1996, **42**:423–9.
14. Schirm E, Tobil H, Van Puijenbroek EP, Monster-Simons MH, den Berg LTW DJ-v: **Reported adverse drug reactions and their determinants in Dutch children outside the hospital.** *Pharmacoepi Drug Safety* 2004, **13**:159–65.
15. Hawcutt DB, Pramod M, Riordan A, Smyth R, Pirmohamed M: **Reported paediatric adverse drug reactions in the UK 2000–2009.** *Brit JClin Pharmacol* 2012, **73**:437–446.
16. Avery AJ, Anderson C, Bond CM, Fortnum H, Gifford A, Hannaford PC, Hazell J, Krska L, Lee AD, McLernon DJ, Murphy E, Shakir S, Watson MJ: **Evaluation of patient reporting of adverse drug reactions to the UK Yellow Card Scheme: literature review, descriptive and qualitative analyses and questionnaire surveys.** *Health Technol Assess* 2011, **15**(20):33–47.
17. Broyles S, Katzmarzyk PT, Srinivasan SR, Chen W, Bouchard C, Freedman DS, Berenson GS: **The pediatric obesity epidemic continues unabated in Bogalusa, Louisiana.** *Pediatr* 2010, **125**(5):900–905.
18. Wang Y, Monteiro C, Popkin BM: **Trends of obesity and underweight in older children and adolescents in the United States, Brazil, China, and Russia.** *Am J Clin Nutr* 2002, **75**(6):971–977.
19. Poirier P, Giles TD, Bray GA, Hong Y, Stern JS, Pi-Sunyer FX, Eckel RH: **Obesity and cardiovascular disease: pathophysiology, evaluation, and effect of weight loss.** *Arterioscler Thromb Vasc Biol* 2006, **26**(5):968–976. 20.
20. Must A: **Morbidity and mortality associated with elevated body weight in children and adolescents.** *Am J Clin Nutr* 1996, **63**(3 Suppl):445S–447S.
21. Filippatos TD, Derdemezis CS, Gazi IF, Nakou ES, Mikhailidis DP, Elisaf MS: **Orlistat-associated adverse effects and drug interactions: a critical review.** *Drug Safety* 2008, **31**(1):53–65.
22. Acharya NV, Wilton LV, Shakir SA: **Safety profile of orlistat: results of a prescription-event monitoring study.** *Int J Obes* 2006, **30**(11):1645–1652. 23: Gonzalez-Gay MA, Garcia-Porrua C, Lueiro M, Fernandez ML. Orlistat-induced cutaneous leukocytoclastic vasculitis. Arthritis & Rheumatism 2002 Oct 15;47(5):567.
23. Sergeant A, Milne G, Shaffrali F: **Lichenoid eruption associated with orlistat.** *Br J Dermatol* 2006, **154**(5):1020–1021.
24. McDuffie JR, Calis KA, Uwaifo GI, Sebring NG, Fallon EM, Hubbard VS, Yanovski JA: **Three-month tolerability of orlistat in adolescents with obesity-related comorbid conditions.** *Obes Res* 2002, **10**(7):642–650.
25. Ozkan B, Bereket A, Turan S, Keskin S: **Addition of orlistat to conventional treatment in adolescents with severe obesity.** *Eur J Pediatr* 2004, **12**(163(12)):738–741.
26. Norgren S, Danielsson P, Jurold R, Ltborn M, Marcus C: **Orlistat treatment in obese prepubertal children: a pilot study.** *Acta Pædiatr* 2003, **92**(6):666–70.
27. Mohamed IN, Helms PJ, Simpson CR, Milne RM, McLay JS: **Using primary care prescribing databases for pharmacovigilance.** *Br J Clin Pharmacol* 2011, **71**(2):244–249.
28. Mohamed IN, Helms PJ, Simpson CR, McLay JS: **Using primary care prescribing databases for pharmacovigilance.** *Brit J Clin Pharmacol* 2011, **712**:244–249.
29. **Scottish Index of Multiple Deprivation.** http://www.scotland.gov.uk/Topics/Statistics/SIMD Accessed 01 04 2013.
30. **Read Code User Guide Dr. Lesley Graham, Ann Ward, Gerry Mulvenna. ISD Scotland July 2000.** https://www.google.co.uk/search?q=Read+Code+User+Guide+Dr.+Lesley+Graham,+Ann+Ward,+Gerry+Mulvenna.+599+ISD+Scotland+July+2000.&ie=utf-8&oe=utf-8&rls=org.mozilla:en-US:official&client=firefox-a&channel=sb&gws_rd=cr&ei=SakZU8iFLaWS7AaliYA4 Accessed 23/07/2013).
31. **Database review by PCCIU.** http://www.abdn.ac.uk/iahs/uploads/files/PCI.pdf. Accessed 25 06 2013.
32. Whitelaw FG, Nevin SL, Milne RM, Taylor RJ, Taylor MW, Watt AH: **Completeness and accuracy of morbidity and repeat prescribing records held on general practice computers in Scotland.** *B J G P* 1996, **46**(404):181–186.
33. Cole TJ, Freeman JV, Preece MA: **Body mass index reference curves for the UK, 1990.** *Arch Dis Child* 1995, **73**(1):25–29.
34. *British National Formulary*, Volume No 64. BMJ and Pharmaceutical Press; 2012. ISBN 978 0 85711 065 7.
35. Mohamed IN, Helms PJ, Simpson CR, McLay JS: **Using routinely collected prescribing data to determine drug persistence for the purpose of pharmacovigilance.** *J Clin Pharmacol* 2011, **51**(2):279–284.
36. Viner RM, Hsia Y, Neubert A, Wong ICK: **Rise in antiobesity drug prescribing for children and adolescents in the UK: a population-based study.** *Br J Clin Pharmacol* 2009, **68**(6):844–851.
37. Tebbi CK: **Treatment compliance in childhood and adolescence.** *Cancer* 1993, **71**(10 Suppl):3441–3449.

38. Friedman IM, Litt IF: **Adolescents' compliance with therapeutic regimens. Psychological and social aspects and intervention.** *J Adolescent Health Care* 1987, **8**(1):52–67.
39. Tebbi CK, Cummings KM, Zevon MA: **Compliance of pediatric and adolescent cancer patients.** *Cancer* 1986, **58**(5):1179–1184.
40. Tucker CM, Fennell RS, Pedersen T, Higley BP, Wallack CE, Peterson S: **Associations with medication adherence among ethnically different pediatric patients with renal transplants.** *Pediatr Nephrol* 2002, **17**(4):251–256.
41. Claxton AJ, Cramer J, Pierce C: **A systematic review of the associations between dose regimens and medication compliance.** *Clin Ther* 2001, **23**(8):1296–1310.
42. Kinra S, Nelder RP, Lewendon GJ: **Deprivation and childhood obesity: a cross sectional study of 20,973 children in Plymouth, United Kingdom.** *J Epidemiol Community Health* 2000, **54**(6):456–460.
43. Strauss RS, Knight J: **Influence of the home environment on the development of obesity in children.** *Pediatr* 1999, **103**(6):e85.
44. Goldblatt PB, Moore ME, Stunkard AJ: **Social factors in obesity.** *JAMA* 1965, **192**:1039–1044.
45. Sobal J, Stunkard AJ: **Socioeconomic status and obesity: a review of the literature.** *Psychol Bull* 1989, **105**(2):260–275.
46. Yanovski JA, Krakoff J, Salaita CG, McDuffie JR, Kozlosky M, Sebring NG, Reynolds JC, Brady SM, Calis KA: **Effects of metformin on body weight and body composition in obese insulin-resistant children: a randomized clinical trial.** *Diabetes* 2011, **60**(2):477–485.
47. Burgert TS, Duran EJ, Goldberg-Gell R, Dziura J, Yeckel CW, Katz S, Tamborlane WV, Caprio S: **Short-term metabolic and cardiovascular effects of metformin in markedly obese adolescents with normal glucose tolerance.** *Pediatr Diabetes* 2008, **9**(6):567–576.
48. Atabek ME, Pirgon O: **Use of metformin in obese adolescents with hyperinsulinemia: a 6-month, randomized, double-blind, placebo-controlled clinical trial.** *J Pediatr Endocrinol* 2008, **21**(4):339–348.
49. Srinivasan S, Ambler GR, Baur LA, Garnett SP, Tepsa M, Yap F, Ward GM, Cowell CT: **Randomized, controlled trial of metformin for obesity and insulin resistance in children and adolescents: improvement in body composition and fasting insulin.** *J Clinl Endocrinol Metab* 2006, **91**(6):2074–2080.
50. Freemark M, Bursey D: **The effects of metformin on body mass index and glucose tolerance in obese adolescents with fasting hyperinsulinemia and a family history of type 2 diabetes.** *Pediatr* 2001, **107**(4):E55.
51. Love-Osborne K, Sheeder J, Zeitler P: **Addition of metformin to a lifestyle modification program in adolescents with insulin resistance.** *J Pediatr* 2008, **152**(6):817–822.
52. Murray ML, de Vries CS, Wong IC: **A drug utilisation study of antidepressants in children and adolescents using the General Practice Research Database.** *Arch Dis Child* 2004, **89**(12):1098–1102.
53. Zito JM, Safer DJ, Sai D, Gardner JF, Thomas D, Coombes P, Dubowski M, Mendez-Lewis M: **Psychotropic medication patterns among youth in foster care.** *Pediatr* 2008, **121**(1):e157–63.
54. Mustillo S, Worthman C, Erkanli A, Keeler G, Angold A, Costello EJ: **Obesity and psychiatric disorder: developmental trajectories.** *Pediatr* 2003, **111**(4 Pt 1):851–859.
55. Atlantis E, Baker M: **Obesity effects on depression: systematic review of epidemiological studies.** *Int J Obes* 2008, **32**(6):881–891.
56. Revah-Levy A, Speranza M, Barry C, Hassler C, Gasquet I, Moro MR, Falissard B: **Association between Body Mass Index and depression: the "fat and jolly" hypothesis for adolescents girls.** *BMC Public Health* 2011, **11**:649.
57. Chanoine J, Hampl S, Jensen C, Boldrin M, Hauptman J: **Effect of orlistat on weight and body composition in obese adolescents: a randomized controlled trial.** *JAMA* 2005, **293**(23):2873–83.
58. Singh A, Sarkar SR, Gaber LW, Perazella MA: **Acute oxalate nephropathy associated with orlistat, a gastrointestinal lipase inhibitor.** *Am J Kidney Dis* 2007, **49**(1):153–157.
59. Weir MA, Beyea MM, Gomes T, Juurlink DN, Mamdani M, Blake PG, Wald R, Amit MPH, Garg X: **Orlistat and acute kidney injury: an analysis of 953 patients.** *Arch Intern Med* 2011, **171**(7):703–4.
60. **MHRA orlistat drug analysis print.** http://www.mhra.gov.uk/Safetyinformation/Howwemonitorthesafetyofproducts/Medicines/TheYellowCardScheme/YellowCarddata/Druganalysisprints/index.htm?secLevelIndexChar=Oq%20-%20Ou#retainDisplay Accessed 22.01.2014.
61. **Highlights of prescribing information-Xenical.** http://www.accessdata.fda.gov/drugsatfda_docs/label/2012/020766s029lbl.pdf Accessed 19/06/2013).
62. The World Health Organisation: **Pharmacovigilance toolkit. pharmacovigilance methods.** http://www.pvtoolkit.org/index.php?option=com_content&view=article&id=6&Itemid=10 Accessed 20. 07 2013.

6

Preclinical and clinical phase I studies of a new recombinant Filgrastim (BK0023) in comparison with Neupogen®

Davide Crobu[1*], Gaia Spinetti[2], Rodolfo Schrepfer[1], Giancarlo Tonon[1], Gloria Saccani Jotti[5], Pierluigi Onali[3], Simona Dedoni[3], Gaetano Orsini[1] and Andrea Di Stefano[4]

Abstract

Background: Filgrastim or methionyl-granulocyte colony-stimulating factor (Met-G-CSF), is a recombinant therapeutic protein widely used to treat severe neutropenia caused by myelosuppressive drugs in patients with nonmyeloid malignancies. In addition to its role in the regulation of granulopoiesis, treatment with G-CSF is considered the standard approach to mobilize CD34 positive ($CD34^+$) mononuclear cells for reconstituting hemopoietic ability for bone marrow transplantation. An intended biosimilar filgrastim (coded BK0023) was produced in GMP conditions by *E.coli* fermentation according to an original recombinant process and showed physico-chemical properties and purity profile similar to Neupogen®, a commercial preparation of filgrastim. The aim of the present study was to demonstrate the comparability of BK0023 to Neupogen® in terms of both *in vitro* biological activities and *in vivo* toxicology, pharmacokinetics and pharmacodynamics.

Methods: Cell proliferation and radioligand binding assays were conducted in NFS-60 cells to compare the biological activity and functional interaction with the G-CSF receptor *in vitro*, while preclinical *in vivo* studies, including pharmacokinetics and pharmacodynamics after repeated dose were performed in normal and neutropenic rats. A phase I study was carried out in healthy male volunteers treated by multiple-dose subcutaneous administration of BK0023 and Neupogen® to evaluate their pharmacodynamic effects as well as their pharmacokinetic and safety profile and to demonstrate their pharmacodynamic equivalence and pharmacokinetic bioequivalence.

Results: The results reported in this work demonstrate that BK0023 is comparable in terms of biological activity, efficacy and safety to Neupogen®.

Conclusions: BK0023 has the same pharmacokinetic profile, efficacy and safety as the reference commercial filgrastim Neupogen® and therefore could be further developed to become a convenient option to treat neutropenia in oncological patients.

Trial registration: Trial registration number (TRN): NCT01933971. Date of registration: Sept 6th 2013.

Keywords: r-Met-G-CSF, BK0023, Biosimilar Filgrastim, Comparability

* Correspondence: davide.crobu@multimedica.it
[1]Bio-Ker S.r.l.-Multimedica Group, Sardinia Scientific and Technological Park, Building 3, I-09010 Pula Cagliari, Italy
Full list of author information is available at the end of the article

Background

Human granulocyte-colony stimulating factor (G-CSF) is a haematopoietic glycoprotein produced by stromal cells, macrophages, endothelial cells, fibroblasts and monocytes which binds with high affinity to the G-CSF receptor expressed on neutrophilic precursor cells in the bone-marrow, inducing them to proliferate and differentiate into infection-fighting neutrophils without significant haemopoietic effects on other lineages of blood cells.

The use of recombinant G-CSF preparations is a well established treatment for accelerating bone marrow recovery, for preventing the onset of severe myelosuppression and its correlated complications and for reducing febrile neutropenia in patients with non-myeloid malignancies under radio- or chemotherapies [1,2]. Moreover, G-CSF is clinically used as bone marrow mobilizer to increase the number of circulating $CD34^+$ progenitor cells [3] employed for hematopoietic cell reconstitution. Besides, since recent preclinical evidences showed a pro-angiogenic potential of $CD34^+$ cells, the use of these cells for regenerative medicine of ischemic diseases is currently under investigation in clinical trials [4]. Other studies suggest that G-CSF is worth investigating as an interesting therapeutical option in cardiovascular field for the prevention of restenosis after percutaneous coronary intervention [5] as well as for its beneficial effect in stroke recovery due to the enhancement of neurogenesis and the stimulation of blood vessel formation [6].

In response to the need of a highly purified protein for medical applications, both glycosylated and non-glycosylated forms of human G-CSF have been manufactured by recombinant DNA technology. Glycosylation appears to increase resistance of G-CSF to proteolysis, but it is not required for receptor binding or biological activity of the protein. In fact, recombinant glycosylated and non-glycosylated G-CSF variants exhibit the same pharmacokinetics and pharmacodynamic profiles [7].

Recombinant Met-G-CSF or filgrastim is a single-chain protein of 175 aminoacids and two disulfide bonds differing from the native G-CSF in that it is not O-glycosylated on threonine 134 and bears an additional N-terminal methionine required for expression in *E. coli*. An original method to produce a biosimilar filgrastim, called BK0023, by high yield bacterial expression of a fusion protein in the form of inclusion bodies was developed. After *in vitro* refolding, the fusion protein was enzymatically cleaved to give functionally active r-Met-G-CSF which was purified and characterized. Finally, we conducted *in vitro* and *in vivo* preclinical studies as well as a clinical phase I study in healthy volunteers to compare the biological, pharmacodynamic, pharmacokinetic and safety profile of BK0023 and Neupogen®.

The results demonstrated the pharmacodynamic equivalence and the pharmacokinetic bioequivalence of BK0023, a recombinant filgrastim produced according to an original process, towards Neupogen®, a proprietary filgrastim approved for clinical use, and support the claim for further assessments of BK0023 as biosimilar drug that, once approved for marketing, could potentially be a useful and cost-effective treatment option for patients requiring G-CSF.

Methods

Cell culture

Murine myeloblastic NFS-60 cells were purchased from Cell Line Service (Eppelheim, Germany). RPMI 1640 medium, fetal bovine serum (FBS), fetal calf serum (FCS), penicillin and streptomycin were provided by Gibco Life Technologies (Monza, Italy). Mouse interleukine 3 (IL-3) was from Sigma-Aldrich (St. Louis, MO, USA) while WST-1 reagent was from Roche (Milan, Italy). Materials for gel electrophoresis were provided by Bio-Rad Laboratories Inc. (Hercules, CA, USA). If not otherwise reported, all other reagents and chemicals were of analytical grade and provided by Sigma Aldrich-Fluka, Merck or Carlo Erba (Milan, Italy).

Test products

Recombinant Met-G-CSF (BK0023) was produced using a Bioker's manufacturing technology at Eurogenetec S.A., Belgium, in GMP conditions by high biomass *E.coli* fermentation according to a previously described protein fusion technology starting from a gene coding for filgrastim bearing an N-terminal enhancer peptidic tag [8]. Briefly, $LacZ_8$-PNP_{20}-Kex-1-Met-G-CSF hybrid fusion protein (where LacZ8 represents the first 8 aminoacids of the LacZ protein fragment [UniProt/SwissProt accession Q37953], PNP_{20} is a sequence coding for the first twenty amino acids of *E.coli* purine nucleoside phosphorylase [9] and the N-terminal methionine residue of filgrastim is immediately preceded by a sequence coding for the short flexible peptide -Glu-Ser-Ser-Met-Ser-Gly-Leu-Phe-Lys-Arg- ending with a Lys-Arg basic dipeptide which *in vitro* is specifically cleaved at C-terminal site of arginine by the endoprotease ss-Kex-1-C_{611} to leave the mature sequence of filgrastim) was expressed in *E.coli* as cytoplasmic inclusion bodies. After isolation of inclusion bodies, the fusion protein was dissolved in 7 M guanidine, renaturated by dilution, dialyzed and cleaved by treatment with the patented recombinant endoprotease ss-Kex1-C_{611} [10] and the released filgrastim was purified to homogeneity by column chromatography to obtain a clinical grade preparation coded BK0023. Bulk BK0023 in pH 4.5 buffered solution, was sterile filtrated, formulated in glass vials containing for each milliliter 300 μg filgrastim, 50 mg sorbitol, 0.04 mg polysorbate 80, 0.59 g acetate ions 0.83 mg sodium ions and stored at 2-8°C. The reference filgrastim was

Neupogen® 300 μg/ml, (Dompé Biotec, Italy) purchased from a pharmacy.

Sodium dodecyl sulphate polyacrylamide gel electrophoresis (SDS-PAGE) and Western Blotting

SDS-PAGE was carried out in reducing and non-reducing conditions on polyacrylamide gels (4% stacking gel, 12% running gel) prepared according to Laemmli [11]. Samples were diluted 1:1 v/v with 62.5 mM Tris–HCl-pH 6.8-25% glycerol-2% SDS-0.01% Bromophenol Blue ± 5% 2-mercaptoethanol buffer and heated for 5 min at 95°C. Ten microliters samples (3–5 μg of protein) were loaded in the gels which, after the electrophoretic migration, were stained with Coomassie Brilliant Blue R 250 and washed with 10% v/v acetic acid-15% v/v ethanol solution.

Western Blotting was carried out, after SDS-PAGE separation and electrophoretic transfer, using anti-G-CSF rabbit polyclonal antibody (PeproTech, Hamburg, Germany) as primary antibody and anti-rabbit goat antibody HRP conjugate (Santa Cruz Biotechnology, Heidelberg, Germany) as secondary antibody.

Reversed Phase-High Pressure Liquid Chromatography (RP-HPLC)

BK0023 purity and contamination with its oxidized forms were detected by RP-HPLC of 3–5 μg/10 μl samples performed on a Symmetry C18 300 Å column, 2.1 × 150 mm, 3.5 μm (Waters Corp., Milford Massachusetts, USA) with a HP 1100 liquid chromatography system (Agilent Technologies, Waldbronn, Germany) equipped with automatic sample injection and UV detection at 215 nm. The column was equilibrated in 46.3% buffer A (HPLC grade H_2O containing 0.1% trifluoroacetic acid) and 53.7% buffer B (acetonitrile containing 0.08% trifluoroacetic acid). Gradient elution was carried out at a flow rate of 0.285 ml/min and 53°C as follows: from 53.7% to 58.3% buffer B in 8 min; from 58.3% to 63,3.6% buffer B in 8 min; from 63.3% to 72.7% buffer B in 6 min.

Size-Exclusion High-Pressure Liquid Chromatography (SE-HPLC)

BK0023 contamination with its aggregated forms was detected by SE-HPLC of 5 μl samples performed on a TSKgel Super SW2000, 4 μm, 4.6 × 30 cm column (Tosho Bioscience, Stuttgart, Germany) with a HP 1100 liquid chromatography system and UV detection at 214 nm. The column was equilibrated and isocratically eluted with 63 mM phospate-pH 7- 3% isopropanol mobile phase at a flow-rate of 250 μl/min and 25°C.

Amino acid sequence analysis and peptide mapping

Amino acid sequences of BK0023 and Neupogen® were compared by NH_2-terminal amino acid sequence analysis of the first 15 residues by standard Edman degradation procedure on an automated Procise 610A Protein Sequencer (Applied Biosystems, Foster City CA, USA) and by peptide mapping after proteolysis in non-reducing and reducing conditions with endoprotease Glu-C from *S aureus* followed by RP-HPLC separation of resulting peptides and MS/MS identification. Mass spectrometry was performed in positive ion mode on a MALDI-TOF Reflex III instrument (Bruker, Bremen, Germany).

Assay of process derived contaminants

Endotoxin contamination of formulated BK0023 was assayed by Lymulus Amoebocyte Lysate (LAL) test using Pyrochrome LAL kit (Cape Code Inc, Falmouth, MA, USA), while residual *E.coli* proteins were detected by immunoenzymatic method assay using an *E.coli* HCP Elisa kit (Cygnus Technologies. Wrentham, MA, USA). Both tests were performed according to the manufacturers' instructions.

Quantization of host/vector DNA contamination has been performed under Good Laboratory Practice conditions by an external contractor (NewLab Bioquality AG, Erkrath, Germany).

Stability study

A three months stability study of formulated BK0023 was performed maintaining aliquots of product solutions at 5 ± 3°C and 25 ± 2°C. At time intervals, samples were assayed by RP- and SE-HPLC to detect the appearance of new minor degradation peaks.

In vitro cell proliferation

Cell proliferation effect of BK0023 in comparison to Neupogen® was measured on a murine myeloblastic NFS-60 cell line according to a described colorimetric method [12]. Briefly, NFS-60 cells were cultured at a confluence of 5×10^5 cells/ml in RPMI 1640 medium containing 200 mM L-glutamine, 1 mM Na-pyruvate, 10% FBS and 33 IU/ml of mouse IL 3 at 37°C, under a 5% CO2 humidified atmosphere. After a starvation period of 17 hours without serum, 1×10^4 cells/well were seeded in triplicate in microtiter plates and incubated for 48 hours with samples in concentration ranging from 0.0015 to 5 ng/ml. At the end of incubation, 20 μl of WST-1 cell proliferation reagent were added and, after 4 hours of incubation, the formation of soluble formazan dye was estimated by reading the absorbance at 450 nm with an ELISA plate reader. EC_{50} of BK0023 and Neupogen were calculated from the sigmoidal concentration-response curve using the GraphPad Prism program (GraphPad Software, San Diego, CA, USA). Raw data for the parallel line method were processed according to the European Pharmacopoeia [13] and the results were expressed as rate of BK0023 towards Neupogen®'s potency.

Radioligand binding assay

The potencies of BK0023 and Neupogen® in displacing ^{125}I-radiolabelled h-G-CSF (Amersham Biosciences, Amersham, UK) bound to the G-CSF receptor were determined using NFS-60 cell line as described [14]. The experiments were carried out in duplicate by incubating 2.5×10^6 cells for 1 hour at 37°C in 150 μl of RPMI 1640 medium containing 10% FCS, 20 mM Hepes-NaOH (pH 7.3), 500 pM [^{125I}]G-CSF and increasing concentrations of either BK0023 or Neupogen®.

After the incubation, the tubes were chilled on ice and the mixtures were layered over 400 μl of phtalate oil (dibutylphtalate: dioctylphtalate 3:2) in 1.5 ml Eppendorf tubes and centrifuged at 6,000 g for 10 min at 4°C. Following aspiration of the aqueous and organic supernatants, the pellets were solubilized and mixed with Formula-989 liquid scintillation cocktail (Perkin-Elmer, Monza, Italy). The radioactivity was determined by liquid scintillation counting in a TRI-CARB 1600TR liquid scintillation counter (Canberra-Packard, Cassina de' Pecchi, Italy) with an efficiency of 70%. Nonspecific binding was determined in the presence of 500 nM unlabeled r-G-CSF. Assays were performed in duplicate.

Immunoenzymatic analysis

BK0023 and Neupogen® concentrations were measured in rat plasma samples by an ELISA method using the commercial kit G-CSF Instant ELISA (Bender Med. System, Vienna, Austria) according to the the manifacture's instructions.

Preclinical studies

Care and handling of animals used for preclinical studies were in accordance with the provisions of the European Economic Community Council Directive 86/209 recognized and adopted by the Italian Government with the Ministerial Decree No. 230/95-B and the NIH publication No. 85–23, revised in 1985.

Seven-nine week old Cr:CD Sprague Dawley rats and 13–18 week old New Zealand White female rabbits were purchased from Charles River Srl (Calco, Italy) and stabulated for acclimatization for about 4 and 2 weeks, respectively, under thorough observation by a veterinarian.

Local tolerability of BK0023 in rabbits

Local tolerability after a single subcutaneous, intravenous (into ear vein) or intramuscular injection of 300 μg/ml/rabbit of formulated BK0023 was studied using 6 female rabbits for each administration route.

The reaction to treatment was assessed by visual inspections on the day of treatment and on the day after in the first 3 animals of each group and for 14 days in the remaining animals. For microscopic evaluation, three animals from each group were killed 48 hours after treatment, while the remaining animals from each group were killed 14 days after dosing.

Repeated dose toxicity in rats

Rats of both sexes (10 males and 10 females for each group) were treated for 4 weeks by daily subcutaneous injection of formulated BK0023 or Neupogen® at dosage of 20, 100 and 500 μg/kg/day. Upon treatment completion, the animals were observed for a further 4 week recovery period.

All the animals were submitted to routine clinical observations (local tolerance, clinical signs, body weight, food and water consumption and ophthalmoscopic examination), standard laboratory analyses (blood chemistry, haematology and urinalysis) and post-mortem examinations (autopsy, organ weight and histology).

The pharmacodynamic parameters (white blood cells and neutrophil counting) were determined by withdrawing blood samples into tubes containing EDTA as anticoagulant before the start of treatment, at days 14 and 28 and upon completion of the recovery period. Blood samples were stored at 4°C and used for counting white blood cells (WBC) and neutrophils (ANC) on a Animal Blood Counter ABC (ABX Diagnostic, Montpellier, France) according to manufacturer's instructions.

The toxicokinetic parameters were determined by collecting serum samples at 1, 2, 4, 8 and 24 hours post-dose on day 1 and on day 14 from all the treated animals. The serum h-G-CSF concentration was measured using an ELISA technique. The formation of anti-G-CSF antibodies was also evaluated by competitive ELISA assay to examine whether a relationship existed between antibody response and toxicokinetics.

Pharmacodynamics and pharmacokinetics in neutropenic and non-neutropenic rats

Male Crl:CD rats were allocated in 12 groups of 10 animals, while one group of 6 animals was used as a control. 6 groups of 10 animals were treated by intraperitoneal administration at day –1 with a single 50 mg/kg dose of cyclophosphamide to induce a marked increase of neutropenia, lasting for several days and of comparable severity to WHO grade III neutropenia in humans [15]. All animals were then treated for 4 consecutive days by subcutaneous injections of 10, 30 and 100 μg/kg of BK0023 and Neupogen® while control group was administered the vehicle alone.

The pharmacodynamic parameters (WBC and ANC) were determined on blood samples withdrawn from the tail vein of the first 6 rats taken from each group at the following time points: pre-dose, 1, 2, 3, 4, 5, 6, 8, 10 and 12 days after the first dose.

In addition, pharmacokinetics was investigated by collecting serum samples at 6 time points (pre-dose, 1, 2, 4, 8 and 24 hours after dosing) on day 1 of administration from the remaining 4 animals of each treatment group.

The sera were stored frozen pending the determination of G-CSF concentration with a commercial ELISA kit.

Phase I clinical study

Evaluation of pharmacodynamic equivalence and pharmacokinetics bioequivalence of BK0023 to Neupogen® were assessed by an external Clinical Research Organization in healthy male volunteers after single and multiple-dose subcutaneous administration according to an experimental protocol authorized by Canton Ticino Ethical Committee and by the Swiss Central Health Authority.

Healthy men were treated with formulated BK0023 or Neupogen® by subcutaneous injections at the following doses according to a cross-over design in 2 consecutive study periods, separated by a wash-out period of at least 28 days.

Group 1 (16 subjects): 2.5 μg/kg/day for 7 consecutive days;
Group 2 (16 subjects): 5 μg/kg/day for 7 consecutive days;
Group 3 (16 subjects): 10 μg/kg/day for 5 consecutive days.

The primary clinical phase I study endpoints were as follows:

1) Equivalence in terms of pharmacodynamic effects of BK0023 versus Neupogen® assessed on baseline adjusted increase of ANC.
2) Bioequivalence of pharmacokinetic profile of BK0023 and Neupogen® assessed as peak concentration of G-CSF (Cmax) and area under the curve ($AUC_{0\text{-}24\ hours}$) for BK0023 and Neupogen at both day 1 and at steady-state (last treatment day).

The secondary clinical phase I study endpoints were as follows:

1) Equivalence in terms of induction of $CD34^+$ cells of BK0023 versus Neupogen® assessed on CD34+ peak concentration and AUC_{CD34+} versus time from day 1 to 10 (2.5 and 5 μg/kg/day dose groups) or from day 1 to 8 (10 μg/kg/day dose group)
2) Bioequivalence in terms of G-CSF peak concentration of BK0023 and Neupogen® at both day 1 and at steady-state (last treatment day)
3) Bioequivalence of pharmacokinetic parameters of BK0023 and Neupogen® at both day 1 and at steady-state (last treatment day) assessed as T_{max} (time to peak concentration), $t_{1/2}$ (half life) and clearance.
4) Safety and tolerability of BK0023 as compared to Neupogen®

The study was designed as a group sequential clinical trial in order to recalculate the correct sample size necessary to obtain statistically acceptable pharmacodynamic and pharmacokinetic results for each group, based on the intra subject variability, to achieve the primary study objectives.

Consequently, the study was conducted in two parts:

Part 1: 16 subjects per dose group were enrolled and treated with both drug products in cross-over. The pharmacodynamic and pharmacokinetic primary parameters, that is the AUC of ANC, the maximal attained ANC and the serum filgrastim AUC on day 1 and at steady state were calculated after the end of the second period of each dose group. A pharmacokineticist, independent from the clinical study management and from the sponsor, temporarily broke the blind with the aim of evaluating intra-subject variability. The biostatistician re-calculated the sample size with the actual study *ad interim* results in order to verify whether additional subjects were needed to obtain statistically valid results.
Part 2: On the basis of sample size re-calculation, an additional number of subjects for each dose group was enrolled: 16 subjects in the Group 1 (2.5 μg/kg/day), 20 subjects in the Group 2 (5 μg/kg/day) and 6 subjects in the Group 3 (10 μg/kg/day).

The pharmacodynamic effects of both BK0023 and Neupogen® were determined by ANC performed on whole blood samples with a fully automated laser ADVIA 120 Haematology System (Bayer) which incorporates flow cytometric principles and cytochemistry and by evaluating the count of peripheral blood CD34 positive ($CD34^+$) hematopoietic stem cells by flow cytometric analysis as described [16]. In fact, beside regulating granulopoiesis, G-CSF is also able to mobilize $CD34^+$ cells from the marrow to the blood enabling the use of stem cell enriched peripheral blood in hematopoietic transplantation in lieu of bone marrow cells [17].

The pharmacokinetic profile of filgrastim was determined in serum samples withdrawn after the 1st and the last dose and stored frozen until the determination of G-CSF concentration with a commercial ELISA kit

Statistical analysis of clinical and preclinical data

Results were analyzed using SAS® version 9.1.2 for Windows software. The AUC of ANC and $CD34^+$ cells and their maximal attained counts were compared based on analysis of variance for a cross-over design: the 95% CI for the ratio of the averages (population geometric means, if parameters are log-transformed) of the values for the test and reference and the two onesided t-tests of Schuirmann at the level of significance of 2.5%. Criteria for equivalence on ANC parameters were that the 95% CI of the ratio between treatment means fell within 85%-115% (or 85%-118% when parameters are log-transformed). AUC and peak concentration of serum filgrastim were compared based on Latin-square analysis of variance for a cross-over design: the 90% CI for the ratio of the averages (population geometric means) of the values for the test and reference and the two one-sided t-tests of Schuirmann at the level of significance of 5%. Criteria for bioequivalence were that the 90% CI of the treatment means ratio fell within the range of 80 to 125%. Pharmacokinetic data were calculated using Kinetica™ Version 4.4.1 software (Thermo Electron Corporation, USA); the area under the blood concentration-time curve (AUC) was calculated using the trapezoidal rule.

Experimental data of in vitro inhibition of radioactive G-CSF binding by BK0023 and Neupogen to cell expressing G-CSF receptor were analyzed by using the GraphPad Prism Program (San Diego, USA).

Information was given in both oral and written form to each volunteer. Before being admitted to the clinical study subjects expressed their consent to participate singing copy of the written informed consent form.

Results

Analysis of physico-chemical properties

Purified BK0023 was characterized by a panel of chemico-physical methods, including amino acid sequence analysis of NH2-terminal residues, RP-HPLC/MS mapping of proteolytic products, MALDI-TOF-MS, SDS-PAGE and Western blotting. The results showed the absolute comparability to the clinically used filgrastim commercialized under the brand name of Neupogen® as well as levels of process- and product-related contaminations within the limits accepted by regulatory authorities (Tables 1, 2 and 3).

The result of the stability study of formulated BK0023 are reported in Table 4. While the drug product appeared stable at +5°C over a three month period, protein degradation and aggregation occurred to a limited extent when the product was stored at 25°C. Consequently, all BK0023 preparations were stored refrigerated as also recommended for Neupogen®.

In vitro studies

Two studies, namely a cell proliferation assay and a radioligand binding assay using the murine myeloblastic NFS-60 cell-line were carried out to compare the *in vitro* biological activity of BK0023 and Neupogen®.

The results of proliferation assay indicated that BK0023 and Neupogen displayed *in vitro* the same biological potency as demonstrated by very close EC_{50} values (respectively 43.90 ng/ml ± 1.16 S.E.M. and 38.59 ng/ml ± 1.24 S.E.M.) overlapping at 95% confidence intervals (with respective range of 31.97-60.29 and 24.61-60.41 ng/ml).

The radioreceptor assay also showed the same competition for BK0023 and Neupogen® towards radiolabelled r-h-G-CSF bound to G-CSF receptors in NFS-60 cells with estimated IC_{50} respectively of 4.52 ± 0.65 and 5.89 ± 0.49 ng/ml with no statistically significant difference (Figure 1).

Local tolerability studies

Local tolerability was assessed in rabbits by a single intravenous, subcutaneous and intramuscular administration of 300 μg of BK0023, which is the highest concentration given in humans as a bolus injection. Slight erythemas or oedemas, which were rapidly and completely reversible, were seen at sites of intravenous and subcutaneous injections while no significant reaction was observed in animals treated by intramuscular route. In any case, no abnormality was detectable by microscopy examination as well as no clinical abnormal signs were seen in any animal. These results indicate that BK0023 is well tolerated locally.

Toxicity studies in rats

A repeated-dose toxicity study was performed in rats to compare the toxicological profile of BK0023 and Neupogen® administered subcutaneously for 4 weeks at

Table 1 Analytical comparison between BK0023 and Neupogen®

Parameter	Analysis	Results and notes
Structural and conformational characterisation	First 15 N-terminal residues by automatic Edman degradation	Results agree with the expected sequence
	Reducing and non-reducing Glu-C proteolysis and RP-HPLC/MS mapping	Primary structure and disulfide bridge positions according to the expected sequence
	MALDI-TOF-MS	According to the calculated value
	SDS-PAGE	Migration profile comparable to Neupogen®
	SE-HPLC	Elution profile comparable to Neupogen®
Identity	Western blotting	Binding to specific antibody as Neupogen®
	RP-HPLC	Elution profile comparable to Neupogen®

Table 2 Product related impurities of purified bulk BK0023 preparations

Impurity	Method	Result
BK0023 oxydized forms	RP-HPLC	< 1%
BK0023 aggregate forms	SE-HPLC	< 1%

dosages of 20, 100 and 500 μg/kg/day, corresponding to 2–4, 10–20 and 50–100 times the clinical dose in humans (5–10 μg/kg/day), respectively. In the same study we compared the pharmacodynamic and the immunotoxicologic profiles of the two products after 28 days of daily subcutaneous administration. The study also included a comparison of the toxicokinetic profiles after 14 days of treatment and an assessment following a 4-week recovery period.

The results showed that administration of BK0023 and Neupogen® produced a comparable significant dose-related increase in neutrophils and white blood cells with respect to the control group (data not shown) indicating that the animals received systemic exposure to both products in a dose-related manner.

As regards the blood chemistry analyses, serum alkaline phosphatase concentration significantly increased in all the treated animals according to a dose-related trend (Table 5). This effect may be correlated to osteoblast and osteoclast cell function which, in turn, is indicative of BK0023 and Neupogen® activity [18] .

Statistically significant increases in urea and creatinine levels in females and decreases in chloride levels in males were also observed in animals receiving the highest dose of Neupogen®, while other statistically significant changes were sporadically recorded in animals receiving the lower doses of BK0023 and Neupogen®. However, these differences were considered too small to be toxicologically meaningful and were therefore considered to have no toxicological implication.

No difference in body weight or food consumption and no ophthalmic lesions were observed during the study. The only anomalous *in vivo* observation was a swelling of the lower hind limbs in both BK0023 and Neupogen treated rats, which is an already described G-CSF treatment related effect possibly due to induction of fluid retention [19]. Of note, all changes observed during treatment were no longer detected following the 4-week recovery period, thereby confirming complete reversibility. The immunogenic response to BK0023 was comparable to that of Neupogen® for anti-G-CSF immunoglobulins were detected in 3 serum samples out of 120 (1 male and 1 female rat treated with 20 and 500 μg/kg/day of BK0023 and 1 female rat treated with 500 μg/kg/day of Neupogen®) at the end of recovery period. Moreover, in a separate study in rats, no specific antibodies against r-h-G-CSF were detected following daily administration of BK0023 at a concentration of 200 μg/kg/day over a 4-week period. The toxicokinetics of BK0023 and Neupogen® assessed by comparing the pharmacodynamic parameters after 1, 14 and 28 days of treatment as well as at the end of 4-week recovery period did not show any significant difference (data not shown).

Table 3 Process related impurities of formulated BK0023 preparations

Impurity	Method	Result
Bacterial endotoxins	LAL test	< 5 EU/mg
Host proteins (ECP)	Immunoenzymatic assay	< 20 ppm
Host/vector DNA	Hybridation to degenerated probe	< 100 pg/mg

EU Endotoxin unit, *ppm* part per million parts, *pg* picograms.

Pharmacodynamic and pharmacokinetic studies in normal and neutropenic rats

Since G-CSF stimulates the production of bone marrow cells interacting with a specific surface receptor, the increase of ANC is a direct biochemical index of efficacy. Thus, white blood cell count and ANC were determined during 4 consecutive days of subcutaneous administrations to normal and cyclophosphamide treated neutropenic rats at the doses of 10, 30 and 100 μg/kg of BK0023 and Neupogen®. The dose range was selected to induce a marked dose–response effect in terms of degree and duration of neutrophil production stimulation in order to detect any difference between BK0023 and Neupogen®.

Pharmacodynamic evaluations demonstrated that both BK0023 and Neupogen® boosted the proliferation of white blood cells (WBC) and in particular of neutrophil cells, which appeared hypersegmented, indicating complete activation.

While both products yielded a comparable and dose–related increase in total WBC and ANC, no difference was observed regarding the other blood cells (lymphocytes, eosinophils, basophils, monocytes and large unstained cells) in either the neutropenic or normal rats (data not shown). In normal rats, neutrophil levels increased during the first day of treatment and returned to normal values approximately 2 days after the last treatment (Figure 2). Differently from normal rats, neutropenic rats exhibited a consecutive cycle of increasing and decreasing of the neutrophil level in response to either BK0023 or Neupogen® (Figure 3). The first increase may be due to the mobilisation of the residual pool of neutrophils after cyclophosphamide administration, while the subsequent decrease may be related to the cyclophosphamide-dependent reduction of neutrophil production by the bone marrow blasts. The second increase could depend on the effect of BK0023 and

Table 4 Stability of formulated BK0023 maintained at 5 and 25°C. Aliquots of samples were assayed at time 0, 1 and 2 months by RP-HPLC and SE-HPLC

Assay	Storage time	Temperature 5°C			Temperature 25°C		
		BK0023 mg/ml	Main peak%	Sum of impurities%	BK0023 mg/ml	Main peak%	Sum of impurities%
RP-HPLC	0	0.29	99.6	0.4	0.29	99.6	0.4
	1 month	0.29	99.6	0.4	0.28	99.6	0.3
	3 months	0.28	99.6	0.4	0.28	99.1	0.9
SE-HPLC	0	0.28	99.6	0.4	0.29	99.6	0.4
	1 month	0.27	99.6	0.4	0.28	99.6	0.3
	3 months	0.28	99.6	0.4	0.28	99.1	0.9

Aliquots of samples were assayed at time 0, 1 and 2 months by RP-HPLC and SE-HPLC. Peak purity and total impurities (or aggregates in the case of SE-HPLC analysis) are reported as percentage of total peak areas.

Neupogen® leading to an increase of cells from the myeloid series.

The results of the pharmacokinetics study on day 1, summarized in Table 6, showed that filgrastim was systemically absorbed in both non-neutropenic and neutropenic rats after both BK0023 and Neupogen® and that the animals were similarly exposed to drugs; some sporadic differences between treatments, shown in Table 6, can be ascribable to the intrinsic animal variability or to different drug absorption after subcutaneous administration.

Summarizing, preclinical *in vivo* studies showed that BK0023 and Neupogen® increased the proliferation of neutrophil cells in normal rats in a similar dose-dependent manner while in neutropenic rats, both products were capable of controlling myelotoxicity with the same dose-dependent recovery of WBC and neutrophil counts. In addition, pharmacokinetic parameters indicated that filgastim was well absorbed in non-neutropenic and neutropenic rats and cleared from blood according to a comparable pharmacokinetic profile after both BK0023 and Neupogen®.

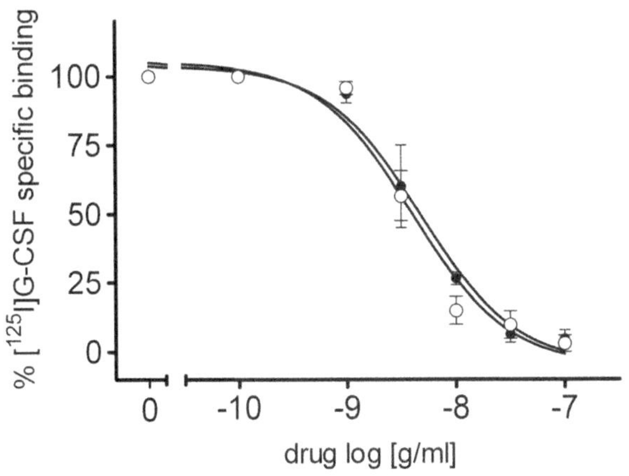

Figure 1 Concentration-dependent inhibition of [^{125}I]-G-CSF binding by BK0023 (black circle) and Neupogen® (open circle) in NFS-60 cells expressing G-CSF receptor. Data are reported as percent of specific binding at each concentration of displacer and are the means ± S.E.M. of four separate experiments. Statistical analysis by Student's t-test did not show any significant difference between BK0023 and Neupogen®.

Phase I clinical study

A phase I clinical study was performed in healthy male volunteers treated with BK0023 and Neupogen® by subcutaneous injection of 2.5 and 5 μg/kg/day for 7 consecutive days and of 10 μg/kg/day for 5 consecutive days in order to assess the equivalence between the two products in terms of pharmacodynamic effect and the bioequivalence in terms of pharmacokinetic profile. The count of neutrophils and $CD34^+$ cells were quite similar in both the rate and extent after a single injection of the two products on day 1 and after a multiple injection treatment of 5 days as shown, for example, in Figure 4 which refers to ANC. Concerning the CD34+ cell concentration, the baseline corrected values measured in 22 subjects up to day 8 after a 5-day treatment with daily injection of 10 μg/kg of BK0023 or Neupogen were respectively of 93,37 ± 35,33 and 95,40 ± 42,59 (mean $CD34^+_{max}$/μL ± SD) and of 8166 ± 2917 and 8670 ± 3797 (mean AUC_{CD34+}/μL x h ± SD). Data analysis performed for each dose group showed no statistically difference for ANC and $CD34^+$ cell count as well as for areas under the curve of both cell types (data not shown). In other words, BK0023 was equivalent to Neupogen® in terms of both AUC and maximal attained level of ANC and $CD34^+$ cells.

Time-dependent serum concentration profile of filgrastim measured by immunoenzymatic assay at day 1 and at last day of subcutaneous treatment with BK0023 and Neupogen at dose levels of 2.5, 5 and 10 μg/kg/day are reported in Figure 5 which shows that pharmacokinetic profiles of serum filgrastim were superimposable both at day 1 (after a single administration) and at steady-state conditions (after 7 daily injections of 2.5 and 5.0 μg/kg/day or 5 daily injections of 10.0 μg/kg/day).

The corresponding calculated pharmacokinetic parameters Cmax and $AUC_{0\text{-}24\ hours}$ for BK0023 and Neupogen at both day 1 and at steady-state (last treatment day)

Table 5 Alkaline phosphatase (U/liter) assayed in blood of both female and male rats treated subcutaneously for 28 days with 20, 100 or 500 μg/kg/day with BK0023 or Neupogen®

Dose	Control		BK0023		Neupogen®	
	Males	Females	Males	Females	Males	Females
0 μg/kg/day	440 ± 110	264 ± 69				
20 μg/kg/day	-	-	669* ± 130	429 ± 135	773** ± 90	400** ± 50
100 μg/kg/day	-	-	1365** ± 303	747** ± 212	1022** ± 127	855** ± 166
500 μg/kg/day	-	-	2109.** ± 538	1227** ± 268	2378.** ± 647	1005** ± 367

Data are reported as mean values ± SD.
* = mean value of group is significantly different from the control group at P < 0.05.
** = mean value of group is significantly different from the control group at P < 0.01.
Statistical analysis was performed according to Dunnett's test.

showed that parameters of BK0023 treated subjects were similar to those of the Neupogen treated ones (Table 7). For both products, a significant reduction of serum levels of G-CSF (Cmax) and AUC was observed at the last day of treatment versus that obtained at day 1. This effect, which was already described for filgrastim, is due to the enhanced G-CSF clearance through receptor binding, internalization and degradation by the increased neutrophil population [20].

Statistical evaluation of the pharmacokinetic bioequivalence was also demonstrated by verifying that the 90% confidence interval for the ratio of the means of AUCday1, AUCSS (steady-state AUC), Cmaxday1 and CmaxSS (steady-state Cmax) between treatments met the acceptance interval 80-125% and that the two one-sided t-tests of Schuirmann did not detect any difference at the level of significance of 5% [21].

Pharmacokinetics of filgrastim following treatment with BK0023 and Neupogen® was proved not to differ significantly also when other parameters (like elimination half-life t½, time of peak concentration Tmax and systemic clearance Cl/body weight) were compared at day 1 of treatment and at last day of subcutaneous treatment by the non-parametric Kruskal-Wallis test [22].

In the whole clinical study, adverse effects were reported for 70/102 subjects after treatment with BK0023, as compared with 67/102 subjects after treatment with Neupogen® for a total of 235 and 261 treatment-related adverse effects for BK0023 and Neupogen treated subjects, respectively.

The most frequent adverse effect was back pain of mild to moderate intensity which reached a frequency of 65% of subjects with BK0023 at the dose of 5 μg/kg/day. followed by bone pain which reached a frequency of 47% of subjects after treatment with Neupogen® at the dose of 10 μg/kg/day. Headache frequency between 8 and 16% of patients treated with at 2.5 to 10 μg/kg/day of BK0023 and Neupogen was also observed. When compared by χ^2 test, no significant statistical difference was detected in either the number of subjects experimenting any adverse affect and the total number of treatment-related adverse effects reported during the study. All observed treatment-related adverse effects were expected since they are linked to the mechanism of action of G-CSF and were already described for filgrastim [23,24]. It is worth noting that all observed adverse effects were transient, resolved spontaneously and did not lead to discontinuation or treatment withdrawal.

Discussion and conclusion

We report the preclinical and phase I clinical comparison of an intended biosimilar filgrastim or r-Met-G-CSF (coded BK0023), produced according to an original recombinant process, with the brand filgrastim product

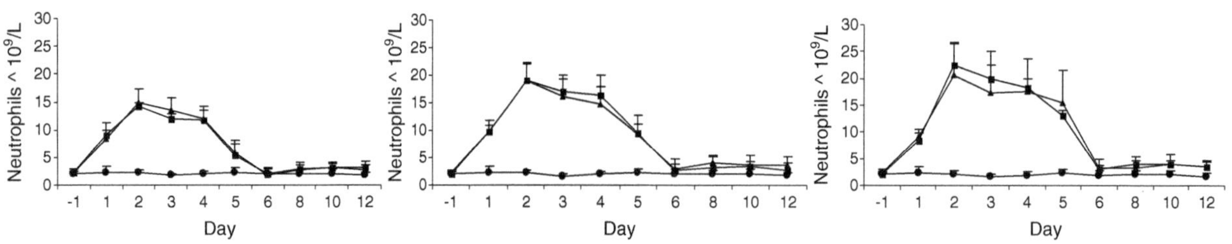

Figure 2 Mean neutrophile counts (× 10⁹/l) obtained in groups of 10 normal rats treated for 4 days by subcutaneous injections of 10, 30 and 100 μg/kg/day of BK0023 and Neupogen® are respectively shown in left, central and right panels where full circles, squares and triangles are respectively referred to control rat, BK0023 and Neupogen. No significant difference was found between BK0023 and Neupogen treated groups analysed by Student's test. Significant differences between treated and control groups analyzed by Dunnet's test were found at P < 0.05 (*) or P < 0.01 (**).

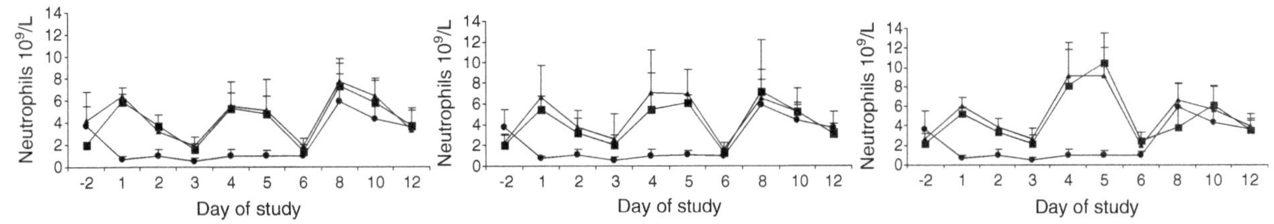

Figure 3 Mean neutrophile counts (× 10^9/l) ± SD obtained in groups of 10 neutropenic rats treated for 4 days by subcutaneous injections of 10, 30 and 100 μg/kg/day of BK0023 and Neupogen® are respectively shown in left, central and right panels where full circles, squares and triangles are respectively referred to control rats, BK0023 and Neupogen. No significant difference was found between BK0023 and Neupogen treated groups analysed by Student's test. Significant differences between treated and control groups analysed by Dunnet's test were found at P < 0.05 (*) or P < 0.01 (**).

Neupogen®, which is largely used for decreasing the duration of febrile neutropenia in oncological patients treated with myelosuppressive anticancer drugs. Due to the same analytical and structural profile, BK0023 is expected to display the same tolerability and toxicity profile of Neupogen® as well as the same efficacy as Neupogen® in controlling myelotoxicity induced by chemotherapy during treatment of solid and haematological tumors

The results reported in this paper confirm that BK0023 and Neupogen® display similar *in vitro* biological potency in terms of both stimulation of proliferation of the G-CSF dependent NFS-60 cell line and competition with radiolabeled r-h-G-CSF for binding to G-CSF receptor in NFS-60 cells. BK0023, when locally

Table 6 Major pharmacokinetic parameters for BK0023 and Neupogen® administered to normal and cyclophosphamide neutropenic rats following a single subcutaneous administration of 10, 30 and 100 μg/kg

		Normal rats			
Product	Nominal dose μg/kg	Cmax ng/ml	Tmax hour	AUC ng · h/ml	t½ hour
BK0023	10	51	2	179	1.5
	30	64	2	377	2.6
	100	377	2	1582	2.6
Neupogen®	10	14	1	65	1.8
	30	68	2	369	2.4
	100	272	1	1121	2.2
		Neutropenic rats			
BK0023	10	27	2	134	1.9
	30	84	2	410	1.7
	100	444	2	1558	1.8
Neupogen®	10	31	2	132	2.0
	30	87	2	485	2.5
	100	309	2	1620	2.4

Abbreviations: *AUC* Area under the serum concentration-time curve from time zero to infinity, C_{max} Maximum observed serum concentration, T_{max} time to C_{max}, $t_{(1/2)}$ Elimination half-life associated with terminal shape (λ_2) of a semilogarithmic concentration-time curve.

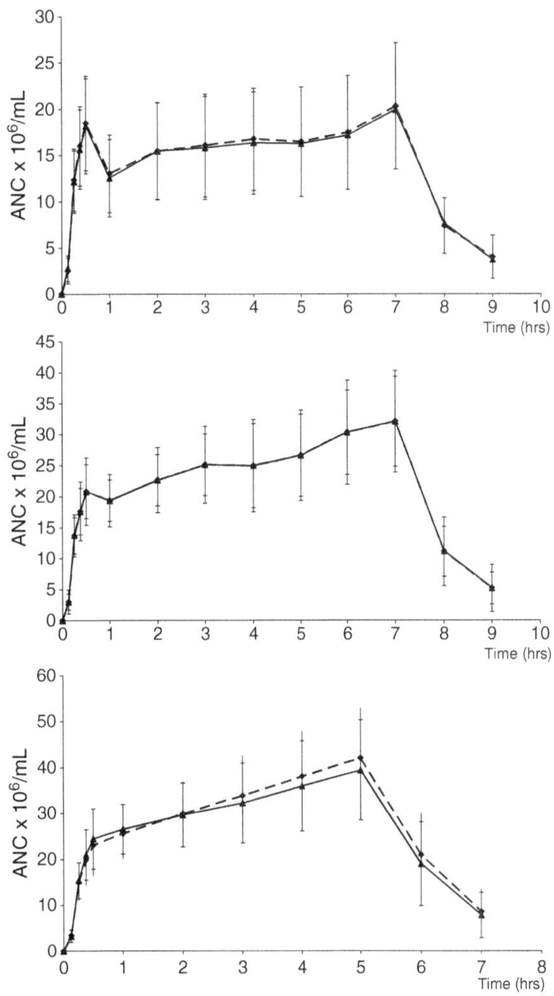

Figure 4 Mean neutrophil counts (× 10^3/μl) ± SD measured in human healthy volonteers treated for 7 days by subcutaneous injections of BK0023 (triangles) and Neupogen® (circles) at dosage of 2.5 μg/kg/day (upper panel) and 5.0 μg/kg/day (central panel) and for 5 days by subcutaneous injections of BK0023 and Neupogen® at dosage of 10.0 μg/kg/day (lower panel).

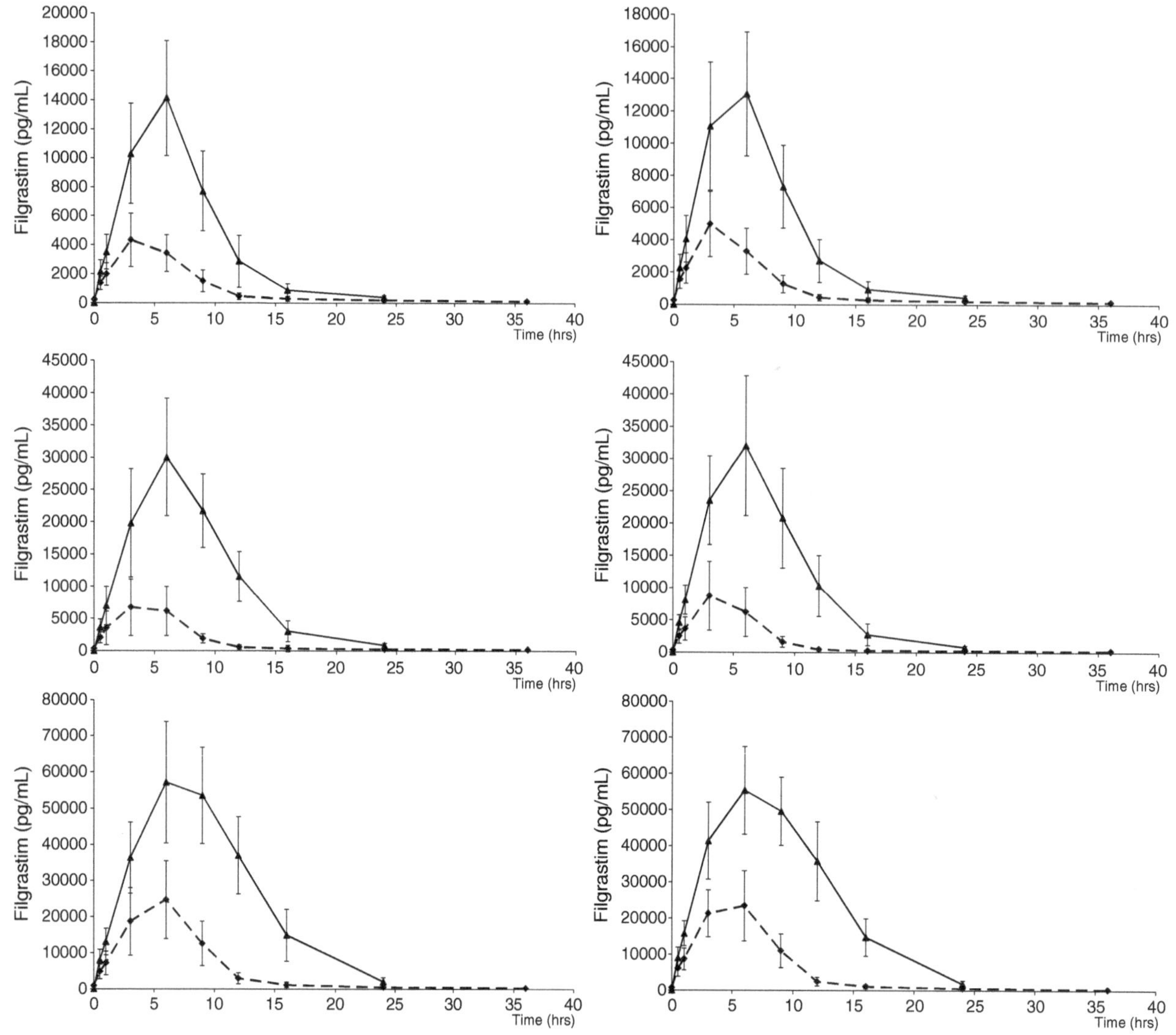

Figure 5 Plasma level profiles of G-CSF (pg/ml) measured by immunoenzymatic assay at day 1 (solid lines) and at the last day of treatment (dashed lines) for BK0023 2.5 µg/kg/day (A); Neupogen 2.5 µg/kg/day (B); BK0023 5 µg/kg/day (C); Neupogen 5 µg/kg/day (D); BK0023 10 µg/kg/day (E); Neupogen 10 µg/kg/day (F).

Table 7 Pharmacokinetic parameters (mean ± SD) calculated at day 1 and after the last day of treatment (steady-state) for human healthy volonteers treated for 7 days with subcutaneous injections of 2.5 and 5.0 µg/kg/day of BK0023 and Neupogen® and for 5 days with subcutaneous injections of 10.0 µg/kg/day of BK0023 and Neupogen®

Product and dosages	First treatment		Steady-state	
	Cmax ng/ml	$AUC_{0\text{-}24\ hours}$ ng/ml · hour	Cmax ng/ml	$AUC_{0\text{-}24\ hours}$ ng/ml · hour
BK0023 2.5 µg/kg/day	14.1 ± 1.4	113.6 ± 30.8	4.7 ± 1.6	32.8 ± 8.5
Neupogen 2.5 µg/kg/day	13.4 ± 3.9	111.9 ± 30.3	5.1 ± 2.0	33.7 · 9.6
BK0023 5 µg/kg/day	30.1 ± 9.1	276.7 ± 71.6	7.9 ± 4.4	51.2 ± 23.7
Neupogen 5 µg/kg/day	32.2 ± 10.7	295.0 ± 86.8	9.0 ± 5.2	55.3 ± 27.0
BK0023 10 µg/kg/day	60.1 ± 16.7	670.0 ± 154.9	25.1 ± 10.3	189.4 ± 69.7
Neupogen 10 µg/kg/day	56.5 ± 11.8	671.5 ± 122.5	25.1 ± 9.0	188.4 ± 52.2

administered to rabbits at the maximal concentration expected to be used clinically as a bolus injection, is well tolerated without onset of systemic toxicity after single intravenous, subcutaneous or intramuscular injection. In this study, the subcutaneous and intravenous administration routes have been chosen since these are the most common administration routes of filgrastim in humans while the intramuscular route has been included in consideration of accidental product exposure.

BK0023 and Neupogen® were also compared in a subchronic toxicity study by subcutaneous administration in rats, which are a relevant animal model for toxicological studies since r-h-Met-G-CSF is pharmacologically active in this species. In fact, data from literature show that r-h-Met-G-CSF not only increases neutrophil counts in peripheral blood but also enhances neutrophil functions in rats [15].

The results of repeated dose toxicity in rats treated for 28 days with 20, 100 and 500 μg/kg/day (which correspond respectively to 2–4, 10–20 and 50–100 times the clinical dose of 5–10 μg/kg/day) showed for the two products comparable toxicokinetic and immunotoxicologic profiles. Besides, no treatment-related effects were observed at the post-treatment recovery period of 4 weeks so that the maximal administered dose of 500 μg/kg/day may be considered as No Observed Adverse Effect Level (NOAEL) for both BK0023 and reference Neupogen®. Altogether, the results obtained in this study indicate the pharma-toxicological comparability of BK0023 and Neupogen®.

The *in vivo* studies on neutropenic and non-neutropenic rats showed that both BK0023 and Neupogen® boosted the proliferation of neutrophil cells in normal rats in a dose-dependent manner while in neutropenic rats both products are capable of controlling myelotoxicity with dose-dependent recovery of neutrophils and white blood cells. In preclinical studies, no significant difference between the two products was observed. Our data clearly demonstrate that the biological activity in animal models of BK0023 is comparable to that of Neupogen®.

Phase I clinical trial in healthy subjects was carried out according to a multiple-dose, randomised, two-period, cross-over design since there are 2 types of pharmacokinetic non-linearity (non-proportional increase with dose and time dependent non-linearity). Dose levels of 2.5 and 5 μg/kg/day were chosen for the pharmacodynamic study since data in the literature show a clear dose–response relationship in terms of the pharmacodynamic parameters over this range [23] while the dose of 10 μg/kg/day was chosen to ensure that the investigated dose range was relevant to the clinical indications and because it is usual in the praxis for filgrastim. The subcutaneous administration was chosen for the pharmacokinetic and pharmacodynamic bioequivalence study since this one is the administration route most commonly used in the clinical setting.

Pharmacodynamic, pharmacokinetic and safety of BK0023 and Neupogen® were compared according to a cross-over design in 2 consecutive periods with a wash-out of at least 28 days between the last injection of period I and the first of period II.

The results showed that BK0023 has the same pharmacokinetic profile, efficacy and safety as the reference commercial filgrastim Neupogen® and therefore could be further developed to become a convenient option to treat neutropenia in oncological patients.

Finally, the demonstration of bioequivalence between BK0023 and commercial filgrastim enabled the preparation of a new long lasting site-specific monopegylated filgrastim derivative as described elsewhere [25].

Competing interests

Bioker srl, is a biotech company located in the Scientific and Technological Park of Sardinia (Italy) fully owned by Multimedica Holding. GS is a IRCCS Multimedica employee; GT is CEO of Bioker srl while DC, RS and GO are Bioker's employees. ADS is employed at Cross Research SA, a CRO which performed the clinical study. Part of preclinical study were performed by GSJ (University of Parma) and PO and SD (University of Cagliari).
GT and GO are coinventors of the granted patents EP1334183B1 and US7,241,609B reported as references in the manuscript.

Authors' contributions

D.C. was responsible of study development and manuscript writing. G.T. was responsible of the research project. R.S. and G.O. were involved in experimental design and studies supporting. P.O. and S.D. were involved in preclinical experiments and results elaboration. G.S. and G.S.J. were involved in the development of the clinical study and drafting of the manuscript. A.D.S. was responsible of clinical development. All authors were involved in experiment planning, results interpretation and discussion and final manuscript revision. All authors read and approved the final manuscript.

Acknowledgements

We acknowledge the Scientific and Technological Park of Sardinia that financed the article-processing charge but had no role in study design, preparation of the manuscript or decision to publish it.
We acknowledge RTC s.p.a. (Research Toxicology Centre, Roma) for its involvement in toxicological studies execution.

Author details

[1]Bio-Ker S.r.l.-Multimedica Group, Sardinia Scientific and Technological Park, Building 3, I-09010 Pula Cagliari, Italy. [2]IRCCS MultiMedica, Laboratory of Diabetological Research, Milan, Italy. [3]Department of Biomedical Sciences, Laboratory of Cellular and Molecular Pharmacology, University of Cagliari, 09042 Monserrato Cagliari, Italy. [4]CROSS Research S.A, Phase I Unit, via F. A. Giorgioli 14, CH-6864 Arzo, Switzerland. [5]Department of Biomedical, Biotechnological and Traslational Science (S.Bi.Bi.T.), University of Parma, via Volturno 39, 43121 Parma, Italy.

References

1. Frampton JE, Lee CR, Faulds D: **Filgrastim. A review of its pharmacological properties and therapeutic efficacy in neutropenia.** *Drugs* 1994, 48:731–760.
2. Garcia-Carbonero R, Mayordomo JI, Tornamira MV, Lopez-Brea M, Rueda A, Guillem V, Arcediano A, Yubero Ribera AF, Gomez C, Tres A, Perez-Gracia JL, Lumbreras C, Hornedo J, Cortes-Funes H, Paz-Ares L: **Granulocyte colony-**

stimulating factor in the treatment of high-risk febrile neutropenia: a multicenter randomized trial. *J Natl Cancer Inst* 2001, **93**:31–38.
3. To LB, Haylock DN, Simmons PJ, Juttner CA: **The biology and clinical uses of blood stem cells.** *Blood 89* 1997, **7**:2233–2258.
4. Mackie AR, Losordo DW: **CD34-positive stem cells: in the treatment of heart and vascular disease in human beings.** *Tex Heart Inst J* 2011, **38**(5):474–485.
5. Hollingshead LM, Goa KL: **Recombinant granulocyte colony-stimulating factor.** *A review of its pharmacological properties and prospective role in neutropenic conditions, Drugs* 1991, **42**:300–330.
6. Schäbitz W, Schneider A: **New targets for established proteins: exploring G-CSF for the treatment of stroke.** *Trends Pharmacol Sci* 2007, **28**:157–161.
7. Tanaka H, Tanaka Y, Shinigawa K, Yamagishi Y, Ohtaki K, Asano K: **Three types of recombinant human granulocyte colony-stimulating factor have equivalent biological activities in monkeys.** *Cytokine* 1997, **9**:360–369.
8. Pozzuolo S, Breme U, Salis B, Taylor G, Tonon G, Orsini G: **Efficient bacterial expression of fusion proteins and their selective processing by a recombinant Kex-1 protease.** *Protein Expr Purif* 2008, **59**:334–341.
9. Zuffi G, Ghisotti D, Oliva I, Capra E, Frascotti G, Tonon G, Orsini G: **Immobilized biocatalysts for the production of nucleosides and nucleoside analogues by enzymatic transglycosylation reactions.** *Enz Microb Technol* 2004, **35**:309–314.
10. Vanoni M, Tortora P, Tonon G, Taylor G, Orsini G: **Novel soluble endoproteases for the in vitro processing of recombinant proteins.** 2006:EP 1334183B1.
11. Laemmli UK: **Cleavage of structural proteins during the assembly of the head of bacteriophage T4.** *Nature* 1970, **227**:680–685.
12. Mosmann T: **Rapid colorimetric assay for cellular growth and survival: application to proliferation and cytotoxicity assays.** *J Immunol Meth* 1983, **65**:55–63.
13. European Directorate for the quality of medicines Strasburg (F): *Statistical analysis of results of biological assays and tests.* 60th edition. European Pharmacopeia; 2008. Chapter 5.3.
14. Fukunaga R, Ishizaka-Ikeda E, Nagasta S: **Purification and characterization of the receptor for murine granulocyte colony-stimulating factor.** *J Biol Chem* 1990, **265**:14008–14015.
15. Nohynek GJ, Plard JP, Wells MY, Zerial A, Roquet F: **Comparison of the potency of glycosylated and nonglycosylated recombinant human granulocyte colony-stimulating factors in neutropenic and non neutropenic CD rats, Cancer Chemother.** *Pharmacol* 1997, **3**:259–266.
16. Tanaka R, Matsudaira T, Aizawa J, Ebihara Y, Muraoka K, Tsuji K, Ikebuchi K, Kodama K, Takaku F, Nakahata T: **Characterization of peripheral blood progenitor cells (PBPC) mobilized by filgrastim (rHuG-CSF) in normal volunteers: dose-effect relationship for filgrastim with the character of mobilized PBPC.** *Br J Haematol* 1996, **92**:795–803.
17. Welte K, Gabrilove J, Bronchud MH, Platzer E, Morstyn G: **Filgrastim (r-metHuG-CSF): the first 10 years.** *Blood* 1996, **88**:1907–1929.
18. Christopher MJ, Link DC: **Granulocyte colony-stimulating factor induces osteoblast apoptosis and inhibits osteoblast differentiation.** *J Bone Miner Res* 2008, **3**:1765–1774.
19. *Neupogen Prescribing Information.* http://www.neupogen.com.
20. Sarkar CA, Lowenhaupt K, Horan T, Boone TC, Tidor B, Lauffenburger DA: **Rational cytokine design for increased lifetime and enhanced potency using pH-activated 'histidine switching.** *Nature Biotechnol.* 2002, **20**:908–913.
21. Schuirmann DJ: **A comparison of the two one-sided tests procedure and the power approach for assessing the equivalence of average bioavailability.** *J Pharmacokin Biopharmac.* 1987, **15**:657–680.
22. Theodorsson-Norheim E: **Kruskal-Wallis test: BASIC computer program to perform nonparametric one-way analysis of variance and multiple comparisons on ranks of several independent samples.** *Comp Meth Programs Biomed* 1986, **23**:57–62.
23. Borleffs JC, Bosschaert M, Vrehen HM, Schneider MM, van Strijp J, Small MK, Borkett KM: **Effect of escalating doses of recombinant human granulocyte colony-stimulating factor (filgrastim) on circulating neutrophils in healthy subjects.** *Clin Ther* 1998, **20**:722–736.
24. Yoshioka T, Takahashi M, Shiba Y, Suzuki C, Morimoto H, Izawa A, Ise H, Ikeda U: **Granulocyte colony-stimulating factor (G-CSF) accelerates reendothelialization and reduces neointimal formation after vascular injury in mice.** *Cardiovascular Res.* 2006, **70**:61–69.
25. Scaramuzza S, Tonon G, Olianas A, Messana I, Schrepfer R, Orsini G, Caliceti P: **A new site-specific monoPEGylated filgrastim derivative prepared by enzymatic conjugation: production and physicochemical characterization.** *J Control Release* 2012, **164**:355–363.

7

Skin sensitizers differentially regulate signaling pathways in MUTZ-3 cells in relation to their individual potency

Ann-Sofie Albrekt[1*], Henrik Johansson[1], Anna Börje[2], Carl Borrebaeck[1] and Malin Lindstedt[1]

Abstract

Background: Due to the recent European legislations posing a ban of animal tests for safety assessment within the cosmetic industry, development of *in vitro* alternatives for assessment of skin sensitization is highly prioritized. To date, proposed *in vitro* assays are mainly based on single biomarkers, which so far have not been able to classify and stratify chemicals into subgroups, related to risk or potency.

Methods: Recently, we presented the Genomic Allergen Rapid Detection (GARD) assay for assessment of chemical sensitizers. In this paper, we show how the genome wide readout of GARD can be expanded and used to identify differentially regulated pathways relating to individual chemical sensitizers. In this study, we investigated the mechanisms of action of a range of skin sensitizers through pathway identification, pathway classification and transcription factor analysis and related this to the reactive mechanisms and potency of the sensitizing agents.

Results: By transcriptional profiling of chemically stimulated MUTZ-3 cells, 33 canonical pathways intimately involved in sensitization to chemical substances were identified. The results showed that metabolic processes, cell cycling and oxidative stress responses are the key events activated during skin sensitization, and that these functions are engaged differently depending on the reactivity mechanisms of the sensitizing agent. Furthermore, the results indicate that the chemical reactivity groups seem to gradually engage more pathways and more molecules in each pathway with increasing sensitizing potency of the chemical used for stimulation. Also, a switch in gene regulation from up to down regulation, with increasing potency, was seen both in genes involved in metabolic functions and cell cycling. These observed pathway patterns were clearly reflected in the regulatory elements identified to drive these processes, where 33 regulatory elements have been proposed for further analysis.

Conclusions: This study demonstrates that functional analysis of biomarkers identified from our genomics study of human MUTZ-3 cells can be used to assess sensitizing potency of chemicals *in vitro*, by the identification of key cellular events, such as metabolic and cell cycling pathways.

Keywords: Pathways in skin sensitization, Skin sensitizer, *in vitro* assay, Signaling pathways, Metabolic pathways

Background

Allergic contact dermatitis (ACD) is an inflammatory skin disease characterized by eczema and recurrent episodes of itching [1]. Hundreds of chemicals are known to cause skin sensitization, making ACD the most common immunotoxic condition in humans. ACD affects a significant proportion of the population. In a recent populations-based investigation, it was demonstrated that the prevalence of ACD is increasing, from 7.2% to 12.9% in the study population [2]. According to the REACH (Registration, Evaluation, and Authorization of Chemicals) regulation [3], chemicals within the EU that are produced or imported (>1 ton/year) must be tested for human hazardous effects. Historically, new chemicals have been tested on animals. For cosmetic ingredients, animal testing is now prohibited [4], even if validated alternative assays are unavailable.

* Correspondence: ann-sofie.albrekt@immun.lth.se
[1]Department of Immunotechnology, Lund University, Medicon Village building 406, 223 81 Lund, Sweden
Full list of author information is available at the end of the article

The Local Lymph Node Assay (LLNA) [5], which is currently the gold standard in hazard classification for sensitization, has been shown to have an accuracy of prediction of 72% relative to human data, the same as for the Guinea Pig Maximization Test (GPMT) [6]. Taken together, the ethical aspects of animal testing, the need for monitoring of hazardous effects and the discrepancy between animal and human immune mechanisms makes the need for *in vitro* tests urgent.

Recently, we presented an *in vitro* test, Genomic Allergen Rapid Detection (GARD), based on MUTZ-3 cells [7,8], that was able to accurately classify compounds as sensitizers or non-sensitizers, using a genomic biomarker signature [9,10]. Furthermore, we reported that sensitizers induced a heterogeneous transcriptional response in MUTZ-3 cells, indicating that different sensitizers affect different pathways. The OECD guidelines on adverse outcome pathways [11] attempts to summarize the biochemical pathways that are associated with skin sensitization, listing the activation of inflammation and cellular stress related pathways as critical events. However, transcriptional data from MUTZ-3 cells indicate that the regulation of biochemical pathways might be more diverse than previously described. This led us to further investigate the signaling pathways in relationship to the chemical reactivity properties of each individual skin sensitizer. Consequently, the aim of the current study was to identify adverse outcome pathways associated with different sensitizers, stratified into various chemical reactivity groups, in order to enhance the understanding of the skin sensitization processes in relation to sensitizer potency.

Methods

Transcriptional data set

A panel of 40 chemical compounds, consisting of 20 sensitizers and 20 non-sensitizers were used for cell stimulations of the human myeloid leukemia-derived cell line MUTZ-3 (DSMZ, Braunschweig, Germany), as detailed earlier in [10]. RNA was isolated, processed to cDNA and hybridized to microarrays (Affymetrix®, Santa Clara, CA) [12]. In short, RNA from un-stimulated and chemically stimulated MUTZ-3 cells, from triplicate experiments, were extracted and analyzed. The preparation of labeled sense DNA was performed, according to Affymetrix® GeneChip® Whole Transcript (WT) Sense Target Labeling Assay (100 ng Total RNA Labeling Protocol), using the recommended kits and controls (Affymetrix®). Hybridization, washing and scanning of the Human Gene 1.0 ST Arrays were performed according to the manufacturer's protocol (Affymetrix®). 18 of the 20 sensitizing chemicals [13-18] passed QC test after array analysis and were subsequently used for functional analysis (Figure 1). The complete data set consisting of 137 samples has been deposited to ArrayExpress with the accession number [E-MTAB-670].

Microarray data analysis and statistical methods

The microarray data set was normalized and quality checked, using the RMA algorithm in the Affymetrix® Expression Console software (Affymetrix®). Sensitizers were assigned to at least one of the following chemical reactivity mechanisms; addition/elimination to carboxylic acid derivatives (Add/El), coordination bonds (Koor), Michael addition or 1,4-addition to a/b unsaturated carbonyl (MA), nucleophilic aromatic substitution (NAR), Schiff's base reaction (SB), biomolecular nucleophilic substitution (SN2), Prehapten (PreH) and Prohapten (ProH). In the present cohort of sensitizers, 9 different groups of chemical reactivity combinations were identified, as shown in Figure 1. The 9 reactivity groups were statistically tested against a pool of non-sensitizing stimulations and vehicle controls (83 samples in total), using ANOVA. The top 1000 genes from each statistical test were identified, and the significance level at which these top genes were found was recorded. All filtering and statistical tests were performed in Qlucore Omics Explorer 2.3 (QOE; Qlucore AB, Lund, Sweden).

Functional analysis of chemical reactivity groups in IPA®

Each of the 9 gene lists identified with statistical testing was used as input in Ingenuity Pathways Analysis ver. 12710793, as of June 2012 (IPA®; Ingenuity Systems Inc., Redwood City, CA), using fold change and p-values as decision values for significance and enrichment calculations. For each data set the significant canonical pathways, significant transcription regulators and cellular functions identified by IPA® Core Analysis of Human data using default settings were exported and analyzed further in QOE. Hierarchical Cluster Analysis (HCA) was performed using non-normalized data with maximum linkage.

Pathway annotation and grouping for assessment of biological functions

All pathways were named according to the terminology used by IPA®. In addition to pathway names, we also grouped pathways into functional groups, according to the grouping used by IPA® (apoptosis signaling, cell cycle regulation etc.) with all pathways being classified as either signaling or metabolic pathways or both. When a pathway was ambiguously assigned we chose the first listing, according to alphabetical order. Findings were confirmed, using MetaCore™ (Thomson Reuters, NY).

Availability of supporting data

The microarray data set used was deposited at Array Express with the accession number [E-MTAB-670].

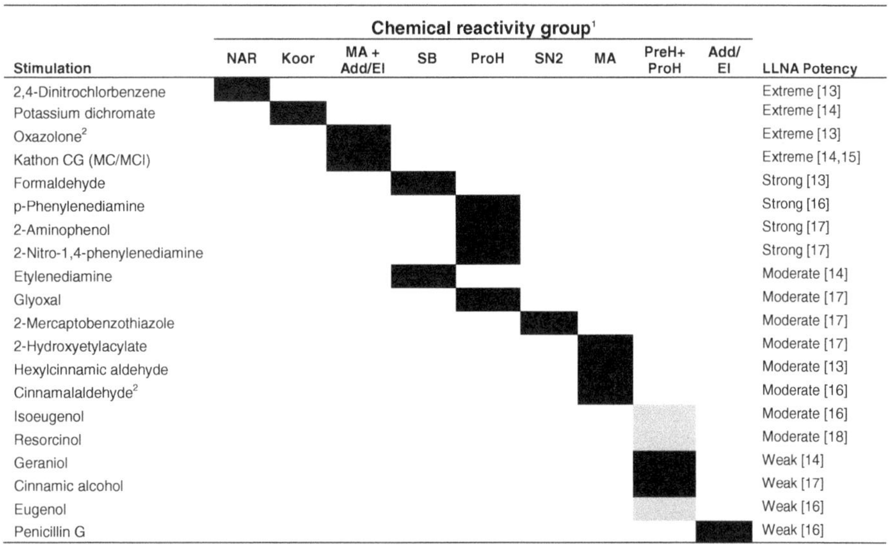

Figure 1 Stratification of chemical sensitizers into reactive mechanism groups. 1) Black: classification generally acknowledged. Grey: possibly ambiguous classification. 2) Indicated stimulations did not pass QC tests and were removed from analysis. Chemical reactivity abbreviations: Add/El: Addition/elimination to carboxylic acid derivatives; Koor: Coordination bonds; MA: Michael addition or 1,4-Addition to a/b unsaturated carbonyl; NAR: nucleophilic aromatic substitution, PreH: Prehapten; Chemical activation (outside the skin); ProH: Prohapten; Enzymatic activation; SB: Schiff's Base reaction; SN2: bimolecular nucleophilic substitution.

Results and discussion

MUTZ-3 transcriptional profiling and stratification of sensitizers into chemical reactivity groups

The transcriptome of MUTZ-3 cells stimulated with skin sensitizers and non-sensitizers was analyzed, using DNA microarray technology, with triplicate samples of 40 individual stimulations [10]. Due to insufficient array quality, 2 out of 20 sensitizers were removed from further analysis, leaving 18 triplicates of sensitizers and 20 triplicates of non-sensitizers for analysis in this study. The relationship between the sensitizers' potency, according to the Local Lymph Node Assay, and the designation of these into different chemical reactivity groups are summarized in Figure 1.

A Principal Component Analysis (PCA) analysis of the complete expression data set visualized that the studied chemical reactivities were indeed quite distinct, as shown in Figure 2. Though there is a certain overlap between the groups there are also clear differences, which is a strong indicator that the 9 chemical groups may trigger different biological activities, while the effects of non-sensitizing samples are homogenous. The PCA plot in Figure 2 was based on the 26 most significant genes in the data set from an ANOVA, comparing sensitizers with non-sensitizers. However, the observed pattern is clearly visible also in the complete data set, where no statistical test has guided the PCA. To further ensure that this is a biological finding, randomization and permutation of data was performed, comparing the original data set to randomized and permuted data sets. Statistical significance was only found in the original data set, which shows that the observed patterns are not seen due to random effects in multidimensional data.

The apparent differences in transcriptional profiles among different reactivity groups led us to further explore the differential engagement of signaling and metabolic pathways and the upstream regulators initiating such pathways. To this end, each chemical reactivity group was compared to the set of non-sensitizers in an ANOVA, yielding 9 lists of differentially regulated genes. These 9 gene lists were subsequently imported into IPA® for further analysis.

Using the Core Analysis of the pathway software IPA®, a number of regulated pathways were identified. In total, 387 regulated pathways were detected in the 9 different chemical reactivity groups. By applying a cut-off of three times, the default IPA® significance ($-\log(\text{p-value}) \leq 3.9$), 33 pathways were selected for a comprehensive investigation. The differential engagement patterns of the 33 pathways, related to sensitizer reactivity, are summarized in Figure 3, and detailed in Additional file 1. In addition, Figures 4 and 5 indicate the direction of regulation, as well as the level of significance at which the IPA® input gene lists were identified. When studying the 33 selected pathways, it is evident that increasing potency correlates with enhanced pathway involvement in terms of number of regulated genes, as well as a shift towards down regulation of the pathways components.

Finally, to identify the drivers in relation to potency, analysis of upstream regulators was performed. In Figure 3,

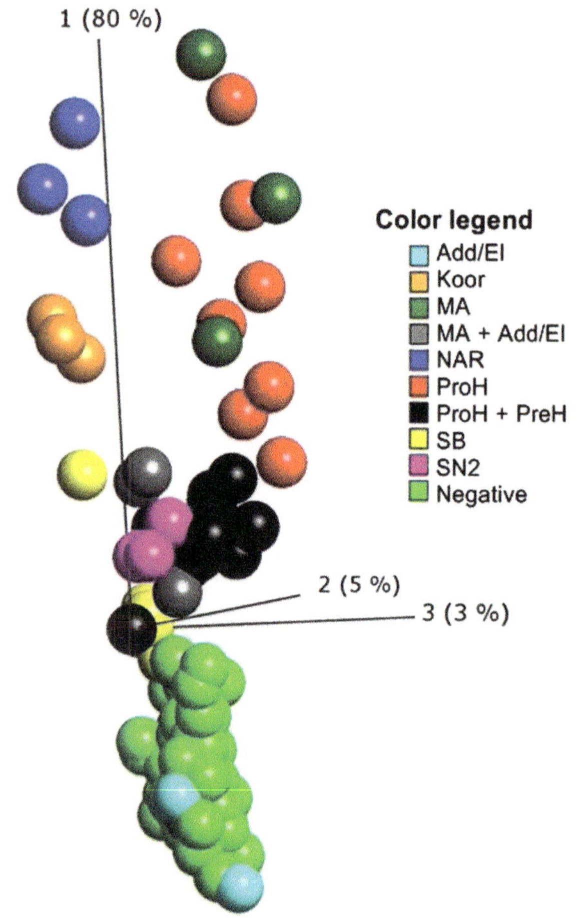

Figure 2 Principal component analysis (PCA) plot of sensitizers and non-sensitizers. The PCA plot shows the 26 most significant genes, based on p-value from an ANOVA comparing sensitizers with non-sensitizers. Triplicate samples of 18 sensitizers and 20 non-sensitizers are shown. The coloring shows the different chemical reactivity groups included. The sensitizers are centered in the top of the plot and the non-sensitizers in the bottom of the plot. Add/El: Addition/elimination to carboxylic acid derivatives; Koor: Coordination bonds; MA: Michael addition or 1,4-Addition to a/b unsaturated carbonyl; NAR: nucleophilic aromatic substitution, PreH: Prehapten; Chemical activation (outside the skin); ProH: Prohapten; Enzymatic activation; SB: Schiff's Base reaction; SN2: bimolecular nucleophilic substitution.

the common regulatory elements for all nine groups are summarized. The significance calculations include a predicted activation or inhibition status, which takes regulation of connected molecules into account. Only upstream regulators predicted to be significantly up or down regulated in four or more chemical groups were reported here. The regulatory elements were studied for their relationship to each other, using the MetaCore™ database. These findings were summarized in Figure 6. A complete list of all regulatory elements predicted is found in the Supplementary materials (Additional file 2).

Prominent pathways and biological functions

The overall impression is that more genes, associated with various pathways, are down-regulated than up-regulated in MUTZ3 cells stimulated with sensitizers. The sensitizers act mainly on cell cycling, cellular stress and injury, and metabolic pathways, in that order. Relevant identified sub functions are apoptosis, cellular growth and development, cellular immune response, intracellular and second messenger signaling, and metabolism and biosynthesis of glycan, lipids, vitamins and co-factors and nucleotides. The general trend is that both metabolic and cell cycle associated pathways are engaged gradually and in correlation with potency. Oxidative stress related pathways are another group of highly engaged pathways. However, these do not correlate with potency in the same manner as the other pathways do. For example, the NRF2-mediated oxidative stress response pathway shows a reversed pattern compared to the other pathways presented in this study. The overall impression of the NRF2 pathway is that phase I and II enzymes, as well as antioxidant proteins, are up-regulated, for an example see Additional file 3. While these trends are quite weak we still think it deserves further investigation. Pathways regulating metabolism and biosynthesis processes are regulated to a lesser extent but still show the same pattern as seen in the cell cycling pathways. Finally, we report 33 potential key regulators of the skin sensitization process found in the analyses. For a complete list of pathways and regulation patterns see Figures 3, 4, and 5. One more pathway has a pattern similar to the one observed in NRF2-mediated oxidative stress response pathway, namely Sphingolipid metabolism. The less potent chemical reactivity groups seem to engage this pathway to a larger extent than the more potent ones.

A few metabolic pathways are generally regulated. These are the nucleotide and lipid metabolism pathways. Chemicals belonging to the nucleophilic aromatic substitution (NAR) and coordination bonds (Koor) group down regulate nucleotide metabolism the most. As the current chemical selection includes only highly potent sensitizers from the Koor and NAR group, we cannot extrapolate these findings to less potent ones. Also, the NAR group constitutes a somewhat odd case, since this is a small group of highly experimental allergens with limited clinical relevance. The other metabolic pathways are regulated in a more mixed fashion, but again, amino acid metabolism is gradually down-regulated with increasing chemical potency. The Glutathione metabolism pathway is interesting in that it goes from clear up regulation by the less potent chemicals to clear down regulation by the NAR group. While the division of pathways into signaling or metabolic pathways is a somewhat arbitrary matter, we still believe it reflects the major cellular

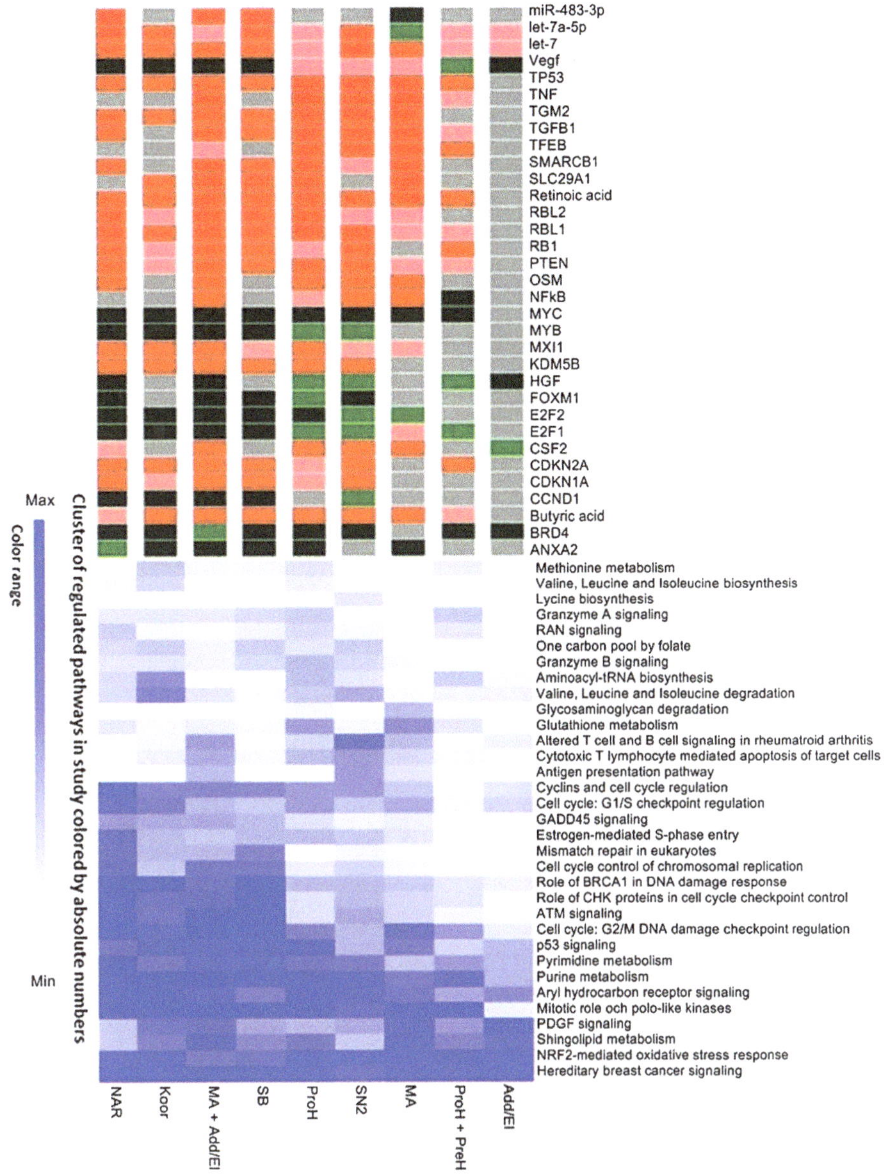

Figure 3 Hierarchical cluster analysis of pathway and regulatory elements. This hierarchical cluster analysis shows the regulatory elements predicted to have a general activity in the data set, i.e. in at least 4 of the 9 groups. Regulatory elements are colored according to the activation state. Red color indicates activation, while green color indicates inhibition. Dark and pale red/green colors indicate high and low significance of change, respectively. 33 pathways were found to be significantly regulated by the chemicals. These were clustered and colored from white to blue according to the involvement grade of the pathway, as estimated by the number of regulated molecules. The chemical groups were ordered according to their Local Lymph Node Assay potency with the most potent to the left and least potent to the right in the picture. The complete data set is given in Additional file 1.

functions quite well. We have followed the KEGG standard [19] at the time, adopted from the IPA® software.

The pathways of cell cycle regulation are also gradually down-regulated with increasing potency. This could indicate that these chemicals induce cell cycle arrest. As discussed later this seems to be connected to activation state of the up-stream regulators identified in the analyses, especially the *let-7* microRNAs.

The apoptosis pathway Aryl hydrocarbon receptor (AHR) signaling is also among the frequently regulated. As seen from Figure 3, its usage does increase with potency, but the base level is among the highest observed. Several caspases in the AHR signaling are highly up-regulated by many of the chemical groups. Caspases are both involved in cell death processes, like cell shrinkage, membrane blebbing, DNA fragmentation and DNA repair,

Pathway group (IPA®)	Signaling pathway[1]	Chemical reactivity group								
		NAR	Koor	MA+Add/El	SB	ProH	SN2	MA	ProH+PreH	Add/El
Apoptosis	Aryl hydrocarbon receptor signaling	↓	↓	MIX	MIX	MIX	MIX	MIX	MIX	MIX
Cancer	Role of BRCA1 in DNA damage response	↓	↓	↓	↓	MIX	↓	MIX	↓	(↑)
	Hereditary breast cancer signaling	↓	↓	↓	↓	MIX	MIX	MIX	MIX	↓
	p53 signaling	MIX	MIX	MIX	MIX	MIX	MIX	MIX	MIX	↓
Cell cycle regulation	Cell cycle control of chromosomal replication	↓	↓	↓	↓	(↓)	↓	(↓)	(↓)	(↑)
	Mitotic role of polo-like kinases	↓	↓	↓	↓	↓	↓	↑	MIX	(↓)
	Cyclins and cell cycle regulation	↓	↓	MIX	↓	MIX	↓	MIX	(↓)	↓
	Estrogen-mediated S-phase entry	↓	↓	MIX	↓	MIX	↓	MIX	(↓)	(↓)
	Cell cycle : G2/M DNA damage checkpoint regulation	↓	MIX	↓	↓	MIX	↓	↑	(MIX)	(MIX)
	Cell cycle: G1/S checkpoint regulation	↓	↓	MIX	↓	MIX	↓	MIX	(↓)	↓
	GADD45 signaling	↓	MIX	MIX	↓	MIX	(MIX)	(MIX)	(↑)	(↓)
	Role of CHK proteins in cell cycle checkpoint control	↓	↓	↓	↓	MIX	MIX	MIX	↓	(↓)
	ATM signaling	↓	↓	↓	↓	↑	MIX	↑	(MIX)	(MIX)
Cellular growth, proliferation and development	RAN signaling	↓	(↓)	(↓)	↓	↓	(↓)	(↓)	↓	(↓)
	PDGF Signaling	MIX	MIX	MIX	MIX	MIX	↓	MIX	MIX	↑
Cellular immune response	Antigen presentation pathway	(↓)	NC	MIX	(↑)	(↑)	↓	↑	(↑)	(↑)
	Granzyme A signaling	(↓)	(↓)	↓	↓	↓	(↓)	(↓)	↓	(↓)
	Cytotoxic T lymphocyte mediated apoptosis of target cells	(MIX)	MIX	MIX	(↑)	MIX	↓	↑	(MIX)	(↑)
	Altered T cell and B cell signaling in rheumatroid arthritis	(↑)	(↑)	MIX	(↑)	↑	MIX	MIX	(↓)	(MIX)
	Granzyme B signaling	MIX	MIX	(MIX)	MIX	MIX	↓	(MIX)	(↓)	NC
Cellular stress and injury	NRF2-mediated oxidative stress response	↓	↓	MIX	MIX	MIX	MIX	↑	MIX	MIX
	Mismatch repair in eukaryotes	↓	↓	↓	↓	NC	(↓)	(MIX)	(↓)	NC
p-value cut-off for 1000* best genes		8e-9	8e-14	5e-4	3e-3	4e-6	2e-4	2e-4	3e-4	3e-3
q-value cut-off for 1000* best genes		2e-7	2e-12	2e-2	10e-2	1e-4	5e-3	4e-3	8e-3	9e-2

Figure 4 Signaling pathways identified to be significantly regulated. The figure shows signaling pathways and general regulation patterns observed in these, as identified by analysis of each chemical reactivity group. Chemical reactivity abbreviations: Add/El: Addition/elimination to carboxylic acid derivatives; Koor: Coordination bonds; MA: Michael addition or 1,4-Addition to a/b unsaturated carbonyl; NAR: nucleophilic aromatic substitution, PreH: Prehapten; Chemical activation (outside the skin); ProH: Prohapten; Enzymatic activation; SB: Schiff's Base reaction; SN2: bimolecular nucleophilic substitution. * most significant genes in t-test of negative samples versus given chemical reactivity group. 1) Only pathways where at least one group gives a contribution of 2 times the significance threshold from IPA® were reported. ↑: 80% of transcripts or more up regulated, regulated transcripts ≥5. (↑): 80% of transcripts or more up regulated, regulated transcripts <5. ↓: 80% of transcripts or more down regulated, regulated transcripts ≥5. (↓): 80% of transcripts or more down regulated, regulated transcripts <5. MIX: a mix of up and down regulation, regulated transcripts ≥5. (MIX): a mix of up and down regulation, regulated transcripts <5. NC: No significant change compared to non-sensitizers.

Pathway group (IPA®)	Metabolic pathway[1]	Chemical reactivity group								
		NAR	Koor	MA+Add/El	SB	ProH	SN2	MA	ProH+PreH	Add/El
Amino acid metabolism	Lysine biosynthesis	(↓)	(↓)	NC	(↓)	(MIX)	↓	(↑)	(↓)	NC
	Valine, Leucine and Isoleucine biosynthesis	(↓)	↓	(↓)	(↓)	(↓)	(↓)	NC	(↓)	(MIX)
	Valine, Leucine and Isoleucine degradation	↓	↓	↓	(↓)	MIX	↓	MIX	(↓)	(↑)
	Methionine metabolism	NC	↓	(↓)	(↓)	↓	(↓)	(MIX)	(MIX)	NC
	Aminoacyl-tRNA biosynthesis	↓	↓	(↓)	NC	↓	↓	(↑)	↓	(↓)
	Glutathione metabolism	↓	(MIX)	(MIX)	(MIX)	↑	(MIX)	MIX	↑	(↑)
Glycan Bio-synthesis and Metabolism	Glycosaminoglycan degradation	NC	NC	(↑)	(↑)	(↑)	NC	MIX	(↑)	NC
Lipid metabolism	Sphingolipid metabolism	MIX	MIX	MIX	MIX	↑	MIX	MIX	MIX	↓
Metabolism of cofactors and vitamins	One carbon pool by folate	↓	↓	↓	↓	↓	↓	NC	(↓)	NC
Nucleotide metabolism	Pyrimidine metabolism	↓	↓	MIX	↓	MIX	MIX	MIX	↓	MIX
	Purine metabolism	↓	↓	MIX	↓	MIX	↓	MIX	↓	MIX
p-value cut-off for 1000* best genes		8e-9	8e-14	5e-4	3e-3	4e-6	2e-4	2e-4	3e-4	3e-3
q-value cut-off for 1000* best genes		2e-7	2e-12	2e-2	10e-2	1e-4	5e-3	4e-3	8e-3	9e-2

Figure 5 Metabolic pathways identified to be significantly regulated. The figure shows metabolic pathways and general regulation patterns observed in these, as identified by analysis of each chemical reactivity group. Chemical reactivity abbreviations: Add/El: Addition/elimination to carboxylic acid derivatives; Koor: Coordination bonds; MA: Michael addition or 1,4-Addition to a/b unsaturated carbonyl; NAR: nucleophilic aromatic substitution, PreH: Prehapten; Chemical activation (outside the skin); ProH: Prohapten; Enzymatic activation; SB: Schiff's Base reaction; SN2: bimolecular nucleophilic substitution. * most significant genes in t-test of negative samples versus given chemical reactivity group. 1) Only pathways where at least one group gives a contribution of 2 times the significance threshold from IPA® were reported. ↑: 80% of transcripts or more up regulated, regulated transcripts ≥5. (↑): 80% of transcripts or more up regulated, regulated transcripts <5. ↓: 80% of transcripts or more down regulated, regulated transcripts ≥5. (↓): 80% of transcripts or more down regulated, regulated transcripts <5. MIX: a mix of up and down regulation, regulated transcripts ≥5. (MIX): a mix of up and down regulation, regulated transcripts <5. NC: No significant change compared to non-sensitizers.

and in processes of post-translational modifications, protein degradation and synthesis [20]. There are also connections between apoptosis and cell cycle regulators. Caspase 6, for example, is known to interact directly with the transcription factor Rb [21], which is a key regulator of the Cell Cycle Control of Chromosomal Replication pathway. As described previously, a shift towards down regulation of pathway members is observed with increasing potency. For a detailed list of the molecules in the AHR signaling pathway, see Additional file 4.

Finally, lipid metabolism is generally affected by all the chemical groups. For instance, addition/elimination to carboxylic acid derivatives (Add/El) clearly down regulates Sphingolipid metabolism and the remaining chemical groups show a mixed or up-regulated pattern.

Biological activity of specific chemical groups

From the pathway analysis it is clear that various chemical reactivity groups stimulate pathway activation or inhibition differentially. This selective effect is e.g. observed for chemicals of the Michael addition or 1,4-Addition to a/b unsaturated carbonyl (MA) group, which up regulate several of the signaling pathways, as well as chemicals of the addition/elimination to carboxylic acid derivatives (Add/El). The groups prehapten (Chemical activation outside the skin; PreH) + prohapten (enzymatic activation; ProH) and Add/El (addition/elimination to carboxylic acid derivatives) both show a very limited activity in most pathways studied.

Considering the activity levels and changes of transcription observed and summarized in Figures 3, 4, and 5, we conclude that there is no single mechanism of action of skin sensitizing chemicals. On the contrary, a range of functions are triggered at different levels by the studied chemical groups. Some chemical groups, notably the most potent ones, down regulate most or all pathways studied. Others, like MA, up regulate relatively many pathways, while e.g. addition/elimination to carboxylic acid derivatives (Add/El) and prohapten +

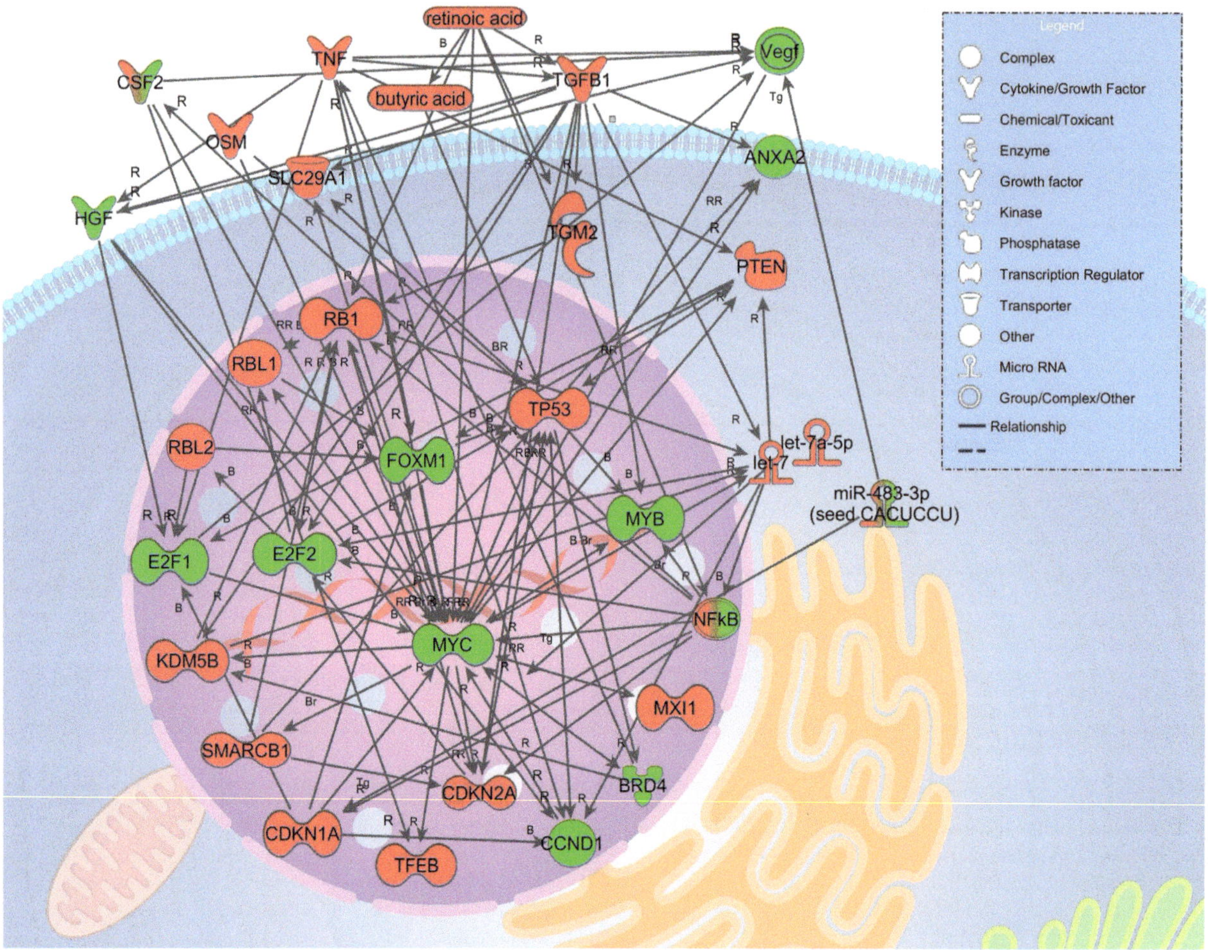

Figure 6 Network of interactions between transcription regulators observed or predicted in the IPA® analysis of the 9 chemical reactivity groups. Observed expression patterns were analyzed using IPA® in order to predict upstream regulation. The prediction was based on the expression patterns of the chemical groups and only the most significant predictions were included here. The network shows the known interactions between the regulatory elements identified to be up or down regulated in the analysis. Red color indicates a observed/predicted activation and green color indicates a observed/predicted inhibition of the molecule or complex of molecules. All interactions are based on experimental evidence from the scientific literature. Arrow directions show which way the regulation is directed, if known. R: regulation; B: binding; Br: binding regulated by target; RR: bidirectional regulation; Tg: target. The network was extracted from the MetaCore™ database (Thomson Reuters). For details about observation/prediction state, see Additional files 2, 3, 4 and 5.

prehapten(ProH + PreH) show a quite limited activity except for a few pathways that seem to always be highly regulated. The method also shows promising results in the detection of pre- and prohapten activation as a grouped class of chemical reactivity. However, it does not distinguish between these two activation routes. In the literature cinnamic alcohol is classified as a prohapten [22,23], but recently it has been shown that cinnamic alcohol autoxidize very rapidly [24], making the older classifications uncertain. Therefore, further investigation into the use of methods for separation of these two classes of chemical reactivity is needed. Especially for prohaptens, it is also crucial to confirm purity levels stated by suppliers as even small amounts of impurities may change the reactivity patterns.

It should be noted that all samples in this study are collected at single concentrations and single time-points. Most likely, the observed differences between chemical groups depend in some instances on a varying reactivity speed. As an example, investigations of transcription factors, connecting directly to selected cell cycle pathways, show that the activity level of the pathway molecules can depend on temporal factors. Those chemicals that did not show a great deal of activity in the pathway did indeed have a relatively higher activity level among the upstream regulators of these pathways. Thus, there may be pathways that are more consistently regulated than is observed in this study, although such similarities may be masked by varying reactivity of the chemical sensitizers.

Upstream regulators

Next, the significantly predicted upstream regulators were investigated. Figure 6 shows the known and experimentally verified interactions in the dataset. The network was manually built, in the IPA® software using molecules predicted to be up or down regulated based on analysis of the expression patterns of the nine chemical reactivity groups studied. The molecular interactions were studied in detail using the MetaCore™ software for pathways analyses focusing on uni- or bidirectional binding and regulation actions of the included molecules. All interactions shown in Figure 6 have been experimentally verified elsewhere and are described in the scientific literature. Several of the transcription regulators included in the network bind to each other, e.g. MYC and ANXA2, RB1 and E2f2 and NFkB and E2f2. Central to the network of Figure 6 is a microRNA group named *let-7* (*lethal-7*). The de-regulation of *let-7* miRNAs has previously been described in association to cancer, where the *let-7* family members act as tumor suppressors acting e.g. through MYC and E2f2 [25]. Both MYC and E2f2 were predicted to be down regulated by a majority of the chemical reactivity groups in this study. The microRNA group *let-7* and specifically the member *let-7a-5p* was predicted to be significantly activated in six out of the nine groups, with very high activation scores (z-score 2.6 to 6.6) and regulated with borderline detection in the three remaining groups (z-score 1.3 to 1.8 in ProH, ProH + PreH and Add/El). This finding fits well with the known down regulation of *let-7* by MYC, through binding of MYC to the transcription start site of the *let-7 g pri-miRNA* [26]. *let-7* is known to be active in cell cycle regulation, DNA replication, cell division, apoptosis and development [27]. In the current study, cell cycle, apoptosis, and nucleotide metabolism pathways were found to be down-regulated. This situation is comparable to many forms of cancer, in which low levels of *let-7* have been observed, giving rise to loss of cell cycle control. In our case, down regulation of cell cycle functions is evident for the majority of the chemical reactivity groups studied, while *let-7* was predicted to be up regulated. In a review by Hou et al. [28], *let-7* RNAs were described as heavily down regulated by environmental chemicals, cigarette smoke and up-regulated by others, such as hexahydro-1,3,5-triazine (RDX). *let-7* up-regulation has also been demonstrated in skin samples from psoriasis patients compared to healthy controls [29], suggesting these microRNAs to be key players in skin pathogenesis. Two other, specific, microRNAs were also predicted to be significantly regulated namely *let-7a-5p* and *mir-483-3p*. We propose that these microRNAs may have similar functions, as described above, in skin, when chemically challenged. For details about molecular interactions found see Additional file 5.

let-7 is known to inhibit a number of molecules: ABCC10, BACH1, BLIMP1 (PRDI-BF1), Bax, CCR7, Dicer, EZH2, HMGA2, HMGI/Y, HOXA9, IL-6, NAV1.9, PGHD, SOCS1, UHRF2, and MYC that are all found regulated in the data set. BCL2L1 and DICER1 were found to be up-regulated while all other were down-regulated. Among the transcription regulators MYC and *let-7* miRNAs are known to bind and interact bi-directionally. Furthermore, *let-7* is regulated by a number of other molecules, several of which were seen regulated in the present analysis, namely PPARA, DROSHA, XPO5, and KDM5B. Finally, *let-7* binds to the predicted activated transcription regulator TGFB1.

The ascribed biological functions of the upstream regulators were extracted from the IPA® database. Many of them have known relevant functions in skin and skin disorders, including CDKN1A, CDKN2A, CCND1, CSF2, MYC, PTEN, SMARCB1, TGM2, TP53, E2F2, Retinoic acid, NFkB, TGFB1, TNF-α and *let-7*. Of particular interest, CSF2, NFkB, TGFB1, TNF-α and TP53 have been associated with hypersensitivity and allergy reactions. BRD4, CCND1, CDKN2A, E2F1, FOXM1, HGF, KDM5B. MYB, MYC, NFkB2, PTEN, RB1, RBL1/2, SMARCB1, TGFB1, TP53, Butyric acid and *let-7* are all regulators of the cell cycle. In addition, a majority of these molecules are associated with various forms of cancer, as many carcinomas act through disruption of the cell cycle. Of interest, many of the predicted elements, such as CDKN2A, E2F1, E2F2, MYC, SMARCB1, TP53, TGM2, TNF-α, Retinoic acid, NFkB and TGFB1 are known regulators or members of the Aryl Hydrocarbon Receptor signaling pathway.

The NFkB complex was also predicted to be activated in this study. This extensively studied nucleic protein has a wide range of functions. Of interest to this study is mainly its involvement in pathways of Xenobiotics Metabolism, Production of Nitric Oxide and Reactive Oxygen Species in Macrophages and Toll like receptor signaling. NFkB showed a heterogeneous pattern, with up regulation in four groups (MA + Add/El, MA, SN2 and ProH) and down regulation in one (ProH + PreH). This may be a relevant finding given the role this molecule plays in epithelial cells where it on one hand maintains immunological homeostasis and on the other induces inflammatory processes [30]. NFkB has been shown to be able both to activate and inhibit inflammatory pathways in skin [31], a finding that might explain the mixed pattern seen in this study.

Implications of the results

Activation of MUTZ-3 cells with skin sensitizers resulted in regulation of a number of previously known, as well as novel, canonical pathways. The 33 most significantly regulated pathways were studied in detail. After stratification of sensitizing chemicals into chemical reactivity groups, it was evident that pathway engagement and the number of regulated molecules within such pathways were linked to the sensitizing potency of the stimulatory agent. For instance, cell cycle associated pathways were engaged gradually in correlation with the sensitizing potency of the chemicals used for cell stimulations. These observations can be utilized when designing tools for assessment of sensitizing potency of chemicals in predictive assays. Currently, the primary prediction call obtained from GARD is binary, i.e. compounds are classified as sensitizers or non-sensitizers. However, this readout can now for the first time be complemented with a potency call based on mechanistic information obtained through pathway analysis. While implementation of such classifications are not straight-forward, similar attempts have been done within cancer research, where pathway activity has successfully been associated with subtypes of cancer and progression of disease [32-34].

Oxidative stress related pathways are also in the group of highly engaged pathways. These do not correlate with potency to the same extent that cell cycle pathways do. For example, the NRF2-mediated oxidative stress response pathway shows a higher engagement by less potent chemical groups compared to more potent ones. This may be a consideration when studying more clinically relevant allergens, as these are rarely in the strong to extreme but rather in the week to medium range of potency.

Pathways regulating metabolism and biosynthesis processes constitute the third large group of canonical pathways identified to be regulated in skin sensitization. These pathways are regulated to a lesser extent but still show the same pattern as seen in the cell cycling pathways.

No canonical pathway was unanimously regulated within each data set. The importance of this fact becomes apparent when considering the design of various proposed tests for animal-free assessment of sensitization, which today are mainly based on analysis of single biomarkers. It is evident that excessively simplistic tests lack the power to accurately assess compounds as sensitizers or non-sensitizers, if the target chemical domain is wide. Recognition of the specific subtype of chemicals to be tested based on reactive mechanism or otherwise, will be crucial in order to train and configure predictive models accurately.

Conclusions

In the present transcriptional profiling study, we have shown that skin sensitizers trigger a large number of signaling and metabolic pathways in MUTZ-3 cells. Among these, we found examples of well-known pathways, as well as pathways previously not described in relation to chemical sensitization. Importantly, a majority of the pathways described show a clear correlation with both chemical reactivity and sensitizing potency.

The strongest correlation between pathway usage and potency is found in the cell cycle, nucleotide metabolism and cancer pathways. As these groupings are obviously rather arbitrary it is probably more correct to say that functions involving cell cycle regulation and cell cycle control both in healthy and diseased conditions correlate very well with chemical potency. Nucleotide metabolism is tightly connected to the cell cycle and consequently a down regulation of nucleotide metabolism in parallel to a down regulation of cell cycle functions is expected. The apoptosis pathway Aryl Hydrocarbon Receptor signaling is a novel finding with regard to potency prediction. This pathway is among the highly regulated ones but still shows a decrease in activity with decrease in potency.

Finally, transcription regulation of the sensitization process was investigated, by prediction of activation and inhibition of upstream regulators. A network of regulatory elements that seemed to be generally involved was identified. These seemed to be centered on the transcription regulator MYC and the miRNA *let-7*.

The presented results have implications for the design of predictive *in vitro* test for assessment of sensitization potency. Few chemicals appear to induce identical responses *in vitro*, indicating that excessively simplistic assays will fail to correctly classify unknown samples. Subdivisions among sensitizers, by reactive domain or otherwise, should be considered with caution and predictive models should be trained accordingly. In brief, we demonstrate for the first time that genomic approaches contain valuable mechanistic information associated with potency assessment of chemicals, which is in line with the current demand of evidence based toxicology.

Additional files

Additional file 1: Table of gene involvement shown per reactivity group and per pathway, used for Figure 3. For each pathway described in Figure 3 the exact numbers of molecules involved are given in this table. No distinction is made between up or down regulated molecules.

Additional file 2: Table of upstream regulators predicted to be up or down regulated in the IPA® analysis. Predictions were based on expression data from the nine chemical reactivity groups studied.

Additional file 3: NRF2 Oxidative Stress Pathway map for Michael addition or 1,4-Addition to a/b unsaturated carbonyl reactive chemicals. The pathway map shows the NRF2 Oxidative Stress Pathway with expression data from the 1000 most significant genes regulated by MA. Red shows up regulation and green down regulation of a given molecule. The less significantly regulated molecules were not shown in this figure, indicated here as white molecule symbols.

Additional file 4: A detailed list of molecules in the Aryl Hydrocarbon Receptor (AHR) signaling pathway. The file shows all the molecules included in the AHR signaling pathway, as defined by IPA®. Common identifiers are included to enable analysis in any software.

Additional file 5: All upstream regulators identified in pathway analysis in IPA®. This file contains the complete result from the prediction analysis of the expression patterns seen in the nine data sets, one from each chemical reactivity group studied. The upstream regulators were predicted from the pattern of up or down regulated target molecules. Significance of finding is given as z-scores for each upstream regulator and an attached predicted activation status shows if the molecule is predicted to be up or down regulated. Molecules measured on the microarrays (observed) are recognized by a value in the fold change column.

Abbreviations

ACD: Allergic contact dermatitis; Add/El: Addition/elimination to carboxylic acid derivatives; AHR: Aryl Hydrocarbon Receptor; HCA: Hierarchical cluster analysis; Koor: Coordination bonds; LLNA: Local Lymph Node Assay; MA: Michael addition or 1,4-Addition to a/b unsaturated carbonyl; NAR: Nucleophilic aromatic substitution; PCA: Principal component analysis; PreH Prehapten: Chemical activation (outside the skin); ProH Prohapten: Enzymatic activation; SB: Schiff's Base reaction; SN2: Bimolecular nucleophilic substitution.

Competing interests

The authors declare no conflicts of interests.

Authors' contributions

ML and CB designed the sensitization study strategy. HJ and ML set up and optimized the cell-based assay. HJ performed the cellular stimulations with chemicals. AA, HJ and ML designed the analysis strategy. AA performed the data analysis and prepared the text and figures. AB contributed with chemical knowledge and data set stratification guidelines. AA, HJ and ML drafted the manuscript. All authors revised and approved the manuscript. All authors read and approved the final manuscript.

Acknowledgements

This work was supported by grants from the Swedish Fund for Research Without Animal Experiments, Faculty of Engineering (LTH), the Swedish Research Council, Swedish Research Council Formas and the European Commission as part of the Integrated project 'Novel Testing Strategies for *in vitro* Assessment of Allergens; Sens-it-iv'. We would like to thank Ann-Charlott Olsson for excellent technical support and microarray sample preparation.

Author details

[1]Department of Immunotechnology, Lund University, Medicon Village building 406, 223 81 Lund, Sweden. [2]Department of Chemistry and Molecular Biology, Dermatochemistry and Skin Allergy, University of Gothenburg, SE-412 96 Gothenburg, Sweden.

References

1. Akhavan A, Cohen SR: **The relationship between atopic dermatitis and contact dermatitis.** *Clin Dermatol* 2003, **21**(2):158–162.
2. Mortz CG, Bindslev-Jensen C, Andersen KE: **Prevalence, incidence rates and persistence of contact allergy and allergic contact dermatitis in The Odense Adolescence Cohort Study: a 15-year follow-up.** *Br J Dermatol* 2013, **168**(2):318–325.
3. The European Parliament and the Council of the European Union: **Regulation (EC) No 1907/2006 of the European Parliament and of the Council of 18 December 2006 concerning the Registration, Evaluation, Authorisation and Restriction of Chemicals (REACH), establishing a European Chemicals Agency, amending Directive 1999/45/EC and repealing Council Regulation (EEC) No 793/93 and Commission Regulation (EC) No 1488/94 as well as Council Directive 76/769/EEC and Commission Directives 91/155/EEC, 93/67/EEC, 93/105/EC and 2000/21/EC.** 2006:1–849.
4. The European Parliament and the Council of the European Union: *Directive 2003/15/EC of the European Parliament and of the Council of 27 February 2003 amending Council Directive 76/768/EEC on the approximation of the laws of the Member States relating to cosmetic products.* 2003:1–10.
5. Basketter DA, Evans P, Fielder RJ, Gerberick GF, Dearman RJ, Kimber I: **Local lymph node assay - validation, conduct and use in practice.** *Food Chem Toxicol* 2002, **40**(5):593–598.
6. Haneke KE, Tice RR, Carson BL, Margolin BH, Stokes WS: **ICCVAM evaluation of the murine local lymph node assay. Data analyses completed by the National Toxicology Program Interagency Center for the Evaluation of Alternative Toxicological Methods.** *Regul Toxicol Pharmacol* 2001, **34**(3):274–286.
7. Masterson AJ, Sombroek CC, De Gruijl TD, Graus YM, van der Vliet HJ, Lougheed SM, van den Eertwegh AJ, Pinedo HM, Scheper RJ: **MUTZ-3, a human cell line model for the cytokine-induced differentiation of dendritic cells from CD34+ precursors.** *Blood* 2002, **100**(2):701–703.
8. Larsson K, Lindstedt M, Borrebaeck CA: **Functional and transcriptional profiling of MUTZ-3, a myeloid cell line acting as a model for dendritic cells.** *Immunology* 2006, **117**(2):156–166.
9. Johansson H, Albrekt AS, Borrebaeck CA, Lindstedt M: **The GARD assay for assessment of chemical skin sensitizers.** *Toxicol In Vitro* 2012, **27**(3):1163–9.
10. Johansson H, Lindstedt M, Albrekt AS, Borrebaeck CAK: **A genomic biomarker signature can predict skin sensitizers using a cell-based *in vitro* alternative to animal tests.** *BMC Genomics* 2011, **12**:399.
11. Environment Directorate Organisation for Economic Co-operation and Development: **The adverse outcome pathway for skin sensitisation initiated by covalent binding to proteins.** *OECD Environment, Health and Safety Publications* 2012, **168**:1–59.
12. Lindstedt M, Schiott A, Bengtsson A, Larsson K, Korsgren M, Greiff L, Borrebaeck CA: **Genomic and functional delineation of dendritic cells and memory T cells derived from grass pollen-allergic patients and healthy individuals.** *Int Immunol* 2005, **17**(4):401–409.
13. Kimber I, Basketter DA, Butler M, Gamer A, Garrigue JL, Gerberick GF, Newsome C, Steiling W, Vohr HW: **Classification of contact allergens according to potency: proposals.** *Food Chem Toxicol* 2003, **41**(12):1799–1809.
14. Gerberick GF, Ryan CA, Kern PS, Schlatter H, Dearman RJ, Kimber I, Patlewicz GY, Basketter DA: **Compilation of historical local lymph node data for evaluation of skin sensitization alternative methods.** *Dermatitis* 2005, **16**(4):157–202.
15. Lasko TA, Bhagwat JG, Zou KH, Ohno-Machado L: **The use of receiver operating characteristic curves in biomedical informatics.** *J Biomed Inform* 2005, **38**(5):404–415.
16. Roberts DW, Patlewicz G, Kern PS, Gerberick F, Kimber I, Dearman RJ, Ryan CA, Basketter DA, Aptula AO: **Mechanistic applicability domain classification of a local lymph node assay dataset for skin sensitization.** *Chem Res Toxicol* 2007, **20**(7):1019–1030.
17. Warbrick EV, Dearman RJ, Basketter DA, Kimber I: **Influence of application vehicle on skin sensitization to methylchloroisothiazolinone/methylisothiazolinone: an analysis using the local lymph node assay.** *Contact Dermatitis* 1999, **41**(6):325–329.
18. Gerberick GF, Robinson MK, Ryan CA, Dearman RJ, Kimber I, Basketter DA, Wright Z, Marks JG: **Contact allergenic potency: correlation of human and local lymph node assay data.** *Am J Contact Dermat* 2001, **12**(3):156–161.
19. **KEGG.** http://www.genome.jp/kegg/pathway.html.
20. Kohler C, Orrenius S, Zhivotovsky B: **Evaluation of caspase activity in apoptotic cells.** *J Immunol Methods* 2002, **265**(1–2):97–110.
21. Lemaire C, Godefroy N, Costina-Parvu I, Rincheval V, Renaud F, Trotot P, Bouleau S, Mignotte B, Vayssiere JL: **Caspase-9 can antagonize p53-induced apoptosis by generating a p76(Rb) truncated form of Rb.** *Oncogene* 2005, **24**(20):3297–3308.
22. Basketter DA: **Skin Sensitization to Cinnamic Alcohol - the Role of Skin Metabolism.** *Acta Derm-Venereol* 1992, **72**(4):264–265.
23. Cheung C, Hotchkiss SAM, Pease CKS: **Cinnamic compound metabolism in human skin and the role metabolism may play in determining relative sensitisation potency.** *J Dermatol Sci* 2003, **31**(1):9–19.
24. Niklasson IB, Delaine T, Islam MN, Karlsson R, Luthman K, Karlberg AT: **Cinnamyl alcohol oxidizes rapidly upon air exposure.** *Contact Dermat* 2013, **68**(3):129–138.
25. Rovira C, Guida MC, Cayota A: **MicroRNAs and other small silencing RNAs in cancer.** *IUBMB life* 2010, **62**(12):859–868.
26. Chang TC, Yu D, Lee YS, Wentzel EA, Arking DE, West KM, Dang CV, Thomas-Tikhonenko A, Mendell JT: **Widespread microRNA repression by Myc contributes to tumorigenesis.** *Nat Genet* 2008, **40**(1):43–50.
27. Barh D, Malhotra R, Ravi B, Sindhurani P: **MicroRNA *let-7*: an emerging next-generation cancer therapeutic.** *Curr Oncol* 2010, **17**(1):70–80.

28. Hou L, Wang D, Baccarelli A: **Environmental chemicals and microRNAs.** *Mutat Res* 2011, **714**(1–2):105–112.
29. Zibert JR, Lovendorf MB, Litman T, Olsen J, Kaczkowski B, Skov L: **MicroRNAs and potential target interactions in psoriasis.** *J Dermatol Sci* 2010, **58**(3):177–185.
30. Wullaert A, Bonnet MC, Pasparakis M: **NF-kappaB in the regulation of epithelial homeostasis and inflammation.** *Cell Res* 2011, **21**(1):146–158.
31. Sur I, Ulvmar M, Toftgard R: **The two-faced NF-kappaB in the skin.** *Int Rev Immunol* 2008, **27**(4):205–223.
32. Chuang HY, Rassenti L, Salcedo M, Licon K, Kohlmann A, Haferlach T, Foa R, Ideker T, Kipps TJ: **Subnetwork-based analysis of chronic lymphocytic leukemia identifies pathways that associate with disease progression.** *Blood* 2012, **120**(13):2639–2649.
33. Kim S, Kon M, DeLisi C: **Pathway-based classification of cancer subtypes.** *Biol Direct* 2012, **7**:21.
34. Lee E, Chuang HY, Kim JW, Ideker T, Lee D: **Inferring pathway activity toward precise disease classification.** *PLoS Comput Biol* 2008, **4**(11):e1000217.

8

Pharmacokinetics and biodistribution of the cyclin-dependent kinase inhibitor -CR8- in mice

Hatem Sallam[1], Ibrahim El-Serafi[1], Laurent Meijer[2] and Moustapha Hassan[1,3,4*]

Abstract

Background: CR8 is a second generation inhibitor of cyclin-dependent kinases derived from roscovitine. CR8 was shown to be 50–100 fold more potent than roscovitine in inducing apoptosis in different tumor cell lines. In the present investigation, we have established an analytical method for the quantification of CR8 in biological samples and evaluated its bioavailability, biodistribution and pharmacokinetics in mice.

Methods: A liquid chromatography method utilizing UV-detection was used for the determination of CR8. CR8 was administered either orally (100 mg/kg) or i.v. (50 mg/kg) and the animals were sacrificed at different time points. Blood samples and organs were collected, after which the pharmacokinetic parameters were calculated for plasma and organs.

Results: CR8 was eluted at 5 minutes in the high performance liquid chromatography system used. The LLOQ detection was 0.10 μg/ml and linearity was observed within the 0.10-10 μg/ml range ($r^2 > 0.998$). The accuracy and precision were >86%, while the recovery from plasma was >95%. CR8 was stable for 2 months at room temperature in both solution and plasma. CR8 pharmacokinetics was fitted to a two-compartment open model after oral administration and to a one compartment model after i.v. injection. The elimination half-life was about 3 hours. Organ exposure to CR8 (expressed as % AUC organ vs. AUC plasma) was highest in liver (205%), adipose tissue (188%) and kidney (150%) and low in bone marrow (30%) and brain (15%) as compared to plasma. The oral bioavailability of CR8 was found to be essentially 100%.

Conclusions: We have developed a rapid and simple method for the analysis of CR8. CR8 pharmacokinetics pattern showed 100% bioavailability, long half-life and limited distribution to brain and bone marrow, which may allow systemic exposure higher than the IC_{50} reported for cell death in tumor cell lines. CR8 displays favorable pharmacological properties and is therefore a good candidate for future clinical studies.

Keywords: Roscovitine, CR8, Pharmacokinetics, Cyclin-dependent kinase inhibitors, Kinase inhibitors, Biodistribution, HPLC

Background

Roscovitine is a selective cyclin-dependent kinase (CDK) 1, 2, 5, 7, and 9 inhibitor [1-4] shown to be effective against several tumors. At present, roscovitine is undergoing Phase II clinical trials in cancer patients (non-small cell lung cancer, nasopharyngeal cancer). The drug has limited side effects and toxicity compared to conventional chemotherapy [5]. However, roscovitine is shown to have a short elimination half-life and rapid metabolism, which leads to suboptimal exposure in clinical trials. Recently, 2-(*R*)-(1-Ethyl-2-hydroxyethylamino)-6-(4-(2-pyridyl)benzyl)-9-isopropylpurine (CR8; Figure 1) was introduced as a second generation cyclin-dependent kinase inhibitor derived from roscovitine [6]. CR8 is shown to be about 50-fold more potent compared to roscovitine in inducing apoptosis in different tumor cell lines including ALL and CLL [7].

Several *in-vivo* and *in-vitro* studies have reported promising results due to the high efficacy of CR8. Bukanov et al. show CR8 to be effective against autosomal dominant polycystic kidney disease by blocking the renal and hepatic cystogenesis in mice [8]. Another study reports that CR8 can induce apoptotic tumor cell death in the neuroblastoma cell line, which is one of the

* Correspondence: moustapha.hassan@ki.se
[1]Experimental Cancer Medicine (ECM), Laboratory Medicine, Karolinska Institutet, 141 86, Stockholm, Sweden
[3]Experimental Cancer Medicine (ECM), Clinical Research Center, Novum, Karolinska University Hospital-Huddinge, 141 86, Stockholm, Sweden
Full list of author information is available at the end of the article

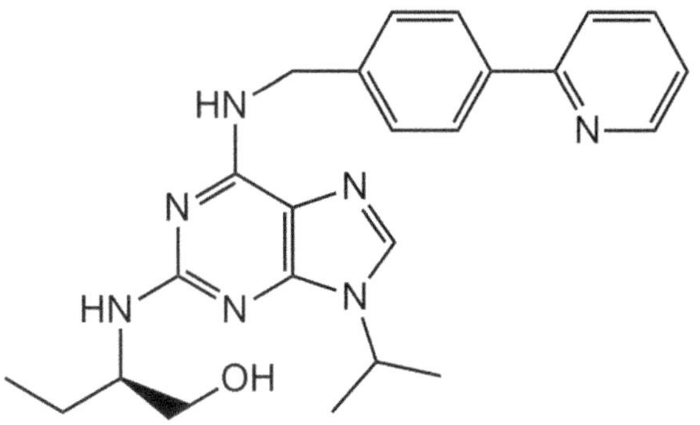

Figure 1 CR8: 2-(*R*)-(1-Ethyl-2-hydroxyethylamino)-6-(4-(2-pyridyl) benzyl)-9-isopropylpurine (CR8).

most frequent solid tumors in children [9]. CR8 is also proven to be a neuro-protector in experimental traumatic brain injury and has significantly reduced the lesion volume in rats subjected to moderate spinal cord contusion injury [10,11]. Moreover, CR8 is shown to increase the number of surviving neurons after spinal cord injury and to decrease the posttraumatic elevation of biochemical markers of apoptosis in an animal model [12].

Generally, the final effects of drugs *in-vivo* are influenced by many factors, such as systemic exposure, distribution in various organs, metabolism, lipophilicity, and protein binding. Bettayeb et al. show the optimal concentrations of CR8 needed to obtain a desirable pharmacological effect *in-vitro* in different cell lines to be about 0.7 μM [7], which is far below that reported for roscovitine (14.6 μM) [4].

Despite these results obtained in cell cultures, the pharmacokinetic profile of CR8 needs to be analyzed prior to further preclinical and possibly clinical investigations. In the present investigation we have established and validated an analytical method for the quantitative determination of CR8 according to standard bioanalytical guidelines. We have also investigated the pharmacokinetics profile and the tissue distribution of CR8 in mice. The present results are encouraging in terms of further development of CR8 as a drug candidate.

Methods

Chemicals and reagents

Tetrahydrofuran and methanol of high performance liquid chromatography (HPLC) grade were obtained from Merck (Darmstadt, Germany), Tween20 and dimethyl sulfoxide (DMSO) from Sigma-Aldrich (Stockholm, Sweden). All other reagents and solvents were of HPLC analytical grade. S-CR8 was dissolved in DMSO as a 75 mg/ml stock solution and was stored at −20°C. Serial dilutions were prepared from the main stock for the calibration curves, as quality control samples and for administration to mice. (R)-roscovitine and (S)-CR8 were synthesized as described previously [13].

Instrumentation and chromatographic conditions

The HPLC system consisted of a Gilson 234 auto-injector equipped with a 100 μl loop, an LKB 2150 pump (Pharmacia inc., Sweden), an "LDC analytical spectromonitor 3200" UV-detector (USA) and a CSW 32 chromatography station integrator. Separation was performed on a Zorbax SB-CN column (3.5 μm × 4.6 mm × 150 mm) from Agilent (USA), while the column was maintained at room temperature during analysis.

The mobile phase consisted of tetrahydrofuran: 25 mM phosphate buffer pH = 2.6, ionic strength = 0.022 (20:80, v/v). Flow rate was set at 0.9 ml/min, running time at 8 min for standard curve and quality controls and at 15 min for animal samples to elute all the metabolites. Injection volume was 50 μl and the UV wavelength used was 305 nm. Standard curves were prepared from spiked pooled human plasma, and were linear in the range of 0.1 - 10 μg/ml.

Standard solutions and controls

Pooled heparin plasma from healthy donors was obtained from the Blood Transfusion Center, Karolinska University Hospital. Serial standard dilutions in 50 mM Hydrochloric acid were prepared from the stocks for the calibration curves and for the quality controls.

Working standard solutions of CR8 in plasma at 10, 8, 6, 5, 4, 3, 2, 1, 0.5, 0.25 and 0.1 μg/ml were prepared by adding 50 μl from the standard stocks to 950 μl plasma to reach 1 ml containing the final concentrations. The calibrators were prepared on the day of each run.

Four quality control samples at concentrations of 0.75, 1.5, 3.5 and 7.0 μg/ml were also prepared in triplicate and stored at room temperature, +4°C and −20°C for stability testing.

The quality control samples were repeated using mouse plasma in triplicate using the same concentrations as in human plasma.

Sample preparation from plasma

70 μl plasma was added to 140 μl methanol and vortexed for 15 sec. Samples were centrifuged at 10000 g for 10 minutes, and 50 μl from the supernatant were injected into the HPLC system.

Bioanalytical method validation

Selectivity

A selective method should involve no interference from endogenous compounds, metabolites and/or different degradation products related to the drug [14]. We confirmed that our method involved no such interference by running blank biological samples from untreated mice and mice receiving only the drug vehicle [15].

Calibration curve

A calibration curve was constructed from eight standard points of CR8 at concentrations ranging from 0.1 - 10 μg/ml, including lower limit of quantification (LLOQ). The peak areas of CR8 were plotted against the concentrations. Linearity was assessed by a weighted least-squares regression analysis and a correlation coefficient (r^2) of 0.99 or better was deemed acceptable. The LLOQ was set as the lowest measurable concentration with acceptable accuracy and precision not more than 20% of the expected values [16].

Precision and accuracy

The precision of the method was defined as the percent relative standard deviation (% SD) calculated from triplicate measurements [(standard deviation)/mean value] × 100. The accuracy was defined as the percent relative error (% E) of the mean of the replicate measurements in relation to the theoretical values [(measured value - nominal value)/nominal value] × 100 [16,17]. Precision and accuracy were determined by analyzing quality control samples (QCs) prepared at four concentrations (0.75, 1.5, 3.5 and 7.0 μg/ml) in pentaplicate on three consecutive days [18].

Recovery

Absolute recovery is defined as percentage of reference compound that is measured to the exact amount of compound added to a blank buffer [15]. Recovery was computed by comparing responses in triplicate of extracted low, middle and high QCs (0.75, 1.5 and 7.0 μg/ml, respectively) samples with those of extracted solvent to which CR8 has been added at the same nominal concentration [14].

Relative recovery is defined as percentage of the amount of drug measured from the plasma compared to the amount measured from pure solvent e.g. 50 mM hydrochloric acid (HCl) [15]. The low, medium and high controls (0.75, 1.5 and 7.0 μg/ml, respectively) were prepared in pooled plasma and in 50 mM HCl. Samples were run in triplicate and recovery was calculated as the percentage of (plasma peak area/methanol peak area) × 100.

Stability

The stability of CR8 was determined in plasma samples using concentrations of 0.75, 1.5, 3.5 and 7.0 μg/ml (in triplicate). The samples were kept at room temperature, +4°C and −20°C and analyzed twice weekly for 2 months. Peak areas of all the samples were compared to peak areas obtained at time zero.

Animals

All experiments in this study were approved by the Stockholm Southern Ethics Committee for Animal Research and were conducted in accordance with the Animal Protection Law, the Animal Protection Regulation and the Regulation for the Swedish National Board for Laboratory Animals.

Female BALB/c mice 8–10 weeks old and weighing 18–21 g were obtained from Scanbur, Sollentuna, Sweden. The mice were allowed to acclimatize to their surroundings for one week before starting treatment. The mice were fed pelleted food and water *ad libitum*.

CR8 was dissolved in DMSO: 50 mM HCl (10:90 v/v). The first group of mice received i.v. doses of CR8 (50 mg/kg body weight), the second received oral doses of CR8 (100 mg/kg body weight) and three control mice received vehicle alone. Three mice were sacrificed at each time point and blood samples were collected by cardiac puncture into heparinized tubes at 10, 20, 30, 60 min, 2, 4, 6, 8 h post administration. Blood samples were centrifuged immediately after collection at 3000 g for 5 min at 4°C and the plasma was prepared as mentioned previously. Supernatants were collected and all samples were frozen at −20°C directly after preparation until further analysis by HPLC. Other organs including liver, spleen, kidneys, brain, adipose tissue and lungs were removed, washed and snap frozen immediately in liquid nitrogen. Bone marrow was flushed from both femurs and mononuclear cells were counted and frozen. The samples were stored at -20°C to avoid any metabolic activity.

Tissue sample preparation

Samples from different organs were homogenized by probe sonication in sodium perborate (PBS) (1:3 – 1:5 w:v) for 2 min and vortexed for 1 min. 100 μl of the homogenate was added to 200 μl methanol, vortexed for 1 min and centrifuged at 10000 g for 10 min. 50 μl of the supernatant were injected into the HPLC system.

Femurs were removed and cleaned; bone marrow was flushed with 0.3 ml of PBS and single cell suspension was prepared by gentle flushing through needle and syringe.

Nucleated cells were counted using Türk solution and bone marrow was stored at −20°C until assay.

Quality control samples were run together with the corresponding mouse samples in duplicate.

Pharmacokinetics

Parameters including distribution volume of the central compartment, elimination rate constant, plasma maximum concentration and micro constants were estimated. Clearance (Cl) and distribution volume at the steady state were calculated from the primary parameters. The plasma concentration versus time curves (AUC) were calculated from the model derived parameters, and the elimination half-lives were calculated from the slope of the terminal elimination phase. Bone marrow data were derived after adjustment of concentrations to 10^9 cells (= approx. 1 g of tissue). The pharmacokinetic modeling was performed using WinNonlin version 5.2 (Pharsight, USA).

Oral bioavailability (F) defined as the fraction of the oral administered dose of CR8 that reaches the systemic circulation was calculated according to the following formula:

$$F = \frac{[AUC]_{po} * \ dose_{IV}}{[AUC]_{IV} * \ dose_{po}}$$

Calculations and statistics

The peak areas of CR8 were plotted versus the corresponding nominal concentrations of the standards, and the standard curve was calculated by linear regression. CR8 concentrations in mouse plasma, organs and quality control samples were calculated from the resulting curves. All values are presented as mean ± S.D.

Results

Analysis of CR8

A precise and accurate method was developed to detect the drug in plasma and tissue samples in order to investigate the pharmacokinetics of CR8. CR8 is a lipophilic compound; however, due to the presence of the 2-pyridyl ring attached to the benzyl ring, its lipophilicity is lower than that of the parent analogue roscovitine. DMSO was found to be a suitable solvent for very high concentrations of CR8, and 50 mM HCl was found to be a suitable solvent for standard concentrations. Protein precipitation is the simplest approach for removing most proteins from biological samples. Methanol was shown to be better than acetonitrile in deproteinizing the plasma and extracting CR8 due to lower number of interfering peaks.

UV absorbance

UV absorbance was determined by running a UV-IVIS spectrum scan of CR8 dissolved in 50 mM HCl (10 µg/ml). No interference in the absorption range was detected. The scan revealed good absorption in the UV 210 nm - 310 nm wavelength ranges, and 305 nm was selected as the best measurement wavelength to ensure good selectivity and good sensitivity with a wide range of linear response for construction of the standard curves.

Chromatograms and specificity

The CR8 retention time was around 5.26 ± 0.3 min. Selectivity was confirmed by the absence of significant interfering peaks from endogenous compounds in the blank plasma at this retention time (Figure 2). Also, no interference was found from endogenous compounds in the mouse plasma and tissue samples compared to control samples (Figure 3).

Linearity and limit of quantification

The calibration curve was linear within the ranges of 0.1 µg/ml - 10 µg/ml, and had a correlation coefficient (r^2) ≥ 0.9987 (n = 6). The lower limit of quantification for CR8 was 0.1 µg/ml in human plasma. The precision and accuracy at LLOQ were 3.7 and 13.3%, respectively.

Accuracy and precision

The precision and accuracy between and within batch were always below 13% from the nominal values in all cases. Precision and accuracy fulfilled the standard guiding principles for validation of bioanalytical methods, i.e. < 15% for QCs both between batches and within batches and < 20% for LLOQ [14,16,17,19,20]. No differences were observed between mouse and human plasma concerning concentrations in QCs (Table 1).

Recovery

The absolute recovery of CR8 in plasma was 97 ± 6%, 95 ± 5.0% and 98 ± 4% at the concentrations of 0.75, 1.5 and 7.0 µg/ml, respectively, while the relative recoveries of the drug for the same concentrations in plasma compared to that obtained from 50 mM HCl were 99 ±3, 103 ± 2 and 96 + 5%, respectively. The recovery from plasma was almost completely with low variability. Consequently, plasma could be a suitable matrix for the regular calibrations needed to analyze patient/animal materials in future *in-vivo* experiments [21].

Stability

The drug proved to be highly stable after 2 months at room temperature, +4°C or −20°C, with no significant decrease in the concentration of the QC samples (stability found to be approximately 97 ± 3.5%).

CR8 Metabolites

Five CR8 metabolites were separated and found to absorb UV at the same wavelength as CR8. These metabolites were named M1-M5 and appeared in the chromatogram in the following order: M1 at 4.23 minutes, M2 at 5.79 - minutes, M3 at 8.13 minutes, M4 at 9.95 minutes and M5 at 11.81 minutes (Figure 4). The first and fifth metabolites (M1 & M5) appeared rapidly with maximum concentration at 20 minutes and slowly disappeared until 8 hours. The metabolite M4 increased by time to reach maximum concentration at 60 minutes then disappeared. The metabolites M2 and M3 increased and accumulated with time until 8 hours post administration (Figure 4).

Pharmacokinetics of CR8

To conduct the CR8 pharmacokinetic studies, a simple HPLC-UV method for the determination of CR8 in human plasma was developed and validated. The pharmacokinetics of CR8 were then investigated in mice and

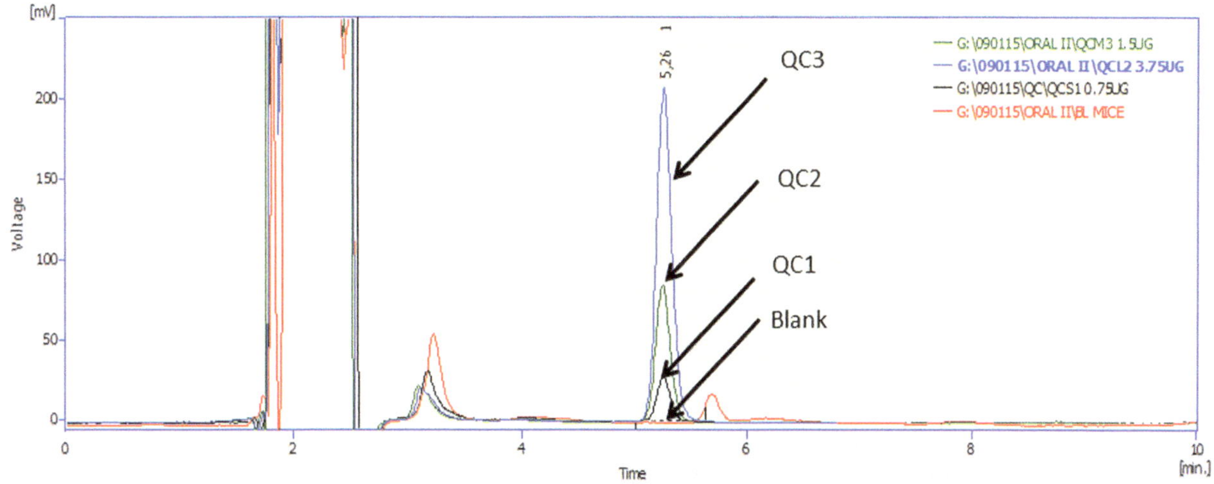

Figure 2 **Quality control samples in human plasma: HPLC chromatograms of blank samples and plasma containing CR8 (QCs) at concentrations of 1.5, 3.75 and 10.75 μg/mL.**

found to fit a two-compartment open model after oral administration and a one compartment bolus model after i.v. administration (Figure 5) using Gauss-Newton criteria.

The CR8 AUC was about 100 μg.hr/ml when 100 mg/kg was administered orally and about 45 μg.hr/ml when 50 mg/kg was administered intravenously. However, the estimated C_{max} was over 100 μg/ml after i.v. administration, which is 4 fold higher compared to that observed after oral administration (Table 2).

Absorption and distribution were rapid and the maximum concentrations were found at 30 min. Most importantly, the elimination half-life was estimated to be about 3 hours.

Exposure to concentrations much higher than the reported average IC_{50} value (0.7 μM) [7] was found to last more than 8–10 hours.

The oral bioavailability of CR8 was calculated to be 108 ± 9%.

Biodistribution of CR8

CR8 was widely distributed into all tissues, and the time - concentration curves (AUCs) were fitted to one compartment for all tissues (Table 3).

Higher exposure was found in the liver (the tissue/plasma exposure ratio was 200%), adipose tissue (180%) and kidneys (150%) compared to that observed as systemic exposure in plasma. Lung and spleen showed a tissue/plasma ratio of 80% and 50%, respectively (Figure 6) as compared to plasma.

CR8 distribution to the bone marrow

Exposure to CR8 was about 30% in bone marrow compared to in plasma when the concentrations were normalized to tissue weight/g (Figure 6).

This exposure is higher than that reported as IC_{50} required for the elimination of leukemic cell lines in about 6 h (data not shown).

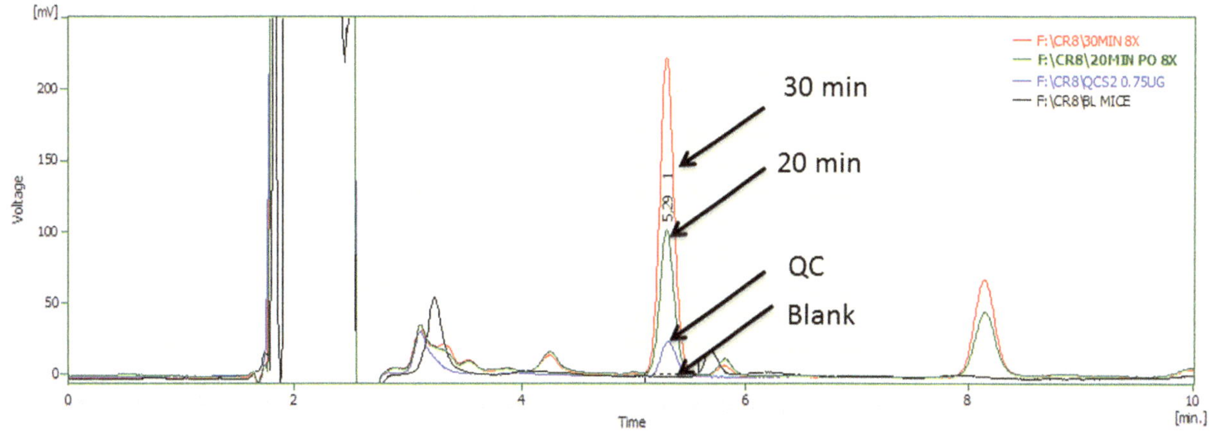

Figure 3 **HPLC chromatograms of mouse plasma: The chromatograms contain blank sample, QC (0.75 μg/mL) and CR8 at 20 and 30 min after oral administration.**

Table 1 Precision and accuracy of the CR8 analysis (n = 3-5 each)

Concentration (μg/ml)		Precision (%)			Accuracy (%)	
Between batch						
0.1 (LLOQ)		3.7			−13.3	
0.75 (QC1)		7.7			−2.0	
1.5 (QC2)		6.9			−3.8	
3.5 (QC3)		4.9			−4.4	
7.0 (QC4)		3.3			−5.3	
Within batch	*Batch1*	*Batch2*	*Batch3*	*Batch1*	*Batch2*	*Batch3*
0.1 (LLOQ)	4.2	3.4	4.8	−16	−15.4	−8.5
0.75 (QC1)	1.4	1.8	1.9	5.5	−12.9	−1.2
1.5 (QC2)	1.5	1.7	0.8	4.3	−6.7	3.0
3.5 (QC3)	0.2	0.6	1.1	−9.1	−9.9	−0.6
7.0 (QC4)	0.8	2	1.3	−3.5	−7.4	−4.1

CR8 distribution to the brain

CR8 was found to pass the blood–brain barrier (BBB) and the concentration in the brain was about 15% of that in plasma. Despite this low tissue/plasma ratio, the concentration reached a value above the reported CDK5/p25 and casein kinase 1 (CK1) inhibitory IC_{50} values for more than 6 hours.

Discussion

Recently, the tri-substituted purine CR8 was introduced as a selective second generation CDK inhibitor analogue of roscovitine [6,7]. *In-vitro* studies have shown that CR8 is 2–4 fold more potent as a CDK inhibitor and 50–100 fold more cytotoxic in tumor cell lines [7]. However, this enhanced *in-vitro* activity of CR8 needs to be confirmed *in-vivo* in animal models prior to further development toward clinical trials in patients. The future investigation and development of this purine requires an accurate analytical method for the quantitative determination of its pharmacokinetics pattern. In the present investigation we have developed and validated a new analytical method for the determination of CR8 in plasma and tissue samples. Our data showed that the method is selective and accurate. The acceptance criteria for the method validation are well in accordance with internationally accepted criteria [15,18]. Moreover, the volume required for the analysis is only 50 μl of plasma, a favorable factor when considering plasma sampling from small laboratory animals.

The present method was employed for studying the pharmacokinetics and biodistribution of the drug in mice. It is of great importance to use a single, suitable analytical method for both pre-clinical and clinical studies of newly introduced drugs, such as CDK inhibitors, that are promising for the treatment of several diseases including cancer. One important factor is that the

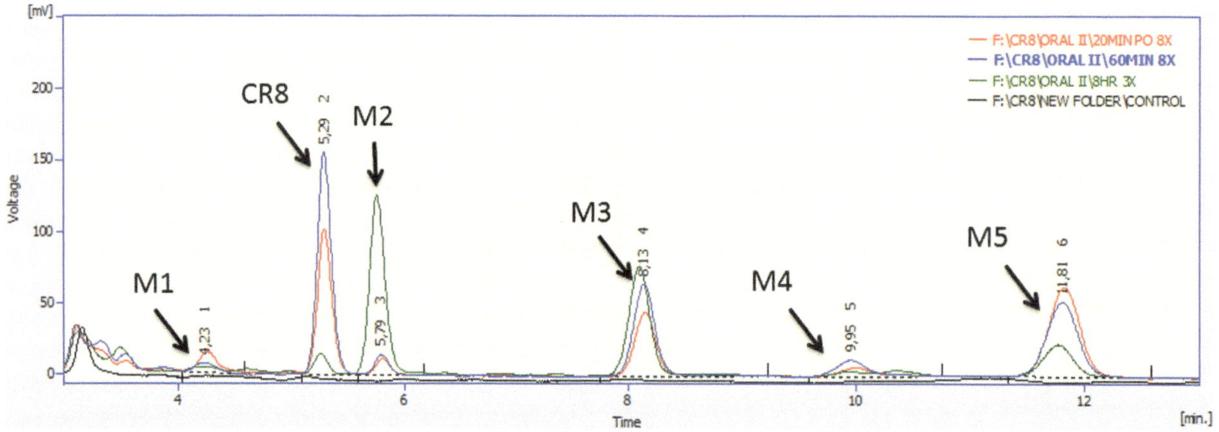

Figure 4 HPLC chromatograms of CR8 and its metabolites. Chromatograms showing CR8 and its five metabolites at different time points after oral administration, (red) 20 minutes post administration, (blue) 60 minutes post administration, (green) 8 hours post administration, (black) blank.

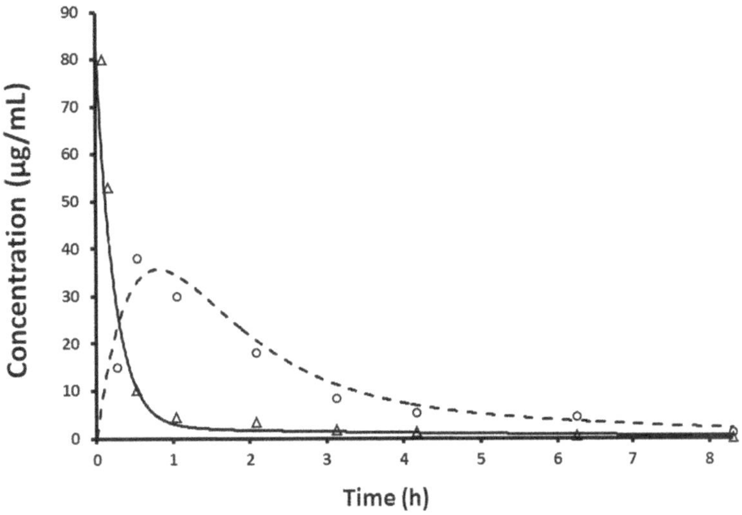

Figure 5 Time–plasma concentration curve after PO and IV CR8 to the mouse. Plasma time concentration curve after the oral administration of 100 mg/kg CR8 where the dashed line is the estimated two compartment model while the open circles are the observed concentrations. The solid line is the estimated one compartment model after the iv administration of 50 mg/kg CR8, while open triangles represent the measured concentrations.

present method does not require work up procedures, a favorable factor for clinical studies where large numbers of samples are generated and speed of analysis is important.

The pharmacokinetics profile (especially the oral bioavailability and the elimination half-life) constitutes a set of critical factors, strongly influencing whether CR8 should enter preclinical and clinical trials as an anti-tumor agent. Good oral absorption and appropriate biological half-life allowing enough exposure to the drug to produce pharmacological activity and anti-tumor effect [22], and sufficient elimination allowing minimal toxicity, are indeed crucial for further development of an anti-cancer drug.

Table 2 PK parameters of CR8 following single oral administration at 100 mg/kg and i.v. bolus administration of 50 mg/kg

PK parameters	Oral	i.v.
AUC (h.µg/ml)	96.34 ± 10.53	44.35 ± 3.3
Tα (h)	1.3 ± 0.43	0.11 ± 0.01
Tβ (h)	3.1 ± 0.35	2.95 ± 0.11
C_{max} (µg/ml)	34.3 ± 1.94	163.9 ± 0.25
Vss (ml)	21 ± 3	44 ± 4
CL (ml/h)	21 ± 2	23 ± 2
Bioavailability	(96.43*50)/(44.35*100)*100 = 108%	

AUC: Area under time plasma concentration curve.
Tα: First elimination half-life.
Tβ: Terminal elimination half-life.
C_{max}: Maximum reached concentration.
Vss: Distribution volume at steady state.
CL: Clearance.

Roscovitine, which was introduced as one of the earliest CDK inhibitors, is at the present time undergoing phase II clinical trials in advanced non-small cell lung cancer and nasopharyngeal cancers [23]. Roscovitine was shown to have good oral bioavailability and low systemic toxicity profile [5,24]. However, the anti-tumor responses observed were modest, most probably a consequence of the drug's short half-life and rapid metabolism to inactive metabolites [25]. Generally, exposure to the drugs is an important factor in the exertion of their anti-tumor activity. It has been shown that the optimum effect of roscovitine and the closely related analogue, N&N1, on tumor cell lines occurs after 8–16 hours of exposure [26-28]. The systemic exposure to roscovitine (expressed as AUC in plasma) in adult animals and humans did not allow a plasma concentration to be maintained above the reported anti-tumor IC_{50} (15–17 µM) for more than 1–2 hours, even when the maximum tolerated doses were administered [5]. The only exception was in young rats, most probably due to immature metabolism [29]. The present results showed that the systemic exposure expressed as plasma AUC of CR8 (after single dose administration of 100 mg/kg) was, for 10 hours, far higher than the anti-tumor IC_{50} values found *in-vitro* (0.3 µg/mL). Thus, second generation analogues of roscovitine might, in addition to increased cell potency, solve the problem of insufficient exposure observed in roscovitine. The higher systemic exposure might in part be explained by the longer half-life (approximately 3 h) found in female BALB/c mice in the present study. In this respect CR8 differs from both roscovitine [27,30] and its close analogue N&N1 [26],

Table 3 Pharmacokinetic parameters of CR8 in different organs following single oral administration of 100 mg/kg

	Plasma	Liver	Adipose tissue	Kidney	Lung	Spleen	Bone marrow	Brain
AUC (μg.hr/g)	96	197	181	145	77	40	34	14
Beta-HL (hr)	3.10	2.43	2.40	2.62	2.58	2.60	1.98	2.12
Cmax (μg/ml)	34.3	52.4	48.7	36.0	19.3	27.7	10.6	4.1
CL/F	21.0	10.2	11.1	13.8	26.2	20.0	29.5	146.0
V2/F	21.0	35.8	38.2	52.2	96.7	74.5	84.5	447.5

which both have a reported half-life of approximately 1 hour when given i.v. at the same dosage.

CR8 was found to have approximately 100% oral bioavailability, which means the drug is suitable for oral route intake and that the first pass effect is negligible.

CR8 distributed rapidly to all the peripheral tissues. The highest tissue distribution, as compared to plasma AUC, was found mainly in elimination organs, namely liver (200%) and kidneys (200%). These results encourage the hope that CR8 could perhaps be used to treat liver and kidney tumors, since it was found to induce apoptotic cell death in both hepatic and renal tumor cell lines [7]. Moreover, CR8 showed high distribution to the adipose tissue (180%) compared to that found in plasma, a factor that should be considered in dose scheduling in obese patients.

Surprisingly, CR8 showed higher distribution to the bone marrow (30%) compared to roscovitine, which was shown to pass the bone marrow barrier by only 1.5% [28] while the biodistribution of CR8 in the spleen was about 40%. Moreover, the cytotoxicity of CR8 against leukemic cell lines has been reported [7]. Altogether, these results suggest the possible use of CR8 in treating leukemia and lymphomas. However, the high biodistribution to the bone marrow may cause myelosuppression, which was not detected in roscovitine [28]. Further studies are currently ongoing in our laboratory to explore the cytotoxic effect of CR8 on normal hematopoietic progenitors. Moreover, we have observed five different metabolites with different polarities that have appeared with different kinetics throughout the CR8 kinetics. Urgent studies are needed to identify and quantify these metabolites, and to establish their pharmacological activates and toxicities.

In the present study, we have also shown that CR8 passes the BBB (concentration reached is 15% of that in plasma) compared to that reported for roscovitine (30%). This exposure of the brain to CR8 is nevertheless higher than that required for inhibition of its neuronal targets like CDK5 and CK1 (IC_{50} values: 0.12 μM and 0.61 μM, respectively) [7]. This fact may benefit the drug during further studies in neurodegenerative animal models and brain tumor models.

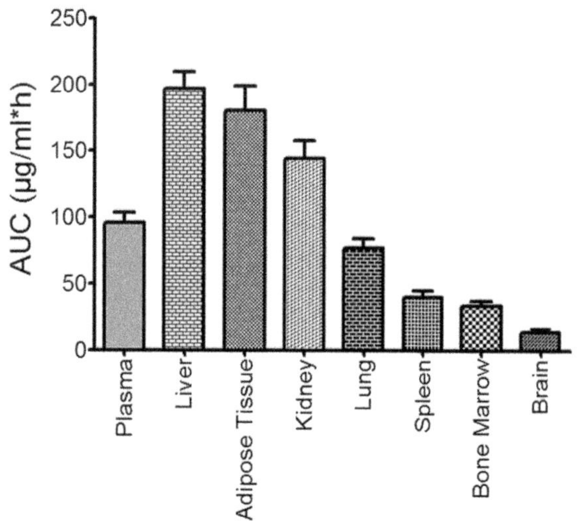

Figure 6 Tissue exposure to CR8 after oral administration of 100 mg/kg to female BALB/c mice. AUC expressed as μg/ml*h in plasma and as μg/g*h in tissues.

Conclusions

We have developed and validated a simple, fast and selective quantitative analytical method which allowed us to analyze the pharmacokinetic profile and tissue distribution of the second generation CDK inhibitor CR8. CR8 was shown to have 100% bioavailability and longer half-life compared to roscovitine, which may allow higher systemic exposure than the IC_{50} values for tumor cell death induction. The drug passes the BBB at a level sufficient to reach concentrations able to inhibit neuronal kinase targets. Bone marrow exposure was about 30% of that found as systemic exposure, a concentration potentially sufficient to eliminate leukemic cells. However, further studies are required to determine the myelosuppressive effect and hematotoxicity of CR8. The present study thus shows favorable pharmacokinetics properties of CR8 compared to its parent analogue roscovitine, encouraging further *in-vivo* studies and consideration of CR8 as a drug candidate.

Competing interests
The authors declare that they have no competing interests.

Authors' contributions
HS: carried out the experiments and drafted the manuscript. I EIS: performed the quality controls, and drafted the manuscript. LM: Provided the drug, drafted the manuscript. MH: Designed the experiment. All authors read and approved the final manuscript.

Acknowledgments
This investigation was supported by grants from the Swedish Childhood Cancer Society (Barncancerfonden) and the Swedish Cancer Foundation (Cancerfonden). This research was also supported by grants from the "Cancéropole Grand-Ouest" (LM), the "Association France-Alzheimer Finistère" (LM), the "Ligue Nationale contre le Cancer (Comité Grand-Ouest)" (LM) and the Polycystic Kidney Disease Foundation (PKD Foundation, USA & France) (LM) and "Association pour la Recherche sur le Cancer" (ARC-1092).

Author details
[1]Experimental Cancer Medicine (ECM), Laboratory Medicine, Karolinska Institutet, 141 86, Stockholm, Sweden. [2]C.N.R.S., 'Protein Phosphorylation and Human Disease' Group, C.N.R.S., Station Biologique, B.P. 74, 29682Roscoff cedex, Bretagne, France. [3]Experimental Cancer Medicine (ECM), Clinical Research Center, Novum, Karolinska University Hospital-Huddinge, 141 86, Stockholm, Sweden. [4]ECM, KFC, Karolinska University Hospital, 141 86, Stockholm, Sweden.

References
1. Bach S, Knockaert M, Reinhardt J, Lozach O, Schmitt S, Baratte B, Koken M, Coburn SP, Tang L, Jiang T, *et al*: **Roscovitine targets, protein kinases and pyridoxal kinase.** *J Biol Chem* 2005, **280:**31208–31219.
2. Meijer L, Borgne A, Mulner O, Chong JP, Blow JJ, Inagaki N, Inagaki M, Delcros JG, Moulinoux JP: **Biochemical and cellular effects of roscovitine, a potent and selective inhibitor of the cyclin-dependent kinases cdc2, cdk2 and cdk5.** *Eur JBiochem* 1997, **243:**527–536.
3. Meijer L, Raymond E: **Roscovitine and other purines as kinase inhibitors. From starfish oocytes to clinical trials.** *Acc Chem Res* 2003, **36:**417–425.
4. Meijer LBK, Galons H: **Roscovitine (CYC202, Seliciclib).** In *Monographs on Enzyme Inhibitors. CDK Inhibitors and their Potential as Anti-Tumor Agents.* Edited by Smith PJ, Yue E. Boca Raton, FL, USA: CRC Press, Taylor & Francis; 2006.
5. Benson C, White J, De Bono J, O'Donnell A, Raynaud F, Cruickshank C, McGrath H, Walton M, Workman P, Kaye S, *et al*: **A phase I trial of the selective oral cyclin-dependent kinase inhibitor seliciclib (CYC202; R-Roscovitine), administered twice daily for 7 days every 21 days.** *Br J Cancer* 2007, **96:**29–37.
6. Oumata N, Bettayeb K, Ferandin Y, Demange L, Lopez-Giral A, Goddard ML, Myrianthopoulos V, Mikros E, Flajolet M, Greengard P, *et al*: **Roscovitine-derived, dual-specificity inhibitors of cyclin-dependent kinases and casein kinases 1.** *J Med Chem* 2008, **51:**5229–5242.
7. Bettayeb K, Oumata N, Echalier A, Ferandin Y, Endicott JA, Galons H, Meijer L: **CR8, a potent and selective, roscovitine-derived inhibitor of cyclin-dependent kinases.** *Oncogene* 2008, **27:**5797–5807.
8. Bukanov NO, Moreno SE, Natoli TA, Rogers KA, Smith LA, Ledbetter SR, Oumata N, Galons H, Meijer L, Ibraghimov-Beskrovnaya O: **CDK inhibitors R-roscovitine and S-CR8 effectively block renal and hepatic cystogenesis in an orthologous model of ADPKD.** *Cell Cycle* 2012, **11:**4040–4046.
9. Bettayeb K, Baunbaek D, Delehouze C, Loaec N, Hole AJ, Baumli S, Endicott JA, Douc-Rasy S, Benard J, Oumata N, *et al*: **CDK inhibitors roscovitine and CR8 trigger Mcl-1 down-regulation and apoptotic cell death in neuroblastoma cells.** *Genes Cancer* 2010, **1:**369–380.
10. Kabadi SV, Stoica BA, Hanscom M, Loane DJ, Kharebava G, Murray Ii MG, Cabatbat RM, Faden AI: **CR8, a selective and potent CDK inhibitor, provides neuroprotection in experimental traumatic brain injury.** *Neurotherapeutics* 2012, **9:**405–421.
11. Wu J, Pajoohesh-Ganji A, Stoica BA, Dinizo M, Guanciale K, Faden AI: **Delayed expression of cell cycle proteins contributes to astroglial scar formation and chronic inflammation after rat spinal cord contusion.** *J Neuroinflammation* 2012, **9:**169.
12. Wu J, Kharebava G, Piao C, Stoica BA, Dinizo M, Sabirzhanov B, Hanscom M, Guanciale K, Faden AI: **Inhibition of E2F1/CDK1 pathway attenuates neuronal apoptosis in vitro and confers neuroprotection after spinal cord injury in vivo.** *PLoS One* 2012, **7:**e42129.
13. Oumata N, Ferandin Y, Meijer L, Galons H: **Practical synthesis of roscovitine and CR8.** *Org Process Res Dev* 2009, **13:**641–644.
14. Bressolle F, Bromet-Petit M, Audran M: **Validation of liquid chromatographic and gas chromatographic methods. Applications to pharmacokinetics.** *J Chromatogr B Biomed Appl* 1996, **686:**3–10.
15. Shah VP, Midha KK, Dighe S, McGilveray IJ, Skelly JP, Yacobi A, Layloff T, Viswanathan CT, Cook CE, McDowall RD: **Analytical methods validation: bioavailability, bioequivalence and pharmacokinetic studies. Conference report.** *Eur J Drug Metab Pharmacokinet* 1991, **16:**249–255.
16. Hartmann C, Smeyers-Verbeke J, Massart DL, McDowall RD: **Validation of bioanalytical chromatographic methods.** *J Pharm Biomed Anal* 1998, **17:**193–218.
17. Karnes HT, March C: **Precision, accuracy, and data acceptance criteria in biopharmaceutical analysis.** *Pharm Res* 1993, **10:**1420–1426.
18. Shah VP, Midha KK, Findlay JW, Hill HM, Hulse JD, McGilveray IJ, McKay G, Miller KJ, Patnaik RN, Powell ML, *et al*: **Bioanalytical method validation–a revisit with a decade of progress.** *Pharm Res* 2000, **17:**1551–1557.
19. Karnes HT, March C: **Calibration and validation of linearity in chromatographic biopharmaceutical analysis.** *J Pharm Biomed Anal* 1991, **9:**911–918.
20. Karnes HT, Shiu G, Shah VP: **Validation of bioanalytical methods.** *Pharm Res* 1991, **8:**421–426.
21. Midha KK, Rawson MJ, Hubbard JW: **Individual and average bioequivalence of highly variable drugs and drug products.** *J Pharm Sci* 1997, **86:**1193–1197.
22. Lin JH, Lu AY: **Role of pharmacokinetics and metabolism in drug discovery and development.** *Pharmacol Rev* 1997, **49:**403–449.
23. Fischer PM, Gianella-Borradori A: **Recent progress in the discovery and development of cyclin-dependent kinase inhibitors.** *Expert Opin Investig Drugs* 2005, **14:**457–477.
24. de la Motte S, Gianella-Borradori A: **Pharmacokinetic model of R-roscovitine and its metabolite in healthy male subjects.** *Int J Clin Pharmacol Ther* 2004, **42:**232–239.
25. McClue SJ, Stuart I: **Metabolism of the trisubstituted purine cyclin-dependent kinase inhibitor seliciclib (R-roscovitine) in vitro and in vivo.** *Drug Metab Dispos* 2007, **36**(3):561–70.
26. Bettayeb K, Sallam H, Ferandin Y, Popowycz F, Fournet G, Hassan M, Echalier A, Bernard P, Endicott J, Joseph B, Meijer L: **N-&-N, a new class of cell death-inducing kinase inhibitors derived from the purine roscovitine.** *Mol Cancer Ther* 2008, **7:**2713–2724.
27. Raynaud FI, Whittaker SR, Fischer PM, McClue S, Walton MI, Barrie SE, Garrett MD, Rogers P, Clarke SJ, Kelland LR, *et al*: **In vitro and in vivo pharmacokinetic-pharmacodynamic relationships for the trisubstituted aminopurine cyclin-dependent kinase inhibitors olomoucine, bohemine and CYC202.** *Clin Cancer Res* 2005, **11:**4875–4887.
28. Song H, Vita M, Sallam H, Tehranchi R, Nilsson C, Siden A, Hassan Z: **Effect of the Cdk-inhibitor roscovitine on mouse hematopoietic progenitors in vivo and in vitro.** *Cancer Chemother Pharmacol* 2007, **60:**841–849.
29. Sallam H, Jimenez P, Song H, Vita M, Cedazo-Minguez A, Hassan M: **Age-dependent pharmacokinetics and effect of roscovitine on Cdk5 and Erk1/2 in the rat brain.** *Pharmacol Res* 2008, **58:**32–37.
30. Nutley BP, Raynaud FI, Wilson SC, Fischer PM, Hayes A, Goddard PM, McClue SJ, Jarman M, Lane DP, Workman P: **Metabolism and pharmacokinetics of the cyclin-dependent kinase inhibitor R-roscovitine in the mouse.** *Mol Cancer Ther* 2005, **4:**125–139.

9

The development of response surface pathway design to reduce animal numbers in toxicity studies

Sagita Dewi[1*], Tore Aune[2], John A Aasen Bunæs[2], Adrian J Smith[3] and Stig Larsen[1*]

Abstract

Background: This study describes the development of Response Surface Pathway (RSP) design, assesses its performance and effectiveness in estimating LD_{50}, and compares RSP with Up and Down Procedures (UDPs) and Random Walk (RW) design.

Methods: A basic 4-level RSP design was used on 36 male ICR mice given intraperitoneal doses of Yessotoxin. Simulations were performed to optimise the design. A *k*-adjustment factor was introduced to ensure coverage of the dose window and calculate the dose steps. Instead of using equal numbers of mice on all levels, the number of mice was increased at each design level. Additionally, the binomial outcome variable was changed to multinomial. The performance of the RSP designs and a comparison of UDPs and RW were assessed by simulations. The optimised 4-level RSP design was used on 24 female NMRI mice given Azaspiracid-1 intraperitoneally.

Results: The *in vivo* experiment with basic 4-level RSP design estimated the LD_{50} of Yessotoxin to be 463 μg/kgBW (95% CI: 383–535). By inclusion of the k-adjustment factor with equal or increasing numbers of mice on increasing dose levels, the estimate changed to 481 μg/kgBW (95% CI: 362–566) and 447 μg/kgBW (95% CI: 378–504 μg/kgBW), respectively. The optimised 4-level RSP estimated the LD_{50} to be 473 μg/kgBW (95% CI: 442–517). A similar increase in power was demonstrated using the optimised RSP design on real Azaspiracid-1 data. The simulations showed that the inclusion of the k-adjustment factor, reduction in sample size by increasing the number of mice on higher design levels and incorporation of a multinomial outcome gave estimates of the LD_{50} that were as good as those with the basic RSP design. Furthermore, optimised RSP design performed on just three levels reduced the number of animals from 36 to 15 without loss of information, when compared with the 4-level designs. Simulated comparison of the RSP design with UDPs and RW design demonstrated the superiority of RSP.

Conclusion: Optimised RSP design reduces the number of animals needed. The design converges rapidly on the area of interest and is at least as efficient as both the UDPs and RW design.

Keywords: Response surface pathway design (RSP), Estimating LD_{50}, Up and down designs, Random walk design, Reduction in animal use

* Correspondence: gitaewi@yahoo.com; Stig.Larsen@nmbu.no
[1]Centre for Epidemiology and Biostatistics, Faculty of Veterinary Medicine and Biosciences, Norwegian University of Life Sciences, P.O. Box 5003, 1432 Ås, Norway
Full list of author information is available at the end of the article

Background

In recent years, acute toxicity studies have been refined to improve animal welfare. In particular, LD_{50} studies are no longer the method of choice in toxicology studies associated with pharmaceutical drug development, or the development of food additives, flavourings, contact materials and cosmetics [1]. In some areas, however, LD_{50} studies cannot yet be replaced by other methods. There is an urgent need for alternative methods, both for ethical reasons and because of the shortcomings of the bioassays, in particular their sensitivity and specificity. *In vitro* methods have been recommended by international expert groups [2]. However, before these can be adopted information on the relative toxicities of all relevant analogues in each toxin group must be obtained, in order to establish toxic equivalency factors (TEFs) [3]. The TEF approach was initially developed to estimate the potential toxicity of mixtures of dioxins, dibenzofurans and PCBs [4-6]. TEF studies of marine algal toxins are based on LD_{50} studies in mice [3]. Ideally, these studies should be performed by exposure via the oral route. However, due to the scarcity of pure toxins in sufficient quantities, LD_{50} studies are performed by intraperitoneal (IP) injections in mice [7]. Until laboratory animal studies can be replaced completely, it is of the utmost importance to optimise trial design, in order to reduce the number of animals used for this purpose [8].

The classical LD_{50} design introduced by Trevan in 1927 requires the use of a large number of animals [9]. The design has been criticised for both ethical and scientific reasons [10,11]. The Organization for Economic Cooperation and Development (OECD) removed the classical LD_{50} (OECD 401) from their acute oral toxicity guidelines in 2002 [12] and recommended OECD 425, the Up and Down Procedure (UDP) to optimise LD_{50} design [13]. The UDP is a sequential procedure that results in rapid convergence on the area of interest, the dose for each animal being adjusted up or down depending on the outcome for the previous animal. This approach was established in 1948 [14] and Bruce proposed the use of the UDP for determination of acute toxicity to chemicals [15]. The UDP in the OECD guidelines uses a calculated dose progression factor based on the antilog of 1 divided by the estimated slope of the dose–response curve and should stay constant during testing. Single animals are dosed until one of three criteria to stop the trial is met [13].

The OECD's UDP can only estimate the point of interest and cannot be used to construct a dose–response curve [9]. Furthermore, the single-animal strategy does not take into account inherent biological variation, or the practical problems that arise from having to test each mouse individually. Tsutakawa introduced a block up and down method known as Random Walk (RW) [16], where every sequence used more than one mouse. This design reduces the number of trials and adds flexibility. The experiment starts with n observations on a given level d_j and continues with n observations, with the dose determined by a procedure for generating the sequences.

In the field of engineering, the term Response Surface is commonly used to obtain the optimal value for one response variable. By combining the philosophy of UDP and the principles of Response Surface methodology [17] the basic Response Surface Pathway (RSP) design was created.

Basic RSP design is based on the theory of stochastic chain models, where the procedure for generating the next step is based on the response at the previous one. The design consists of n levels in which the results obtained on one design level determine the dose to be used on the next. The starting dose used on the first design level is designated m. This dose may be an educated guess made by the responsible toxicologist. If a dose window for the given toxin is known, the mid-dose of this window might be a suitable choice. In order to estimate the LD_{50}, an odd number of laboratory animals is assigned to this starting dose. If more than 50% of the animals die, the dose to be used on the second design level is reduced by $m/2$. If not, the dose is increased by the same amount (Figure 1). The same number of animals is included on the second design level. If 50% die, the second design level dose is reduced by $m/4$ or conversely, if the animals survive, increased by $m/4$ on the third design level. In general, the dose to be used on design level i will be given by the equation:

$$m_i = m_{i-1} \pm \frac{m}{2^{i-1}} \text{ where } m_{i-1} \text{ denotes the dose used on design level } i-1. \tag{1}$$

This basic RSP-design has previously been used in toxicity studies to estimate LD_{50} with satisfactory results [18,19]. However, these studies used a large amount of animals and did not describe in detail the rationale behind the dose steps. Using the data from one of these studies [19], the concept of RSP has been refined and developed using simulation procedures.

The aims of this paper were to introduce and describe the optimisation of RSP design, to assess its performance and effectiveness in estimation of LD_{50} and to compare it with UDPs and RW design using simulations performed on data from an *in vivo* experiment.

Methods

Material

The first in vivo study has been described in detail previously [19], and comprised 36 male ICR mice of SPF quality (16-20 g) divided into 4 equal groups. The study was conducted in 2006 and was authorized by the Norwegian Animal Research Authority, in accordance

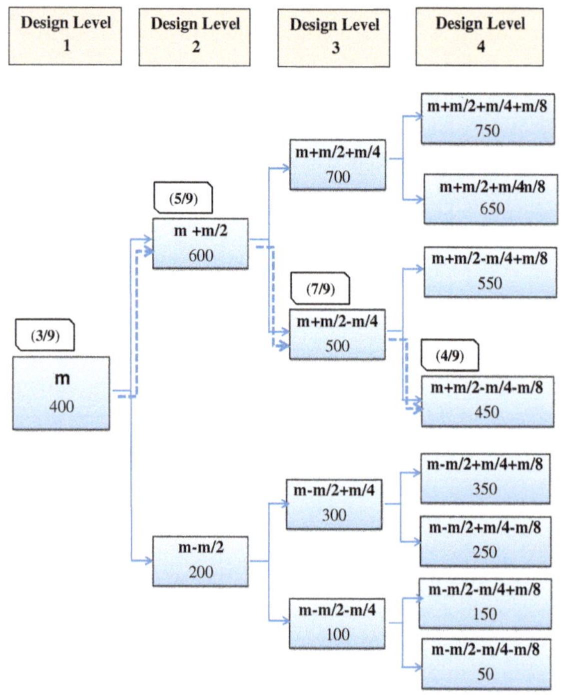

Figure 1 The pathway obtained in the *in vivo* Yessotoxin study using the basic 4-level RSP design. The basic 4-level RSP design in *in vivo* Yessotoxin study used 9 mice on each design level with the binomial outcome. The pathway obtained is indicated by dashed line. The doses are given in µg/kg BW and the numbers given in brackets are the ratios of dead mice.

with the Norwegian Regulation on Animal Experimentation. The mice were given Yessotoxin (YTX) IP at varying concentrations with a predefined LD_{50} dose window of 100–700 µg/kg body weight (BW). The outcome variable was "death" within the 24 hours after injection.

Simulation study: All the simulation studies used the LD_{50} of YTX derived from the material in the *in-vivo* study to estimate the probability of death at a given dose.

The second in vivo study consisted of 24 female NMRI mice of SPF quality (15–21 g), randomly divided into 4 groups comprising 3, 5, 7 and 9 mice per cage, respectively. The mice were supplied 1 week before the experiment for acclimatisation purposes. They were housed on aspen bedding in standard macrolone cages on a 12:12 light/dark cycle at 21-23°C with food and water available *ad libitum*. The mice were nulliparous and were not fasted before treatment. Injection volumes were adjusted for bodyweight to 1 mL/20 g BW. The animals were observed for 24 hours after injection. Symptoms and time to death were recorded. The study was conducted in 2011 with the authorization of the Norwegian Animal Research Authority, application number FOTS ID: 1132), in accordance with the Norwegian Regulation on Animal Experimentation. The mice were given Azaspiracid-1 (AZA1) IP in four different concentrations with a predefined LD_{50} dose window of 25 - 375 µg/kg BW. The outcome variable was the number of dead mice within 24 hours after injection.

Optimisation of the basic RSP design

Some prior information about the toxicity range is always available, and can also be obtained by educated guesswork. The study can then be focused on the area of interest, thereby increasing the amount of useful information and the efficiency of animal use. In basic RSP design, no attention is paid to upper or lower doses.

Let D_U and D_L denote the upper and the lower limits of the dose window, respectively.

Let m denote the mid dose of the dose window, m_i the dose on design level i and k the dose adjustment factor. The dose on the design level i is then given by the equation

$$m_i = m_{i-1} \pm \frac{m}{k^{i-1}}; \, m_{i-1} \textit{denotes the dose used on design level } i-1 \tag{2}$$

Using the formula for the sum of a geometric series [20,21], the upper dose D_U of the window on the highest design level n will be given by:

$$D_U = m\frac{(k^n-1)}{(k^n-k^{n-1})} \tag{3}$$

The dose window of the LD_{50} for YTX was from D_L = 100 µg/kg BW to D_U = 700 µg/kg BW. The middle dose of the window was used as the starting dose, i.e. m = 400 µg/kg BW. Using equation (3) above, the adjustment factor k was:

$$700 = 400\frac{(k^4-1)}{(k^4-k^3)} \rightarrow k = 2.21$$

For AZA1, the predefined dose window of the LD_{50} was from D_L = 25 µg/kg BW to D_U = 375 µg/kg BW which gave a starting dose of 200 µg/kg BW. Using equation (3) above this gives an adjustment factor k of:

$$375 = 200\frac{(k^4-1)}{(k^4-k^3)} \rightarrow k = 2.0$$

Increasing the number of animals with increased design level

The basic RSP design uses an equal number of animals on each design level. The starting dose is either based on an educated guess or on the mid-dose of the dose window. Due to the structure of the design, it is likely to approach the parameter in question with increasing design level. It is therefore unnecessary to use the same number of animals at the starting dose as on the highest design level. By using the lowest possible number of animals at the starting dose and increasing the number at increasing design levels, the total number of animals needed will be reduced without loss of information. One practical solution is to use three animals on the first level, five on the second, seven on the third, nine on the fourth, and so on.

Multinomial outcome variable

In toxicological studies the most common outcome variable is binomial. In the determination of the LD_{50}, the outcome is "dead" or "alive" after a certain time interval. The decision to either increase or decrease the dose on the next design level is based upon whether there were more or less than 50% dead animals on the previous level. However, there is clearly a difference between outcomes where 0, 1, 2 or 3 animals die. It is reasonable to assume that by changing the outcome variable from binomial to multinomial, the amount of information obtained will increase. The binomial outcome variable can be replaced by "the number of dead animals". If none of the animals die, the toxin dose can be increased maximally on the next level. Conversely, if all the animals die on a given level, an equally large decrease in the dose is performed (Table 1).

Comparisons of 3-level RSP design, UDPs and RW design

Simulation of all the four designs was performed on the first *in vivo* material. The 3-level RSP with multinomial outcome was performed with 3, 5, and 7 mice on design levels 1, 2, and 3 respectively. The *k*-adjustment factor in the 3-level situation was calculated to be 2. The UDP simulation was performed using OECD 425 guidelines [13]. The LD_{50} of YTX was assumed to be 400 μg/kg BW with a sigma of 0.25 μg/kg BW and a progression factor of 1.78. The same dose sequence and starting dose for OECD's UDP was used in both simple UDP and RW design, which use 3 mice on each level. The dose was decreased if more than 50% mice died, and increased if less than 50% mice died. If no mice died in the RW design, the dose was increased. If more than 2 mice died, the dose was reduced. If one mouse died, a coin was tossed to decide whether to increase the dose or stay at the same dose. The starting dose was 225 μg/kg BW and the simulations were halted when a total of 15 animals had been included.

Simulation procedure

The YTX *in vivo* study was used to estimate the probability of death at a given dose using logistic regression in a binomial distribution. A total of 10,000 simulated mice samples were generated for each dose. The simulation procedure was repeated 10 times and the average of the 10 outcomes was used as the simulated result. The same procedure was also carried out to compare 3-level RSP Design, UDPs and RW Design. Three pathways within the RSP design were considered to assess its performance, with binomial outcome, k-adjustment factor and either the same number of animals at each design level or increasing numbers at increasing design levels, respectively.

For the optimised 4-level RSP design with multinomial outcome, k-adjustment factor and increasing numbers of mice at increasing design levels, eighteen pathways were created, but only four are of interest.

When assessing the performance of optimised 3-level RSP design with multinomial outcome, k-adjustment factor and increasing number of mice with increasing design level, eight pathways were created. As in the previous

Table 1 The doses assigned on the four design levels using the k-adjustment factor and the dose m_i at level *i*

Design level I (3 animals)	Design level 2 (5 animals)		Design level 3 (7 animals)		Design level 4 (9 animals)	
Outcome	Dose (m_2)	Outcome	Dose (m_3)	Outcome	Dose (m_4)	Outcome
0	$m + m/k$	0	$m_2 + m/k^2$	0	$m_3 + m/k^3$	0
1	$m + m/k^2$	1	$m_2 + m/k^3$	1	$m_3 + m/k^4$	1
2	$m - m/k^2$	2	$m_2 + m/k^4$	2	$m_3 + m/k^5$	2
3	$m - m/k$	3	$m_2 - m/k^4$	3	$m_3 + m/k^6$	3
		4	$m_2 - m/k^3$	4	$m_3 - m/k^6$	4
		5	$m_2 - m/k^2$	5	$m_3 - m/k^5$	5
				6	$m_3 - m/k^4$	6
				7	$m_3 - m/k^3$	7
						8
						9

The dose $m = m_1$ is the starting dose. The number of mice used on the design levels was 3, 5, 7 and 9, respectively.

simulations, the probability of dead mice at a given dose was estimated using logistic regression in a binomial distribution from the YTX *in vivo* study. For each scenario, the mean number of dead mice at the assigned dose in 10,000 simulations was recorded and the outcome was used to simulate the number of dead mice at each design level.

Statistical analysis

The results are expressed with 95% confidence intervals (CIs) using isotonic regression [22] and trimmed Spearman-Karber regression estimation [23]. The isotonic regression was performed using the pooled adjacent-violators algorithm (PAVA) [22]. The CIs were obtained using parametric bootstrap numerical methods [24]. The trimmed Spearman-Karber program originated from Montana State University and was modified at the Duluth and Athens National Exposure Research Laboratories [25]. The LD_{50} in OECD's UDP was analysed by Maximum Likelihood Estimation (MLE) using AOT425 software [26].

Results

Basic RSP design (*in vivo* YTX study)

Three of the nine mice at the starting dose of 400 μg/kg BW died and the dose for the second design level was increased to 600 μg/kg BW (Figure 1). This resulted in the death of five of nine mice, which resulted in a dose of 500 μg/kg BW on the third design level. On this design level, seven of nine mice died and the dose for the fourth design was decreased to 450 μg/kg BW. Four of nine mice died on the fourth and last design level. Based on the data obtained, the LD_{50} of Yessotoxin was estimated to be 463 μg/kg BW (Table 2).

The ways in which the pathways and results from a single simulation study were used in each of the RSP designs to estimate the LD_{50} are described below:

Application of the *k*-adjustment factor (simulated YTX study)

The *k*-adjustment factor of 2.21 was calculated to ensure that the design covered the total predefined dose window (Figure 2). Of the nine simulated mice given 400 μg/kg BW, three died and the dose for the second design level was increased to 581 μg/kg BW. On this design level, five mice died and the dose for the third design level was decreased to 499 μg/kg BW. The simulated results on this design level again resulted in five dead mice and the dose for the fourth and last design level was set to 462 μg/kg BW. Four of the nine mice died. Based on these simulated data, the LD_{50} was estimated to be 481 μg/kg BW (Table 2).

Increasing number of mice with increasing design level (simulated YTX study)

Of the three mice assigned to the first design level given 400 μg/kg BW, one died (Figure 2). The dose for the second design level was increased to 581 μg/kg BW and five mice were included. Four of these five died and the dose for the next design level was reduced to 499 μg/kg

Table 2 The estimated LD_{50} of Yessotoxin (YTX) in different developmental stages of RSP design

Design	Dose (μg/kg BW)	Proportion of dead mice	LD_{50} with 95% CI (μg/kg BW)	
			Isotonic regression	Spearman-Karber
Basic RSP	400	3/9 (0.33)	463 (383 – 535)	457 (400 – 522)
	450	4/9 (0.44)		
	500	7/9 (0.78)		
	600	5/9 (0.56)		
*) Included *k*-adjustment factor	400	3/9 (0.33)	481 (362 – 566)	480 (408 – 565)
	462	4/9 (0.44)		
	499	5/9 (0.56)		
	581	5/9 (0.56)		
*) Optimising use of mice	400	1/3 (0.33)	447 (378 – 504)	444 (379 – 521)
	462	5/9 (0.56)		
	499	5/7 (0.71)		
	581	4/5 (0.80)		
*) Multinomial decision variable with all four design levels	400	1/3 (0.33)	473 (442 – 517)	471 (430 – 516)
	465	3/7 (0.43)		
	468	4/9 (0.44)		
	482	3/5 (0.60)		

The results are expressed with 95% Confidence Intervals. *) Simulated data based on the 36 observations in the basic RSP model.

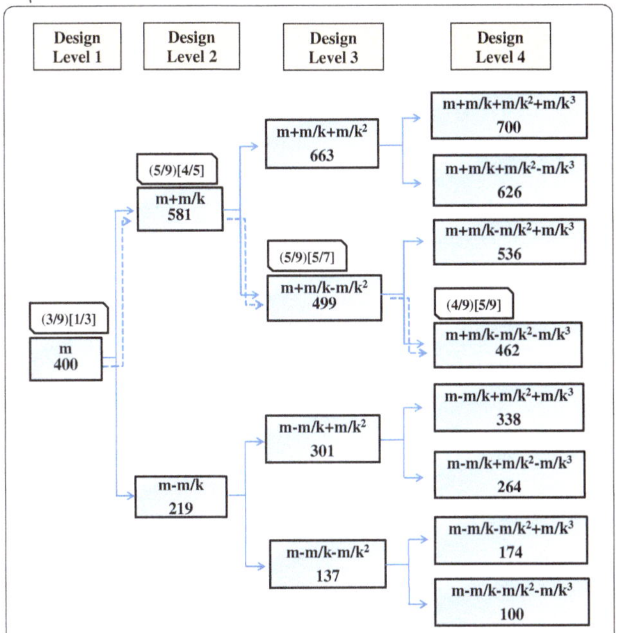

Figure 2 Simulated Yessotoxin studies using 4-level RSP designs with k-adjustment factor with fixed and increasing number of mice. The simulated Yessotoxin pathways obtained in the two 4-level RSP designs. The pathways obtained are shown by dashed line. The doses are given in µg/kg BW. The first design incorporates binomial outcome, k-adjustment factor, and 9 mice at each design level, where the ratios of dead mice are given in bracket. The second design incorporates binomial outcome, k-adjustment factor and increasing number of mice from 3 at the first level to 9 at the fourth, where the ratios of dead mice are given in square brackets [ ].

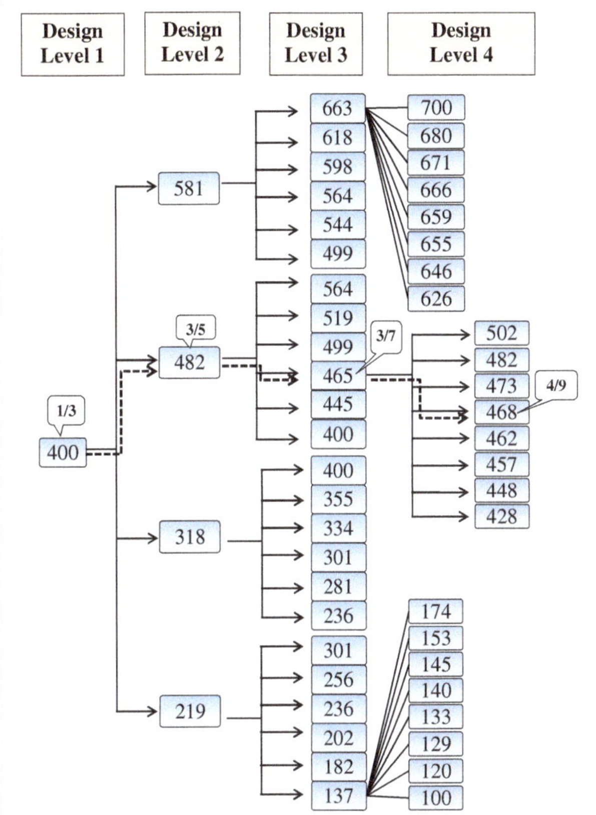

Figure 3 The obtained pathway in the simulated Yessotoxin study using the optimised 4-level RSP design. The optimised 4-level RSP design incorporates multinomial outcome, used k-adjustment factor and increasing number of mice with increasing design levels, and the pathway obtained in the simulation study is shown by dashed line. The doses are given in µg/kg BW and the numbers in the callouts represent the ratios of dead mice.

BW. Of the seven mice on this third design level, five died, which led to a reduction to 462 µg/kg BW for the fourth design level. Nine mice were simulated on this level and 5 died. Based on these simulated data, the LD_{50} was estimated to be 447 µg/kg BW (Table 2).

Number of dead mice as outcome or decision variable (simulated YTX study)

Three mice were assigned in the simulation to 400 µg/kg BW on the first design level and one died (Figure 3). The dose for the second design level was increased to 482 µg/kg BW and three of the five mice died. Consequently, the dose was decreased to 465 µg/kg BW and three of the seven mice died. The dose for the fourth design level was increased to 468 µg/kg BW and four of nine mice died. Based on the simulated data, the LD_{50} was estimated to be 473 µg/kg BW (Table 2).

Performance of the RSP designs

The estimated LD_{50} of YTX with a 95% confidence interval obtained *in vitro* was used as the reference in evaluation of the simulated results of the three RSP designs.

For pathway 01 (Table 3), 24 and 10 scenarios, respectively were created for the 4-level RSP designs with binomial outcome, k-adjustment factor and nine mice on each design level or with increasing number of mice from three on the first level to nine on the fourth. For both of these two RSP designs, all the estimated LD_{50} deviated with a maximum of 10% from the *in vitro* reference. The estimated LD_{50} from pathway 02 was higher than the reference value. For the RSP design with binomial outcome, k-adjustment factor and nine mice at each level, three of the 12 scenarios deviated with a maximum of 10% from the *in vitro* reference. By increasing the number of mice from three on the first design level to nine on the fourth, two of six scenarios fulfilled the same demands. All the scenarios in pathway 03 estimated the LD_{50} to be below the *in vitro* reference value. Simulation of the optimised 4-level RSP design with multinomial outcome, k-adjustment factor and increasing numbers of mice from three to nine on the last level, estimated the LD_{50} in 11 of 18 pathways with a deviation of at most 10% from the *in vitro* reference (Figure 4).

Table 3 Mean values of estimated LD_{50} of Yessotoxin in different pathways using 4-level RSP designs

Pathway	Dose on design level 1	Dose on design level 2	Dose on design level 3	Dose on design level 4	Mean LD50 (μg/kgBW)	95% CI of Mean LD50 (μg/kgBW)
4-Level RSP design with binomial outcome, k-adjustment factor and 9 animals at each design level						
01	400 M = 3.29	581 M = 6.23	499 M = 5.01	462 M = 4.38	457	449 – 466
02	400 M = 3.29	581 M = 6.23	499 M = 5.01	536 M = 5.07	513	510 – 516
03	400 M = 3.29	219 M = 0	301 M = 1.05	338 M = 1.97	391	389 – 392
4-Level RSP design with binomial outcome, k-adjustment factor and increasing number of mice with increasing design levels						
01	400 M = 1.10	581 M = 3.35	499 M = 3.9	462 M = 4.41	464	449 – 479
02	400 M = 1.10	581 M = 3.35	499 M = 3.9	536 M = 5.57	510	501 – 520
03	400 M = 1.10	219 M = 0	301 M = 0.82	338 M = 1.96	379	374 – 384
4-Level RSP design with multinomial outcome, k-adjustment factor and increasing number of mice with increasing design levels						
01	400 M = 1.10	482 M = 2.45	499 M = 3.87	502 M = 5.06	501	498 – 503
02	400 M = 1.10	482 M = 2.45	499 M = 3.87	496 M = 4.97	490	470 – 510
03	400 M = 1.10	482 M = 2.45	465 M = 3.48	468 M = 4.51	470	432 – 508
04	400 M = 1.10	482 M = 2.45	465 M = 3.48	462 M = 4.41	455	353 – 557

The results are expressed with 95% Confidence interval. M represents the mean of dead mice based on 10,000 simulations on the assigned dose.

Comparison of the optimised 3- and 4-level RSP design resulted in similar estimation of LD_{50} (Figure 4). A total of eight pathways were formed with the optimised 3-level RSP design and the estimated LD_{50} deviated with a maximum of 10% from the *in vitro* reference in 50% of the cases.

Application of the complete RSP design (*in vivo* AZA1 study)

Three mice were given the starting dose of 200 μg/kg BW and all died within 24 hours (Figure 5). In accordance with the design, the dose for the second design level was decreased to 100 μg/kg BW, but all five mice died. The dose for the third design level was decreased to 50 μg/kg and all seven mice survived 24 hours after the injection. By only including data up to the third level, the LD_{50} of AZA-1 was estimated to be 76.3 μg/kg BW and 70.7 μg/kg BW using isotonic regression and the Spearman-Karber method, respectively. For the fourth design level, the dose was increased to 75 μg/kg BW, where four of the nine mice died. Inclusion of all four design levels resulted in estimation of the LD_{50} of AZA1 to be 77.5 μg/kg BW (95% CI: 68 – 88 μg/kg BW) using isotonic regression and 74 μg/kg BW (95% confidence interval: 66 – 83 μg/kg BW) using the Spearman-Karber method.

Comparisons of 3-level RSP, UDPs and RW design

In the 3-level RSP design, three mice were given a starting dose of 400 μg/kg BW (Table 4). One of the three mice died and 500 μg/kg BW was then given to 5 mice. Three of the 5 mice died and the 7 mice on the third design level were given 475 μg/kg BW. Four of the seven mice died and the LD_{50} of YTX was estimated to be 453 μg/kg BW. The length of the CI was 133 μg/kg BW.

The simulation of OECD's UDP was started by including one mouse given a dose of 225 μg/kg BW. The mouse survived. The next mouse was assigned to 400 μg/kg BW and survived. The third mouse died at 710 μg/kg BW and the dose was then decreased again to 400 μg/kg BW. The fourth mouse survived this dose and the fifth mouse was given a dose of 710 μg/kg BW. The fifth mouse died and the dose for the next mouse was decreased again to 400 μg/kg BW. This sixth mouse survived. The study was stopped after six mice since one criterion for this had been met and the LD_{50} was estimated to be 400 μg/kg BW (Table 4). The length of the CI was 779 μg/kg BW.

In the simple UDP, none of three mice given a starting dose 225 μg/kg BW died. In the second simulation sequence a dose of 400 μg/kg BW was given and 2 of 3 mice died. The dose was decreased to 225 μg/kg BW and all the mice survived. Consequently, a dose of 400 μg/kg BW was again assigned and one of 3 mice

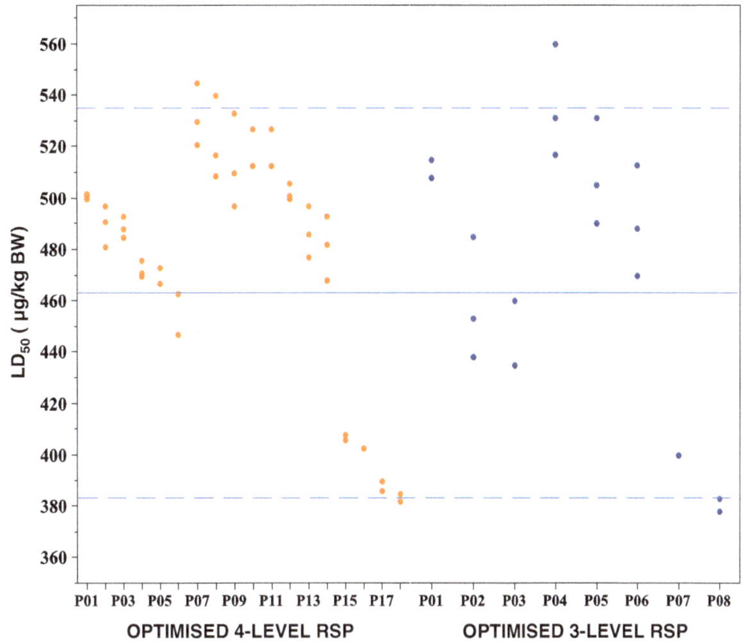

Figure 4 The estimation of LD_{50} using the optimised 3- and 4-level RSP designs. The optimised 3-level and 4-level RSP designs incorporate multinomial outcome, using k-adjustment factor and increasing number of mice with increasing design levels. The numbers of pathways are given along the x-axis, where the orange dots represent estimated value for 4-level RSP design and blue dots estimated value for 3-level RSP design.

died. The dose was then increased to 710 µg/kg BW and 2 of 3 mice died.

In the RW design, three mice were given a dose of 225 µg/kg BW and all survived. In the next sequence, three mice were allocated a dose of 400 µg/kg BW and two mice died. The dose was decreased again, and three mice survived at 225 µg/kg BW. The dose was again increased to 400 µg/kg BW and one of 3 mice died. A coin was tossed to decide whether to increase or stay at the same dose: the dose was increased to 710 µg/kg BW and 2 of 3 mice died. The LD_{50} of YTX was estimated to be 400 µg/kg BW both in the simple UDP and RW design (Table 4), and the length of the CI was 514.8 µg/kg BW.

Comparison of the four designs showed that OECD's UDP, simple UDP, and RW design resulted in CIs that were 4.9, 2.9, and 2.9 times larger, respectively, than the RSP design.

Discussion

When designing a classical LD_{50} study, the dose window is divided into fixed dose intervals of equal range that cover the dose window. In the present example with a dose window of 100–700 µg/kg BW, the classical LD_{50} study with four dose levels would entail the same number of animals being assigned to doses of 100, 300, 500, and 700 µg/kg BW, respectively. A comparison of the classical LD_{50} design and RSP design demonstrates the strength of RSP. Only one of the doses chosen for a classical LD_{50} study is close to the real LD_{50}. In the present study where the LD_{50} was estimated from the basic RSP design and the four simulated studies using optimised RSP design, the dose assignments ranged from 400 to 581 µg/kg BW. The lowest dose assigned, which was in the simulation of 4-level RSP design with k-adjustment factor, a fixed number of mice on each design level or increasing numbers with increasing design level, was 218 µg/kg BW. However the probability for assigning this dose in real life is minimal. Assigning doses based on the number of dead animals, as was done in the optimised RSP design, gave an opportunity to allocate a more appropriate dose.

To our knowledge, no rational procedure for choosing the size of the increase or decrease in dose has been described for UDP and the change in dose is the same regardless of the dose level. OECD recommends that the dose adjustment or progression factor in UDP design is based on the estimated slope of the dose–response curve and should remain constant throughout the test. If no information about this slope is available, a constant adjustment factor of 3.2 should be used [13]. In the basic RSP design an attempt is made to solve this problem by using a fixed but chosen dose adjustment factor of 2. Moreover, the size of the increase and decrease in dose depends on the design level. Toxicologists have quite often a predefined dose window for the toxin to be investigated. By using a chosen dose adjustment factor or predefined incremental procedure, doses outside the dose window are less likely to be included. This may reduce the amount of information in the basic RSP design

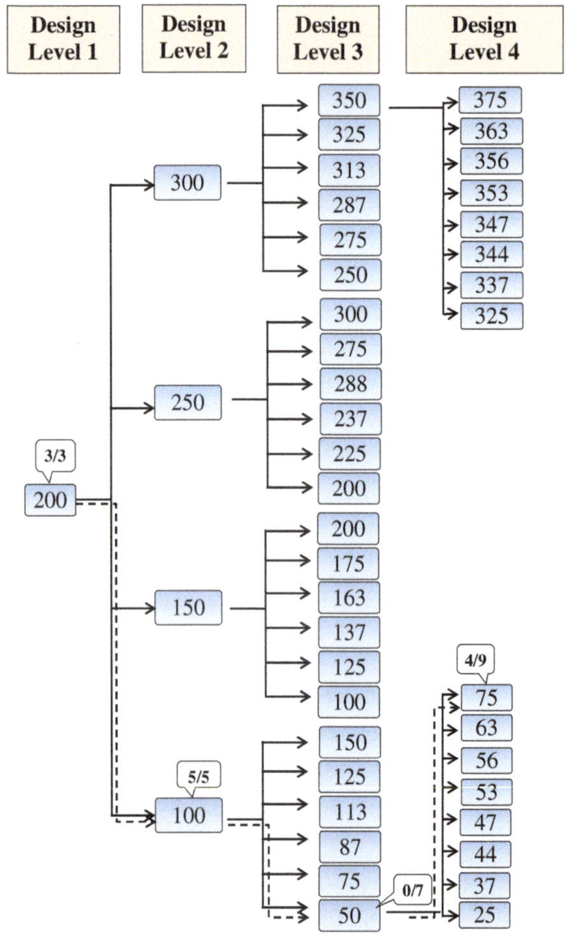

Figure 5 The obtained pathway in the *in-vivo* Azaspiracid-1 study using the optimised 4-level RSP design. The optimised 4-level RSP design incorporates multinomial outcome, using k-adjustment factor and increasing number of mice with increasing design levels, the pathway obtained is shown by dashed line. The doses are given in μg/kg BW and the numbers in the callouts represent the ratios of dead mice.

and result in failures. In order to increase the power of the basic RSP design, the fixed dose adjustment factor of 2 has therefore been amended in our study to an adjustment factor *k* dependent upon the predefined dose window. This factor is related to the number of levels in the design and is calculated by a simple procedure to ensure that all the values in the dose window will be covered. Intuitively, this will increase the power of the design, even though this was not clearly demonstrated by the results of the simulations in the present study.

The choice of the middle of the dose window as a starting point is based on an assumption that this dose is more likely to be the LD_{50}. Using the mid-dose and the procedure for calculation of the *k*-adjustment ensures both the upper limit (D_U) and the lower limit (D_L) of the dose window will be covered. The predefined dose window for

Table 4 Comparisons of optimised 3-level RSP Design, UDPs and Random Walk Design in estimation of LD_{50} of YTX

Design	Dose (μg/kg BW)	Proportion of dead mice	LD_{50} with 95% CI (μg/kg BW)
Multinomial outcome variable with 3-level RSP design	400	1/3	453 (380 - 513)
	475	4/7	
	500	3/5	
UDP of OECD	225	0/1	400 (198 - 977)
	400	0/3	
	710	2/2	
Simple UDP	225	0/6	400 (65.2 - 580)
	400	3/6	
	710	2/3	
Random walk design	225	0/6	400 (65.2 - 580)
	400	3/6	
	710	2/3	

The results are expressed with 95% Confidence Intervals.

AZA toxin was 25–375 μg/kg BW. No information was available on where in the window the value of LD_{50} was likely to be. The LD_{50} was assumed to be 200 μg/kg BW. However, the true LD_{50} turned out to be close to the lower part of the dose window. The design made a pathway directly to the area of interest after inclusion of only 3 animals.

The number of animals used in these studies was quite small. Maximum Likelihood Estimation (MLE) does not seem to be suitable in design analysis when the sample size is small [27]. The Trimmed Spearman-Karber method [23], which was used in the present study, requires at least one mortality rate that is less than or equal to 50% and at least one that is greater or equal to 50%. This method is recommended because it is freely available and it is a simple program for those who are not highly skilled in statistical analysis. Non-parametric modified isotonic regression may be a more optimal method and is recommended for small samples [22]. It is slightly more complicated, but can easily be calculated manually. Furthermore, this method assumes that the chance of toxicity does not decrease over the set of possible dosages. The analysis of the present data gave similar results with these two statistical methods.

A reduction in the number of laboratory animals is a central aim of UDPs, RW and RSP design. The UDP [15] actually recommends that only one animal is used on each dose level. The single-animal strategy used in OECD's UDP might at first sight appear advantageous in reducing the number of animals in the study, but it does not take into account the inherent biological variation in an animal model. The probability of changing the dose on the next level in the wrong direction is high and may affect the study. Simple UDP and RW address this problem by including more than one animal on each level. As in the simple UDP and RW design, basic RSP-design uses more than one animal, with equal numbers on each dose level. Due to the structure of the design, the dose always converges on the end result with increasing dose level. It seems therefore apparent that it is unnecessary to use the same number of animals at the starting dose as on the last dose level. By using the lowest possible number of animals at the starting dose and increasing the number of animals on increasing dose levels, the total number of animals will be reduced. In order to avoid the problem of biological variation that is not addressed in OECD's UDP, the procedure should be to start with 3 animals at the first dose level and continue with 5, 7 and 9 animals, respectively, on subsequent levels. This reduces the total number of animals from 36 to 24. The present simulation indicated that the ability of the modified RSP designs to estimate LD_{50} values was equally good as the basic RSP design.

A large disadvantage of most of the designs that have been proposed for this area is the binomial outcome variable. So far, this has also been the case for the basic RSP design. However, the decision variable can easily be changed from "more or less than 50% dead mice" to "the number of dead mice". If none or only one of the three mice on the first design level dies, the dose for the next design level has to be increased, otherwise it is decreased. A similar procedure is used on the next design level. The simulation of this procedure in the present paper clearly demonstrated a substantial increase in the power of the RSP design. From the simulated results it seems that the increase in information in the model is so large that the fourth level of the design can be omitted. The number of animals can therefore be reduced from the initial 36 in the basic RSP design to 24 by including the *k*-adjustment dose factor and by increasing the number of animals at increasing design levels. The simulation results also indicated that the optimised 3-level RSP design estimated the LD_{50} as well as all the other 4-level RSP variants. By reducing the number of levels in the design from 4 to 3, only 15 animals are needed. The optimised RSP design created more pathways, estimated LD_{50} slightly higher and performed better than the other two RSP designs.

The RSP design should be performed sequentially and the dose to be used on the next design level is not available until the experiment on the previous level has ended. This may result increase the duration of the study as a whole. Furthermore, experimental conditions such as the weight of the animals, the composition of the test compound, variations in the time to death and environmental factors may differ between design levels and influence the results. A reduction from four to three design levels is therefore an advantage for many reasons.

The complete optimised RSP design was used in the AZA1 toxicity study. In this experiment, the predefined dose window of AZA1 was quite large and the dose used on the first design level proved to be far from the end result. The study demonstrated the power of the design and that the area of interest was already detected by the third design level. This underlines the fact that the fourth design level of the 9 mice was not needed and 15 mice would have been sufficient. If the AZA1 study had been performed using optimised 3-level RSP design, the k-adjustment factor would have been 1.78 and the estimated LD_{50} would not have been different from the value estimated by using the optimised 4-level RSP design. In order to simulate an optimal 3-level RSP for estimation of the LD_{50} of AZA1, the results obtained in the prospective 4-level study were used. All the three mice at the first design level died, which led to a dose of 88 μg/kg being assigned on the second level, where 3 of 5 mice died. The dose for the third design level was then reduced to 68 μg/kg and 3 of 7 mice died. This simulation estimated the LD_{50} of AZA1 to be 76.3 (95% CI: 38.5 - 101.58) and 75.7 μg/kg BW (95% CI 49.4 – 116.2) using isotonic regression and the Spearman-Karber method, respectively. The confidence intervals were, as expected, larger compared to those in the prospective 4-level RSP design study, but they still support the use of only 3 dose levels.

The simulated comparison between 3-level RSP, UDPs and RW design showed that the RSP reduced the number of study sequences compared to the other two designs. One way of comparing the information from the three designs is to compare the length of the CI for the parameter in question. If this is done, the RSP design was clearly superior to both the RW and the UDPs. Both the simulation and the results from the AZA1 study showed that the RSP designs rapidly converge on the area of interest. The RSP design was found to increase the information that could be obtained and it was possible to develop a dose–response curve.

The optimized 3-level RSP-design has recently been used in two other studies (manuscripts in preparation). However, further studies are needed to confirm the performance of the 3-level RSP design.

The dose to be used on a given design level in the RSP design is derived mathematically and may in some cases be impossible to titrate or administer in the laboratory. In these cases the dose must be adjusted to the nearest practicable value.

The determination of LD_{50} in the present paper was merely used to demonstrate how the RSP design was optimised. The designs can also be used to estimate the LD_X, where 50% is replaced by x%. This design can also be used in other areas of medicine. The most relevant of these may be dose-finding studies, but the RSP design is also applicable to studies where the primary aim is estimation of quantile response.

Conclusions

The RSP is a sequential design, which can reduce the number of animals needed to a minimum without loss of information. The design takes into account the variation in response between animals, using prior knowledge and information obtained during the study and it converges rapidly on the area of interest. It is as least as efficient as both the UDPs and RW designs.

Competing interest

The authors declare that they have no competing interests.

Author's contributions

All the authors participated in development of the manuscript. The Response Surface Pathway design has mainly been developed by SD and SL who also performed the statistical analyses and wrote the initial draft of the manuscript. The laboratory work was performed or designed by AS, TA and JAAB. All the authors have participated in the literature review and development of the manuscript, and have approved the final version.

Acknowledgements

The authors wish to thank Meabco AS for financial support, Prof. Steen Lindkaer-Jensen for scientific advice and Brit Heidenreich for technical assistance with the animal experiments. The *in vivo* part of the project was financed by the Norwegian Research Council (NFR), project nr 172561/S40 and support was also obtained from the ASTOX2-project (Grant-Aid Agreement No PBA/AF/08/001(01)) under the Sea Change strategy with the support of the Irish Marine Institute and the Marine Research Sub-Programme of the National Development Plan 2007–2013, co-financed under the European Regional Development Fund.

Author details

[1]Centre for Epidemiology and Biostatistics, Faculty of Veterinary Medicine and Biosciences, Norwegian University of Life Sciences, P.O. Box 5003, 1432 Ås, Norway. [2]Department of Food Safety and Infection Biology, Faculty of Veterinary Medicine and Biosciences, Norwegian University of Life Sciences, P.O. Box 5003, 1432 Ås, Norway. [3]Norecopa, c/o Norwegian Veterinary Institute, P.O. Box 750, Sentrum 0106 Oslo, Norway.

References

1. Seidle T, Robinson S, Holmes T, Creton S, Prieto P, Scheel, Chlebus M: **Cross-sector review of drivers and available 3Rs approaches for acute systemic toxicity testing.** *Toxicol Sci* 2010, **116**:382–396.
2. Hess P, Grune B, Anderson DB, Aune T, Botana LM, Caricato P, Van Egmond HP, Halder M, Hall S, Lawrence JF, Moffat C, Poletti R, Richmond J, Rossini GP, Seamer C, Vilageliu JS: **Three Rs Approaches in Marine Biotoxin Testing. The Report and Recommendations of a joint ECVAM/DG SANCO Workshop (ECVAM Workshop 54).** *Altern Lab Anim* 2006, **34**:193–224.
3. Alexander J, Benford D, Boobis A, Ceccatelli S, Cravedi J, Domenico AD, Doerge D, Dogliotti E, Edler L, Farmer P, Filipic M, Fink-Gremmels J, Fürst P, Guerin T, Knutsen HK, Machala M, Schlatter J, Mutti A, Schlatter J, Leeuwen RV, Verger P: **Opinion of the Scientific Committee/Scientific Panel, Marine biotoxins in shellfish - Summary on regulated marine biotoxins.** *EFSA journal* 2009, **7**:1–23.
4. Barnes D, Alford-Stevens A, Birnbaum L, Kutz FW, Wood W, Patton D: **Toxicity equivalency factors for PCBs?** *Qual Assur* 1991, **1**:70–81.
5. Barnes DG: **Toxicity equivalents and EPA's risk assessment of 2,3,7,8-TCDD.** *Sci Total Environ* 1991, **104**:73–86.
6. Safe SH: **Comparative Toxicology and Mechanism of Action of Polychlorinated Dibenzo-P-Dioxins and Dibenzofurans.** *Annu Rev Pharmacol Toxicol* 1986, **26**:371–399.
7. Aune T, Sorby R, Yasumoto T, Ramstad H, Landsverk T: **Comparison of oral and intraperitoneal toxicity of yessotoxin towards mice.** *Toxicon* 2002, **40**:77–82.
8. Rusche B: **The 3Rs and animal welfare - conflict or the way forward?** *ALTEX* 2003, **20**:63–76.
9. Rispin A, Farrar D, Margosches E, Gupta K, Stitzel K, Carr G, Greene M, Meyer W, McCall D: **Alternative methods for the median lethal dose (LD(50)) test: the up-and-down procedure for acute oral toxicity.** *ILAR J* 2002, **43**:233–243.
10. Lorke D: **A new approach to practical acute toxicity testing.** *Arch Toxicol* 1983, **54**:275–287.
11. Zbinden G, Flury-Roversi M: **Significance of the LD50-test for the toxicological evaluation of chemical substances.** *Arch Toxicol* 1981, **47**:77–99.
12. Botham PA: **Acute systemic toxicity–prospects for tiered testing strategies.** *Toxicol In Vitro* 2004, **18**:227–230.
13. *OECD Guideline for the testing of chemical 425, Acute oral toxicity- Up-and-Down Procedure (UDP).* [http://www.oecd-ilibrary.org/content/book/9789264071049-en]
14. Dixon WJ, Mood AM: **A Method for Obtaining and Analyzing Sensitivity Data.** *J Am Stat Assoc* 1948, **43**:109–126.
15. Bruce RD: **An Up-and-Down Procedure for Acute Toxicity Testing.** *Toxicol Sci* 1985, **5**:151–157.
16. Tsutakawa RK: **Random Walk Design in Bio-Assay.** *J Am Stat Assoc* 1967, **62**:842–856.
17. Myer RH, Montgomery DC: *Response Surface Methodology: Process and Product Optimization Using Designed Experiments.* New Jersey: John Wiley and sons; 2002.
18. Aune T, Larsen S, Aasen JAB, Rehmann N, Satake M, Hess P: **Relative toxicity of dinophysistoxin-2 (DTX-2) compared with okadaic acid, based on acute intraperitoneal toxicity in mice.** *Toxicon* 2007, **49**:1–7.
19. Aune T, Aasen JAB, Miles CO, Larsen S: **Effect of mouse strain and gender on LD50 of yessotoxin.** *Toxicon* 2008, **52**:535–540.
20. Fisher G: *Series and Sequences.* Phoenix Education: Putney; 1996.
21. Finney RL, Thomas GB: *Calculus.* 1st edition. Reading: Addison-Wesley Publishing Company; 1990.
22. Stylianou M, Flournoy N: **Dose Finding Using the Biased Coin Up-and-Down Design and Isotonic Regression.** *Biometrics* 2002, **58**:171–177.
23. Hamilton MA, Russo RC, Thurston RV: **Trimmed Spearman-Karber method for estimating median lethal concentrations in toxicity bioassays.** *Environ Sci Technol* 1977, **11**:714–719.
24. Stylianou M, Proschan M, Flournoy N: **Estimating the probability of toxicity at the target dose following an up-and-down design.** *Statist Med* 2003, **22**:535–543.
25. *Lethal Concentration, 50% (LC50).* [http://sdi.odu.edu/model/lc50.php]
26. *Acute Oral Toxicity (AOT) Up-And-Down-Procedure.* [http://www.epa.gov/oppfead1/harmonization/]
27. Silvapulle MJ: **On the Existence of Maximum Likelihood Estimators for the Binomial Response Models.** *J R Stat Soc Series B Stat Methodol* 1981, **43**:310–313.

10

Modeling of chemical inhibition from amyloid protein aggregation kinetics

José Antonio Vázquez

Abstract

Backgrounds: The process of amyloid proteins aggregation causes several human neuropathologies. In some cases, *e.g.* fibrillar deposits of insulin, the problems are generated in the processes of production and purification of protein and in the pump devices or injectable preparations for diabetics. Experimental kinetics and adequate modelling of chemical inhibition from amyloid aggregation are of practical importance in order to study the viable processing, formulation and storage as well as to predict and optimize the best conditions to reduce the effect of protein nucleation.

Results: In this manuscript, experimental data of insulin, Aβ42 amyloid protein and apomyoglobin fibrillation from recent bibliography were selected to evaluate the capability of a bivariate sigmoid equation to model them. The mathematical functions (logistic combined with Weibull equation) were used in reparameterized form and the effect of inhibitor concentrations on kinetic parameters from logistic equation were perfectly defined and explained. The surfaces of data were accurately described by proposed model and the presented analysis characterized the inhibitory influence on the protein aggregation by several chemicals. Discrimination between true and apparent inhibitors was also confirmed by the bivariate equation. EGCG for insulin (working at pH = 7.4/T = 37°C) and taiwaniaflavone for Aβ42 were the compounds studied that shown the greatest inhibition capacity.

Conclusions: An accurate, simple and effective model to investigate the inhibition of chemicals on amyloid protein aggregation has been developed. The equation could be useful for the clear quantification of inhibitor potential of chemicals and rigorous comparison among them.

Keywords: Protein fibrillation kinetics, Mathematical modeling, Sigmoid bivariate equation

Background

The aggregation and fibrillation of proteins has been commonly associated with numerous degenerative disorders in humans including Alzheimer's, Parkinson's, prion's, diabetes type II and Huntington's diseases [1-5]. These proteins, called amylodogenics, are also involved in production, purification and formulation interferences of biotechnology and pharmacologic processes [6,7]. The phenomenon of protein aggregation, led by nucleation-dependent polymerization mechanism, consists in the formation of amyloid fibrils formulated with β-sheet structures in cross-β-sheet arrangement producing insoluble aggregates [8-10]. For example, insulin peptide also generates fibrillar structures under specific conditions such as low pH, high temperatures or organic solvents dilution [11-13]. Those phase transformations are not observed *in vivo* but are very common, for example, in the clinical preparations of insulin for diabetics [14]. Human amyloid proteins (Aβ) are peptides of rather 39-42 residues. Aβ40 contains 40 amino acids and Aβ42 is the major isoform in the Aβ peptides with 42 residues polypeptide chain and it is the responsible of amyloid plaques generated in Alzheimer's disorder [15,16].

In general, much of the success in the future application of chemicals to inhibit the *in vivo* formation of such fibrils is dependent on the correct modelling and evaluation of *in vitro* kinetic data in order to establish protocols of action, effectiveness of molecules and dose-optimization of compounds. The kinetic description of amyloid protein aggregation based on mechanistic and thermodynamic approaches have been extensively studied [17-22] and an ample number of plausible mechanisms of nucleation and fibrillation have been proposed [23,24]. So remarkable,

Correspondence: jvazquez@iim.csic.es
Grupo de Reciclado e Valorización de Residuos (REVAL), Instituto de Investigacións Mariñas (IIM-CSIC), C/ Eduardo Cabello 6, CP36208 Vigo, Spain

two new and similar proposal: "Ockham's razor"/minimalistic and Crystallization-like Model, have been recently developed. Both have solid biophysical basis and they were successfully applied to describe and explain the experimental data of different amyloid protein aggregation [25-28]. However, the combined effect of anti-aggregation protein agents, *e.g.* surfactants, osmolytes and food additives, on time-dependent responses has not been modelled by that way or by means of empirical equations.

Although the use of empirical sigmoid equations, mainly the logistic equation, does not provide a direct explanation of the molecular steps that underlie in the generation of fibrils, it is a robust tool to examine protein aggregation kinetic data and to address all the phases of the process [4,29,30]. In addition, other authors assimilated the parameters from logistic [20] to those obtained by an autocatalytic mechanism [23,27]. Nonetheless, that equation is always formulated without the parameters (fibrillation rate and lag phase) in an explicit form hindering the estimation of their statistical error.

In the present work, the capability of fit and experimental data predictability of a sigmoid bivariate model that simulates the growth of aggregation process on different proteins along with the effects of inhibitory chemicals on the kinetic parameters is explored in selected cases obtained from the literature. The results reveal its efficacy and validity to analyze the most relevant parameters that describe geometrically and macroscopically the mentioned process.

Methods

Experimental data

Amyloid protein aggregation data were collected from results previously reported in the bibliography and digitized from the published curves using GetData Graph Digitizer 2.24. The kinetics of insulin inhibition induced by (–)-epigallocatechin-3-gallate (EGCG) were selected from Wang et al. [31], methylglyoxal effects were collected from Oliveira et al. [32] and those produced by 1,2-diheptanoyl-sn-glycero-3-phosphocholine (di-C7-PC) were described in Wang et al. [33]. Two conditions of EGCG affecting to fibrillation kinetics were used: EGCG_1 (case 1) studied at pH = 2.0/T = 60°C and EGCG_2 (case 2) at pH = 7.4/T = 37°C.

On the other hand, the aggregation kinetics of Aβ42 amyloid protein inhibited by apigenin and taiwaniaflavone were selected from Thapa et al. [16] and the data affected by ectoine and hydroxyectoine from Kanapathipillai et al. [15]. Finally, apomyoglobin fibrillation experiments were published in Vilasi et al. [34]. The datasets were obtained by the two most common methods used to probe amyloid formation in vitro, the increment in light scattering of the protein solution due to insolubilization, and the increase in ThT fluorescence due to amyloid binding.

Mathematical modelling

The model developed to simulate the process of aggregation and hence insulin fibrillation was defined by a bivariate equation. Such model is based on the combination of Weibull function as chemical-concentration model [35,36] modifying the most important parameters of the reparameterized logistic equation [37] used for aggregation description. This expression (1) has been successfully used, in recent works, to evaluate the inhibitory effect of organic acids and heavy metals on the growth of various bacteria [38,39]. Its mathematical form is as follows (see also Appendix section):

$$X = \frac{X_{m\bullet}}{1 + \exp\left[2 + \frac{4v_{m\bullet}}{X_{m\bullet}}(\lambda_{\bullet} - t)\right]} \quad ; \text{ where :} \qquad (1)$$

$$X_{m\bullet} = X_m\left\{1 - K_x\left[1 - \exp\left(-\ln 2\left(\frac{C}{m_x}\right)^{a_x}\right)\right]\right\}$$

$$v_{m\bullet} = v_m\left\{1 - K_v\left[1 - \exp\left(-\ln 2\left(\frac{C}{m_v}\right)^{a_v}\right)\right]\right\}$$

$$\lambda_{\bullet} = \lambda\left\{1 + K_\lambda\left[1 - \exp\left(-\ln 2\left(\frac{C}{m_\lambda}\right)^{a_\lambda}\right)\right]\right\}$$

where, v_m is the maximum aggregation rate, X_m is the maximum aggregation growth, λ is the lag phase and C is the chemical concentration. The meanings of other symbolic notations as well as the corresponding units are summarized in Table 1. In the experimental data chosen, the dependent variable of response or time-dependent signals (X) to detect amyloid protein aggregation were absorbance at 600 nm (data obtained from Wang et al. [31]), relative ThT fluorescence intensity (%) (data from Wang et al. [33]) and ThT fluorescence intensity at 482 nm or 490 nm (data obtained from Thapa et al. [16]; Kanapathipillaia et al. [15]; Oliveira et al. [32] and Vilasi et al. [34]).

Additionally, a global parameter ($EC_{50,\tau}$) was also selected for the overall description of chemical effects on fibrillation growth studies according the algebraic steps previously described [38]. This parameter was defined as the chemical concentration (in mM) that reduces the aggregation by 50% compared to that produced by the control without agent at time (τ) which also reduces the maximum aggregation by 50%.

Numerical methods and statistical analysis

The fitting procedures and parametric estimates from the experimental results were performed by minimizing the sum of quadratic differences between the observed and model-predicted values using the nonlinear least-

Table 1 Symbolic notations used and corresponding units

Insulin aggregation kinetics measured by absorbance or fluorescence	
X :	Amyloid aggregation growth measured as absorbance at 600 nm, relative ThT fluorescence intensity (%) and ThT fluorescence intensity at 482 nm or 490 nm. Units: absorbance units (AU) or (%).
t :	Time. Units: h or d
X_m :	Maximum aggregation growth. Units: AU or %
v_m :	Maximum aggregation rate. Units: AU h^{-1}, AU d^{-1} or % h^{-1}
λ :	Lag phase. Units: h or d
$X_{m^\bullet}$:	Maximum insulin aggregation affected by chemical agent. Units: AU or %
$v_{m^\bullet}$:	Maximum insulin aggregation rate affected by chemical agent. Units: AU h^{-1}, AU d^{-1} or % h^{-1}
$\lambda_\bullet$:	Lag phase affected by chemical agent. Units: h or d
Concentration effects on insulin aggregation kinetics	
C :	Concentration of chemical agent. Units: mM or μM
K_x :	Maximum response affecting on X_m. Dimensionless
m_x :	Concentration corresponding to the semi-maximum response affecting on X_m. Units: mM or μM
a_x :	Shape parameter affecting on X_m. Dimensionless
K_v :	Maximum response affecting on v_m. Dimensionless
m_v :	Concentration corresponding to the semi-maximum response affecting on v_m. Units: mM or μM
a_v :	Shape parameter affecting on v_m. Dimensionless
K_λ :	Maximum response affecting on λ. Dimensionless
m_λ :	Concentration corresponding to the semi-maximum response affecting on λ. Units: mM or μM
a_λ :	Shape parameter affecting on λ. Dimensionless

squares (quasi-Newton) method provided by the '*Solver*' macro from Microsoft Excel spreadsheet. The confidence intervals of the best-fit values for the parametric estimates (Student's t test, $\alpha = 0.05$), consistency of the mathematical models (Fisher's F test; $p < 0.05$) and covariance and correlation matrices were calculated using the '*SolverAid*' macro, which is freely available from Levie's Excellaneous website http://www.bowdoin.edu/~rdelevie/exellaneous/. An example of the type of Excel spreadsheet used for modeling (Ab42amyloid apigenin case) was provided as Additional file 1. These statistical procedures and residual analysis (Durbin-Watson test) were confirmed and evaluated, respectively, by DataFit 9 (Oakdale Engineering, Oakdale, PA). Moreover, bias and accuracy factors of fittings (B_f and A_f, respectively) were calculated according to the expressions reported by Ross [40].

Results and discussion

Characteristics and simulations of bivariate model

In the description of amyloidogenic fibrillation growths, the logistic equation used to formalize their kinetic profiles is always formulated through an explicit expression based on the time required to reach 50% of the maximal aggregation (x_0) and a time parameter (τ), although the initial lag phase and the aggregation rate are commonly the most important parameters that need to be calculated [30]. In this work, the logistic equation was reparameterized to make the lag phase (λ) and the maximum aggregation rate (v_m), which represents the overall aggregation process rate, explicit (Figure 1). This last coefficient more adequately characterizes the reaction rate of fibrillation than the parameter conventionally used (k_{app}, defined as specific or apparent rate) because it is less sensitive to experimental error and because it is a more efficient to describe the global rate of the kinetic process [41]. Additionally, the v_m calculated from the experimental data obtained by Sabaté et al. [42] for yeast prion proteins follows the Arrhenius dependence with temperature (data not shown).

In contrast, the fit using the reparameterized functions can be used to easily calculate the confidence intervals of the parameters. The algebraic steps required to obtain the corresponding reparameterization of λ and v_m from the logistic equation are detailed in the Appendix. Thus, the parameters from this equation define all of the aggregation kinetic phases [19]: pre-nucleation, which is characterized by λ, post-nucleation, which is represented by v_m or τ, and elongation, which is determined by X_m.

The absolute correlation between the lag phase and the aggregation growth was recently demonstrated in several sets of protein data [43]. Indeed, this relationship is obvious because the specific or apparent rate (k_{app} or k_g, depending on the authors) is inversely proportional to the lag phase based the following expression when the logistic model (1) is applied [44]:

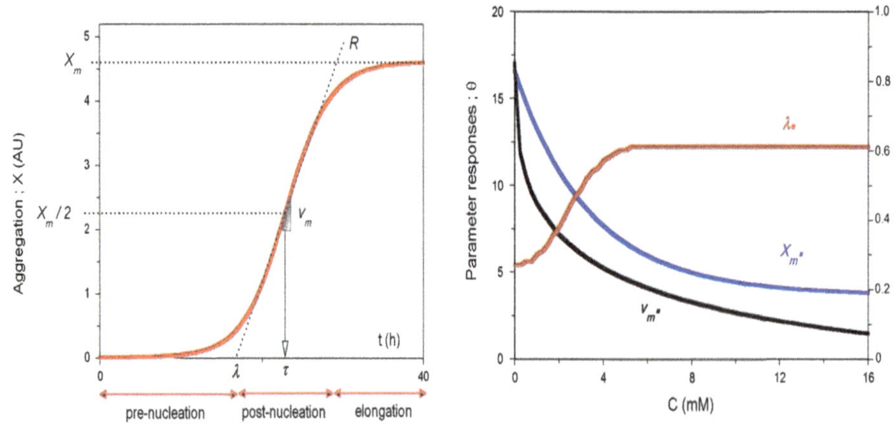

Figure 1 Left, Graphical description of the kinetic parameters (X_m, λ, v_m and τ) from the logistic equation (A.8) and the corresponding aggregation phases: pre-nucleation, post-nucleation and elongation. Right, Simulations of the most common profiles for the parameters ($X_m{\bullet}$, $\lambda{\bullet}$, $v_m{\bullet}$), affected by chemical concentration, using the Weibull equations (A.15).

$$\lambda = \tau - \frac{2}{k_{app}}$$

Figure 2 shows an illustrative set of simulations that were developed under the numerical conditions described in Table 2. In these simulations, all of the possible sigmoid effects of the chemical concentration on the logistic parameters are defined. Weibull's equation, which was adequately configured to simulate the dose-response trends, is a mathematical tool that provides excellent predictions for varied experimental profiles from different scientific fields [45,46]. In the present context, the flexibility of this equation to describe different chemical-concentration relationships as linear, sigmoid, exponential, or hyperbolic curves depending on the numerical values of the parameters is particularly valuable. The combination of both of these mathematical resources (1) generates a wide variety of theoretical casuistries that will be verified using the experimental data selected below.

Inhibitory effect of EGCG on insulin aggregation

The representation of the experimental data from selected cases and surfaces predicted by equation (1) are depicted in Figure 3A and B. The results of the parameter estimations and the statistical analysis of the fit for the EGCG influence on insulin fibrillation are summarized in Table 3. Both datasets were accurately fitted with equation (1) to obtain R^2_{adj} values greater than 0.98. Moreover, the *p*-values obtained from Fisher's F test indicated the complete consistency and robustness of the equation to the adjustment of the experimental patterns. The residual analysis through the Durbin-Watson test revealed a lack of residual autocorrelation and therefore a random distribution (data not shown).

At an acidic pH and a high temperature, the effect of EGCG on the kinetic parameters was not significant for the maximum aggregation rate but statistically significant for X_m and the lag phase. As can be observed in Figure 3A, the slopes of the sigmoid curves were parallel to the influence of the EGCG concentration, and the surface can be assimilated to that simulated in Figure 2D but with less effect on X_m. These results show a longer pre-nucleation phase, which indicates that EGCG blocks the formation of the seeding nuclei without changing the fibril elongation rate (post-nucleation). This behaviour is consistent with the definition reported by Martins [26] who denominates the compounds that modify kinetic parameters (for instance in the present case, v_m and/or λ) as true inhibitors.

In contrast, different surface and parametric responses were observed for EGCG_2 up to a concentration of 0.2 mM polyphenol with only significant modifications in the maximum aggregation growth parameter (Figure 3B). Under experimental conditions of higher pH and lower T, EGCG acts as an apparent inhibitor that only alters the thermodynamic properties of aggregation process [26]. Higher concentrations of EGCG (from 0.35 to 0.7 mM) led to an increase in the fibrillation response more than the inhibition of the amyloid process [31]. These experimental points were deleted in this mathematical analysis because biphasic aggregation data with profiles of decreasing and increasing values of X_m cannot be fitted by the proposed equation or by any other simple equation.

The global description of chemical inhibition was calculated by means of a single index: $EC_{50,\tau}$ (Table 3). This parameter can be defined as a summary of all of the effects on the aggregation kinetics observed at the time required to reach the semi-maximum aggregation growth. Thus, the obtained value of this parameter can be used

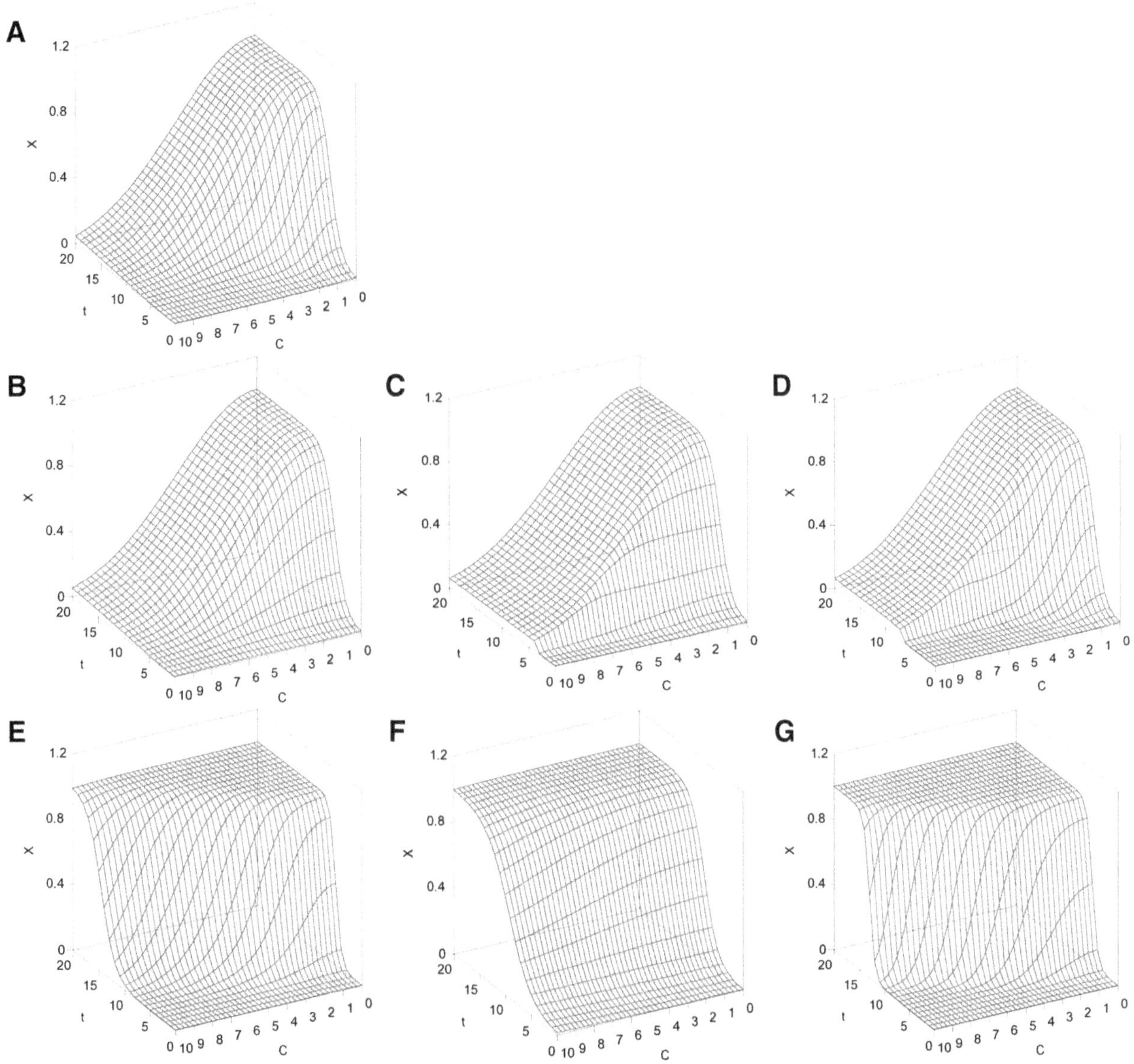

Figure 2 Profiles obtained by simulation under the numerical conditions specified in Table 2 using the equation (1) and that representing all the theoretical kinetics of protein aggregation process. **A**: all the parameters from logistic equation (X_m, v_m and λ) are affected by chemical concentration; **B**: parameters (X_m and v_m) are modified by chemical; **C**: only the parameter X_m is affected by chemical; **D**: parameters (X_m and λ) are modified by chemical; **E**: parameters (v_m and λ) are affected by chemical; **F**: only the parameter v_m is modified by chemical; **G**: only the parameter λ is affected by chemical. In all cases, time (t), aggregation response (X) and chemical concentration (C) are simulated with arbitrary units.

for the comparison and the evaluation of the application of chemicals to reduce the protein fibrillation. The results demonstrated that the most inhibitory conditions for EGCG are established at neutral pH and a lower temperature (case 2), but these conditions require a longer time (τ) to achieve the parameter $EC_{50,\tau}$.

Inhibitory effect of di-C7-PC and methylglyoxal on insulin aggregation

Figure 3C displays the surface described by equation (1) and data on the insulin kinetics in the presence of a surfactant. The parameter values and the statistical characteristics of the modeling were also determined (Table 3). All of the statistical results revealed good agreement and accuracy between the observed and the predicted values, the consistency of the equation, and a lack of bias during the fitting process.

Regarding the effects, the two kinetic parameters v_m and X_m were significantly affected by di-C7-PC, whereas the lag phase was not modified by the surfactant (Student's t test, $\alpha = 0.05$), as determined in the simulated conditions defined by Figure 2B. This result is in agreement with data

Table 2 Arbitrary numerical values defined for the simulations of Figure 1 (A, B, C, D, E, F and G) according to the parameters defined in the equation (1)

Parameters		Simulation conditions A	B	C	D	E	F	G
Aggregation growth	X_m	1.00	1.00	1.00	1.00	1.00	1.00	1.00
	v_m	0.25	0.25	0.25	0.25	0.50	0.20	0.50
	λ	3.00	3.00	3.00	3.00	4.00	5.00	4.00
Effect on X_m	K_x	1.00	1.00	1.00	1.00	-	-	-
	m_x	5.00	5.00	5.00	5.00	-	-	-
	a_x	2.00	2.00	2.00	2.00	-	-	-
Effect on v_m	K_v	1.00	1.00	-	-	0.60	0.60	-
	m_v	4.00	4.00	-	-	3.00	8.00	-
	a_v	2.00	2.00	-	-	2.00	2.00	-
Effect on λ	K_λ	1.00	-	-	1.00	4.00	-	4.00
	m_λ	2.00	-	-	2.00	10.00	-	10.00
	a_λ	2.00	-	-	2.00	2.00	-	2.00

reported for different systems of effector/protein, such as copper/β-amyloid [47] or glutathione/hen egg-white lysozyme, although these data were obtained using a non-mathematical approach [48]. The value of $EC_{50,\tau}$ was similar to that obtained for EGCG (case 1) for a lower initial concentration of insulin, but a much longer time was required to obtain this parametric value (150.68 h).

Similar inhibitory responses were also observed with methylglyoxal; thus, v_m and X_m were the kinetic parameters inhibited by this aldehyde form of pyruvic acid (Table 3 and Figure 3D). Under an initial insulin concentration (3 g/L) that was higher than the initial EGCG concentration, methylglyoxal effectively reduced the aggregation growth (0.33 mM) within a shorter time (3.9 h). Both chemicals (di-C7-PC and methylglyoxal), under the experimental conditions assayed, showed similar features of true inhibitors [26]. The application of the proposed methodology may help the design of optimal strategies for the reduction of the fibril deposition of insulin in commercial preparations.

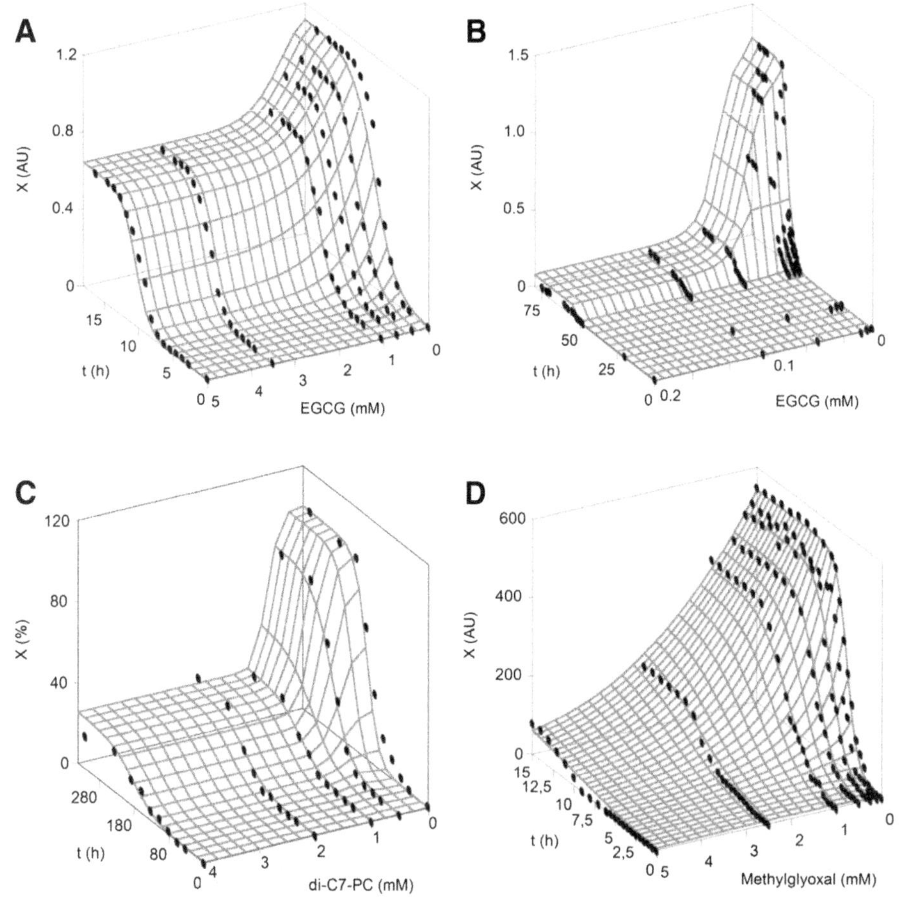

Figure 3 Insulin fibrillation kinetics at different concentrations of EGCG, di-C7-PC and methylglyoxal (points) and fittings to equation (1) (surface). *X*: aggregation data measured by absorbance at 600 nm (AU), ThT fluorescence intensity at 482 nm (AU) or ThT fluorescence intensity (%). **A**: experimental data of EGCG obtained at pH = 2.0 and T = 60°C. **B**: experimental data of EGCG obtained at pH = 7.4 and T = 37°C. **C**: di-C7-PC data. **D**: methylglyoxal data.

Table 3 Parametric estimates and confidence intervals (α = 0.05) from the equation (1) applied to the aggregation insulin increased data influenced by EGCG_1, EGCG_2, di-C7-PC and methylglyoxal concentrations

Parameters		EGCG_1	EGCG_2	di-C7-PC	Methylglyoxal
Aggregation model	X_m (AU or %)	1.12±0.03	1.28±0.06	99.85±4.91	541.20±11.38
	v_m (AU h^{-1} or % h^{-1})	0.18±0.01	0.25±0.04	1.55±0.27	219.68±20.98
	λ (h)	4.78±0.28	53.34±0.28	124.62±5.86	2.92±0.12
Effect on X_m	K_x	0.43±0.03	0.94±0.02	0.75±0.05	1.00±0.44
	m_x (mM)	0.68±0.08	0.01±0.00	0.65±0.12	1.80±1.25
	a_x	1.65±0.45	0.96±0.20	4.04±2.37	0.99±0.23
Effect on v_m	K_v	NS	NS	0.86±0.04	0.99±0.01
	m_v (mM)	NS	NS	0.47±0.06	0.42±0.07
	a_v	NS	NS	2.51±2.35	0.74±0.08
Effect on λ	K_λ	0.81±0.10	NS	NS	NS
	m_λ (mM)	0.50±0.08	NS	NS	NS
	a_λ	0.98±0.24	NS	NS	NS
	$EC_{50,\tau}$ (mM)	0.44	0.006	0.47	0.33
	τ (h)	7.65	55.02	150.68	3.92
	p-value	<0.001	<0.001	<0.001	<0.001
	B_f	0.88	0.80	1.00	1.04
	A_f	1.23	1.40	1.18	1.15
	R^2_{adj}	0.992	0.977	0.984	0.974

Statistical values of adjusted coefficient of multiple determination (R^2_{adj}) and p-values from Fisher's F-test (α = 0.05). B_f and A_f are the bias and accuracy factor, respectively. NS: non-significant.

Inhibitory effect of mono and biflavonoids on Aβ42 amyloid protein

The dependence of the kinetic parameters of fibrillation on the apigenin and taiwaniaflavone concentrations is represented in Figures 4A and B. Both response surfaces were similar to that defined by the simulation shown in Figure 2A. The three parameters (v_m, X_m, and λ) were clearly and significantly modified by these chemical doses (Table 4), which show a longer pre-nucleation phase, a lower elongation rate (post-nucleation), and a lower elongation stage. Such responses confirmed their chemical features of true inhibitors, being the only case in which both kinetic parameters (v_m and λ) significantly affected aggregation process [26]. All of the statistical tests corroborated the perfect agreement between the experimental and the theoretical data (*e.g.*, $R^2_{adj} > 0.99$). The bias and accuracy factors (B_f and A_f) were also indicative of the good fitting quality obtained with model (1).

The numerical values of $EC_{50,\tau}$ confirmed the superior antifibrillogenic capacity of the biflavonoid taiwaniaflavone ($EC_{50,\tau}$ = 0.91 μM) compared with the monoflavonoid apigenin ($EC_{50,\tau}$ = 2.45 μM). However, the time τ was quite similar in both cases. This affirmation is consistent with the conclusions reported in the original work conducted by Thapa et al. [16].

Inhibitory effect of osmolytes on Aβ42 amyloid protein

Different types of molecules have been recently suggested as drug candidates for the treatment of neurodegenerative disorders caused by the anti-aggregation properties of amyloid proteins [49]. One of the most interesting candidates are osmolytes (compounds that protect against the osmotic stress), such as the ectoines that are obtained from aerobic heterotrophic bacteria [50]. The response surface for hydroxyectoine (Figure 4C) shows a behavior that is similar to that obtained with the simulation shown in Figure 2B. Based on the numerical fittings summarized in Table 4, it was statistically demonstrated that osmolytes inhibited the maximum aggregation rate and the maximum fibrillation growth. In contrast, no significant changes in the lag phase were observed. Therefore, both osmolytes effectively blocked the post-nucleation and the elongation stages but not the pre-nuclei formation. In addition, ectoine was much more effective as an antineurotoxic ($EC_{50,\tau}$ = 0.96 mM) than hydroxyectoine ($EC_{50,\tau}$ = 2.20 mM).

Inhibition of apomyoglobin fibrils formation by trehalose

The effect of trehalose on the apomyoglobin aggregation kinetics was also studied using model (1), and excellent statistical results were obtained from the modeling and the description of the experimental data (Figure 4D and

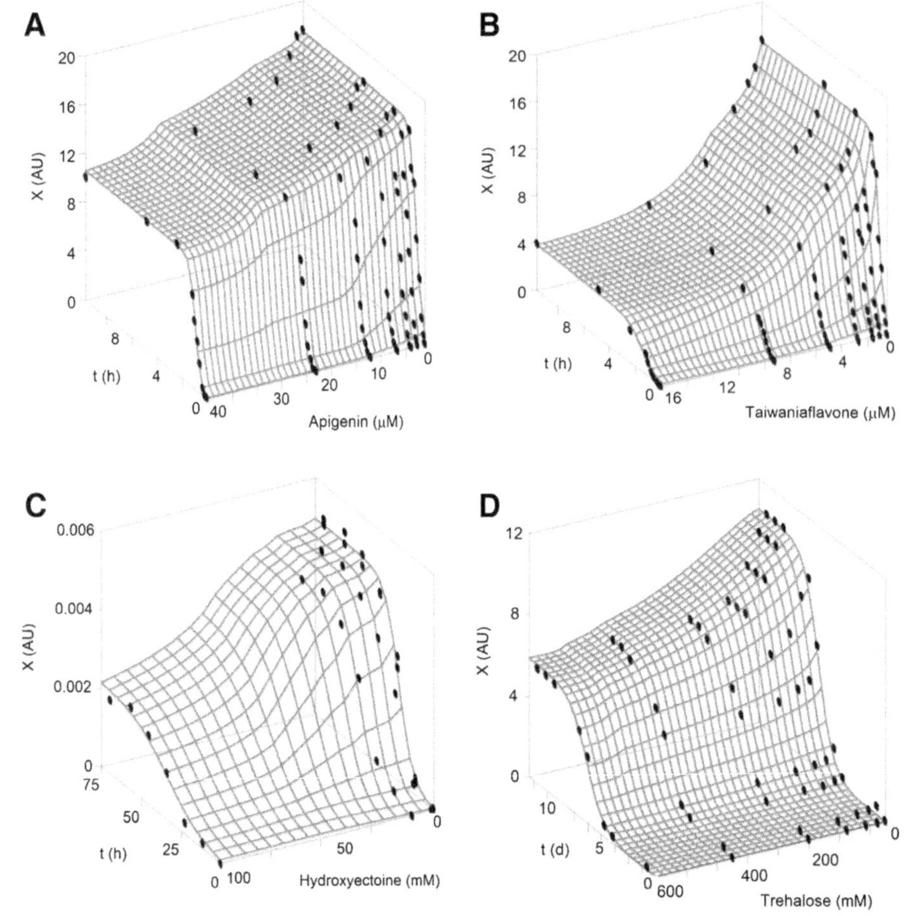

Figure 4 Amyloid protein aggregation kinetics at different concentrations of apigenin, ectoine, taiwaniaflavone and trehalose (points) and fittings to equation (1) (surface). *X*: aggregation data measured by ThT fluorescence intensity at 482 nm or 490 nm (AU). **A**: experimental data of apigenin. **B**: taiwaniaflavone data. **C**: experimental data of hydroxyectoine. **D**: data of trehalose affecting apomyoglobin kinetics.

Table 4). As in the previous case, the disaccharide significantly inhibited the two kinetic parameters v_m and X_m without affecting the pre-nucleation phase (λ). Nevertheless, its relative efficacy was obtained at a much higher concentration (21.43 mM), and much longer times (6.5 d) were required than compared with the other cases studied.

Conclusions

In summary, a general bivariate model that combines the logistic equation for the description of kinetics and the Weibull equation for the chemical-concentration response has been proposed for the characterization of the inhibitory effects produced by several chemicals on the growth of the aggregation of amyloid proteins. In all cases, the inhibitory effects on the kinetic parameters were established, and the theoretical response surfaces were in perfect agreement with the selected data. In addition, the recent definition of true and apparent inhibitors reported by Martins [24] can be also evaluated and validated. EGCG at pH 7.4 and a temperature of 37°C was the best option for the reduction of the formation of insulin fibrils ($EC_{50,\tau} = 6$ μM) but the shortest time (τ) was obtained with methylglyoxal. For the Aβ42 amyloid protein, the biflavonoid taiwaniaflavone produced the highest inhibition response at the lowest dose (0.91 μM) and the shortest time (0.65 h). The bivariate equation was validated using data obtained by two methods based on different chemical phenomena. Although this model can not define the mechanisms of action of chemical inhibitors on protein aggregation, it provides a consistent tool for the comparison of the ability of such compounds in the inhibition of the protein fibrillation process, regardless of the method used for its determination, and is a first step for the optimization of the *in vitro* application of them. Further experiments and corresponding modeling should be done to establish its validity for *in vivo* applications of anti-aggregation chemicals.

Table 4 Parametric estimates and confidence intervals (α = 0.05) from the equation (1) applied to the aggregation of Aβ42-amyloid protein increased data influenced by apigenin, ectoine, hidroxyectoine and taiwaniaflavone concentrations

Parameters		Apigenin	Ectoine	Hidroxyectoine	Taiwaniaflavone	Trehalose
Aggregation model	X_m (AU)	17.43±0.50	(5.07±0.23) × 10^{-3}	(4.96±0.24) × 10^{-3}	16.55±0.55	10.49±0.28
	v_m (AU h^{-1} or AU d^{-1})	16.10±1.49	(0.24±0.05) × 10^{-3}	(0.30±0.08) × 10^{-3}	17.01±2.09	3.31±0.33
	λ (h or d)	0.25±0.03	11.60±2.26	13.50±2.31	0.27±0.06	5.76±0.14
Effect on X_m	K_x	0.41±0.06	1.00±0.99	1.00±0.90	0.78±0.05	0.44±0.03
	m_x (mM or μM)	6.52±1.93	11.82±11.03	66.70±65.78	2.32±0.38	51.58±7.27
	a_x	0.91±0.25	0.19±0.13	0.43±0.43	0.98±0.16	1.36±0.31
Effect on v_m	K_v	0.38±0.12	0.83±0.06	0.86±0.16	1.14±0.60	0.53±0.08
	m_v (mM or μM)	9.29±5.35	0.33±0.32	1.35 (NS)	1.88±1.73	33.22±17.26
	a_v	1.35±1.13	0.36±0.14	0.34±0.20	0.40±0.21	0.66±0.33
Effect on λ	K_λ	1.76±0.70	NS	NS	1.27±1.13	NS
	m_λ (mM or μM)	2.16±0.29	NS	NS	2.53±1.45	NS
	a_λ	2.39±0.99	NS	NS	2.33±2.31	NS
	$EC_{50,\tau}$ (mM or μM)	2.45	0.96	2.20	0.91	21.43
	τ (h or d)	0.75	17.31	20.52	0.65	6.54
	p-value	<0.001	<0.001	<0.001	<0.001	<0.001
	B_f	0.99	1.04	1.00	1.02	1.03
	A_f	1.06	1.09	1.18	1.11	1.08
	R^2_{adj}	0.995	0.988	0.984	0.990	0.995

The case of apomyoglobin affected by trehalose is also shown. Statistical values of adjusted coefficient of multiple determination (R^2_{adj}) and p-values from Fisher's F-test (α = 0.05). B_f and A_f are the bias and accuracy factor, respectively. NS: non-significant.

Appendix

Reparameterization of logistic equation

It is well-known the autocatalytic origin of the logistic equation based on the following differential equation:

$$\frac{dX}{dt} = k_{app}X\left(1-\frac{X}{X_m}\right) \qquad (A.1)$$

which, integrated between $X_0 \rightarrow X$ and $0 \rightarrow t$ gives the explicit form of aggregation growth as a function of the time:

$$X = \frac{X_m}{1+\exp\left[\ln\left(\frac{X_m-X_0}{X_0}\right)-k_{app}t\right]} \qquad (A.2)$$

The parameter τ is defined as the time required to obtain the semimaximum fibrillation growth (when $X = X_m/2$):

$$\frac{X_m}{2} = \frac{X_m}{1+\left(\frac{X_m-X_0}{X_0}\right)\exp\left[-k_{app}\tau\right]} \Rightarrow \tau = \frac{1}{k_{app}}\ln\left(\frac{X_m-X_0}{X_0}\right) \qquad (A.3)$$

The inflection point ($t = t_i$) can be obtained when the second derivative from (A.1) is equal to zero and the abscissa is isolated [31]:

$$t_i = \tau = \frac{1}{k_{app}}\ln\left(\frac{X_m-X_0}{X_0}\right) \qquad (A.4)$$

The value of aggregation when $t = t_i$ is:

$$X(t_i) = \frac{X_m}{2} \qquad (A.5)$$

The slope in the inflection point (v_m) is defined by the following operation:

$$v_m = \frac{dX}{dt}\Big|_{t=t_i} = \frac{X_m k_{app}\exp\left[\ln\left(\frac{X_m-X_0}{X_0}\right)-k_{app}t_i\right]}{\left[1+\exp\left[\ln\left(\frac{X_m-X_0}{X_0}\right)-k_{app}t_i\right]\right]^2} = \frac{X_m k_{app}}{4} \qquad (A.6)$$

The lag phase (λ) or pre-nucleation phase is defined as the intersection of the tangent at the inflection point with the abscissa (Figure 1):

$$R = X(t_i) + v_m(L-t_i)$$

with $L = \lambda$ when $R = 0$:

$$\lambda = t_i - \frac{X(t_i)}{v_m} = \tau - \frac{X_m}{2v_m} = \tau - \frac{2}{k_{app}} \tag{A.7}$$

Reorganizing terms, two reparameterized functions can be defined:

$$X = \frac{X_m}{1 + \exp\left[2 + \frac{4v_m}{X_m}(\lambda - t)\right]} \tag{A.8}$$

$$X = \frac{X_m}{1 + \exp\left[\frac{4v_m}{X_m}(\tau - t)\right]} \tag{A.9}$$

When parameters from both equations are influenced by chemical agent concentration, they can be rewritten as follows:

$$X = \frac{X_{m\bullet}}{1 + \exp\left[2 + \frac{4v_{m\bullet}}{X_{m\bullet}}(\lambda_\bullet - t)\right]} \tag{A.10}$$

$$X = \frac{X_{m\bullet}}{1 + \exp\left[\frac{4v_{m\bullet}}{X_{m\bullet}}(\tau_\bullet - t)\right]} \tag{A.11}$$

On the other hand, the calculation of the time τ for $EC_{50,\tau}$ is obtained by the following formula:

$$\frac{X_{m\bullet}}{4} = \frac{X_{m\bullet}}{1 + \exp\left[\frac{4v_{m\bullet}}{X_{m\bullet}}(\tau_\bullet - \tau)\right]} \Rightarrow \tau = \tau_\bullet - \frac{X_{m\bullet}\ln 3}{4v_{m\bullet}} \tag{A.12}$$

Weibull equation and bivariate model (1)

The most interesting form of Weibull equation for dose-response modelling is expressed as follows [35]:

$$Y = Y_m\left\{1 - \exp\left[-\ln 2\left(\frac{C}{m}\right)^a\right]\right\} \tag{A.13}$$

where, Y is the response and Y_m the maximum response, m is the concentration corresponding to the semi-maximum response, C is the concentration and a is a shape parameter related to the maximum slope of the response.

This equation can be modified according with the graphical tendencies of chemicals effects (Figure 1) on the aggregation parameters [38]:

$$\theta = \theta_0(1 - Y_\theta) \quad \text{or} \quad \theta = \theta_0(1 + Y_\theta) \tag{A.14}$$

Thus, decrease of v_m and X_m and increase of λ and τ were the characteristic responses observed for the inhibition of amyloid protein fibrillation kinetics induced by chemicals:

$$\begin{aligned}
X_{m\bullet} &= X_m\left\{1 - K_x\left[1 - \exp\left(-\ln 2\left(\frac{C}{m_x}\right)^{a_x}\right)\right]\right\}\\
v_{m\bullet} &= v_m\left\{1 - K_v\left[1 - \exp\left(-\ln 2\left(\frac{C}{m_v}\right)^{a_v}\right)\right]\right\}\\
\lambda_\bullet &= \lambda\left\{1 + K_\lambda\left[1 - \exp\left(-\ln 2\left(\frac{C}{m_\lambda}\right)^{a_\lambda}\right)\right]\right\}\\
\tau_\bullet &= \tau\left\{1 + K_\tau\left[1 - \exp\left(-\ln 2\left(\frac{C}{m_\tau}\right)^{a_\tau}\right)\right]\right\}
\end{aligned} \tag{A.15}$$

When the equations (A.15) are inserting directly on equation (A.10) or (A.11), the bivariate model (1) is obtained.

Additional file

Additional file 1: Excel spreadsheet used for modeling the Ab42amyloid apigenin case.

Competing interests

The author declares that he has no competing interests.

Acknowledgements

The authors also thank the Unit of Information Resources for Research (URICI-CSIC) for the co-financing of this publication in Open Access.

References

1. Bucciantini M, Giannoni E, Chiti F, Baroni F, Formigli L, Zurdo J, Taddei N, Ramponi G, Dobson CM, Stefani M: **Inherent toxicity of aggregates implies a common mechanism for protein misfolding diseases.** *Nature* 2002, **416**:507–511.
2. Chiti F, Dobson CM: **Protein misfolding, functional amyloid, and human disease.** *Annu Rev Biochem* 2006, **75**:333–366.
3. Stefani M, Dobson CM: **Protein aggregation and aggregate toxicity: new insights into protein folding, misfolding diseases, and biological evolution.** *J Mol Med* 2003, **81**:678–699.
4. Uversky VN, Fink AL: **Conformational constraints for amyloid fibrillation: the importance of being unfolded.** *Biochim Biophys Acta* 2004, **1698**:131–153.
5. Wang SSS, Good TA: **An overview of Alzheimer's disease.** *J Chin Inst Chem Eng* 2005, **36**:533–559.
6. Cromwell MEM, Hilario E, Jacobson F: **Protein aggregation and bioprocessing.** *AAPS J* 2006, **8**:E572–E579.
7. Rosenberg AS: **Effects of protein aggregates: an immunologic perspective.** *AAPS J* 2006, **8**:E501–E507.
8. Knowles TP, Fitzptrick AW, Meehan S, Mott HR, Vendruscolo M, Dobson CM, Welland ME: **Role of intermolecular forces in defining material properties of protein nanofibrils.** *Science* 2007, **318**:1900–1903.
9. Nelson R, Eisenberg D: **Recent atomic models of amyloid fibril structure.** *Curr Opin Struct Biol* 2006, **16**:260–265.
10. Ross CA, Poirier MA: **What is the role of protein aggregation in neurodegeneration?** *Nat Rev Mol Cell Biol* 2005, **6**:891–898.
11. Mauro M, Craparo EF, Podesta A, Bulone D, Carrotta R, Martorana V, Tiana G, San Biagio PL: **Kinetics of different processes in human insulin amyloid formation.** *J Mol Biol* 2007, **366**:258–274.
12. Loksztejn A, Dzwolak W: **Vortex-induced formation of insulin amyloid superstructures probed by time-lapse atomic force microscopy and circular dichroism spectroscopy.** *J Mol Biol* 2010, **395**:643–655.
13. Slusky V, Tamada JA, Klibanov AM, Langer R: **Kinetics of insulin aggregation in aqueous solutions upon agitation in the presence of hydrophobic surfaces.** *Proc Natl Acad Sci U S A* 1991, **88**:9377–9381.
14. Dische FE, Wernstedt C, Westermark GT, Westermark P, Pepys MB, Rennie JA, Gilbey SG, Watkins PJ: **Insulin as an amyloid-fibril protein at sites of repeated insulin injections in a diabetic patient.** *Diabetol* 1988, **31**:158–161.

15. Kanapathipillaia M, Lentzenb G, Sierksa M, Parka CB: **Ectoine and hydroxyectoine inhibit aggregation and neurotoxicity of Alzheimer's β-amyloid.** *FEBS Lett* 2005, **579**:4775–4780.
16. Thapa A, Woo ER, Chi EY, Sharoar MG, Jin HG, Shin SY, Park IS: **Biflavonoids are superior to monoflavonoids in inhibiting amyloid-β toxicity and fibrillogenesis via accumulation of nontoxic oligomer-like structures.** *Biochem* 2011, **50**:2445–2455.
17. Andrews JM, Roberts CJ: **A Lumry-Eyring nucleated polymerization model of protein aggregation kinetics: 1. Aggregation with pre-equilibrated unfolding.** *J Phys Chem B* 2007, **111**:7897–7913.
18. Bernacki J, Murphy RM: **Model discrimination and mechanistic interpretation of kinetic data in protein aggregation studies.** *Biophys J* 2009, **96**:2871–2887.
19. Ghosh P, Kumar A, Datta B, Rangacharim V: **Dynamics of protofibril elongation and association involved in Aβ42 peptide aggregation in Alzheimer's disease.** *BMC Bioinformatics* 2010, **11**(Suppl 6):S24.
20. Lee CC, Nayak A, Sethuraman A, Belfort G, McRae GJ: **A three-stage kinetic model of amyloid fibrillation.** *Biophys J* 2007, **92**:3448–3458.
21. Roberts CJ: **Kinetics of irreversible protein aggregation: Analysis of extended Lumry-Eyring models and implications for predicting protein shelf life.** *J Phys Chem B* 2003, **107**:1194–1207.
22. Ruzafa D, Conejero-Lara F, Morel B: **Modulation of the stability of amyloidogenic precursors by anion binding strongly influences the rate of amyloid nucleation.** *Phys Chem Chem Phys* 2013, **15**:15508–15517.
23. Ruzafa D, Morel B, Varela L, Azuaga AI, Conejero-Lara F: **Characterization of oligomers of heterogeneous size as precursors of amyloid fibril nucleation of an SH3 domain: an experimental kinetics study.** *Plos One* 2012, **7**:e49690.
24. Morris AM, Watzky MA, Finke RG: **Protein aggregation kinetics, mechanism, and curve-fitting: a review of the literature.** *Biochim Biophys Acta* 2009, **1794**:375–397.
25. Crespo R, Rocha FA, Damas AM, Martins PM: **A generic crystallization-like model that describes the kinetics of amyloid fibril formation.** *J Biol Chem* 2012, **287**:30585–30594.
26. Martins PM: **True and apparent inhibition of amyloid fibril formation.** *Prion* 2013, **7**:136–139.
27. Morris AM, Watzky MA, Agar JN, Finke RG: **Fitting neurological protein aggregation kinetic data via a 2-step, minimal/"Ockham's Razor" model: the Finke-Watzky mechanism of nucleation followed by autocatalytic surface growth.** *Biochem* 2008, **47**:2413–2427.
28. Morris AM, Finke RG: **α-Synuclein aggregation variable temperature and variable pH kinetic data: a re-analysis using the Finke–Watzky 2-step model of nucleation and autocatalytic growth.** *Biophys Chem* 2009, **140**:9–15.
29. Naiki H, Hasegawa K, Yamaguchi I, Nakamura H, Gejyo F, Nakakuki K: **Apolipoprotein E and antioxidants have different mechanisms of inhibiting Alzheimer's β-Amyloid fibril formation in vitro.** *Biochem* 1998, **37**:17882–17889.
30. Nielsen L, Khurana R, Coats A, Frokjaer S, Brange J, Vyas S, Uversky VN, Fink AL: **Effect of environmental factors on the kinetics of insulin fibril formation: elucidation of the molecular mechanism.** *Biochem* 2001, **40**:6036–6046.
31. Wang SH, Dong XY, Sun Y: **Effect of (−)-epigallocatechin-3-gallate on human insulin fibrillation/aggregation kinetics.** *Biochem Eng J* 2012, **63**:38–49.
32. Oliveira LMA, Lages A, Gomes RA, Neves H, Família C, Coelho AV, Quintas A: **Insulin glycation by methylglyoxal results in native-like aggregation and inhibition of fibril formation.** *BMC Biochem* 2011, **12**:41.
33. Wang SSS, Liu KN, Han TC: **Amyloid fibrillation and cytotoxicity of insulin are inhibited by the amphiphilic surfactants.** *Biochim Biophys Acta* 2010, **1802**:519–530.
34. Vilasi S, Iannuzzi C, Portaccio M, Irace G, Sirangelo I: **Effect of trehalose on W7FW14F apomyoglobin and insulin fibrillization: new insight into inhibition activity.** *Biochem* 2008, **47**:1789–1796.
35. Murado MA, Vázquez JA, Rial D, Beiras R: **Dose-response modeling with two agents: application to the bioassay of oil and shoreline cleaning agents.** *J Hazardous Materials* 2011, **185**:807–817.
36. Riobó P, Paz B, Franco JM, Vázquez JA, Murado MA, Cacho E: **Mouse bioassay for palytoxin. Specific symptoms and dose-response against dose-death time relationships.** *Food Chem Toxicol* 2008, **46**:2639–2647.
37. Vázquez JA, Murado MA: **Mathematical tools for objective comparison of microbial cultures Application to evaluation of 15 peptones for lactic acid bacteria productions.** *Biochem Eng J* 2008, **39**:276–287.
38. Rial D, Vázquez JA, Murado MA: **Effects of three heavy metals on the bacteria growth kinetics: a bivariate model for toxicological assessment.** *Appl Microbiol Biotechnol* 2011, **90**:1095–1109.
39. Vázquez JA, Durán A, Rodríguez-Amado I, Prieto MA, Rial D, Murado MA: **Evaluation of toxic effects of several carboxylic acids on bacterial growth by toxicodynamic modelling.** *Microb Cell Fact* 2011, **10**:100.
40. Ross T: **Indices for performance evaluation of predictive models in food microbiology.** *J Appl Bacteriol* 1996, **81**:501–508.
41. Vázquez JA, Murado MA: **Unstructured mathematical model for biomass, lactic acid and bacteriocin production by lactic acid bacteria in batch fermentation.** *J Chem Technol Biotechnol* 2008, **83**:91–96.
42. Sabaté R, Villar-Piqué A, Espargaró A, Ventura S: **Temperature dependence of the aggregation kinetics of Sup35 and Ure2p yeast prions.** *Biomacromolecules* 2012, **13**:474–483.
43. Fändrich M: **Absolute correlation between lag time and growth rate in the spontaneous formation of several amyloid-like aggregates and fibrils.** *J Mol Biol* 2007, **365**:1266–1270.
44. Vázquez JA, Lorenzo JM, Fuciños P, Franco D: **Evaluation of non-linear equations to model different animal growths with mono and bisigmoid profiles.** *J Theor Biol* 2012, **314**:95–105.
45. Murado MA, González MP, Vázquez JA: **Dose-reponse relationships. An overview a generative model and its application to the verification of descriptive models.** *Enz Microb Technol* 2002, **31**:439–455.
46. Riobó P, Paz B, Franco JM, Vázquez JA, Murado MA: **Proposal for a simple and sensitive haemolytic assay for palytoxin. Toxicological dynamics, kinetics, ouabain inhibition and thermal stability.** *Harmful Algae* 2008, **7**:415–429.
47. Shimanouchi T, Onishi R, Kitaura N, Umakoshi H, Kuboi R: **Copper-mediated growth of amyloid β fibrils in the presence of oxidized and negatively charged liposomes.** *J Biosc Bioeng* 2011, **112**:611–615.
48. Wang SSS, Chou SW, Liu KN, Wu CH: **Effects of glutathione on amyloid fibrillation of hen egg-white lysozyme.** *Int J Biol Macromol* 2009, **45**:321–329.
49. Arora A, Ha C, Park CB: **Inhibition of insulin amyloid formation by small stress molecules.** *FEBS Lett* 2004, **564**:121–125.
50. Vorob'eva LI: **Stressors, stress reactions, and survival of bacteria: a review.** *Appl Biochem Microbiol* 2004, **40**:261–269.

Distinct single cell signal transduction signatures in leukocyte subsets stimulated with khat extract, amphetamine-like cathinone, cathine or norephedrine

Therese Bredholt[1†], Elisabeth Ersvær[1,2†], Bjarte Skoe Erikstein[1], André Sulen[1], Håkon Reikvam[1,3], Hans Jørgen Aarstad[4,5], Anne Christine Johannessen[5,6], Olav Karsten Vintermyr[5,6], Øystein Bruserud[1,3] and Bjørn Tore Gjertsen[1,3*]

Abstract

Background: Amphetamine and amphetamine derivatives are suggested to induce an immunosuppressive effect. However, knowledge of how amphetamines modulate intracellular signaling pathways in cells of the immune system is limited. We have studied phosphorylation of signal transduction proteins (Akt, CREB, ERK1/2, NF-κB, c-Cbl, STAT1/3/5/6) and stress sensors (p38 MAPK, p53) in human leukocyte subsets following *in vitro* treatment with the natural amphetamine cathinone, the cathinone derivatives cathine and norephedrine, in comparison with a defined extract of the psychostimulating herb khat (*Catha edulis* Forsk.). Intracellular protein modifications in single cells were studied using immunostaining and flow cytometry, cell viability was determined by Annexin V-FITC/Propidium Iodide staining, and T-lymphocyte proliferation was measured by ^{3}H-thymidine incorporation.

Results: Cathinone, cathine and norephedrine generally reduced post-translational modifications of intracellular signal transducers in T-lymphocytes, B-lymphocytes, natural killer cells and monocytes, most prominently affecting c-Cbl (pTyr700), ERK1/2 (p-Thr202/p-Tyr204), p38 MAPK (p-Thr180/p-Tyr182) and p53 (both total p53 protein and p-Ser15). In contrast, the botanical khat-extract induced protein phosphorylation of STAT1 (p-Tyr701), STAT6 (p-Tyr641), c-Cbl (pTyr700), ERK1/2 (p-Thr202/p-Tyr204), NF-κB (p-Ser529), Akt (p-Ser473), p38 MAPK (p-Thr180/p-Tyr182), p53 (Ser15) as well as total p53 protein. Cathinone, cathine and norephedrine resulted in unique signaling profiles, with B-lymphocytes and natural killer cells more responsive compared to T-lymphocytes and monocytes. Treatment with norephedrine resulted in significantly increased T-lymphocyte proliferation, whereas khat-extract reduced proliferation and induced cell death.
(Continued on next page)

* Correspondence: bjorn.gjertsen@med.uib.no
†Equal contributors
[1]Department of Clinical Science, University of Bergen, Bergen, Norway
[3]Department of Internal Medicine, Haukeland University Hospital, Bergen, Norway
Full list of author information is available at the end of the article

(Continued from previous page)

Conclusions: Single-cell signal transduction analyses of leukocytes distinctively discriminated between stimulation with cathinone and the structurally similar derivatives cathine and norephedrine. Cathinone, cathine and norephedrine reduced phosphorylation of c-Cbl, ERK1/2, p38 MAPK and p53(Ser15), and norephedrine induced T-lymphocyte proliferation. Khat-extract induced protein phosphorylation of signal transducers, p38 MAPK and p53, followed by reduced cell proliferation and cell death. This study suggests that protein modification-specific single-cell analysis of immune cells could unravel pharmacologic effects of amphetamines and amphetamine-like agents, and further could represent a valuable tool in elucidation of mechanism(s) of action of complex botanical extracts.

Keywords: Signal transduction, Leukocytes, Single-cell modification-specific flow cytometry, Natural amphetamine, Cathinone, Khat-extract

Background

The herbal drug khat (*Catha edulis* Forsk.) is chewed for its psychostimulating effects by millions of people [1,2]. The alkaloid cathinone represents its main psychoactive compound, with a structure and pharmacological profile similar to the synthetic drug amphetamine [3]. Cathinone represents a labile precursor for cathine and norephedrine [3], being metabolized primarily to norephedrine *in vivo* [4]. In addition to cathinone and its derivates, khat contains other bioactive constituents, including tannins, ascorbic acid, the phenylalkylamine meruchatine [5], catheduline alkaloids [6], flavonoids and triterpenoids [3,7].

During khat chewing, cathinone, cathine and norephedrine are extracted into saliva, and the oral buccal mucosa plays a major role in absorption [8]. Like amphetamine, cathinone induces release of dopamine, serotonin (5-hydroxytryptamine, 5-HT) and noradrenaline from presynaptic neuronal terminals, and has further been suggested to inhibit neurotransmitter reuptake [3]. Cathinone, cathine and norephedrine have been shown to act as substrates at the noradrenaline and dopamine transporters, to bind α_2-adrenergic receptors [9,10], and cathinone has in addition been reported to bind 5-HT receptors [10,11]. The β_1-adrenergic receptor was suggested to mediate khat-induced increase in systolic blood pressure and pulse rate [12], whereas the α_1-adrenergic receptor has been implicated in bladder dysfunction following khat chewing [13].

Leukocytes express transporters and receptors for dopamine and serotonin, and several types of immune cells store these neurotransmitters (reviewed in [14,15]). It has further been suggested that lymphocytes are capable of producing dopamine [16,17]. Leukocytes are known to express adrenergic receptors, and expression of the noradrenaline transporter has also been reported [18]. Various drugs that influence neurotransmitter transport, including anti-depressants and amphetamines, have demonstrated immunosuppressive effects *in vivo* (reviewed in [14,19]). Several studies have suggested that at least part of the immunosuppression could be due to direct impact of such pharmacological substrates on immune cells. For instance, House et al. reported that amphetamine could suppress B-lymphocyte proliferation and IL-2 secretion from T-lymphocytes *in vitro* [20]. Amphetamine was further seen to reduce zymosan-induced phagocytosis both *in vitro* and *in vivo* [21].

Intracellular signal transduction proteins and cell stress sensors have been linked to activation of adrenergic, dopaminergic and serotonergic receptors, which represent G-protein coupled receptors. The β-adrenergic/G stimulatory/protein kinase A pathway was reported to induce phosphorylation of mitogen-activated protein kinase (MAPK) p38 in activated B-lymphocytes [22] and in T-lineage cells [23]. 5-HT_7 receptor stimulation on naïve T-lymphocytes has been suggested to induce activation of extra-cellular regulated kinase 1/2 (ERK1/2) [24]. Further, stimulation of dopaminergic D2-like receptors was reported to reduce phosphorylation of cyclic AMP response element binding (CREB) protein in T-lymphocytes [25].

In this study we exposed peripheral blood leukocytes *in vitro* to cathinone, cathine, norephedrine, and to physiological relevant concentrations of khat-extract, and investigated the impact on selected signaling and stress sensor proteins. The distinct signatures of protein modifications detected in the leukocyte subsets indicate cellular effects and mechanism(s) of action of the khat-derived alkaloids, and further demonstrate that the cellular signaling response diverge from treatment with a complex botanical khat-extract.

Results

Peripheral blood mononuclear cells (PBMCs) from healthy donors (n = 6) were treated with khat-extract (10^{-3} and 3.16×10^{-4} dilutions), cathinone, cathine and norephedrine (10^{-4} M concentrations) for 4, 10 and 15 minutes, *in vitro*. Based on cathinone, cathine and norephedrine concentrations in the khat-extract, the experimental dilutions should be comparative to local concentrations of khat constituents *in vivo* during khat chewing (Table 1) [26]. The impact on signal transduction proteins and stress sensors in T-lymphocytes, B-

Table 1 Cathinone, cathine and norephedrine concentrations in the khat-extract stock solution, and in experimental cell cultures

	Cathinone		Cathine		Norephedrine	
	Mw 150.1		Mw 152.1		Mw 152.1	
	mg ml^{-1}	M	mg ml^{-1}	M	mg ml^{-1}	M
khat-extract stock solution	2.5	1.7×10^{-2}	3.0	2.0×10^{-2}	0.3	2.0×10^{-3}
10^{-3} dilution	2.5×10^{-3}	1.7×10^{-5}	3×10^{-3}	2.0×10^{-5}	3×10^{-4}	2.0×10^{-6}
3.16×10^{-4} dilution	7.9×10^{-4}	5.4×10^{-6}	9.5×10^{-4}	6.3×10^{-6}	9.5×10^{-5}	6.3×10^{-7}

The stock solution concentrations were determined based on HPLC-MS-MS analyses [30].

lymphocytes, natural killer (NK) cells and monocytes was assessed using modification-specific antibodies and flow cytometric analyses (Figure 1A).

Fold change values based on median fluorescence intensity (MFI) measurements were used as basis for data analyses, and signal transduction signatures for the leukocyte subsets are displayed as heatmaps of statistical significant changes (Figure 1B, 2A, 3A, 4A), and as cluster analyses (Figure 1C, 2B, 3B, 4B). The levels of phosphorylated (p) signal transducer and activator of transcription (STAT) 5, p-CREB, and p53 acetylated (ac)-Lysine (Lys)382 were not significantly altered by any stimulus (Additional file 1: Table S1) and were excluded from the heatmaps (Figure 1B, 2A, 3A, 4A) but included in the cluster analyses of signaling responses (Figure 1C, 2B, 3B, 4B). Cathinone did not induce significant signaling responses at the concentration and exposure times tested.

Signal transduction in T-lymphocytes

For T-lymphocytes (Figure 1B), treatment with the lowest khat-extract concentration induced p-STAT1, p-p38 MAPK, p-STAT6 and p-AKT; the highest khat-extract concentration induced p-c-Cbl, p-ERK1/2, p-p38 MAPK, p53 p-Serine (Ser)15 and total p53; cathine reduced p-c-Cbl, p-ERK1/2, p-p38 MAPK, p53 p-Ser15 and total p53; the combination norephedrine/cathinone reduced p-c-Cbl and p53 p-Ser15. The time-points and p-values for these changes are listed in Additional file 1: Table S1.

The cluster analysis of signal transduction in T-lymphocytes following 15 minutes of stimulation present significant and non-significant changes (Figure 1C). Khat-extract generally increased protein phosphorylation, in contrast to cathinone, cathine and norephedrine, which reduced phosphorylation of several proteins. Cathinone and its derivatives clustered separately from khat-extract, indicating different pharmacological properties of the complex extract compared to the pure khat components.

Signal transduction in B-lymphocytes

For B-lymphocytes (Figure 2A), treatment with the lowest khat-extract concentration induced p-STAT1, p-p38 MAPK, p-STAT6, p-AKT and p53 p-Ser37; the highest concentration of khat-extract induced p-STAT1, p-c-Cbl, p-ERK1/2, p-STAT3, p-NF-κB, p-p38 MAPK, p53 p-Ser15 and total p53. In contrast, cathine reduced p-c-Cbl, p-ERK1/2, p-p38 MAPK, p53 p-Ser15 and total p53; the combination norephedrine/cathinone reduced p53 p-Ser15. The time-points and p-values for these changes are listed in Additional file 1: Table S1.

The cluster analysis of signal transduction in B-lymphocytes (15 minutes) displays significant and non-significant changes (Figure 2B). As in T-lymphocytes, khat-extract induced protein phosphorylation, whereas cathinone and its derivatives decreased phosphorylation levels. In particular, p-c-Cbl, p-ERK1/2, p-p38- MAPK and p53 p-Ser15 were prominently reduced, and these phosphorylation responses clustered together.

Signal transduction in natural killer cells

For NK cells (Figure 3A), treatment with the lowest khat-extract concentration induced p-STAT1, p-STAT3, p-NF-κB, p-STAT6, p-AKT and total p53; the highest khat-extract concentration induced p-c-Cbl, p-ERK1/2, p-STAT3, p-NF-κB, p-p38 MAPK, p53 p-Ser15 and total p53; norephedrine induced p-STAT3; cathine reduced p-c-Cbl, p-ERK1/2, p-p38 MAPK and p53 p-Ser15. The time-points and p-values for these changes are listed in Additional file 1: Table S1. The cluster analysis of signal transduction in NK cells (15 minutes) displays significant and non-significant changes (Figure 3B). In NK cells, cathinone and its derivatives both induced and decreased protein phosphorylation.

Signal transduction in monocytes

For monocytes (Figure 4A), treatment with the lowest khat-extract concentration induced p-STAT1, p-p38 MAPK, p-STAT6 and p-AKT; the highest khat-extract concentration induced p-c-Cbl, p-ERK1/2, p-p38 MAPK, p53 p-Ser15 and total p53; cathine reduced p-c-Cbl and p53 p-Ser15. The cluster analysis of signal transduction in monocytes (15 minutes) indicates significant and non-significant changes (Figure 4B). Cathinone and its derivatives gave a less pronounced reduction in phosphorylation levels in the monocyte subset.

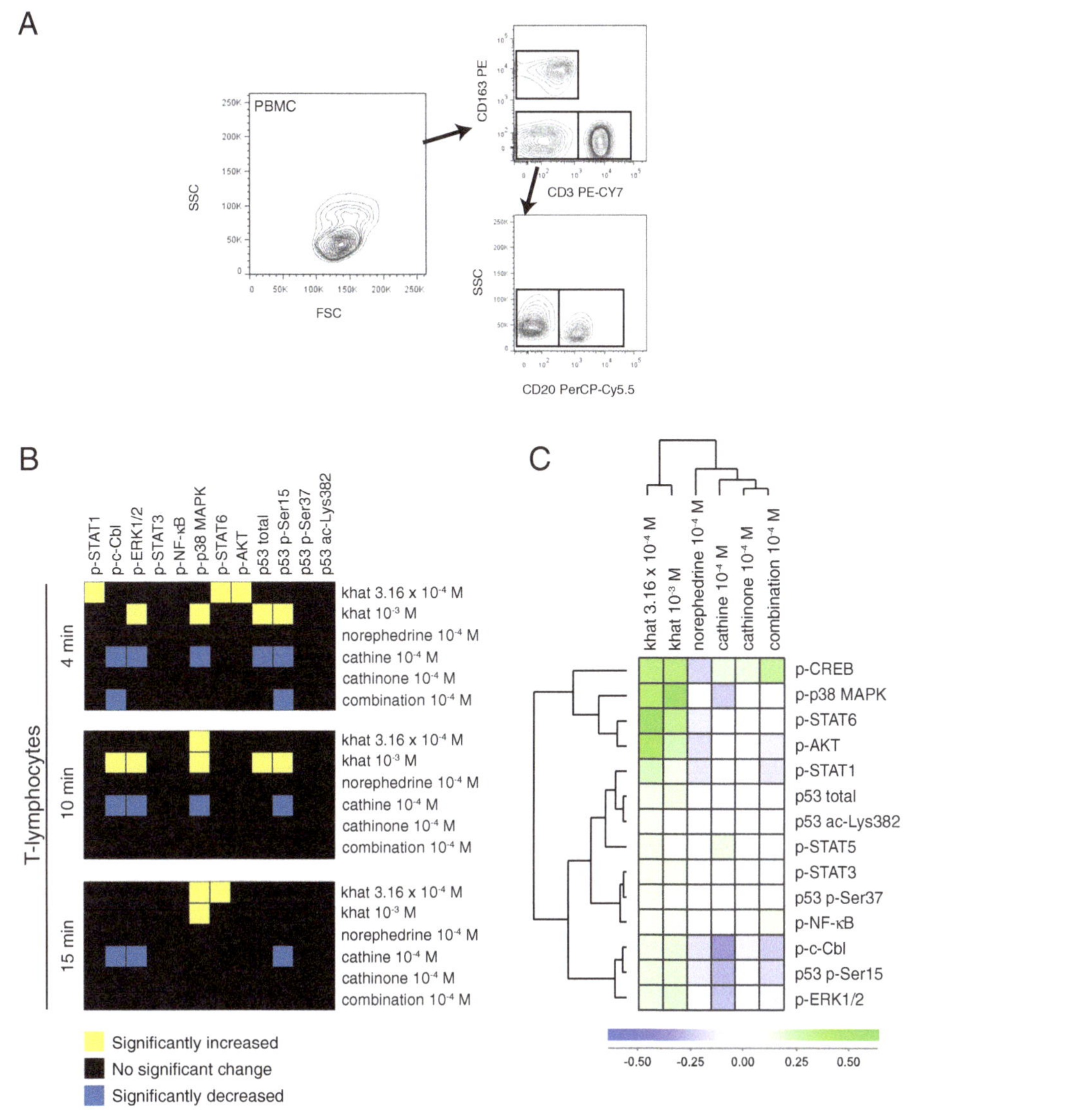

Figure 1 Gating strategies and signal transduction in T-lymphocytes. PBMCs ($n = 6$) were stimulated with khat-extract (10^{-3} and 3.16×10^{-4} dilutions), cathinone, cathine, norephedrine (10^{-4} M) and a combination of cathinone and norephedrine (combination: 2×10^{-4} M) for 4, 10 and 15 minutes, *in vitro*. **(A)** The PBMCs were fixed, permeabilized, stained with antibodies against specific cell surface markers and modification-specific antibodies and analyzed by flow cytometry. The PBMCs were identified as T-lymphocytes ($CD3^+$ $CD20^-$ $CD163^-$), B-lymphocytes ($CD3^-$ $CD20^+$ $CD163^-$), NK cells ($CD3^-$ $CD20^-$ $CD163^-$) and monocytes ($CD3^-$ $CD20^-$ $CD163^+$). **(B)** Heatmaps of statistical significant changes in protein-modification levels and total protein levels in T-lymphocytes. The analysis is based on fold change values for the modification-specific antibodies calculated from MFI measurements: $MFI_{stimulated}/MFI_{control}$. ANOVA of the mean was used to determine statistical significant changes. **(C)** Unsupervised hierarchical clustering analysis of the different stimuli and signal transduction proteins in T-lymphocytes following 15 minutes of stimulation. The mean fold changes were calculated, and log(2) converted before the unsupervised hierarchical clustering analysis was performed.

Alterations in p53 post-translational modifications

Based on MFI values for total p53, p53 p-Ser15, p53 p-Ser37 and p53 ac-Lys382, fold change values of p53 post-translational modifications relative to total p53 level were calculated (Figure 5). Significant changes in phosphorylation/acetylation of p53 were seen for all leukocyte subsets. For details on time-points and p-values, see Additional file 2: Table S2.

For T-lymphocytes, the highest khat-extract concentration reduced p-Ser37; cathine, cathinone and the combination norephedrine/cathinone reduced p-Ser15. For B-lymphocytes, cathine, cathinone and norephedrine/cathinone reduced p-Ser15, while cathine increased p-Ser37. For NK cells, the highest khat-extract concentration reduced p-Ser37 and ac-Lys382; cathine, cathinone and norephedrine/cathinone all reduced p-Ser15. In

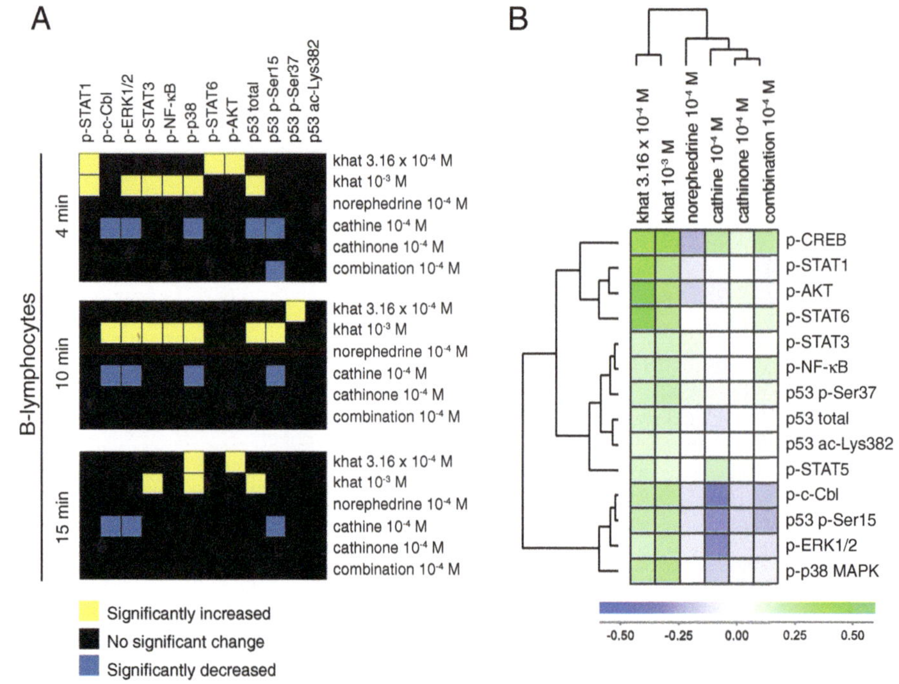

Figure 2 Signal transduction in B-lymphocytes. (A) Heatmap of statistical significant changes in protein-modification levels and total protein levels in B-lymphocytes. **(B)** Unsupervised hierarchical clustering analysis of the different stimuli and signal transduction proteins in B-lymphocytes following 15 minutes of stimulation.

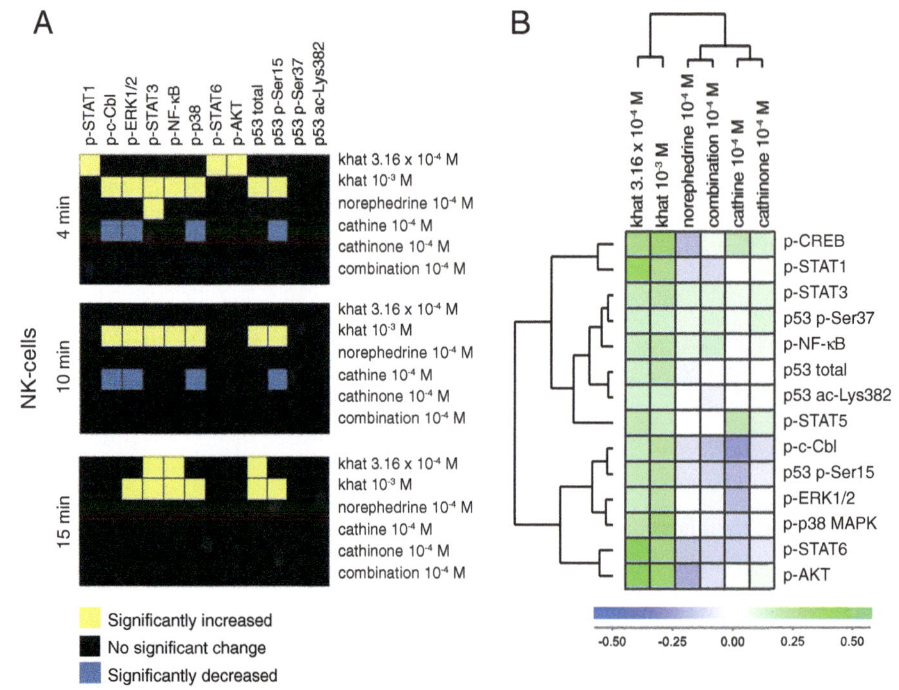

Figure 3 Signal transduction in NK cells. (A) Heatmap of statistical significant changes in protein-modification levels and total protein levels in NK-cells. **(B)** Unsupervised hierarchical clustering analysis of the different stimuli and signal transduction proteins in NK-cells following 15 minutes of stimulation.

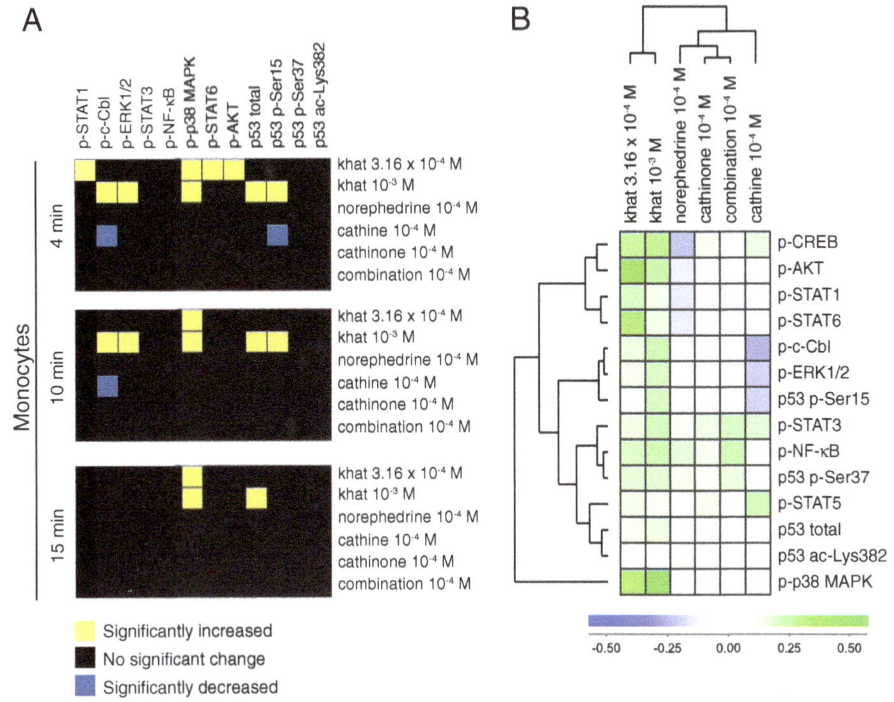

Figure 4 Signal transduction in monocytes. (A) Heatmap of statistical significant changes in protein-modification levels and total protein levels in monocytes. **(B)** Unsupervised hierarchical clustering analysis of the different stimuli and signal transduction proteins in monocytes following 15 minutes of stimulation.

monocytes, the highest khat-extract concentration reduced ac-Lys382; cathine reduced p-Ser15. The observations of modifications of central signal transduction pathways and stress proteins were extended with analyses of effects on cell death and proliferation in an attempt to connect early signal transduction responses with later functional effects on leukocytes.

Khat, cathinone and its derivatives affected leukocyte viability and proliferation

Levels of apoptosis were determined after 6 hours of stimulation, using Annexin V-fluorescein isothiocyanate (FITC) and propidium iodide (PI) staining followed by flow cytometric analyses (Figure 6A). The highest khat-extract concentration significantly reduced the levels of viable PBMCs, whereas the lower khat-extract concentration, cathinone, cathine and norephedrine had no significant effects.

Effects on T-lymphocyte proliferation were assessed following 4 days of stimulation, based on ^{3}H-thymidine incorporation (Figure 6B). The highest khat-extract concentration inhibited proliferation by approximately 50%. Treatment with cathinone and cathine gave elevated CPMA values, and norephedrine significantly increased T-lymphocyte proliferation ($p < 0.008$).

Discussion

Single-cell profiling of signal transduction using modification-specific antibodies and flow cytometry represents a powerful method in analyses of signaling networks [27-29]. Here we used this method to investigate the impact on signal transduction in leukocyte subsets following short-time exposure (4, 10 and 15 minutes) to the natural khat-derived amphetamine-like cathinone, its derivatives cathine and norephedrine, and a partly characterized khat-extract, *in vitro*. Functional implications were assessed based on determination of cell death induction and T-lymphocyte proliferation following long-time exposure (4 days). A summary of our present and previous findings regarding in vitro cellular effects of khat-extract is presented in Figure 7, and the present findings regarding cathinone and its natural derivatives is presented in Figure 8.

Cathinone and its natural derivatives generally suppressed basal phosphorylation of the examined signal transducers and stress sensors, while khat-extract induced protein post-translational modifications (Figures 1, 2, 3 and 4). The different impact on signal transduction proteins in the leukocytes was reflected in the functional assays, demonstrating khat-induced cell death and reduced T-lymphocyte proliferation, whereas no cytotoxic effects were detected for cathinone, cathine and norephedrine (Figure 6). Toxic

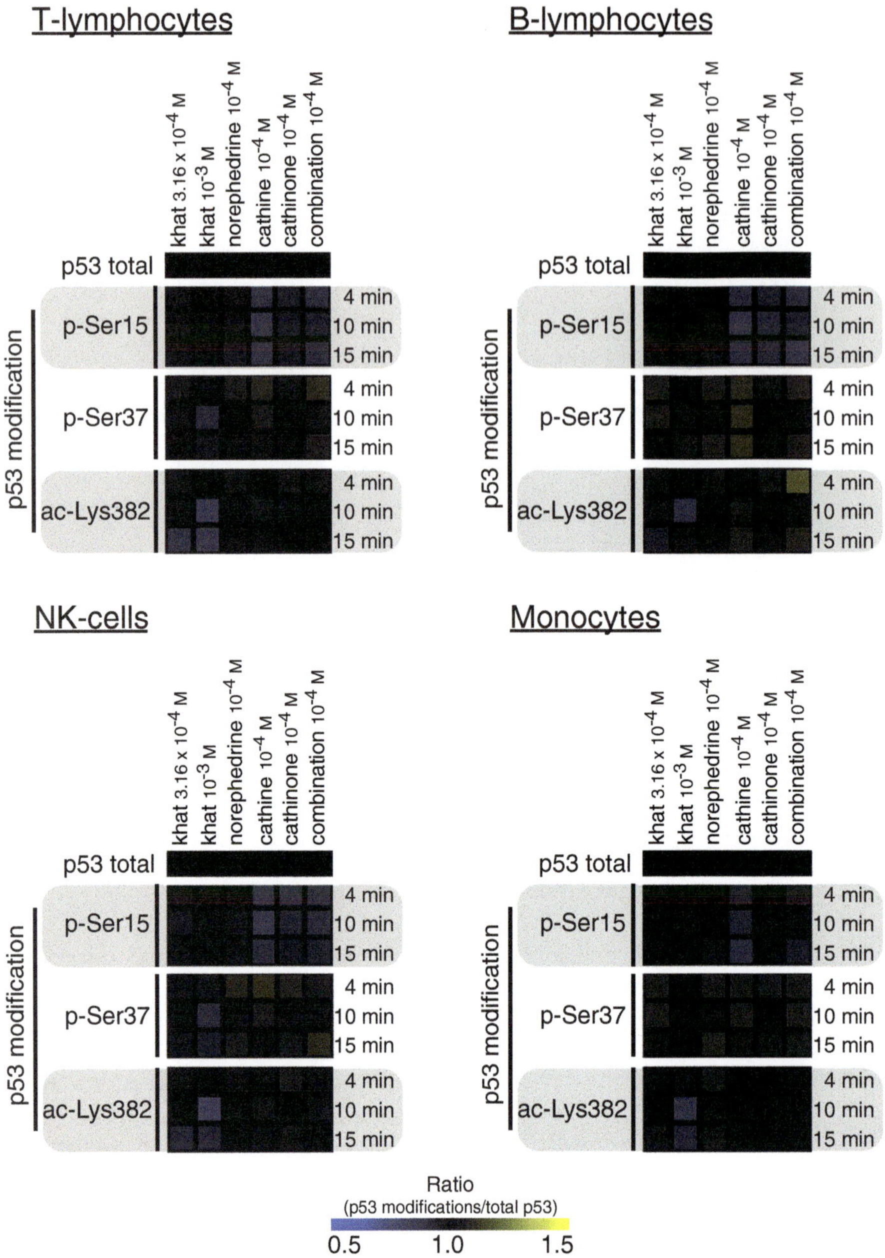

Figure 5 p53 post-translational modifications relative to total p53. Experiments and flow cytometry analyses as in the legend to Figure 1. Based on MFI values the median ratio of p-Ser15, p-Ser37 and ac-Lys382 relative to total p53 levels were determined for the various stimuli and time-points for the different leukocyte subsets.

effects by khat have been reported in *in vivo* and *in vitro* studies [3,30-32]. We have previously shown that khat induce caspase-dependent apoptosis in myeloid cells and keratinocytes [30,31,33]. Khat-induced apoptosis may involve induction of reactive oxygen species [31] (see also Aleruyani et al. for review [34]), which is described to function upstream of p53 and p38 in some model systems, while in others ROS production could be a downstream effect of p53 activation [35,36]. We therefore anticipated that single cell signalling analysis of total and modified p53 and phosphorylated p38 MAPK should reveal the mechanisms involved in khat toxicity when compared with cathinone and its natural derivatives.

There are conflicting results regarding toxic effects by cathinone and its natural derivatives [20,26,33]. Here we observed that norephedrine significantly increased T-lymphocyte proliferation after long-time exposure. A study by House and co-workers, comparing synthetic amphetamines and cathinone, demonstrated

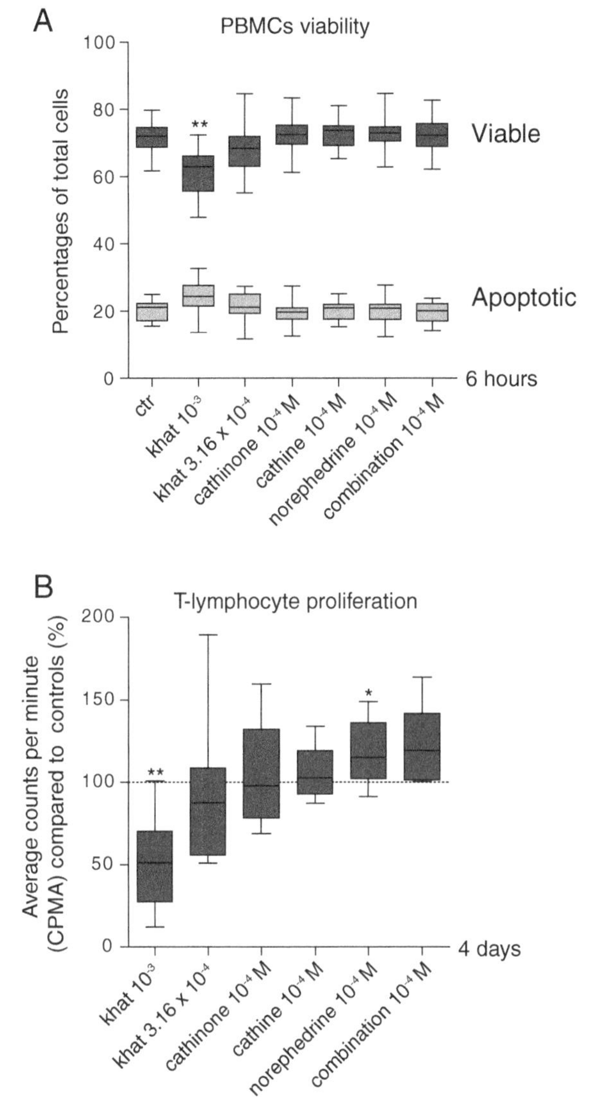

Figure 6 Functional effects: cell death and T-lymphocyte proliferation. (A) PBMCs were treated with khat (k 10^{-3} and 3.16×10^{-4} dilutions), 10^{-4} M of cathinone, cathine, norephedrine ($n = 14$), and a combination of the latter three ($n = 7$) for 6 hours. The PBMCs were stained with Annexin V-FITC and PI, and analyzed by flow cytometry. The results are expressed as percentages viable (Annexin V^-PI^-) and apoptotic (Annexin V^+PI^-) cells of the total cell number analyzed. **(B)** PBMCs were treated with khat (10^{-3} and 3.16×10^{-4} dilutions) and 10^{-4} M of cathinone, cathine, norephedrine ($n = 14$) and a combination of the latter three ($n = 7$). Nuclear radioactivity following ^{3}H-thymidine incorporation was assayed by liquid scintillation counting after four days. Results are expressed as percent average counts per minute (CPMA) in treated cells relative to the CPMA in control cells. * denotes $p < 0.008$ and ** denotes $p < 0.001$.

that cathinone induced B-lymphocyte proliferation, cytotoxic T-lymphocyte induction and IL-2 production [20]. As far as we know, a cell proliferative effect by norephedrine has not previously been demonstrated *in vitro*.

We have previously reported that khat-extract induced the tumor suppressor and cellular stress sensor p53 in normal oral keratinocytes and fibroblasts [26]. Here we demonstrate that p53 protein accumulates in leukocytes following khat-extract treatment, accompanied by, in particular, increased Ser15 phosphorylation (Figures 1, 2, 3 and 4). In contrast to khat-extract, cathinone and its derivatives generally reduced total p53 levels, p53 Ser15 phosphorylation (Figures 1, 2, 3 and 4) and Ser15 phosphorylation was further seen reduced relative to total p53 (Figure 5).

Cathine significantly reduced p38 MAPK phosphorylation in the various leukocyte subsets, whereas khat-extract mediated a significant increase in phosphorylation of this cell stress protein. In agreement with our observations, khat was recently reported to induce p38 MAPK phosphorylation in PBMCs *in vitro*, and khat-treatment was seen to induce cell death by apoptosis [32]. p38 is probably acting upstream of p53, and may be pivotal in khat-induced abnormal differentiation of *in vitro*-reconstructed human normal buccal mucosa [37]. Additionally, our data indicate that in particular cathine attenuated c-Cbl, ERK1/2 and p53 Ser15 phosphorylation in the various subsets, further including p-STAT6 and p-Akt reduction in T-lymphocytes (Figure 1). Interestingly, c-Cbl was recently reported to play an important role in trafficking of the 5-HT$_{2A}$ receptor in human embryonic kidney cells [38], whereas de-phosphorylation of AKT was observed following stimulation of striatal class D2 dopamine receptors [39,40].

Our results suggest that cathinone and its derivatives generally reduced basal phosphorylation levels of the proteins analysed, but as an exception, norephedrine was seen to significantly induce phosphorylation of STAT3 in NK cells. STAT3 is known to induce both proliferative and anti-proliferative effects, but a recent study suggested that STAT3 could mediate an immunosuppressive effect in NK cells [41]. Further, even if not statistical significant, cathine and cathinone indicated elevated p-CREB levels in all leukocyte subsets, whereas norephedrine reduced basal phosphorylation of CREB. Our results may indicate that the alkaloids cathine and cathinone induce CREB phosphorylation as has been shown for e.g. ephedrine. Ephedrine, an alkaloid chemically similar to cathinone, has been suggested to induce PKA-mediated CREB phosphorylation through β-adrenergic receptor/cyclic AMP/PKA/DARPP-32 signaling pathway [42]. Taken together these observations show that cathinone, cathine and norephedrine resulted in distinct signaling signatures, even if the compounds are closely related structurally.

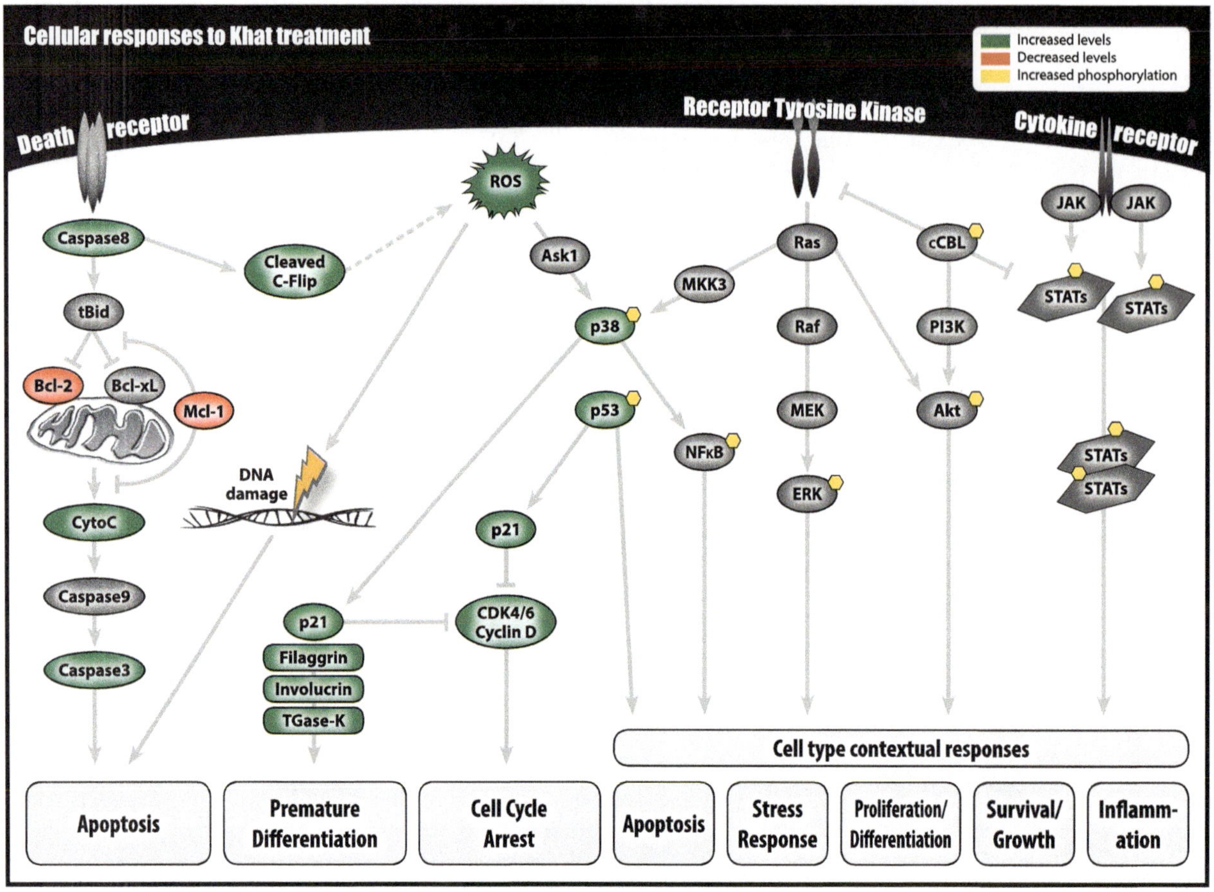

Figure 7 A summary of previous and present findings of cellular effects of khat-extract. Our studies have shown that exposure of various cell types (i.e. leukemic cell lines, normal oral keratinocytes and fibroblasts, normal peripheral leukocytes) to khat-extract *in vitro* affects various proteins involved in cell death, cell stress, cell cycle regulation, differentiation and cell signaling [26,30,31,33,37].

The leukocyte subsets differed in their signaling responses to the various treatments, and B-lymphocytes and NK cells were generally seen as more responsive compared to T-lymphocytes and monocytes. This observation could relate to varying levels or different repertoires of monoamine transporters and receptors on the immune cells. For instance, T-lymphocytes and monocytes were reported to exhibit a low expression of dopamine receptors when compared to B-lymphocytes and NK cells, which displayed a higher and more consistent expression [43]. The mechanism(s) behind the different responses to khat-extract, cathinone and its derivatives seen in the various leukocyte subsets should be addressed in future studies.

In recent years, synthetic cathinone derivatives have been designed, being widely distributed as recreational drugs. The use of these drugs has been reported with harmful health effects, and has been suspected to be involved in several deaths [44]. Signal transduction studies and functional assays of synthetic cathinone derivatives and other amphetamine-like agents, like the ones performed here, could be useful in evaluation of potential harmful short term and long term effects on various immune cells. In this study we observed significant changes in phosphorylation levels for several of the investigated signal transduction and cell stress proteins, but the changes were still modest. In order to evaluate more fully the impact of pharmacological substrates on cells of the immune system, the approach should be extended and involve analyses of immune cells following *in vivo* studies with experimental animals.

Conclusions

We report that the khat-derived cathinone and its derivatives generally reduced the levels of activating protein modifications of signal transducers and stress sensors in leukocytes, and that norephedrine increased *in vitro* T-lymphocyte proliferation. The closely structurally related compounds cathinone, cathine and norephedrine were seen to induce unique signaling signatures in leukocytes. Further, this study

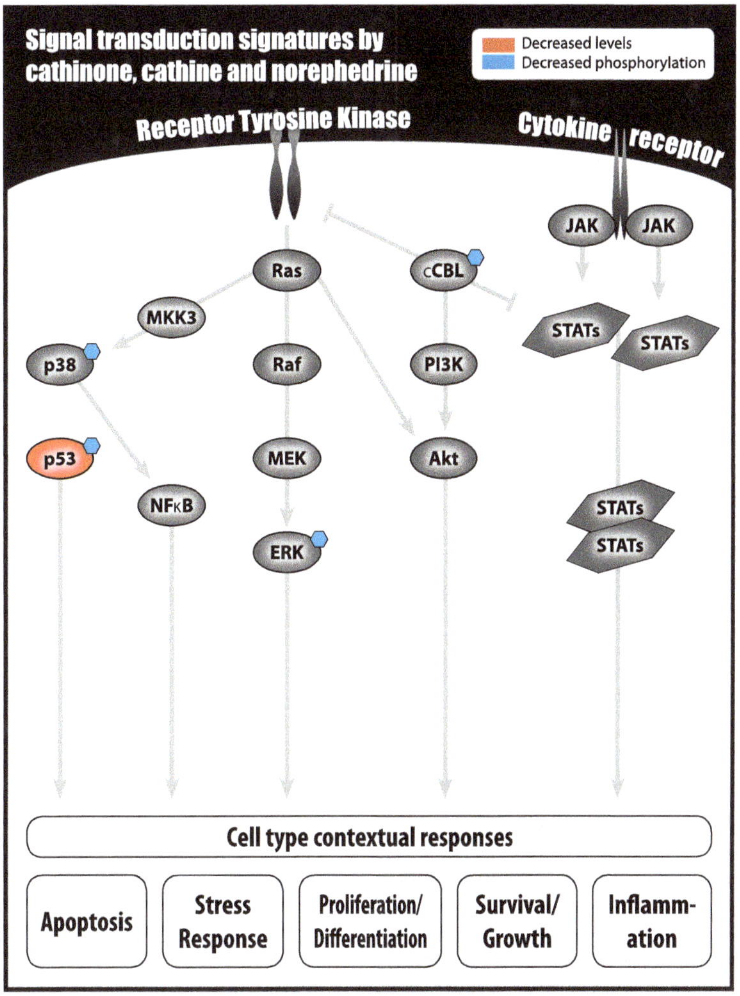

Figure 8 A summary of our present findings of cell signal transduction signatures in leukocytes stimulated with amphetamine-like cathinone, cathine or norephedrine.

confirmed that compounds in a botanical khat-extract activated cell stress sensors in immune cells and induced cytotoxic effects. Our results suggest that single-cell flow cytometric analysis of intracellular signaling pathways may be an informative and feasible approach when elucidating pharmacological effects and mechanisms of action in immune cells.

Methods

Blood donors

Blood was obtained from healthy donors from Department of Immunology and Transfusion Medicine, Haukeland University Hospital, Bergen, Norway. The blood donors used in the signal transduction analyses were 6 healthy individuals (4 females, 2 males) with a mean age of 38.2 years (range: 24–59). The use of blood for research purposes was approved by the local ethics committee REK (Regionale komiteer for medisinsk og helsefaglig forskningsettikk), Haukeland University Hospital, and samples collected after written consent by the blood donors, in accordance with the Declaration of Helsinki.

Cathinone, cathine and norephedrine

S-(−)-cathinone, (1S,2S)-(+)-norpseudoephedrine (cathine) and (1R,2S)-(−)-norephedrine were purchased from Sigma-Aldrich, and dissolved in DMSO (Sigma-Aldrich). These compounds were used in cell cultures at the concentration 10^{-4} M, and import and experiments were performed after written permission from The Norwegian Medicines Agency.

Khat-extract

Khat (asili cultivate) from the Meru district in Kenya was purchased in Nairobi, transported at 4°C under moist conditions, and the material was extracted within 48 hrs of harvest with methanol [30,33]. The khat-extract was prepared from approximately 200 g of khat, using the leaves and the soft parts of the twigs, which were chopped into pieces of approximately 5 mm length and submerged in methanol. The methanol extract was dried using a rotary evaporator, the semi-solid residue dissolved at a concentration of 0.2 g/ml in dimethylsulphoxide (DMSO; Sigma, St. Louis, MO, USA) and the stock solution stored at −80°C.

The stock solution was diluted in Roswell Park Memorial Institute (RPMI)-1640 medium (Sigma-Aldrich) with 10% fetal bovine serum (FBS), 2 mM L-glutamine and antibiotics (100 IU ml^{-1} penicillin and 100 µg ml^{-1} streptomycin; Gibco, Grand Island, NY, USA), and precipitates removed by centrifugation (10 000 g, 15 minutes, 4°C) [30]. The khat-extract supernatant was added experimental cell cultures giving final dilutions of 10^{-3} and 3.16×10^{-4}, based on previous studies [30]. All experimental cell cultures contained 0.1% DMSO.

Cathinone is relatively unstable, being transformed to cathine upon wilting of khat leaves, while being metabolized predominantly to norephedrine *in vivo* [3,4]. Cathinone, cathine and norephedrine are therefore suited as reference substances, indicating the freshness of the khat sample and the stability of the khat-extract. The concentrations of cathinone, cathine and norephedrine in the khat-extract were determined using high pressure liquid chromatography and mass spectrometry (HPLC-MS-MS), as previously described [30], and the values are displayed in Table 1, together with experimental cell culture concentrations.

In order to import and study khat, classified as an illegal narcotic substance in Norway, written permission was obtained from The Norwegian Medicines Agency (permission 01/705 of 2002-07-08).

Peripheral blood mononuclear cells

Peripheral blood mononuclear cells (PBMCs) were isolated from buffy coats using density gradient separation (Lymphoprep; Nycomed, Oslo, Norway; specific density 1.077), and resuspended at: (i) 1×10^6 cells ml^{-1} in X-vivo10® culture medium (BioWhittaker, Walkersville, MA, USA) with 100 µg ml^{-1} gentamicin for use in proliferation studies, (ii) 1×10^6 cells ml^{-1} in RPMI-1640 medium (10% FBS, L-glutamine, antibiotics) for studies on signal transduction, or (iii) 200 000 cells ml^{-1} in RPMI-1640 medium (10% FBS, L-glutamine, antibiotics) when determining apoptosis.

Annexin V-fluorescein isothiocyanate (FITC)/propidium iodide (PI) staining

When determining apoptosis, the PBMCs were stained with Annexin V-FITC and PI, using the Apoptest™ kit from Nexins Research (Hoeven, the Netherlands) according to the manufacturer's protocol. Data were collected on a FACS Calibur flow cytometer (Becton Dickinson, BD, Immunocytometry Systems, San Jose, CA, USA) and analyzed with FlowJo 7.2.5 software (TreeStar Inc., Ashland, OR, USA).

Table 2 Antibodies used in this study

Antigen	Epitope	Clone	Conjugate	Manufacturer
AKT	p-Ser473	F29-763	Alexa Fluor® 647	BD
CREB	p-Ser133	J151-21	Alexa Fluor® 647	BD
p38	p-Thr180/p-Tyr182	36/p38	Alexa Fluor® 488	BD
ERK1/2	p-Thr202/p-Tyr204	20A	Alexa Fluor® 488	BD
STAT1	p-Tyr701	4a	Alexa Fluor® 647	BD
STAT3	p-Tyr705	4/P-STAT3	Alexa Fluor® 488	BD
STAT5	p-Tyr694	47	Alexa Fluor® 647	BD
STAT6	p-Tyr641	18/P-STAT6	Alexa Fluor® 647	BD
p53	aa 1-45	DO-7	FITC	BD
p53	p-Ser37	J159-641.79	Alexa Fluor® 647	BD
p53	p-Ser15	16G8	Alexa Fluor® 488	Cell Signaling Technologies
p53	ac-Lys382	L82-51	Alexa Fluor® 647	BD
NF-κB	p-Ser529	K10-895.12.50	Alexa Fluor® 488	BD
c-Cbl	p-Tyr700	47/c-Cbl	Alexa Fluor® 488	BD
CD3	CD3	SK7	PE-Cy7	BD
CD20	CD20	H1(FB1)	PerCP-Cy 5.5	BD
CD163	CD163	Mac2-158	PE	Trillium Diagnostics

^{3}H-thymidine proliferation assay

The assay used to determine *in vitro* lymphocyte proliferation is based on a whole blood protocol [45]. Experiments were performed in triplicates in 96-well plates, and each well added (i) 5 × 10^4 PBMCs; (ii) CD3 antibody (mouse IgE Moab; CLB-T3/4.E), final concentration 316 ng ml^{-1}; (iii) CD28 antibody (mouse IgG1 Moab, CLB-CD28/1), final concentration 842 ng ml^{-1}; and (iv) test compound (cathinone, cathine, norephedrine, khat-extract) or control medium. The cell cultures were incubated (37°C, 5% CO_2) for 3 days, added ^{3}H-thymidine (37 kBq per well; TRA 310, Amersham International, Amersham, UK), and nuclear radioactivity assayed on day four by liquid scintillation counting. Results are expressed as percent average counts per minute (CPMA) in treated cells relative to CPMA in controls: ($CPMA_{treated}$/$CPMA_{control}$) × 100. All CPMA values were >1000, indicating proliferating cells.

Intracellular staining of proteins and flow cytometric analyses

PBMCs were fixed in 1.6% paraformaldehyde, permeabilized with 100% methanol and stored at −80°C until flow cytometric analysis. To achieve high-throughput and to reduce costs, the PBMCs were barcoded [29], and intracellular proteins stained as previously described [46]. Data were collected on a FACS Fortessa (BD) and analyzed with Stanford CytoBank software (http://cytobank.stanford.edu/public/openid/). Median fluorescence intensity (MFI) values were used as basis for data analyses. Antibodies used are listed in Table 2.

Statistical and bioinformatical approaches

Heatmaps: Statistical comparisons were made using GraphPad PRISM (version 5.0, GraphPad Software, Inc., USA) software, with one-way analysis of variance (ANOVA) and Tukey's multiple comparison post-tests to determine significant differences. A Student's unpaired or paired t-test was employed when only two groups were compared. *Cluster analyses*: Analysis were performed using J-Express 2011 analysis suite (MolMine AS, Bergen, Norway) [47]. For each protein the mean fold change for the donors was calculated, for each leukocyte subset and each time point. Values were log(2) converted before unsupervised hierarchical clustering analyses were performed using Euclidean correlation with complete linkage.

Additional files

Additional file 1: Table S1. Levels of significance for the observed in vitro induced phosphorylation/acetylation alterations of all target molecules.

Additional file 2: Table S2. Levels of significance for the observed in vitro induced phosphorylation/acetylation alterations of p53.

Competing interests

The authors declare that they have no competing interests.

Authors' contributions

TB and EE conceived, designed and performed experiments, analyzed data and wrote the manuscript. BSE participated during experiments and performed statistical analyses. AS participated during experiments and performed flow cytometric analyses. HR performed statistical analyses. HJA, ACJ, OKV and ØB conceived and guided the study. BTG conceived and guided the study, and wrote the manuscript. All authors read and approved the final manuscript.

Acknowledgements

This work was supported by funding from the following grants: The Norwegian Cancer Society with Solveig and Ole Lunds Legacy, the Western Regional Norwegian Authority (Helse-Vest), and the Norwegian Research Council with Programme in Functional Genomics. The authors would like to thank Kåre Strønen for his valuable contribution to improve the figures.

Author details

[1]Department of Clinical Science, University of Bergen, Bergen, Norway. [2]Institute of Biomedical Laboratory Sciences, Bergen University College, Bergen, Norway. [3]Department of Internal Medicine, Haukeland University Hospital, Bergen, Norway. [4]Department of Head and Neck Surgery, Haukeland University Hospital, Bergen, Norway. [5]Department of Clinical Medicine, University of Bergen, Bergen, Norway. [6]Department of Pathology, Haukeland University Hospital, Bergen, Norway.

References

1. Al-Hebshi NN, Skaug N: **Khat (Catha edulis)-an updated review.** *Addict Biol* 2005, **10**(4):299–307.
2. Al-Motarreb A, Baker K, Broadley KJ: **Khat: pharmacological and medical aspects and its social use in Yemen.** *Phytother Res* 2002, **16**(5):403–413.
3. Kalix P: **Pharmacological properties of the stimulant khat.** *Pharmacol Ther* 1990, **48**(3):397–416.
4. Toennes SW, Kauert GF: **Excretion and detection of cathinone, cathine, and phenylpropanolamine in urine after kath chewing.** *Clin Chem* 2002, **48**(10):1715–1719.
5. Brenneisen R, Geisshulser S, Schorno X: **Merucathine, A New Phenylalkylamine from Catha edulis.** *Planta Med* 1984, **50**(6):531.
6. Crombie L: **The cathedulin alkaloids.** *Bull Narc* 1980, **32**(3):37–50.
7. Halbach H: **Medical aspects of the chewing of khat leaves.** *Bull World Health Organ* 1972, **47**(1):21–29.
8. Toennes SW, Harder S, Schramm M, Niess C, Kauert GF: **Pharmacokinetics of cathinone, cathine and norephedrine after the chewing of khat leaves.** *Br J Clin Pharmacol* 2003, **56**(1):125–130.
9. Cleary L, Docherty JR: **Actions of amphetamine derivatives and cathinone at the noradrenaline transporter.** *Eur J Pharmacol* 2003, **476**(1–2):31–34.
10. Rothman RB, Vu N, Partilla JS, Roth BL, Hufeisen SJ, Compton-Toth BA, Birkes J, Young R, Glennon RA: **In vitro characterization of ephedrine-related stereoisomers at biogenic amine transporters and the receptorome reveals selective actions as norepinephrine transporter substrates.** *J Pharmacol Exp Ther* 2003, **307**(1):138–145.
11. Glennon RA, Liebowitz SM: **Serotonin receptor affinity of cathinone and related analogues.** *J Med Chem* 1982, **25**(4):393–397.
12. Hassan NA, Gunaid AA, El-Khally FM, Al-Noami MY, Murray-Lyon IM: **Khat chewing and arterial blood pressure. A randomized controlled clinical trial of alpha-1 and selective beta-1 adrenoceptor blockade.** *Saudi Med J* 2005, **26**(4):537–541.
13. Nasher AA, Qirbi AA, Ghafoor MA, Catterall A, Thompson A, Ramsay JW, Murray-Lyon IM: **Khat chewing and bladder neck dysfunction. A randomized controlled trial of alpha 1-adrenergic blockade.** *Br J Urol* 1995, **75**(5):597–598.

14. Gordon J, Barnes NM: **Lymphocytes transport serotonin and dopamine: agony or ecstasy?** *Trends Immunol* 2003, **24**(8):438–443.
15. Meredith EJ, Chamba A, Holder MJ, Barnes NM, Gordon J: **Close encounters of the monoamine kind: immune cells betray their nervous disposition.** *Immunology* 2005, **115**(3):289–295.
16. Josefsson E, Bergquist J, Ekman R, Tarkowski A: **Catecholamines are synthesized by mouse lymphocytes and regulate function of these cells by induction of apoptosis.** *Immunology* 1996, **88**(1):140–146.
17. Bergquist J, Silberring J: **Identification of catecholamines in the immune system by electrospray ionization mass spectrometry.** *Rapid Commun Mass Spectrom* 1998, **12**(11):683–688.
18. Mata S, Urbina M, Manzano E, Ortiz T, Lima L: **Noradrenaline transporter and its turnover rate are decreased in blood lymphocytes of patients with major depression.** *J Neuroimmunol* 2005, **170**(1–2):134–140.
19. Boyle NT, Connor TJ: **Methylenedioxymethamphetamine ('Ecstasy')-induced immunosuppression: a cause for concern?** *Br J Pharmacol* 2010, **161**(1):17–32.
20. House RV, Thomas PT, Bhargava HN: **Comparison of immune functional parameters following in vitro exposure to natural and synthetic amphetamines.** *Immunopharmacol Immunotoxicol* 1994, **16**(1):1–21.
21. Freire-Garabal M, Nunez MJ, Balboa JL, Fernandez-Rial JC, Belmonte A: **Effects of amphetamine on the activity of phagocytosis in mice.** *Life Sci* 1992, **51**(15):PL145–PL148.
22. McAlees JW, Sanders VM: **Hematopoietic protein tyrosine phosphatase mediates beta2-adrenergic receptor-induced regulation of p38 mitogen-activated protein kinase in B lymphocytes.** *Mol Cell Biol* 2009, **29**(3):675–686.
23. Lajevic MD, Suleiman S, Cohen RL, Chambers DA: **Activation of p38 mitogen-activated protein kinase by norepinephrine in T-lineage cells.** *Immunology* 2011, **132**(2):197–208.
24. Leon-Ponte M, Ahern GP, O'Connell PJ: **Serotonin provides an accessory signal to enhance T-cell activation by signaling through the 5-HT7 receptor.** *Blood* 2007, **109**(8):3139–3146.
25. Huang Y, Qiu AW, Peng YP, Liu Y, Huang HW, Qiu YH: **Roles of dopamine receptor subtypes in mediating modulation of T lymphocyte function.** *Neuro Endocrinol Lett* 2010, **31**(6):782–791.
26. Lukandu OM, Costea DE, Dimba EA, Neppelberg E, Bredholt T, Gjertsen BT, Vintermyr OK, Johannessen AC: **Khat induces G1-phase arrest and increased expression of stress-sensitive p53 and p16 proteins in normal human oral keratinocytes and fibroblasts.** *Eur J Oral Sci* 2008, **116**(1):23–30.
27. Sachs K, Perez O, Pe'er D, Lauffenburger DA, Nolan GP: **Causal protein-signaling networks derived from multiparameter single-cell data.** *Science* 2005, **308**(5721):523–529.
28. Krutzik PO, Crane JM, Clutter MR, Nolan GP: **High-content single-cell drug screening with phosphospecific flow cytometry.** *Nat Chem Biol* 2008, **4**(2):132–142.
29. Krutzik PO, Nolan GP: **Fluorescent cell barcoding in flow cytometry allows high-throughput drug screening and signaling profiling.** *Nat Methods* 2006, **3**(5):361–368.
30. Bredholt T, Dimba EA, Hagland HR, Wergeland L, Skavland J, Fossan KO, Tronstad KJ, Johannessen AC, Vintermyr OK, Gjertsen BT: **Camptothecin and khat (Catha edulis Forsk.) induced distinct cell death phenotypes involving modulation of c-FLIPL, Mcl-1, procaspase-8 and mitochondrial function in acute myeloid leukemia cell lines.** *Mol Cancer* 2009, **8**:101.
31. Lukandu OM, Costea DE, Neppelberg E, Johannessen AC, Vintermyr OK: **Khat (Catha edulis) induces reactive oxygen species and apoptosis in normal human oral keratinocytes and fibroblasts.** *Toxicol Sci* 2008, **103** (2):311–324.
32. Murdoch C, Aziz HA, Fang HY, Jezan H, Musaid R, Muthana M: **Khat (Catha edulis) alters the phenotype and anti-microbial activity of peripheral blood mononuclear cells.** *J Ethnopharmacol* 2011, **138**(3):780–787.
33. Dimba EA, Gjertsen BT, Bredholt T, Fossan KO, Costea DE, Francis GW, Johannessen AC, Vintermyr OK: **Khat (Catha edulis)-induced apoptosis is inhibited by antagonists of caspase-1 and −8 in human leukaemia cells.** *Br J Cancer* 2004, **91**(9):1726–1734.
34. Aleryani SL, Aleryani RA, Al-Akwa AA: **Khat a drug of abuse: roles of free radicals and antioxidants.** *Drug Test Anal* 2011, **3**(9):548–551.
35. Maillet A, Pervaiz S: **Redox regulation of p53, redox effectors regulated by p53: a subtle balance.** *Antioxid Redox Signal* 2012, **16**(11):1285–1294.
36. Matsuzawa A, Ichijo H: **Redox control of cell fate by MAP kinase: physiological roles of ASK1-MAP kinase pathway in stress signaling.** *Biochim Biophys Acta* 2008, **1780**(11):1325–1336.
37. Lukandu OM, Neppelberg E, Vintermyr OK, Johannessen AC, Costea DE: **Khat alters the phenotype of in vitro-reconstructed human oral mucosa.** *J Dent Res* 2010, **89**(3):270–275.
38. Baldys A, Raymond JR: **Role of c-Cbl carboxyl terminus in serotonin 5-HT2A receptor recycling and resensitization.** *J Biol Chem* 2011, **286**(28):24656–24665.
39. Beaulieu JM, Sotnikova TD, Marion S, Lefkowitz RJ, Gainetdinov RR, Caron MG: **An Akt/beta-arrestin 2/PP2A signaling complex mediates dopaminergic neurotransmission and behavior.** *Cell* 2005, **122**(2):261–273.
40. Beaulieu JM, Sotnikova TD, Yao WD, Kockeritz L, Woodgett JR, Gainetdinov RR, Caron MG: **Lithium antagonizes dopamine-dependent behaviors mediated by an AKT/glycogen synthase kinase 3 signaling cascade.** *Proc Natl Acad Sci U S A* 2004, **101**(14):5099–5104.
41. Bedel R, Thiery-Vuillemin A, Grandclement C, Balland J, Remy-Martin JP, Kantelip B, Pallandre JR, Pivot X, Ferrand C, Tiberghien P, *et al*: **Novel role for STAT3 in transcriptional regulation of NK immune cell targeting receptor MICA on cancer cells.** *Cancer Res* 2011, **71**(5):1615–1626.
42. Jia JJ, Zeng XS, Li Y, Ma S, Bai J: **Ephedrine induced thioredoxin-1 expression through beta-adrenergic receptor/cyclic AMP/protein kinase A/dopamine- and cyclic AMP-regulated phosphoprotein signaling pathway.** *Cell Signal* 2013, **25**(5):1194–1201.
43. McKenna F, McLaughlin PJ, Lewis BJ, Sibbring GC, Cummerson JA, Bowen-Jones D, Moots RJ: **Dopamine receptor expression on human T- and B-lymphocytes, monocytes, neutrophils, eosinophils and NK cells: a flow cytometric study.** *J Neuroimmunol* 2002, **132**(1–2):34–40.
44. Morris K: **UK places generic ban on mephedrone drug family.** *Lancet* 2010, **375**(9723):1333–1334.
45. Wendelbo O, Bruserud O: **Functional evaluation of proliferative T cell responses in patients with severe T lymphopenia: characterization of optimal culture conditions and standardized activation signals for a simple whole blood assay.** *J Hematother Stem Cell Res* 2003, **12**(5):525–535.
46. Irish JM, Anensen N, Hovland R, Skavland J, Borresen-Dale AL, Bruserud O, Nolan GP, Gjertsen BT: **Flt3 Y591 duplication and Bcl-2 overexpression are detected in acute myeloid leukemia cells with high levels of phosphorylated wild-type p53.** *Blood* 2007, **109**(6):2589–2596.
47. Stavrum AK, Petersen K, Jonassen I, Dysvik B: **Analysis of gene-expression data using J-Express.** *Curr Protoc Bioinformatics* 2008:. **Chapter 7**:Unit 7 3.

12

Conditional disruption of interactions between $G\alpha_{i2}$ and regulator of G protein signaling (RGS) proteins protects the heart from ischemic injury

Sergio Parra[1], Xinyan Huang[1], Raelene A Charbeneau[1], Susan M Wade[1], Kuljeet Kaur[1], Boyd R Rorabaugh[2*] and Richard R Neubig[3*]

Abstract

Background: Regulator of G protein signaling (RGS) proteins suppress G protein coupled receptor signaling by catalyzing the hydrolysis of Gα-bound guanine nucleotide triphosphate. Transgenic mice in which RGS-mediated regulation of $G\alpha_{i2}$ is lost (RGS insensitive $G\alpha_{i2}^{G184S}$) exhibit beneficial (protection against ischemic injury) and detrimental (enhanced fibrosis) cardiac phenotypes. This mouse model has revealed the physiological significance of RGS/$G\alpha_{i2}$ interactions. Previous studies of the $G\alpha_{i2}^{G184S}$ mutation used mice that express this mutant protein throughout their lives. Thus, it is unclear whether these phenotypes result from chronic or acute $G\alpha_{i2}^{G184S}$ expression. We addressed this issue by developing mice that conditionally express $G\alpha_{i2}^{G184S}$.

Methods: Mice that conditionally express RGS insensitive $G\alpha_{i2}^{G184S}$ were generated using a floxed minigene strategy. Conditional expression of $G\alpha_{i2}^{G184S}$ was characterized by reverse transcription polymerase chain reaction and by enhancement of agonist-induced inhibition of cAMP production in isolated cardiac fibroblasts. The impact of conditional RGS insensitive $G\alpha_{i2}^{G184S}$ expression on ischemic injury was assessed by measuring contractile recovery and infarct sizes in isolated hearts subjected to 30 min ischemia and 2 hours reperfusion.

Results: We demonstrate tamoxifen-dependent expression of $G\alpha_{i2}^{G184S}$, enhanced inhibition of cAMP production, and cardioprotection from ischemic injury in hearts conditionally expressing $G\alpha_{i2}^{G184S}$. Thus the cardioprotective phenotype previously reported in mice expressing $G\alpha_{i2}^{G184S}$ does not require embryonic or chronic $G\alpha_{i2}^{G184S}$ expression. Rather, cardioprotection occurs following acute (days rather than months) expression of $G\alpha_{i2}^{G184S}$.

Conclusions: These data suggest that RGS proteins might provide new therapeutic targets to protect the heart from ischemic injury. We anticipate that this model will be valuable for understanding the time course (chronic versus acute) and mechanisms of other phenotypic changes that occur following disruption of interactions between $G\alpha_{i2}$ and RGS proteins.

Keywords: G protein coupled receptors, Ischemia-reperfusion, Cre-*LoxP*, Mutation, cAMP inhibition, Regulator of G protein signaling, RGS

* Correspondence: b-rorabaugh@onu.edu; rneubig@msu.edu
[2]Department of Pharmaceutical and Biomedical Sciences, Ohio Northern University College of Pharmacy, Ada, OH 45810, USA
[3]Department of Pharmacology and Toxicology, B440 Life Sciences, Michigan State University, 1355 Bogue St, East Lansing, MI 48824, USA
Full list of author information is available at the end of the article

Background

G protein coupled receptor signaling is mediated by four major families of G proteins ($G\alpha_s$, $G\alpha_{i/o}$, $G\alpha_q$, and $G\alpha_{12}$). $G\alpha_i$ coupled receptors play important roles in regulating inflammation, cardiovascular function, endocrine signaling, drug abuse, and anxiety/depression – related behaviors [1-5]. Three different $G\alpha_i$- isoforms ($G\alpha_{i1}$, $G\alpha_{i2}$, $G\alpha_{i3}$) have been cloned and characterized. Gαi/o-coupled responses can be distinguished from responses mediated by other families of G proteins by their sensitivity to pertussis toxin, but the *in vivo* roles of individual $G\alpha_{i/o}$ isoforms remain obscure.

Signaling through $G\alpha_i$ is suppressed by regulator of G protein signaling (RGS) proteins which terminate $G\alpha_i$ signaling by accelerating the hydrolysis of Gα-bound guanine nucleotide triphosphate (GTP) [6,7]. More than 20 different RGS proteins have been identified. However identifying the physiological roles of individual RGS proteins through selective pharmacological inhibition is not yet possible. Knockout mouse models in which individual RGS proteins have been genetically deleted have been useful in identifying the functions of some RGS proteins, but this approach is complicated by the potential for compensation of the lost RGS protein by other RGS proteins that may have redundant functions. Consequently, we have exploited a mutation in $G\alpha_{i2}$ ($G\alpha_{i2}{}^{G184S}$) that blocks RGS binding and activity [8]. This allows us to define the functions of this individual $G\alpha_i$-isoform and to explore the physiological roles of interactions between $G\alpha_{i2}$ and endogenous RGS proteins [8,9]. Knock-in mice expressing $G\alpha_{i2}^{G184S}$ show enhanced receptor-dependent signaling through $G\alpha_{i2}$ [8,9], and they exhibit a number of interesting cardiac phenotype changes including enhanced carbachol-induced bradycardia, enhanced isoproterenol-induced cardiac fibrosis, and premature death in a dilated cardiomyopathy model [8-12]. Hearts from both homozygous and heterozygous $G\alpha_{i2}{}^{G184S}$ mutant mice also exhibit smaller infarcts and better recovery of cardiac contractile function following an ischemic insult [13]. Genetic disruption of interactions between $G\alpha_{i2}$ and endogenous RGS proteins also produces several noncardiac phenotypic changes including antidepressant-like behavior [5], resistance to high fat diet-induced weight gain, decreased body fat, and protection from the development of insulin resistance [14].

One limitation of this transgenic model is that the $G\alpha_{i2}{}^{G184S}$ mutation is chronically expressed throughout the prenatal and postnatal life of the animal. Thus, it is unclear whether the phenotypes that have been reported result from changes during embryological development and whether the phenotypes require chronic or only acute disruption of interactions between $G\alpha_{i2}$ and endogenous RGS proteins. In the present study, we addressed this issue by creating a conditional knock-in mouse model that conditionally expresses RGS insensitive $G\alpha_{i2}{}^{G184S}$. This study focused on the ability of acute $G\alpha_{i2}{}^{G184S}$ expression to protect the heart from ischemic injury.

Methods

Gene targeting

All protocols and procedures were approved by the University Committee on Use and Care of Animals at the University of Michigan and by the Animal Care and Use Committee of Ohio Northern University. Experimental procedures and animal husbandry were conducted in accordance with NIH guidelines. Animals were housed in a specific pathogen free facility with a 12 hour: 12 hour light: dark cycle and free access to food and water. Mice expressing RGS-insensitive $G\alpha_{i2}{}^{G184S}$ were generated by a "floxed minigene" strategy [15,16]. The targeting construct to create the conditional knock-in of the G184S mutation at $G\alpha_{i2}$ (Figure 1A) was generated from a 129 BAC library in a manner similar to that previously described for the conventional $G\alpha_{i2}{}^{G184S}$ knock-in mutant mice [11]. Elements included: a 6.4 kb 5' homology arm containing the endogenous Gnai2 sequence encompassing exons 2 to 4, a minigene version of the wild type Gnai2 gene composed of the fused exons 5 to 8, intron 8 and exon 9 (this *Gnai2* wild-type minigene was flanked with *loxP* sites allowing its deletion under the action of the Cre recombinase), the mutated exon 5 containing the G184S mutation (GGGC to TAGT mutation in position 85 in exon 5), a neo selection cassette flanked with FRT sites allowing its deletion under the Flp recombinase action, and a 2.4 kb 3' homology arm containing the endogenous Gnai2 sequence encompassing exons 6 to 9 and sequence located downstream of the gene. In addition, AflII and SacI restriction sites were inserted in the 5' homology arm at the BstEII site between Exon 4 and the 5' *loxP* site to be used for Southern blot analysis of the targeted ES cells. A Thymidine Kinase (TK) negative selection marker was inserted upstream of the 5' homology arm. ES cells (5×10^6 cells - SV129 strain) were electroporated (GenOway; Lyon, France) with 40 μg of linearized plasmid and selection started 48 hours later with 200 ug/ml of G418 followed by selection in GANIX to enhance the likelihood of homologous recombination. Targeted cells were identified by 3' genomic PCR. Of the 23 positive clones, five also showed the appropriate presence of the AflII/SacI restriction site on 5' PCR. All five were confirmed by 5' and 3' Southern Blot analysis (13.0 kb EcoNI fragment and 11.5 kb AflII fragment, respectively) (GenOway; Lyon, France).

Mouse generation

Three independent embryonic stem (ES) cell lines with normal karyotype were used for blastocyst injection into C57BL/6J host blastocysts. Highly chimeric males were bred to C57BL/6J female mice and F1 agouti offspring

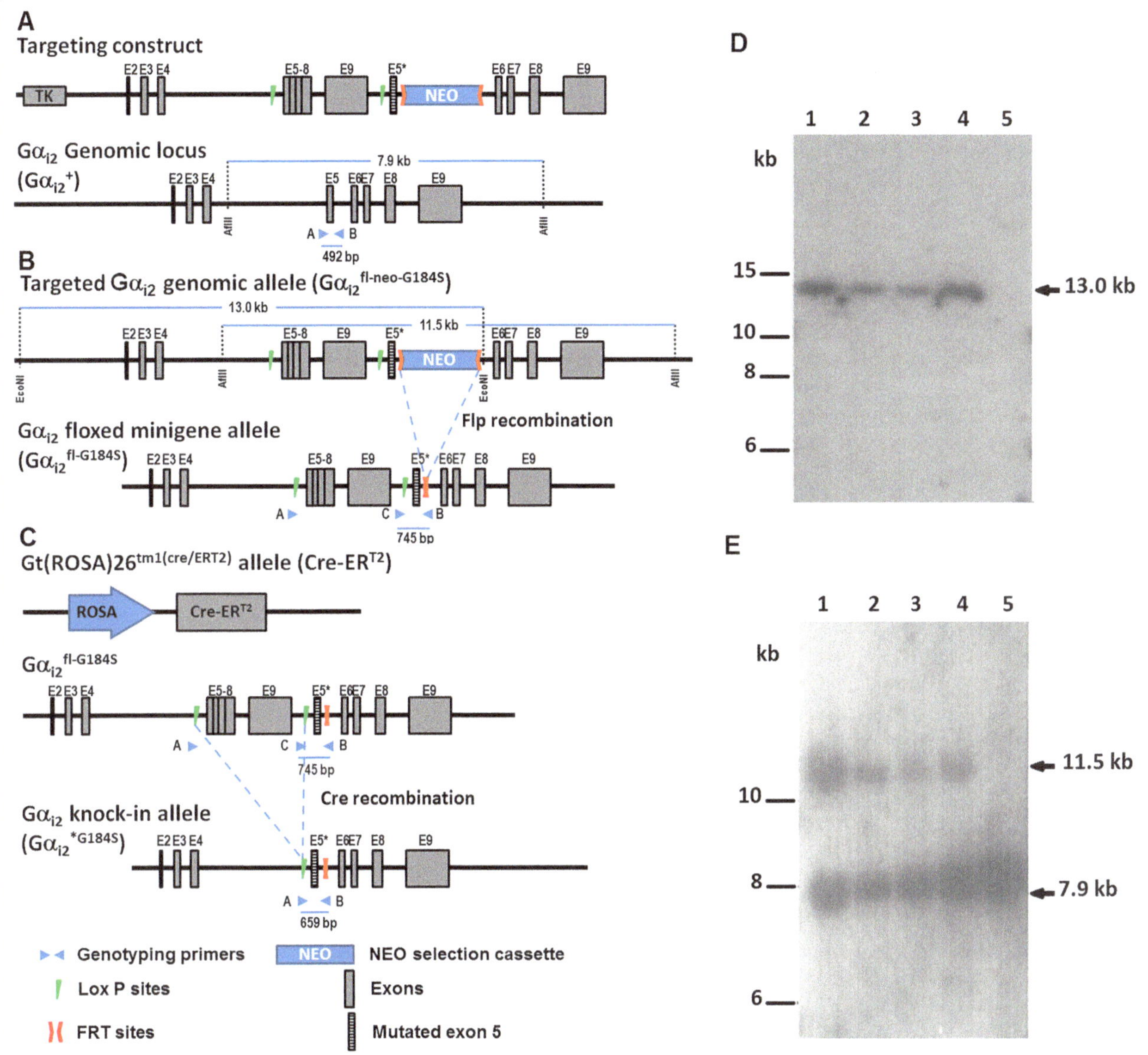

Figure 1 Floxed mini-gene targeting strategy for the generation of conditional "knock-in" of $G\alpha_{i2}^{*G184S}$ allele. A Exon 5 of the genomic locus of the gene Gnai2 was replaced by homologous recombination using a vector containing a G184S mutant Exon 5 (E5*) with a 3′ extension containing Flp Recombinase Target (FRT)-sites (red chevrons) flanking a neo selection cassette and a 5′ extension with Lox P sites (green triangles) flanking a minigene containing wild-type E5-9. **B** After introduction of the targeting vector, the neo marker is removed by breeding the $G\alpha_{i2}^{fl\text{-}neo\text{-}G184S}$ positive mice with transgenic Flp recombinase expressing animals. **C** To generate whole-body $G\alpha_{i2}^{*G184S}$ conditional knock-in mice, transgenic mice carrying tamoxifen-sensitive, Cre-ER^{T2} gene driven by the Gt(ROSA)26Sor^{tm1} (ROSA) promoter were bred with $G\alpha_{i2}^{fl/fl\text{-}G184S}$ mice. After tamoxifen administration there is recombination of genomic Lox P sites which leads to removal of the E5-9 minigene and the mutant E5* is positioned in the normal Gnai2 gene to express the $G\alpha_{i2}{}^{*G184S}$ mutant allele. **D** Southern blot analysis of ES cell genomic DNA following digestion with EcoNI and hybridization with the 5′-Neo probe to screen for 5′ homologous recombination event. **E** Southern blot verification analysis of ES cell genomic DNA following digestion with AflII and hybridization with an external 3′ probe. In figures *d* and *e* lanes 1 to 4 are correctly targeted ES cell clones, lane 5 is a non-targeted (WT) ES cell clone.

mice were genotyped by PCR and Southern blot hybridization to validate germline transmission (GenOway; Lyon, France). To delete the FRT-flanked neo gene, offspring showing the presence of the $G\alpha_{i2}^{+/fl\text{-}neo\text{-}G184S}$ allele by genomic PCR were crossed against beta-actin FLPe mice (from the University of Michigan Transgenic Animal Model Core). Litters from this cross were analyzed for the presence of the FLP transgene as well as $G\alpha_{i2}$ genotypes by genomic PCR. FLP/$G\alpha_{i2}^{+/fl\text{-}G184S}$ mice lacking the neo cassette were backcrossed onto the C57BL/6J strain to eliminate the FLPe gene. To generate whole-body $G\alpha_{i2}^{G184S}$ conditional knock-in mice, transgenic mice carrying the tamoxifen-sensitive, Cre-ER^{T2} gene driven by the ROSA26 promoter (The Jackson Laboratory; Bar

Harbor, ME) were bred with $G\alpha_{i2}{}^{fl\text{-}G184S/fl\text{-}G184S}$ mice. All mice used in this study have been backcrossed for five generations onto the C57BL/6J strain. They were between 8 – 20 weeks old and the number for each experiment is indicated in the figure legends. Animals were maintained in a specific pathogen-free facility with a 12-h light/dark cycle and fed standard laboratory chow and water ad libitum.

Genotyping

Genomic DNA was isolated from mouse tail using the HotSHOT method [17] and analyzed in a single PCR reaction using two forward primers A and C (GAGCCCA TGTTTCTTAAAGAAGCAAGGATA and TCCCACAC CTTAGTGCCACACCT, respectively) and reverse primer B (TGAGGACATGCCTTCCCAACACAAT), which amplify the $G\alpha_{i2}{}^{+}$ (492-bp) and $G\alpha_{i2}{}^{fl\text{-}G184S}$ (745-bp) alleles, respectively.

Tamoxifen preparation and treatment

Tamoxifen (Sigma, T5648) was prepared in peanut oil (Sigma, P2144) containing 10% ethanol at a concentration of 60 mg/ml [16]. Daily doses of 50 mg/kg over five days were given by intraperitoneal injection to induce recombination. Control mice were treated with vehicle (90% peanut oil/10% ethanol) alone.

Blood and tissue collection

Blood was withdrawn from the saphenous vein into dipotassium ethylenediamine tetraacetic acid -coated microtubes before the first and 72 hours after the last dose of tamoxifen and then stored at -80°C until processing for analysis. Mice were euthanized by pentobarbital injection and tissues were quickly removed, snap-frozen in liquid nitrogen, and stored at -80°C until analysis.

Recombination assessment

Qualitative assessment for recombination, before and after tamoxifen treatment, was performed by polymerase chain reaction (PCR) using genomic DNA isolated from whole blood and tissue samples from genotyped mice carrying one copy of the ROSA Cre-ER^{T2} gene and the indicated $G\alpha_{i2}$ alleles ($G\alpha_{i2}{}^{+/+}$or $G\alpha_{i2)}{}^{G184S}$ was amplified by using forward primer A and reverse primer B described above. This PCR reaction generates a 659-bp band only after Cre recombination. PCR reactions for testing genotype and recombination were carried out under the following conditions: 95°C for 5 min, 35 cycles at 95°C, and 64.5°C each for 30 s, followed by extension at 72°C for 1 min and final extension at 72°C for 2 min.

Western blotting

Tissues were dissected and homogenized in a Bullet Blender homogenizer (Next Advance; Averill Park, NY) with RIPA buffer containing protease inhibitors (20 mM Tris-HCl, pH7.4, 150 mM NaCl, 1 mM EDTA, 1 mM β-glycerophospate, 1% Triton X-100, 0.1% SDS, Complete protease inhibitor cocktail (Roche; Pleasanton, CA). Protein concentrations were measured using the BCA Protein Assay kit (Thermo Fisher Scientific; Rockford, IL). Eighty micrograms of protein were separated on a denaturing 12% SDS–PAGE gel and transferred to PVDF membrane. The membranes were washed, blocked (5% milk in PBS-T), and incubated in the appropriate antibodies overnight at 4°C. Antibodies for Western blot analysis: rabbit anti-$G\alpha_{i2}$ (a gift from Dr. Susanne Mumby, University of Texas Southwestern Medical Center) at a dilution of 1:1000 and mouse anti-GAPDH (Cell Signaling Technology, Danvers, MA), as loading control, at a dilution of 1:5000. Secondary antibodies were horseradish peroxidase conjugated. Visualization of the protein bands was done using the Super Signal West Pico chemiluminescent substrate (Thermo Fisher Scientific, Rockford, IL). Films were scanned and quantified using Image J software (NIH, Bethesda, MD). All samples were normalized with GAPDH as a loading control and the amount of $G\alpha_{i2}$ protein in wild type tissue was set to 100%.

Allele ratio conversion

RNA was isolated from whole blood, heart, brain, and kidney using a commercial kit (Qiagen, Valencia, CA), and reverse transcription was carried out using Reverse Transcription reagents (Applied Biosystems). PCR was performed using a set of primers that amplify a 442–base pair segment of $G\alpha_{i2}$ cDNA including both wildtype and $G\alpha_{i2}{}^{G184S}$. The primers used were CCAGCGTGCGGAT GATGCC and GATGAGGAGATGAACCGCATGCAT. The cDNA PCR products obtained for each sample were purified (Qiagen, Valencia, CA), and directly sequenced on an ABI 3730XL using the forward primer used for amplification of $G\alpha_{i2}$ in PCR. The allelic expression ratio of mutant $G\alpha_{i2}{}^{G184S}$ to wildtype $G\alpha_{i2}$ in mice was determined from the chromatogram peak heights of the bases differentiating between the $G\alpha_{i2}{}^{G184S}$ mutant and wildtype $G\alpha_{i2}$ alleles. Peak heights were determined using Image J software and mutant allele expression was calculated using the formula: % mutant allele expression = (T + A + T-peak heights)/((T + A + T-peak heights) + (G + G + C-peak heights)) X 100. If any of the peaks of the mutant or the wild type sequence were not detected in the chromatogram the sample was considered 100% wild type or 100% mutant, respectively.

Adult cardiac fibroblast culture

Adult cardiac fibroblasts (ACF) were isolated from mice as previously described [12,18]. Hearts were quickly isolated, placed in ice-cold perfusion buffer, and then perfused via an aortic cannula for 4 min with calcium-free perfusion buffer (NaCl, 113 mM; KCl, 4.7 mM; $MgSO_4$-$7H_2O$, 1.2 mM; Na_2HPO_4, 0.6 mM; KH_2PO4, 0.6 mM; phenol red, 0.032 mM; HEPES, 10 mM; $NaHCO_3$, 12 mM; $KHCO_3$, 10 mM; taurine, 30 mM; glucose, 5.5 mM; and butanedione monoxime, 10 mM, pH 7.46). Hearts were then perfused for 8 min with the same buffer containing 0.5 mg/ml collagenase II (Worthington Biochemicals, Lakewood) and 1.25 μM $CaCl_2$. Hearts were removed from the apparatus and the ventricles were suspended in perfusion buffer with collagenase and 1.25 μM $CaCl_2$. The tissue was disrupted with fine forceps and by gentle pipetting. Cells were transferred to buffer containing 1.25 μM CaCl2 and 10% serum to stop the digestion. Samples were centrifuged at 180×g for 1 min to remove debris and myocytes. The remaining suspended fibroblasts were centrifuged at 300 × g for 10 min, then resuspended in phosphate buffered saline, centrifuged again, the supernatant was discarded, and the final cell pellet was resuspended in Dulbecco's modified Eagle's medium supplemented with 1% penicillin/streptomycin, insulin/transferrin/selenium (ITS from Sigma) 1X, and 10% fetal bovine serum.

cAMP production in adult cardiac fibroblasts

The effect of lysophosphatidic acid (LPA) on 3′,5′ cyclic adenosine monophosphate (cAMP) production in ACF was determined in 384-well plates using the Lance Ultra cAMP kit (PerkinElmer; Waltham, MA). Briefly, ACF (passage 2) were added at 1,000 cells per well and cAMP accumulation was initiated by adding stimulation buffer containing 0.5 mM isobutyl-1-methylxanthine and 10 μM forskolin with the indicated concentrations of LPA. After 30 min at room temperature, the reaction was stopped by lysing the cells using the buffer supplied with the PerkinElmer kit. Time-resolved fluorescence was measured with a Synergy 2 (BioTek; Winooski, VT) microplate reader.

Langendorff isolated heart preparation and infarct size measurement

Mice were treated with tamoxifen or vehicle for 5 days as described above. Fourteen days after the first injection, mice were anesthetized and heparinized by a single injection containing pentobarbital (100 mg/kg) and heparin (150 mg/kg). Hearts were immediately excised and cannulated while bathed in ice-cold Krebs solution. Krebs solution was perfused through the aortic cannula at a constant pressure of 75 mmHg. Hearts were subjected to 30 minutes of ischemia and 2 hours reperfusion as previously described [13]. Contractile function of the left ventricle was continuously measured using an intraventricular balloon and infarct size was measured by triphenyltetrazolium chloride staining as described previously [13].

Statistical analyses

Data were analyzed using one-way or two-way analysis of variance, followed by a Bonferroni's post test or a Tukey's post test when appropriate. GraphPad Prism version 4.0 (GraphPad Software, San Diego, CA) was used for statistical analysis.

Results

To implement a conditional knock-in strategy, a replacement-type minigene targeting vector was used to modify the Gnai2 gene as depicted in Figure 1A-C. This construct was designed to (1) flank an exon 5 through 9 minigene with *loxP* recombination recognition sites, (2) insert a neomycin selection cassette that was flanked by FRT recombination sites downstream of the floxed wild type $G\alpha_{i2}$ coding and regulatory sequences, and (3) replace the wildtype genomic exon 5 with the G184S mutant version followed by the remainder of the wildtype $G\alpha_{i2}$ sequence in the normal genomic context. Because of size constraints on the cloning vector used to create the targeting construct, exons 5 through 8 were fused and introns 5-7 were deleted. Intron 8 and non-coding exon 9 were retained due to the presence of regulatory elements. The knock-in mutation was introduced into the genomic exon 5 to change the codon for glycine 184 to serine (Figure 1A). Following electroporation of the targeting construct into embryonic stem cells, G418-resistant ES cell clones were screened for gene targeting by PCR and confirmed by Southern blot analysis. Blots were hybridized to 5' and 3' probes. After genomic DNA digestion with EcoNI, the 5' probe hybridized with a 13.0 kb fragment generated from a recombinant $Ga_{i2}{}^{G184S}$ allele (Figure 1D). This was confirmed by blotting with a 3' probe after genomic DNA digestion with AflII. This probe hybridized to a 7.9 kb fragment from the wild type Ga^{i2} allele and an 11.5 kb fragment from a $Ga_{i2}{}^{G184S}$ allele (Figure 1E). One ES cell clone was not targeted (lane 5) and four clones were correctly targeted (lanes 1 to 4). Three targeted ES cell clones with normal karyotype were used to produce germline-competent chimeric mice using standard techniques. After FLP recombinase crosses, mice that were heterozygous for the targeted locus without the neomycin cassette ($^{fl\text{-}G184S}$ allele) were subsequently backcrossed with C57BL/6J mice to eliminate the beta-actin FLP transgene. Figure 2A shows representative results from the PCR screening used to select mice with the desired genotype.

To demonstrate a global, time-dependent, and Cre-mediated conversion of the conditional allele ($^{fl\text{-}G184S}$) to the RGS insensitive allele (^{G184S}), we crossed mice that were homozygous for the fl-G184S allele ($G\alpha_{i2}{}^{fl\text{-}G184S/fl\text{-}G184S}$) mice with a tamoxifen-dependent Cre general deleter mouse line [19-21]. This line expresses a tamoxifen-sensitive Cre (Cre-ER^{T2}) from the ROSA26 locus

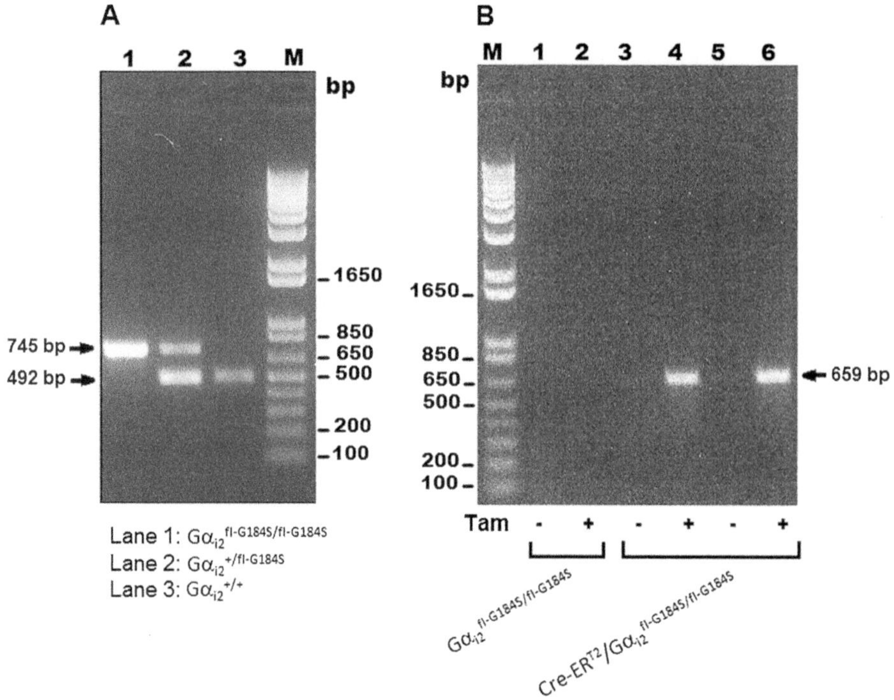

Figure 2 Representative agarose gel images assessing genotypes and recombination in mice. A PCR genotyping was done simultaneously using three primers A, B, and C from Figure 1. A 492-bp band represents the wild-type Gnai2 allele and the 745-bp band represents the Gnai2 fl-G184S conditional allele after removal of the *neo* cassette. **B** Genomic DNA extracted from blood was amplified before and after tamoxifen treatment. Lanes 1 and 2 were from Cre negative $G\alpha^{fl\text{-}G184S/fl\text{-}G184S}$ mice while lanes 3-6 were from Cre-ER^{T2}, $G\alpha_{i2}^{fl\text{-}G184S/fl\text{-}G184S}$ mice. Tamoxifen-induced recombination was evaluated using primers A and B and confirms the in vivo conversion to the *G184S allele for expression of the RGS-insensitive $G\alpha_{i2}$. The 659-bp band was exclusively generated after tamoxifen treatment (Tam). The non-recombined fl-G184S allele is not detected due to the large size of the PCR product (3189-bp).

(Figure 1C). When tamoxifen is administered, its metabolite 4-OH tamoxifen binds to the Cre-ER^{T2} which translocates to the nucleus facilitating recombination of genomic *loxP* sites. As shown in Figure 2B, this removes the E5-9 minigene and positions mutant Exon 5 (E5*) in the normal Gnai2 genomic context to express the mutant $G\alpha_{i2}^{G184S}$ protein. $G\alpha_{i2}^{fl\text{-}G184S/fl\text{-}G184S}$ and Cre-$ER^{T2}/G\alpha_{i2}^{fl\text{-}G184S/fl\text{-}G184S}$ mice are viable and do not show any gross developmental abnormalities.

Reverse transcription-polymerase chain reaction (RT-PCR) analysis was used to amplify a 442-bp cDNA product expressed from the Gnai2 gene to assess the ratio of mutant to wildtype $G\alpha_{i2}$ RNA expression. Only the Cre-$ER^{T2}/G\alpha_{i2}^{+/fl\text{-}G184S}$, or Cre-$ER^{T2}/G\alpha_{i2}^{fl\text{-}G184S/fl\text{-}G184S}$ mice express mutant mRNA after tamoxifen treatment. $G\alpha_{i2}$-specific PCR products from each genotype were sequenced (Figure 3A). This analysis confirmed that the $G\alpha_{i2}$ cDNA sequence from $G\alpha_{i2}^{fl\text{-}G184S/fl\text{-}G184S}$ mice prior to tamoxifen treatment was identical to the previously published mouse cDNA sequence [22,23]. In contrast, the $G\alpha_{i2}$ cDNA sequence from Cre-$ER^{T2}/G\alpha_{i2}^{+/fl\text{-}G184S}$, or Cre-$ER^{T2}/G\alpha_{i2}^{fl\text{-}G184S/fl\text{-}G184S}$ mice revealed the nucleotide changes that were introduced to change the codon for glycine at 184 to serine. Peak heights from the chromatograms were used to quantify the relative amount of mutant mRNA expression in several tissues [24]. In mice that were homozygous for fl-G184S ($G\alpha_{i2}^{fl\text{-}G184S/fl\text{-}G184S}$), we found 60 – 100% conversion to the mutant sequence in most tissues evaluated (Figure 3B). As expected, heterozygous animals ($G\alpha_{i2}^{+/fl\text{-}G184S}$) exhibited lower rates of conversion because they retained one copy of the wildtype allele. The lack of conversion in brain was presumably due to lack of Cre-ER^{T2} expression in post-mitotic neurons, and low brain penetration by tamoxifen [20].

Surprisingly, $G\alpha_{i2}$ protein expression levels were significantly reduced in several organs (heart, brain, and kidney) isolated from $G\alpha_{i2}^{fl\text{-}G184S/fl\text{-}G184S}$ and Cre-$ER^{T2}/G\alpha_{i2}^{fl\text{-}G184S/fl\text{-}G184S}$ mice compared to $G\alpha_{i2}^{+/+}$control animals that do not express Cre or the $G\alpha_{i2}^{G184S}$ mutation (Figure 4). We also assessed whether there were compensatory changes in other G proteins in heart ventricles. We found no detectable levels of $G\alpha_o$, $G\alpha_{i1}$, or $G\alpha_{i3}$ in wildtype ventricles nor were they present in $G\alpha_{i2}^{fl\text{-}G184S/fl\text{-}G184S}$ or Cre-ER^{T2}/

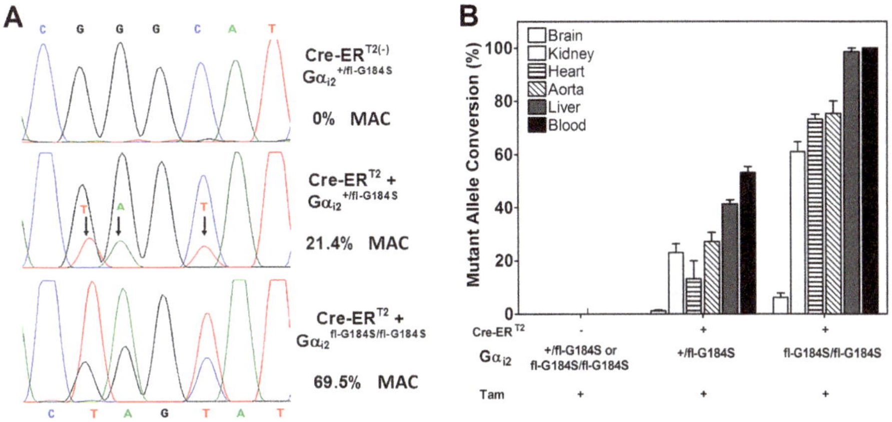

Figure 3 Efficiency and genotype specificity of Cre-induced mutant allele mRNA conversion (MAC) in tissues after tamoxifen treatment in $G\alpha_{i2}^{fl\text{-}G184S}$ mice. A Representative chromatograms of sequenced PCR products from mRNA purified from hearts of tamoxifen-treated mice (50 mg/kg i.p. on five consecutive days). Mice lacking Cre (Cre-ER^{T2-}) showed no evidence of the TAGT sequence expected for G184S mutant mRNA (top chromatogram). For mice expressing Cre (Cre-ER^{T2+}), the percentage conversion to the mutated sequence (% MAC) was higher in mice that were homozygous for the G184S mutation ($G\alpha_{i2}^{fl\text{-}G184S/fl\text{-}G184S}$, lower chromatogram) than in heterozygous ($G\alpha_{i2}^{+/fl\text{-}G184S}$, middle chromatogram) animals. **B** The extent of recombination was higher in blood and liver than in other tissues with heart showing approximately 80% MAC in homozygotes. Values are expressed as the mean (±SE, n = 3) of the percentage of the mutated allele determined from the added peak heights of the three changed bases (see Methods).

$G\alpha_{i2}^{fl\text{-}G184S/fl\text{-}G184S}$ ventricles either before or after tamoxifen treatment (data not shown). This is consistent with previous reports that $G\alpha_{i2}$ is a predominant $G\alpha_i$ isoform in the myocardium [25,26].

We previously demonstrated that embryonic fibroblasts from conventional (i.e. non-conditional) $G\alpha_{i2}^{G184S}$ knock-in mice have enhanced activity in several biochemical and physiological measures of the $G\alpha_i$ signaling pathway [8]. Thus, we investigated the functional consequences of conditional $G\alpha_{i2}^{G184S}$ expression at the cellular level in a cAMP inhibition assay. Adult cardiac fibroblasts from mice treated with tamoxifen (which developed ~90% mutant allele expression, data not shown) were isolated and cultured. cAMP production in these cells was measured following exposure to forskolin (10 μM) and increasing concentrations of lysophosphatidic acid (LPA). Data were compared by two-way ANOVA with genotype and LPA cohcentration as variables. A significant effect of genotype ($P < 0.05$) in the inhibition of cAMP production was observed. Bonferroni's post test revealed that ACF from the conditional knock-in mice (Cre-ER^{T2}/$G\alpha_{i2}$) had significantly ($P < 0.05$) augmented inhibition of cAMP production with the highest concentration of LPA compared to cells from $G\alpha_{i2}^{fl\text{-}G184S/fl\text{-}G184S}$ mice that do not convert to the G184S mutation (Figure 5). These data are consistent with our previous finding that LPA-induced inhibition of adenylate cyclase activity is enhanced in embryonic fibroblasts in the nonconditional $G\alpha_{i2}^{G184S}$ model [13], and they provide evidence that agonist-induced $G\alpha_{i2}$ signaling is enhanced in cardiac fibroblasts that conditionally express the $G\alpha_{i2}^{G184S}$ allele.

We previously demonstrated that the conventional $G\alpha_{i2}^{G184S}$ mutant mice (both heterozygotes and homozygotes) are resistant to ischemia-reperfusion injury [13]. However, it was unclear whether this phenotype resulted from $G\alpha_{i2}^{G184S}$ expression during embryonic development or whether the cardioprotective phenotype requires chronic or acute $G\alpha_{i2}^{G184S}$ expression. In the present study, we found that ischemia-induced infarct size was significantly decreased in tamoxifen-treated Cre-ER^{T2}/$G\alpha_{i2}^{fl\text{-}G184S/fl\text{-}G184S}$ compared to both vehicle-treated Cre-ER^{T2}/$G\alpha_{i2}^{fl\text{-}G184S/fl\text{-}G184S}$ hearts and tamoxifen-treated $G\alpha_{i2}^{fl\text{-}G184S/fl\text{-}G184S}$ without Cre expression (Figure 6). Consistent with reduced myocardial infarct size (Figure 6), hearts isolated from tamoxifen-treated Cre-ER^{T2}/$G\alpha_{i2}^{fl\text{-}G184S/fl\text{-}G184S}$ exhibited significantly enhanced postischemic recovery of developed pressure compared to hearts isolated from either vehicle-treated Cre-ER^{T2}/$G\alpha_{i2}^{fl\text{-}G184S/fl\text{-}G184S}$ mice or tamoxifen-treated $G\alpha_{i2}^{fl\text{-}G184S/fl\text{-}G184S}$ mice that do not express Cre-ER^{T2} (Table 1). Postischemic recovery of + dP/dT and −dP/dT were also enhanced in hearts isolated from tamoxifen treated Cre-ER^{T2}/$G\alpha_{i2}^{fl\text{-}G184S/fl\text{-}G184S}$ animals. Postischemic recovery of end diastolic pressure was nominally lower in tamoxifen-treated Cre-ER^{T2}/$G\alpha_{i2}^{fl\text{-}G184S/fl\text{-}G184S}$ compared to the other groups (Table 1). However, this did not reach statistical significance. These data are consistent with our previous report that nonconditional expression of $G\alpha_{i2}^{G184S}$ protects the heart from ischemic injury [13]. Importantly, they extend our previous findings by demonstrating that the cardioprotective phenotype does not result from embryonic or chronic expression of $G\alpha_{i2}^{G184S}$. Rather, acute

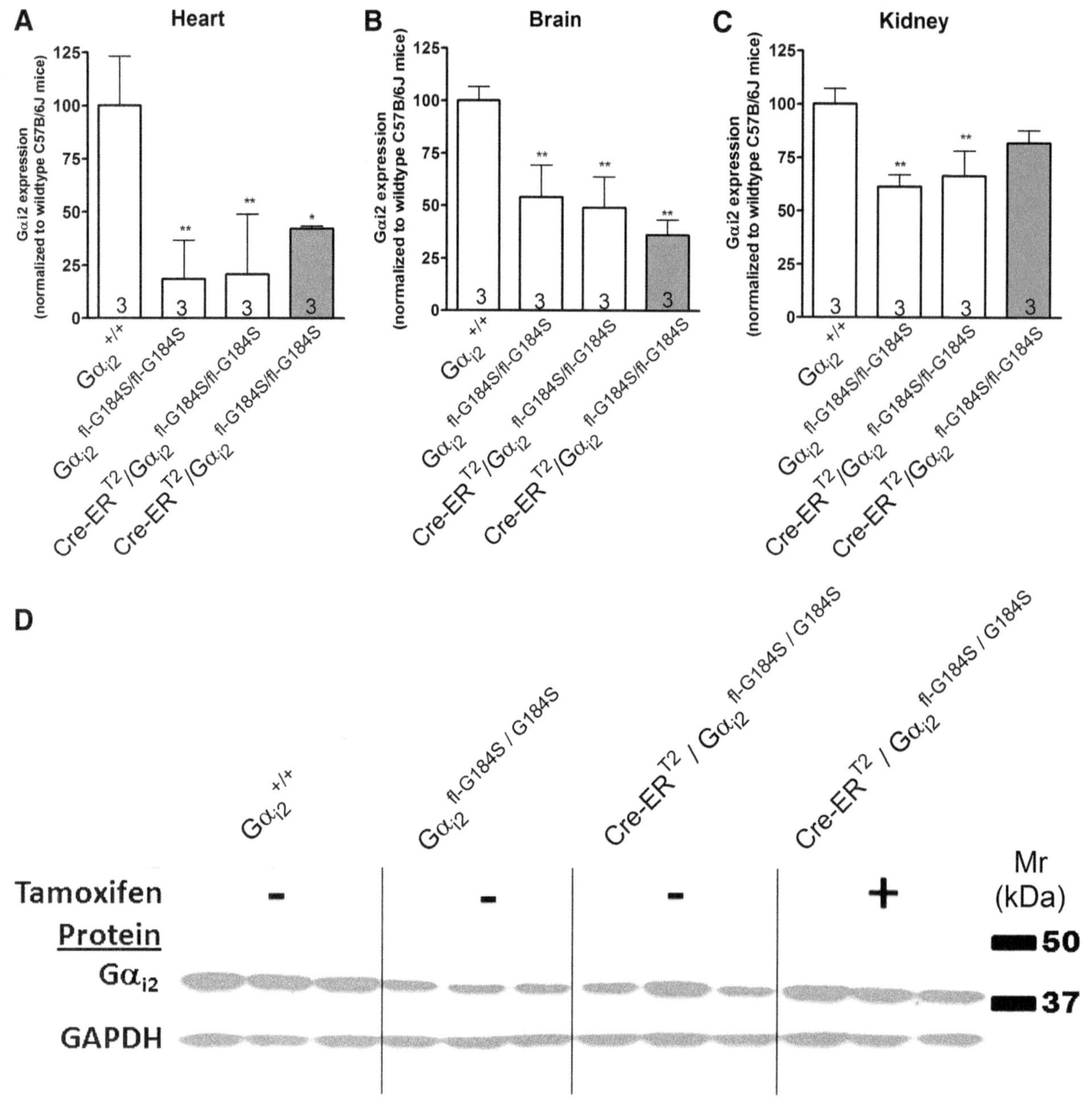

Figure 4 Gα_{i2} protein expression is reduced in mice conditionally expressing Gα_{i2}^{G184S}. Gα_{i2} protein expression was measured by Western blot in hearts **(A)**, brains **(B)**, and kidneys **(C)** isolated from mice treated with tamoxifen (50 mg/kg; shaded bars) or vehicle (nonshaded bars) for 5 consecutive days. The membrane was stripped and reblotted with a GAPDH antibody as a loading control. Values represent the mean ± SE of tissues from three different animals for each genotype. Data are normalized to Gα_{i2} protein expression in tissues from wildtype C57B/6J mice that do not express Cre and do not carry the Gα_{i2}^{G184S} mutation. Panel **D** shows a representative blot of kidneys from three different animals of each genotype. * and ** indicate significant differences ($p < 0.05$ and $p < 0.01$, respectively) relative to control mice ($G_{\alpha i2}^{+/+}$) that do not carry the Cre-ER^{T2} or $G_{\alpha i2}^{fl\text{-}G184S/fl\text{-}G184S}$ genes.

disruption of interactions between Gα_{i2} and endogenous RGS proteins is sufficient to induce cardioprotection.

Discussion

We previously described a mouse model in which signaling by Gα_{i2} was enhanced by introduction of a point mutation (G184S) that blocks negative regulation by RGS proteins [8]. These mice exhibited a number of complex and interesting phenotypes including protection from cardiac ischemia/reperfusion injury [13]. However, it was unclear whether this cardioprotective phenotype resulted from changes in Gα_{i2} signaling during embryonic

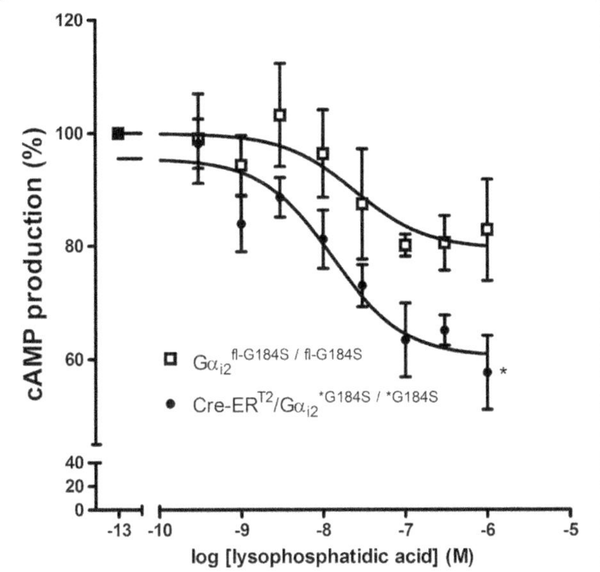

Figure 5 Enhanced inhibition of forskolin-stimulated adenylate cyclase by lysophosphatidic acid following conditional induction of the $G\alpha_{i2}^{G184S}$ mutation in adult cardiac fibroblasts. Concentration-response curves were generated from adult cardiac fibroblasts isolated from three different mice of each genotype after treatment with tamoxifen (50 mg/kg i.p. on five consecutive days). Data from 5 independent determinations for both $G\alpha_{i2}^{fl\text{-}G184S/fl\text{-}G184S}$ and Cre-ER^{T2}/$G\alpha_{i2}^{*G184S/*G184S}$ are shown as mean ± SE. Data are normalized to cAMP production in the presence of 10^{-13} M lysophosphatidic acid. Two way ANOVA revealed a significant effect for genotype [$F = 5.58$ (1,8) $p < 0.05$] and a significant effect for lysophosphatidic acid concentration [$F = 12.09$ (8, 64) $p < 0.0001$]. * indicates a significant difference ($p < 0.05$ compared to $G\alpha_{i2}^{fl\text{-}G184S/fl\text{-}G184S}$ cells treated with 10^{-6}M LPA) using Bonferroni's post test.

development. It was also unknown whether chronic $G\alpha_{i2}^{G184S}$ expression was required or whether acute expression was sufficient to protect the heart from ischemic injury. These are important issues because the potential finding that embryonic or chronic expression of $G\alpha_{i2}^{G184S}$ is required for cardioprotection would likely preclude the use of pharmacological RGS inhibitors from therapeutic use in the treatment of ischemic heart disease. The present study extends our previous findings by demonstrating that acute (days rather than months) disruption of interactions between $G\alpha_{i2}$ and endogenous RGS proteins is sufficient to protect the heart from ischemic injury. These data suggest that RGS proteins might provide novel therapeutic targets to protect the heart from ischemic injury.

Conditional expression of $G\alpha_{i2}^{G184S}$ resulted in a 55% reduction in infarct size relative to hearts isolated from tamoxifen-treated mice that did not express Cre-ER^{T2}, and a 65% reduction in infarct size compared to hearts isolated from mice that expressed Cre-ER^{T2} but were not treated with tamoxifen. By comparison, we previously reported that nonconditional expression of $G\alpha_{i2}^{G184S}$ resulted in 41% and 68% reductions in infarct sizes in hearts isolated from mice that were heterozygous or homozygous for the $G\alpha_{i2}^{G184S}$ mutation, respectively [13]. Recovery of developed pressure, +dP/dT, and -dP/dT were significantly increased in both models of $G\alpha_{i2}^{G184S}$ expression (Table 1 and [13]). Thus, conditional expression of this mutation produced a cardioprotective phenotype that was similar to the phenotype previously observed in the conventional (nonconditional) $G\alpha_{i2}^{G184S}$ knockin model.

Mice expressing the $G\alpha_{i2}^{G184S}$ in a nonconditional fashion also exhibit several noncardiac phenotypic differences including: resistance to high fat diet-induced weight gain and resistance to the development of insulin insensitivity, reduced embryonic viability, elevated neutrophil counts, and antidepressant-like behavior [5,8,14]. We anticipate that the conditional $G\alpha_{i2}^{G184S}$ expression model described here will be helpful in characterizing the temporal requirements (acute versus chronic) of $G\alpha_{i2}^{G184S}$ expression for some of these phenotypes. Our finding that tamoxifen produced very little conversion to the $G\alpha_{i2}^{G184S}$ mutation in the brain suggests that this model may not be useful for characterizing the anxiolytic or antidepressant-like behavior that has been previously reported in nonconditional $G\alpha_{i2}^{G184S}$ mice [5]. On one hand, this represents a significant limitation of this model. However, the observation that the conventional $G\alpha_{i2}^{G184S}$ model, but not the conditional $G\alpha_{i2}^{G184S}$ model, expresses the G184S mutation in the brain might be useful for elucidating the ability of enhanced $G\alpha_{i2}$ signaling in the central nervous system to impact the function of peripheral tissues. The reason for a lack of conversion to the $G\alpha_{i2}^{G184S}$ mutation in the brain is unclear. However, other investigators using the Cre-ER^{T2} system have reported similar results. Seibler et al. confirmed that Cre-ER^{T2} is expressed in the brain and suggested that the lack of recombination may reflect low local concentrations of 4-hydroxytamoxifen [27].

The tamoxifen- and Cre-dependent recombination and expression of mutant mRNA meets the criteria planned for the engineered Gnai2 locus: lack of mutant mRNA expression before tamoxifen treatment with good conversion to the G184S mutation after tamoxifen treatment. We did observe reduced $G\alpha_{i2}$ protein expression in the heart, kidney, and brain of $G\alpha_{i2}{}^{flG184S/fl\text{-}G184S}$ and Cre-ER^{T2}/$G\alpha_{i2}{}^{flG184S/fl\text{-}G184S}$ mice relative to wildtype mice that do not express Cre or carry the G184S mutation, suggesting that the loss of introns in the minigene that carries the wildtype sequence and/or the residual LoxP or FLP recombinase (FRT) sites may perturb regulatory and/or splicing elements. However, the observation that LPA-induced inhibition of cAMP production is augmented in cardiac fibroblasts isolated from Cre-ER^{T2}/$G\alpha_{i2}{}^{flG184S/fl\text{-}G184S}$ mice (Figure 5) indicates that

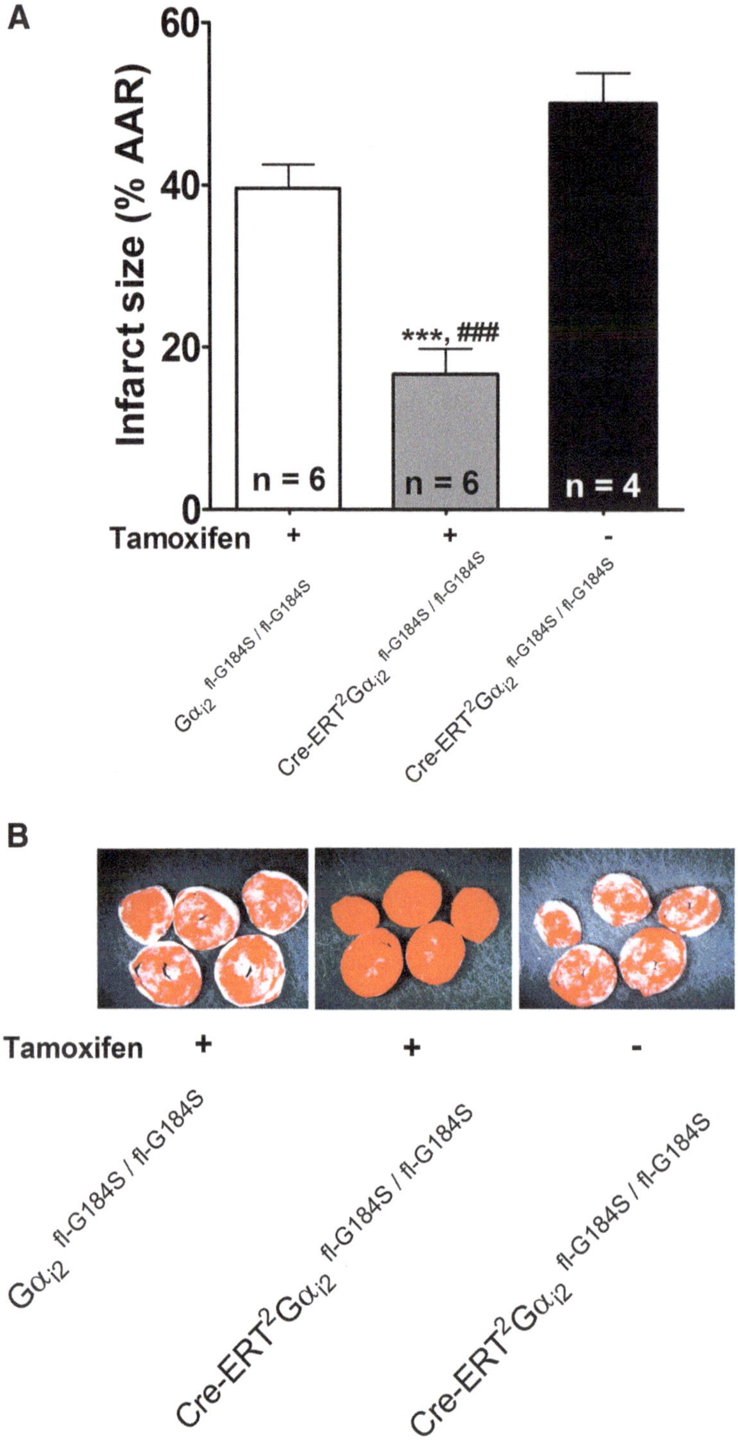

Figure 6 Conditional expression of $G\alpha_{i2}{}^{G184S}$protects the heart from ischemic injury. Conditional expression of $G\alpha_{i2}{}^{G184S}$ significantly ($p < 0.001$) decreased infarct sizes in hearts exposed to 30 min of ischemia **(A)**. Values represent means ± SE. The number of replicates for each group is shown within the bars. Data were compared by one way ANOVA and posthoc Tukey analysis. *** indicates a significant difference ($p < 0.001$) compared to hearts isolated from tamoxifen treated $G\alpha_{i2}{}^{fl\text{-}G184S/fl\text{-}G184S}$ mice, and ### indicates a significant difference ($p < 0.001$) compared to hearts isolated from Cre-ER^{T2}/$G\alpha_{i2}{}^{fl\text{-}G184S/fl\text{-}G184S}$ mice that were treated with vehicle instead of tamoxifen. Photographs of representative triphenyltetrazolium chloride-stained hearts are shown in panel **B**.

Table 1 Preischemic and postischemic recovery of contractile function

	Preischemic			Postischemic recovery		
	$G\alpha_{i2}$ $^{fl\text{-}G184S/fl\text{-}G184S}$ + tamoxifen (n = 6)	Cre-ER^{T2}/$G\alpha_{i2}$ $^{fl\text{-}G184S/fl\text{-}G184S}$ + tamoxifen (n = 6)	Cre-ER^{T2}/$G\alpha_{i2}$ $^{fl\text{-}G184S/fl\text{-}G184S}$ + vehicle (n = 4)	$G\alpha_{i2}$ $^{fl\text{-}G184S/fl\text{-}G184S}$ + tamoxifen (n = 6)	Cre-ER^{T2}/$G\alpha_{i2}$/$^{fl\text{-}G184S/fl\text{-}G184S}$ + tamoxifen (n = 6)	Cre-ER^{T2}/$G\alpha_{i2}$ $^{fl\text{-}G184S/fl\text{-}G184S}$ + vehicle (n = 4)
Developed pressure (mmHg)	130 ± 6	140 ± 8	132 ± 6	45 ± 5	78 ± 8 * #	29 ± 7
+dP/dT (mmHg/sec)	6375 ± 570	6145 ± 621	4587 ± 251	2223 ± 321	3557 ± 521 #	985 ± 258
-dP/dT (mmHg/sec)	-4471 ± 291	-4601 ± 275	-3837 ± 235	-1600 ± 197	-2581 ± 263 * #	-908 ± 243
End diastolic pressure (mmHg)	5.7 ± 1.0	6.2 ± 0.9	5.0 ± 1.0	30 ± 2	21 ± 3	33 ± 7
Coronary flow rate (ml/min)	4.5 ± 0.4	4.1 ± 0.3	4.6 ± 0.4	2.7 ± 0.3	2.6 ± 0.2	2.9 ± 0.4

Preischemic contractile function was measured prior to 30 minutes of ischemia. Postischemic recovery of contractile function was measured following 1 hour of reperfusion. Data from each group were compared by one way ANOVA and posthoc Tukey analysis (preischemic and postischemic values were analyzed separately from one another). There were no significant differences between groups for any parameters of preischemic contractile function. *indicates a significant difference ($p < 0.05$) in postischemic recovery of contractile function compared to hearts isolated from tamoxifen treated $G\alpha_{i2}$ $^{fl\text{-}G184S/fl\text{-}G184S}$ mice. # indicates a significant difference ($p < 0.01$) in postischemic recovery of contractile function compared to hearts isolated from Cre-ER^{T2}/$G\alpha_{i2}$ $^{fl\text{-}G184S/fl\text{-}G184S}$ mice that were treated with vehicle instead of tamoxifen.

agonist-induced signaling via $G\alpha_{i2}$ is actually increased (relative to fibroblasts that do not express the mutation), despite decreased $G\alpha_{i2}$ expression levels. This presumably occurs because the negative regulatory effect of RGS proteins toward $G\alpha_{i2}$ is disrupted in these cells. Many different $G\alpha_i$-coupled receptors are known to protect the heart from ischemia/reperfusion injury. Thus, the finding that conditional expression of $G\alpha_{i2}^{G184S}$ produces a cardioprotective phenotype is also consistent with enhanced $G\alpha_{i2}$ signaling despite decreased $G\alpha_{i2}$ protein expression.

Conclusions

In conclusion, the conditional $G\alpha_{i2}^{G184S}$ knock-in model described here permits the disruption of interactions between $G\alpha_{i2}$ and endogenous RGS proteins in a time-dependent manner. Our data demonstrate that acute (rather than chronic) disruption of interactions between RGS proteins and $G\alpha_{i2}$ is sufficient to protect the heart from ischemic injury. This suggests that the development of chemical inhibitors of RGS proteins or other agents that disrupt interactions between RGS proteins and $G\alpha_{i2}$ might provide new therapeutic tools to protect the heart from ischemic injury. In addition, we anticipate that this transgenic mouse model will provide a valuable tool for characterizing the mechanisms by which disruption of RGS protein-$G\alpha_{i2}$ interactions confers other phenotypes that have been identified in mice expressing $G\alpha_{i2}^{G184S}$.

Abbreviations

ACF: Adult cardiac fibroblast; ES: Embryonic stem; $G\alpha_{i2}^{+/+}$: Wildtype $G\alpha_{i2}$ allele; $G\alpha_{i2}^{G184S}$: $G\alpha_{i2}$ allele with point mutation; PCR: Polymerase chain reaction; RGS: Regulator of G protein signaling.

Competing interests

The authors have no financial or nonfinancial competing interests.

Authors' contributions

RRN, SP, and XH conceived and designed the experiments. SP, BRR, KK, RAC, SMW, and XH performed the experiments. SP, RRN, and BRR analyzed the data and wrote the manuscript. All authors read and approved the final manuscript.

Acknowledgements

This work was supported by NIH R01-GM39561 (R.R.N) and was also supported in part by the Michigan Diabetes, Research, and Training Center (NIH P60 DK20572), and the University of Michigan Comprehensive Cancer Center (NIH P30 CA046592). We thank Dr. Susanne Mumby (UT Southwestern Medical Center) for the specific $G\alpha_{i2}$ antibody, Dr. Thomas Gettys for the specific $G\alpha_{i1}$ and $G\alpha_{i3}$ antibodies, Dr. Thomas Saunders and Elizabeth Hughes (University of Michigan Transgenic Animal Model Core) for providing the FLPe mice and for the ES cells electroporation, respectively. We also thank Dr. Sally Camper, Dr. Thomas Saunders, and the staff at the University of Michigan Transgenic Animal Model Core and the staff at GenOway (Lyon, France) for helpful suggestions regarding the generation of the conditional knock-in mice.

Author details

[1]Department of Pharmacology, University of Michigan, Ann Arbor, Michigan 48109, USA. [2]Department of Pharmaceutical and Biomedical Sciences, Ohio Northern University College of Pharmacy, Ada, OH 45810, USA. [3]Department of Pharmacology and Toxicology, B440 Life Sciences, Michigan State University, 1355 Bogue St, East Lansing, MI 48824, USA.

References

1. Hörnquist CE, Lu X, Rogers-Fani PM, Rudolph U, Shappell S, Birnbaumer L, Harriman GR: **G(alpha)i2-deficient mice with colitis exhibit a local increase in memory CD4+ T cells and proinflammatory Th1-type cytokines.** *J Immunol* 1997, **158:**1068–1077.
2. DeGeorge BR Jr, Gao E, Boucher M, Vinge LE, Martini JS, Raake PW, Chuprun JK, Harris DM, Kim GW, Soltys S, Eckhart AD, Koch WJ: **Targeted inhibition of cardiomyocyte Gi signaling enhances susceptibility to apoptotic cell death in response to ischemic stress.** *Circulation* 2008, **117:**1378–1387.
3. Nagata K, Ye C, Jain M, Milstone DS, Liao R, Mortensen RM: **Galpha(i2) but not Galpha(i3) is required for muscarinic inhibition of contractility and calcium currents in adult cardiomyocytes.** *Circ Res* 2000, **87:**903–909.
4. Inoue Y, Yao L, Hopf FW, Fan P, Jiang Z, Bonci A, Diamond I: **Nicotine and ethanol activate protein kinase A synergistically via G(i) betagamma subunits in nucleus accumbens/ventral tegmental cocultures: the role of dopamine D(1)/D(2) and adenosine A(2A) receptors.** *J Pharmacol Exp Ther* 2007, **322:**23–29.
5. Talbot JN, Jutkiewicz EM, Graves SM, Clemans CF, Nicol MR, Mortensen RM, Huang X, Neubig RR, Traynor JR: **RGS inhibition at G(alpha)i2 selectively potentiates 5-HT1A-mediated antidepressant effects.** *Proc Natl Acad Sci U S A* 2010, **107:**11086–11091.
6. Kimple AJ, Bosch DE, Giguere PM, Siderovski DP: **Regulators of G-protein signaling and their Galpha substrates: promises and challenges in their use as drug discovery targets.** *Pharmacol Rev* 2011, **2011**(63):728–749.
7. Sjogren B, Blazer LL, Neubig RR: **Regulators of G protein signaling proteins as targetes for drug discovery.** *Prog Mol Biol Transl Sci* 2010, **91:**81–119.
8. Huang X, Fu Y, Charbeneau RA, Saunders TL, Taylor DK, Hankenson KD, Russell MW, D'Alecy LG, Neubig RR: **Pleiotropic phenotype of a genomic knock-in of an RGS-insensitive G184S Gnai2 allele.** *Mol Cell Biol* 2006, **26:**6870–6879.
9. Fu Y, Zhong H, Nanamori M, Mortensen RM, Huang X, Lan K, Neubig RR: **RGS-insensitive G-protein mutations to study the role of endogenous RGS proteins.** *Methods Enzymol* 2004, **389:**229–243.
10. Fu Y, Huang X, Piao L, Lopatin AN, Neubig RR: **Endogenous RGS proteins modulate SA and AV nodal functions in isolated heart: implications for sick sinus syndrome and AV block.** *Am J Physiol Heart Circ Physiol* 2007, **292:**H2532–H2539.
11. Fu Y, Huang X, Zhong H, Mortensen RM, D'Alecy LG, Neubig RR: **Endogenous RGS proteins and Galpha subtypes differentially control muscarinic and adenosine-mediated chronotropic effects.** *Circ Res* 2006, **98:**659–666.
12. Kaur K, Parra S, Chen R, Charbeneau RA, Wade SM, Jay PY, Neubig RR: **Galpha(i2) signaling: friend or foe in cardiac injury and heart failure? Naunyn Schmiedebergs.** *Arch Pharmacol* 2012, **38:**443–453.
13. Waterson RE, Thompson CG, Mabe NW, Kaur K, Talbot JN, Neubig RR, Rorabaugh BR: **Galpha(i2)-mediated protection from ischaemic injury is modulated by endogenous RGS proteins in the mouse heart.** *Cardiovasc Res* 2011, **91:**45–52.
14. Huang X, Charbeneau RA, Fu Y, Kaur K, Gerin I, MacDougald OA, Neubig RR: **Resistance to diet-induced obesity and improved insulin sensitivity in mice with a regulator of G protein signaling-insensitive G184S Gnai2 allele.** *Diabetes* 2008, **57:**77–85.
15. Xin HB, Deng KY, Shui B, Qu S, Sun Q, Lee J, Greene KS, Wilson J, Yu Y, Feldman M, Kotlikoff MI: **Gene trap and gene inversion methods for conditional gene inactivation in the mouse.** *Nucleic Acids Res* 2005, **33:**e14.
16. Wingate AD, Martin KJ, Hunter C, Carr JM, Clacher C, Arthur JS: **Generation of a conditional CREB Ser133Ala knockin mouse.** *Genesis* 2009, **47:**688–696.
17. Truett GE, Heeger P, Mynatt RL, Truett AA, Walker JA, Warman ML: **Preparation of PCR-quality mouse genomic DNA with hot sodium hydroxide and tris (HotSHOT).** *Biotechniques* 2000, **29:**52–54.
18. O'Connell TD, Rodrigo MC: **Simpson PC (2007) Isolation and culture of adult mouse cardiac myocytes.** *Methods Mol Biol* 2007, **357:**271–296.

19. Anastassiadis K, Glaser S, Kranz A, Berhardt K, Stewart AF: **A practical summary of site-specific recombination, conditional mutagenesis, and tamoxifen induction of CreERT2.** *Methods Enzymol* 2010, **2010**(477):109–123.
20. Hameyer D, Loonstra A, Eshkind L, Schmitt S, Antunes C, Groen A, Bindels E, Jonkers J, Krimpenfort P, Meuwissen R, Rijswijk L, Bex A, Berns A, Bockamp E: **Toxicity of ligand-dependent Cre recombinases and generation of a conditional Cre deleter mouse allowing mosaic recombination in peripheral tissues.** *Physiol Genomics* 2007, **31**:32–41.
21. Rodríguez CI, Buchholz F, Galloway J, Sequerra R, Kasper J, Ayala R, Stewart AF, Dymecki SM: **High-efficiency deleter mice show that FLPe is an alternative to Cre-loxP.** *Nat Genet* 2000, **25**:139–140.
22. Strathmann M, Wilkie TM: **Simon MI (1989) Diversity of the G-protein family: sequences from five additional alpha subunits in the mouse.** *Proc Natl Acad Sci U S A* 1989, **86:**7407–7409.
23. Sullivan KA, Liao YC, Alborzi A, Beiderman B, Chang FH, Masters SB, Levinson AD, Bourne HR: **Inhibitory and stimulatory G proteins of adenylate cyclase: cDNA and amino acid sequences of the alpha chains.** *Proc Natl Acad Sci U S A* 1986, **83:**6687–6691.
24. Akada H, Yan D, Zou H, Fiering S, Hutchison RE, Mohi MG: **Conditional expression of heterozygous or homozygous Jak2V617F from its endogenous promoter induces a polycythemia vera-like disease.** *Blood* 2010, **115:**3589–3597.
25. Dizayee S, Kaestner S, Kuck F, Hein P, Klein C, Piekorz RP, Meszaros J, Matthes J, Nürnberg B, Herzig S: **Gαi2- and Gαi3-specific regulation of voltage-dependent L-type calcium channels in cardiomyocytes.** *PLoS One* 2011, **6:**e24979.
26. Foerster K, Groner F, Matthes J, Koch WJ, Birnbaumer L, Herzig S: **Cardioprotection specific for the G protein Gi2 in chronic adrenergic signaling through beta 2-adrenoceptors.** *Proc Natl Acad Sci U S A* 2003, **100:**14475–14480.
27. Seibler J, Zevnik B, Kuter-Luks B, Andreas S, Kern H, Hennek T, Rode A, Heimann C, Faust N, Kauselmann G, Schoor M, Jaenisch R, Rajewsky K, Kuhn R, Schwenk F: **Rapid generation of inducible mouse mutants.** *Nucleic Acids Res* 2003, **31:**e11–e13.

Prognosis of concomitant users of clopidogrel and proton-pump inhibitors in a high-risk population for upper gastrointestinal bleeding

Qing Wang[1], Rickard Ljung[1,2], Jesper Lagergren[1,3] and Yunxia Lu[1,4*]

Abstract

Background: It is unclear whether concomitant use of clopidogrel and proton-pump inhibitors (PPIs) increases the risk of recurrence of cardiovascular disease or death in patients at high risk of upper gastrointestinal (GI) bleeding.

Methods: Based on the Swedish Patient Register, a cohort of cardiovascular disease (including acute myocardial infarction, stroke and angina, from 2006 to 2008) was selected from a population with any diagnosis of upper GI bleeding. Data on drug prescription was retrieved from the Prescribed Drug Register. Patients entered into the cohort after their first discharge for cardiovascular disease and were followed up to death, recurrence of cardiovascular disease, or 90 days. A Cox regression model was conducted and hazard ratios (HRs) with 95% confidence intervals (CIs) were estimated to evaluate the risks among users of different drug prescriptions.

Results: Patients who were current users of only PPIs (HR 2.02, 95% CI 1.19-3.44), only clopidogrel (HR 1.14, 95% CI 0.53-2.45) and nonusers of both (HR 2.36, 95% CI 1.39-4.00) were at a higher risk of death compared with patients with a concomitant use. Results were similar among 1779 patients who had any history of upper GI bleeding (HR 2.05, 95% CI 1.18-3.54; HR 1.25, 95% CI 0.57-2.72; HR 2.30, 95% CI 1.33-3.98, respectively).

Conclusion: Among patients at high risk of upper GI bleeding, those with a concomitant use of PPIs and clopidogrel were at a decreased risk of mortality, and possibly also a decreased risk of recurrence of cardiovascular disease.

Keywords: Clopidogrel, Proton-pump inhibitors, Gastrointestinal bleeding, Cardiovascular disease

Background

Clopidogrel is a widely used medication for atherosclerotic diseases [1], particularly in the prevention of thrombotic events in stable cardiovascular disease, and as a secondary prevention after myocardial infarction and stroke [2,3]. Upper gastrointestinal (GI) bleeding is, however, a common and potentially serious adverse event in clopidogrel users [4]. Proton-pump inhibitors (PPIs), drugs that alleviate acid-related symptoms by inhibition of the hydrogen-potassium adenosine triphosphatase enzyme in gastric mucosa [5,6], are often prescribed to prevent such bleedings [5,7-9]. However, there are reports of an increased risk of mortality and recurrence of cardiovascular disease among patients with concomitant use of clopidogrel and PPIs [10-14]. A possible mechanism is that PPIs, which are mainly metabolized by the cytochrome system, might counteract the inhibitory effect of clopidogrel on platelet aggregation [15,16]. Nevertheless, some other studies have failed to find any interaction between clopidogrel and PPIs [17-19], or any increase in the risk of cardiovascular rehospitalizations [20]. There is presently no general consensus on this issue, although the US Food and Drug Administration and the European Medicines Agency have stated that PPIs may reduce the effect of clopidogrel in the prevention of serious cardiovascular events [21,22].

During the past four years, accumulating relevant studies have been published. Few studies, however, have

* Correspondence: yunxia.lu@ki.se
[1]Department of Molecular Medicine and Surgery, Karolinska Institutet, SE-171 76 Stockholm, Sweden
[4]Department of Epidemiology and Biostatistics, Imperial College London, London, United Kingdom
Full list of author information is available at the end of the article

focused on patients with cardiovascular disease at high risk of upper GI bleeding [23]. Most have excluded patients with a history of GI bleeding [14,17,18,20,24] although these patients might be at high risk of a recurrence of severe GI bleeding. Furthermore, these studies have mainly evaluated the combined use of clopidogrel and aspirin together with PPIs which might dilute or mix the real interaction between clopidogrel and PPIs [25,26]. In addition, recurrence of cardiovascular disease is the major measured outcome in most previous studies rather than death. Death, though, is the most important and clearly measured outcome for cardiovascular disease and acute peptic ulcer bleeding. The recurrence of cardiovascular disease is, however, generally difficult to be identified completely.

In this cohort study, we focused on cardiovascular disease with any diagnosis of upper GI bleeding to clarify whether concomitant use of clopidogrel and PPIs increases the risk of recurrence of cardiovascular disease or death, compared with other treatment strategies.

Methods

Study design

Within a population-based cohort of patients (1987 to 2008 in Sweden) with any hospitalization for complicated upper GI ulcer disease (International Classification of Disease 10th revision [ICD] diagnosis codes: K25-K28 with .0 .1 .2 .4 .5 .6), patients were selected for the final study if they had been hospitalized for cardiovascular disease from 2006 until the end of 2008. The entry date into the study cohort was the discharge date of the first cardiovascular disease hospitalization after January 1, 2006 (Figure 1). Patients were followed for 60, 90, 180 and 360 days to assess the outcomes death, re-hospitalization, or revisit to outpatient/primary health care for cardiovascular disease. In this study, we only present the results of the 90-day follow-up. The reason for this is that the short-term drug prescriptions after discharge for cardiovascular disease might more appropriately reflect the treatment in relation to fatality and recurrence. Moreover, restriction of the follow-up to only 60 days, 180 days and 360 days after entry rendered similar results to the 90-day follow-up (data not shown).

Data sources

Data regarding basic patient information (admission date, discharge date, main diagnosis and secondary diagnosis) were retrieved from the *Swedish Patient Register*, which has been completed nationwide since 1987. Information on prescribed drugs and dates of dispatch were retrieved from the similarly complete Swedish Prescribed Drug Register (SPDR), which was initiated in July 1, 2005. This register contains information on age, sex, personal number, prescriber's profession and practice and, particularly, drug utilization and expenditure on prescribed drugs for the entire Swedish population. The defined cohort began on January 1, 2006, in order to ensure drug exposure covering at least half a year. The legally compulsory register of prescribed drugs in Sweden guarantees the complete capture of drugs exposure in this study. Death dates and underlying causes of death were identified from the nationwide complete *Swedish Cause of Death Register* (initiated in 1952), and data on cancer as a co-morbidity was collected from the nationwide complete *Swedish Cancer Register* (initiated in 1958).

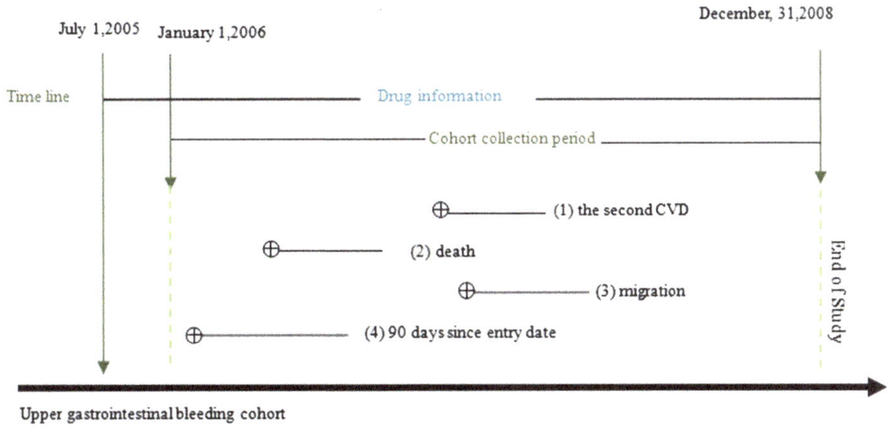

Figure 1 The flow chart for study design. The timeline showed how the cohort was defined. The Swedish Prescribed Drug Register started on July 1st, 2005. This study chose to start on January, 1st 2006 thus at least half-year drug exposure information can be guaranteed. Patients who discharged from hospitalizations for cardiovascular diseases since January, 1st 2006 were included in the cohort. They had been followed up the second cardiovascular event (1), death (2), migration (3), or end of study (4) within 90 days follow-up period. All of the patients had historical upper GI bleeding or they bled during/after the follow up period but before December, 31, 2008. Symbol ⊕ means diagnosis of cardiovascular diseases.

Identification of the study cohort

As we described above in the Study design section, patients with a first hospitalization for cardiovascular disease (including acute myocardial infarction, stroke, and angina) after January 1, 2006, were included in the study. These diseases were identified from the following ICD codes: main diagnosis or co-diagnosis of acute myocardial infarction (I21, I22), main diagnosis or co-diagnosis of ischemic stroke (I63, I64), and main diagnosis of angina (I20). In order to focus on clopidogrel and PPIs, we excluded patients with any filled prescription of aspirin (Anatomical Therapeutic Chemical [ATC] code: B01AC06, N02BA01, A01AD05) during the study period. Patients were also excluded from the final study cohort if they had previous acute myocardial infarction, stroke or angina hospitalizations within one year before entry, if they had emigrated before January 1, 2006, or if they had a cardiovascular rehospitalization or had died less than 7 days after entry.

Drug exposures

Current drug use was categorized into four groups: i) only PPIs, ii) only clopidogrel, iii) both clopidogrel and PPIs and, iv) no PPIs or clopidogrel. All the PPI types available in Sweden were included (omeprazole, pantoprazole, lansoprazole, rabeprazole, esomeprazole). The sample size did not allow separate analyses of single PPI groups. We calculated drug exposures at 30 days before the entry date as some patients might have had leftovers of previous PPIs or clopidogrel prescriptions at hand, which might have met their demands for current medications. We also analyzed the data using drug exposure that started from the entry date, or drug exposure 60 days before the entry. All of the results based on three definitions of exposures were similar. Thus, to make the study more concise, we only used the first definition of drug exposure. In Sweden, the typical prescription for PPIs or clopidogrel is for approximately 90 days or less. The extra 30 days plus 90 days of follow-up ensured enough time to cover any defined drug exposures. The ATC codes for clopidogrel were B01AC04 and B01AC30, and the ATC codes for PPIs were A02BC01-05 and A02BD01-06.

Definition of outcomes

The outcomes under study were: recurrence of acute myocardial infarction (main or secondary diagnosis codes I21 or I22), stroke (main or secondary diagnosis codes I60-I64), angina (main diagnosis code I20), or all-cause mortality. We also specified hemorrhagic stroke and ischemic stroke from the total stroke patients.

Co-morbidities

A co-morbidity score was calculated based on the following concomitant diagnoses: *i)* chronic heart failure (diagnosis code I50); *ii)* diabetes (diagnosis codes E10-E14); *iii)* chronic liver insufficiency (diagnosis codes K702-K704, K709, K717, K72, or K743-K746); *iv)* chronic renal insufficiency (diagnosis codes N18, N19, I132, I200, or I311); *v)* chronic obstructive lung disease (diagnosis codes J42-J44); *vi)* malignancy (diagnosis codes C00-C97). The reason for the selection of these diseases for the calculation of the co-morbidity score is because they are very commonly diagnosed and are composed of the most frequent causes of death in an elderly population [27,28]. The number of co-morbidities was categorized into four groups: no concomitant diagnosis, one concomitant diagnosis, two concomitant diagnoses, three or more concomitant diagnoses. History of cardiovascular disease was defined as any diagnosis of acute myocardial infarction, stroke, or angina at least one year before entry into the study cohort.

Statistical analyses

A proportional risk model was conducted and hazard ratios (HRs) with 95% confidence intervals (CI) were estimated to evaluate the risk of death or cardiovascular disease in users of different categories of drug prescriptions. Current clopidogrel and PPI prescriptions were set as the reference. Patients who were diagnosed as having acute myocardial infarction at entry were analyzed as a subgroup and compared with patients diagnosed as having overall cardiovascular disease including acute myocardial infarction. Analyses were specified for patients who had a hospitalization for upper GI bleeding before or after the cardiovascular disease hospitalizations. The characteristics of patients for the diagnosis of upper GI bleeding were categorized into four groups based on a bleeding episode which happened before, during or after the study period. Group I contained patients who had a history of peptic ulcer bleeding before cohort entry. Group II contained patients who had a bleeding history and who bled again during the study period. Group III contained patients who had no history of bleeding but experienced a bleeding episode during the study period, and Group IV contained patients who did not bleed during but after the defined study period. Compared with the general population, all these patients are apt to have a higher risk of GI bleeding, therefore, reasonable subjects for analysis in a whole group [29,30]. Furthermore, we performed additional analysis for sub-groups. Since there are a limited number of patients in the third and fourth groups, we only did a sub-analysis for patients who had a history of upper GI bleeding (Groups I and II). All of the proportional models were adjusted for age (<65, 65–74, 75–84, ≥85), sex (male, female), history of cardiovascular disease (yes, no), history of bleeding (yes, no), and co-morbidity (0, 1, 2, 3 or more). To assess surveillance bias, additional analyses were conducted after excluding cases that died within 30 days after entry. SAS (the Statistical Analysis System, version 9.2, SAS Institute Inc., Cary, NC, USA) was used for all analyses. The study was approved by the Regional Ethical Review Board in Stockholm.

Results

Study participants

In total, 98 725 cases of peptic ulcer bleeding were ascertained from the Swedish Patient Register. Among them, 2285 first cardiovascular disease events were included in the study. Table 1 shows the baseline characteristics of the study participants at the time of inclusion. Among the patients with cardiovascular disease, we also did a sub-group analysis for acute myocardial infarction (Tables 1 and 2). The cohorts were followed for the outcomes death and recurrence of cardiovascular disease. Of the 2285 cardiovascular disease patients, 1536 (67%) were older than 75 years of age and 1269 (56%) were men. There were 812 (36%) current users of only PPIs, 165 (7%)

Table 1 Characteristics of study participants diagnosed with cardiovascular disease

Characteristics	Death				Re-hospitalization for cardiovascular disease			
	CVD* cohort		AMI** cohort		CVD* cohort		AMI** cohort	
	Number (%)		Number (%)		Number (%)		Number (%)	
Total	2219		673		2285		695	
Men	1227	55%	365	54%	1269	56%	374	54%
Women	992	45%	308	46%	1016	44%	321	46%
Age group, years								
<65	291	13%	57	8%	303	13%	62	9%
65-75	425	19%	95	14%	446	20%	98	14%
75-85	844	38%	280	42%	872	38%	292	42%
> = 85	659	30%	241	36%	664	29%	243	35%
Upper gastrointestinal bleeding								
I. Bleeding before entry	1730	78%	513	76%	1773	78%	527	76%
II. Bleeding before entry and during the follow up	49	2%	22	3%	44	2%	20	3%
III. New bleeding during the follow up period	86	4%	41	6%	71	3%	33	5%
IV. Bleeding after endpoints	354	16%	97	14%	397	17%	115	17%
Cardiovascular disease history								
No	1315	59%	456	68%	1361	60%	475	68%
Yes	904	41%	217	32%	924	40%	220	32%
Comorbidities (number)								
0	1382	62%	328	49%	1426	62%	340	49%
1	628	28%	244	36%	643	28%	250	36%
2	173	8%	81	12%	178	8%	85	12%
≥3	36	2%	20	3%	38	2%	20	3%
Drug exposure								
Current clopidogrel and PPIs§	309	14%	95	14%	403	18%	116	17%
No current PPIs or clopidogrel	861	39%	211	31%	905	40%	226	33%
Current only PPIs	847	38%	316	47%	812	36%	308	44%
Current only clopidogrel	202	9%	51	8%	165	7%	45	6%
Patients with diagnosis of bleeding before entry								
Current clopidogrel and PPIs	252	14%	78	15%	244	13%	77	14%
No current PPIs or clopidogrel	659	37%	154	29%	702	39%	164	30%
Current only PPIs	714	40%	265	50%	713	39%	266	49%
Current only clopidogrel	154	9%	38	7%	158	9%	40	7%
subtotal	1779		535		1817		547	

**CVD* cardiovascular disease; ***AMI* acute myocardial infarction; *§PPIs* proton-pump inhibitors.

Table 2 Risk of death or recurrent cardiovascular events in 90 days follow-up among cardiovascular disease patients

Drug exposures	Cardiovascular disease cohort		Acute myocardial infarction cohort	
	Death	Cardiovascular disease	Death	Cardiovascular disease
	§HR (95% CI)	§HR (95% CI)	§HR (95% CI)	§HR (95% CI)
Total cohort				
*Current clopodogrel and PPI** (reference)*	1.00	1.00	1.00	1.00
No PPI and no clopidogrel	2.36 (1.39-4.00)	1.54 (1.05-2.24)	3.13 (1.47-6.68)	1.77 (0.92-3.41)
Current only PPIs	2.02 (1.19-3.44)	1.11 (0.75-1.65)	1.93 (0.91-4.11)	1.02 (0.52-1.99)
Current only clopidogrel	1.14 (0.53-2.45)	1.80 (1.15-2.83)	1.88 (0.70-5.03)	1.88 (0.85-4.08)
Patients with diagnosis of bleeding before entry*				
Current clopodogrel and PPI(reference)	1.00	1.00	1.00	1.00
No PPI and no clopidogrel	2.30 (1.33-3.98)	1.54 (0.98-2.40)	3.30 (1.47-7.41)	1.65 (0.78-3.47)
Current only PPI	2.05 (1.18-3.54)	1.04 (0.65-1.65)	2.12 (0.95-4.73)	0.80 (0.37-1.72)
Current only clopidogrel	1.25 (0.57-2.72)	1.84 (1.07-3.16)	2.26 (0.82-6.26)	1.78 (0.70-4.57)

*cohort members had history of upper gastrointestinal bleeding before entry into the cohorts. Results for patients who had any other hospitalizations for upper gastrointestinal bleeding were not shown due to the small number of cases.
***PPIs* proton-pump inhibitors.
§*HR* harzard ratio; *CI* confidence interval. All of the proportional models were adjusted for age (<65, 65–74, 75–84, ≥85), sex (male, female), history of cardiovascular diseases (yes, no), history of bleeding (yes, no), and co-morbidity (0, 1, 2, 3 or more).

current users of only clopidogrel, and 403 (18%) current users of concomitant prescriptions of PPIs and clopidogrel. In patients who only used one type of PPI, there were 878 omeprazole users, 162 esomeprazole users, 96 lansoprazole, 95 pantoprazole and 5 rabeprazole users. Among all participants, 245 (11%) died within the 90-day follow-up, 158 (7%) suffered ischemic stroke and 8 (0.3%) hemorrhagic stroke, while among 1817 (80%) patients with a diagnosis of upper GI bleeding before first entry into the cardiovascular disease cohort, 225 (13%) died within 90 days after discharge.

Hazard ratios for different drug exposures in the cardiovascular disease cohort

The HR for risk of death within 90 days of follow-up was 2.02 (95% CI 1.19-3.44) for current users of only PPIs, 1.14 (95% CI 0.53-2.45) for current users of only clopidogrel, and 2.36 (95% CI 1.39-4.00) among patients with no PPI or clopidogrel prescription, compared with patients using PPIs and clopidogrel concomitantly (Table 2). Regarding the risk of recurrent cardiovascular disease, the corresponding HRs were: 1.11 (95% CI 0.75-1.65), 1.80 (95% CI 1.15-2.83), and 1.54 (95% CI 1.05-2.24), respectively.

Hazard ratios for different drug exposures in the acute myocardial infarction cohort

In the acute myocardial infarction cohort, the HR for risk of death was 1.93 (95% 0.91-4.11) for current users of only PPIs, 1.88 (95% 0.70-5.03) for current users of only clopidogrel, and 3.13 (95% CI 1.47-6.68) for patients with no PPI or clopidogrel prescriptions. All the HRs for the risk of recurrent cardiovascular disease after acute myocardial infarction are not statistically different when compared to concomitant use of PPIs and clopidogrel.

Patients with a diagnosis of upper GI bleeding before entry

Patients with any upper GI bleeding diagnosis before entry into the study were analyzed separately. The results were consistent with the main analyses (Table 2). An elevated risk of death (HR 2.05, 95% 1.18-3.54) was detected for current only PPIs, and an increased risk of recurrent cardiovascular disease (HR 1.84, 95% CI 1.07-3.16) was found for current use of only clopidogrel, compared with concomitant use of PPIs and clopidogrel. Restricting the cohort to those who had experienced a bleeding within one year before entry rendered similar results (data not shown).

Discussion and conclusions

This study reveals no evidence of an increased risk of death or recurrence of cardiovascular disease among concomitant users of clopidogrel and PPIs in a population with a high risk of upper GI bleeding. Use of clopidogrel or PPIs alone seems to increase the risk of mortality and recurrent cardiovascular disease compared with concomitant use of these drugs.

Strengths of the study include the large sample size and the data collection from registers with complete nationwide coverage of the drug exposures and outcomes, i.e., recurrent cardiovascular disease and death. The nationwide register-based design counteracts selection and recall bias. Moreover, confounding was reduced by excluding patients with any recorded prescription of aspirin. There are, however, also several weaknesses. Filled prescriptions of PPIs and clopidogrel were regarded as the exposure, but there was no information on whether the patients had actually taken their medications. Also, PPI sub-types could not be analyzed separately due to the limited number, although the safety of pantoprazole has been specifically targeted in some studies [31]. More studies with a large sample size for possibly separating the analysis of PPI subtypes are warranted. In addition, it was not possible to entirely distinguish patients with a filled prescription after hospital admission from patients who still had drugs left from prescriptions filled before the index admission. Furthermore, we had no data on some important risk factors at baseline, such as tobacco smoking and alcohol consumption, which may bias the results [32]. We were, however, able to control for cardiovascular history and other co-morbidity as registered on hospital admission. Finally, confounding by indication could not be avoided completely in this observational study. Reasons for patients lacking any prescriptions might indicate that some completely recovered or that they might have had such severe symptoms that their physicians decided not to use any medication. These two opposite statuses of patients might make the confounding by indication less influential. The reason why some patients had only prescriptions of clopidogrel or only PPIs might be due to the recent reports of the increased risk of concomitant use of these two drugs rather than any specific disease indications. On the other hand, the consistently increased risk of recurrence of cardiovascular disease in clopidogrel only patients compared with the concomitant users may indicate the competing risk of death in this group.

Whether concomitant prescriptions of clopidogrel PPIs are associated with an increased recurrence of cardiovascular events is controversial [33]. Some studies have indicated a concern that the interaction between clopidogrel and PPIs could impair the treatment effect of clopidogrel [10-14,16], but others have not found any association. Instead, an independent cardiovascular risk by PPIs alone has been detected in a few studies. Several relevant meta-analyses have been published since 2010. Hulot and his coworkers initiated a meta-analysis in 2009 focusing on clopidogrel-treated patients with cytochrome P450 2C19*2 loss-of-function allele or the co-administration of PPIs. The results displayed an increased risk of major adverse cardiovascular events in the co-administration of clopidogrel and PPIs [34]. During the same year, the study by Kwok et al. showed that propensity-matched or randomized trial participants had no associated cardiovascular risk with PPIs, whereas other observational studies generally showed a significant association [35]. The same team published an updated study in 2012 with a focus on the potential risk with individual PPIs. They found an elevated risk of PPI therapy alone is associated with an adverse cardiovascular risk. They also admitted that major adverse cardiovascular events were mostly limited by the moderate to substantial heterogeneity of the studies included for meta-analysis. The high possibility of confounding and bias was indicated [31]. Siller-Matula and his colleagues published another meta-analysis in 2010. Their results indicated that concomitant PPI use might be associated with an increased risk of cardiovascular events but does not influence the risk of death. Articles included in these meta-analyses were not completely the same due to different inclusion criteria and time of publication. They further confirmed the presence of significant heterogeneity which might indicate that the evidence is biased, confounded, or inconsistent [36]. The clinical validity or relevance of the hypothesized PPI-clopidogrel interaction, thus, remains questionable.

The present study indicates that the co-administration of clopidogrel and PPIs results in a better effect regarding the prevention of death in patients with a high risk of GI bleeding. The current findings are consistent with some previous studies [17-20,37-40]. For example, a cohort study in the US and Canada which included 18 565 patients with acute coronary syndrome undergoing percutaneous coronary intervention (PCI) found no conclusive evidence of a clopidogrel-PPI interaction, even though there was a slightly increased risk of hospitalization for myocardial infarction. A study from Austria included 300 patients with coronary artery disease who had PCI. The platelet reactivity index was measured in patients with and without PPIs, and no interaction was found between clopidogrel and pantoprazole or esomeprazole [17]. One big cohort study from Denmark found that the apparent association between recurrent myocardial infarction and the use of PPIs with clopidogrel is affected by confounding by indication. The association is not present when confounding is addressed by design [41]. Although indications of reduced antiplatelet activity have been found *in vivo* in the case of PPI administration in clopidogrel users, the interaction between antiplatelet agents and PPIs at the enzymatic level does not seem to result in worse clinical outcomes.

In summary, recent studies have shown conflicting and inconsistent data regarding the adverse interaction of clopidogrel and PPIs. Together with our study, we think clinicians should focus on the potential harm from ulcers or hemorrhage before deciding to omit PPIs in patients taking clopidogrel. In selected patients at high-risk of GI bleeding, clinicians should in fact be very cautious and cannot overlook the life-threatening risk that bleedings represent.

Competing interests

All authors have no competing interests to declare: no support from any organization for the submitted work; no financial relationships with any organizations that might have an interest in the submitted work in the previous three years and no other relationships or activities that could appear to have influenced the submitted work.

Authors' contributions

QW participated in the study design, carried out the statistical analysis and drafted the manuscript. RL collected the data, contributed to data arrangement, data analysis, and interpretation of results and helped to draft the manuscript; JL participated in the study design, contributed to interpretation of the results and drafted the manuscript; LY conceived of the study, contributed to the acquisition of the data, participated in the study design and helped to draft the manuscript. All authors read and approved the final manuscript.

Acknowledgements

We acknowledge financial support from the Swedish Research Council (SIMSAM), the Swedish Medical Society and the Karolinska foundation. None of these funding bodies had any role in any process of the current study.

Author details

[1]Department of Molecular Medicine and Surgery, Karolinska Institutet, SE-171 76 Stockholm, Sweden. [2]Unit of Epidemiology, Institute of Environmental Medicine, Karolinska Institutet, Stockholm, Sweden. [3]Division of Cancer Studies, King's College London, London, United Kingdom. [4]Department of Epidemiology and Biostatistics, Imperial College London, London, United Kingdom.

References

1. Terpening C: **Clopidogrel: a pharmacogenomic perspective on its use in coronary artery disease.** *Clin Med Insights Cardiol* 2010, **4**:117–128. PubMed PMID: 21151850. Pubmed Central PMCID: 2998935. Epub 2010/12/15. eng.
2. Tran H, Anand SS: **Oral antiplatelet therapy in cerebrovascular disease, coronary artery disease, and peripheral arterial disease.** *JAMA* 2004, **292**(15):1867–1874. PubMed PMID: 15494585. Epub 2004/10/21. eng.
3. Rogowski W, Burch J, Palmer S, Craigs C, Golder S, Woolacott N: **The effect of different treatment durations of clopidogrel in patients with non-ST-segment elevation acute coronary syndromes: a systematic review and value of information analysis.** *Health Technol Assess* 2009, **13**(31):1–77. iii-iv, ix-xi, PubMed PMID: 19573471. Epub 2009/07/04. eng.
4. Jackowski L, Stocks N, Rowett D: **Reducing the risk of adverse thrombotic events - The role of aspirin and clopidogrel.** *Aust Fam Physician* 2008, **37**(9):721–723. 5–6. PubMed PMID: 18797530. Epub 2008/09/18. eng.
5. Boparai V, Rajagopalan J, Triadafilopoulos G: **Guide to the use of proton pump inhibitors in adult patients.** *Drugs* 2008, **68**(7):925–947. PubMed PMID: 18457460. Epub 2008/05/07. eng.
6. Madanick RD: **Proton pump inhibitor side effects and drug interactions: much ado about nothing?** *Cleve Clin J Med* 2011, **78**(1):39–49. PubMed PMID: 21199906. Epub 2011/01/05. eng.
7. Furuta T: **Risk and benefit of proton pump inhibitor for patients undergoing anti-platelet therapy including clopidogrel.** *Intern Med* 2009, **48**(21):1847–1848. PubMed PMID: 19881232. Epub 2009/11/03. eng.
8. Moayyedi P, Sadowski DC: **Proton pump inhibitors and clopidogrel - hazardous drug interaction or hazardous interpretation of data?** *Can J Gastroenterol* 2009, **23**(4):251–252. PubMed PMID: 19373416. Pubmed Central PMCID: 2711671. Epub 2009/04/18. eng.
9. Barrison AF, Jarboe LA, Weinberg BM, Nimmagadda K, Sullivan LM, Wolfe MM: **Patterns of proton pump inhibitor use in clinical practice.** *Am J Med Genet* 2001, **111**(6):469–473. PubMed PMID: 11690573.
10. Huang CC, Chen YC, Leu HB, Chen TJ, Lin SJ, Chan WL, Chen JW: **Risk of adverse outcomes in Taiwan associated with concomitant use of clopidogrel and proton pump inhibitors in patients who received percutaneous coronary intervention.** *Am J Cardiol* 2010, **105**(12):1705–1709. PubMed PMID: 20538118. Epub 2010/06/12. eng.
11. Gupta E, Bansal D, Sotos J, Olden K: **Risk of adverse clinical outcomes with concomitant use of clopidogrel and proton pump inhibitors following percutaneous coronary intervention.** *Dig Dis Sci* 2009, **55**(7):1964–1968. PubMed PMID: 19731021. Epub 2009/09/05. eng.
12. Ho PM, Maddox TM, Wang L, Fihn SD, Jesse RL, Peterson ED, Peterson ED, Rumsfeld JS: **Risk of adverse outcomes associated with concomitant use of clopidogrel and proton pump inhibitors following acute coronary syndrome.** *JAMA* 2009, **301**(9):937–944. PubMed PMID: 19258584. Epub 2009/03/05. eng.
13. Juurlink DN, Gomes T, Ko DT, Szmitko PE, Austin PC, Tu JV, Henry DA, Kopp A, Mamdami MM: **A population-based study of the drug interaction between proton pump inhibitors and clopidogrel.** *CMAJ* 2009, **180**(7):713–718. PubMed PMID: 19176635. Pubmed Central PMCID: 2659819. Epub 2009/01/30. eng.
14. Stockl KM, Le L, Zakharyan A, Harada AS, Solow BK, Addiego JE, Ramsey S: **Risk of rehospitalization for patients using clopidogrel with a proton pump inhibitor.** *Arch Intern Med* 2010, **170**(8):704–710. PubMed PMID: 20421557. Epub 2010/04/28. eng.
15. Gilard M, Arnaud B, Cornily JC, Le Gal G, Lacut K, Le Calvez G, Mansourati J, Mottier D, Abgrall JF, Boschat J: **Influence of omeprazole on the antiplatelet action of clopidogrel associated with aspirin: the randomized, double-blind OCLA (Omeprazole CLopidogrel Aspirin) study.** *J Am Coll Cardiol* 2008, **51**(3):256–260. PubMed PMID: 18206732. Epub 2008/01/22. eng.
16. Pezalla E, Day D, Pulliadath I: **Initial assessment of clinical impact of a drug interaction between clopidogrel and proton pump inhibitors.** *J Am Coll Cardiol* 2008, **52**(12):1038–1039. author reply 9. PubMed PMID: 18786491. Epub 2008/09/13. eng.
17. Bhatt DL, Cryer BL, Contant CF, Cohen M, Lanas A, Schnitzer TJ, Shook TL, Lapuerta P, Goldsmith MA, Laine L, Scirica BM, Murphy SA, Cannon CP, COGENT Investigators: **Clopidogrel with or without omeprazole in coronary artery disease.** *N Engl J Med* 2010, **363**(20):1909–1917. PubMed PMID: 20925534. Epub 2010/10/12. Eng.
18. O'Donoghue ML, Braunwald E, Antman EM, Murphy SA, Bates ER, Rozenman Y, Rozenman Y, Michelson AD, Hautvast RW, Ver Lee PN, Close SL, Shen L, Mega JL, Sabatine MS, Wiviott SD: **Pharmacodynamic effect and clinical efficacy of clopidogrel and prasugrel with or without a proton-pump inhibitor: an analysis of two randomised trials.** *Lancet* 2009, **374**(9694):PubMed PMID: 19726078–PubMed PMID: 19726997. PubMed PMID: 19726078.
19. Rassen JA, Choudhry NK, Avorn J, Schneeweiss S: **Cardiovascular outcomes and mortality in patients using clopidogrel with proton pump inhibitors after percutaneous coronary intervention or acute coronary syndrome.** *Circulation* 2009, **120**(23):2322–2329. PubMed PMID: 19933932. Pubmed Central PMCID: 2818789. Epub 2009/11/26. eng.
20. Ray WA, Murray KT, Griffin MR, Chung CP, Smalley WE, Hall K, Hall K, Daugherty JR, Kaltenbach LA, Stein CM: **Outcomes with concurrent use of clopidogrel and proton-pump inhibitors: a cohort study.** *Ann Intern Med* 2010, **152**(6):337–345. PubMed PMID: 20231564. Pubmed Central PMCID: 3176584.
21. Administration. UFaD: *Information for healthcare professionals: update to the labeling of clopidogrel bisulfate (marketed as Plavix) to alert healthcare professionals about a drug interaction with omeprazole (marketed as Prilosec and Prilosec OTC).* U.S. Department of Health and Human Services. 11/17/2009. http://www.fda.gov/Drugs/DrugSafety/PostmarketDrugSafetyInformationforPatientsandProviders/DrugSafetyInformationforHeathcareProfessionals/ucm190787.htm.
22. Juhasz M, Herszenyi L, Tulassay Z: **Current standings of the proton pump inhibitor and clopidogrel co-therapy: review on an evolving field with the eyes of the gastroenterologist.** *Digestion* 2010, **81**(1):10–15. PubMed PMID: 20029203. Epub 2009/12/24. eng.
23. Tsai YW, Wen YW, Huang WF, Chen PF, Kuo KN, Hsiao FY: **Cardiovascular and gastrointestinal events of three antiplatelet therapies: clopidogrel, clopidogrel plus proton-pump inhibitors, and aspirin plus proton-pump inhibitors in patients with previous gastrointestinal bleeding.** *J Gastroenterol* 2011, **46**(1):39–45. PubMed PMID: 20811753.
24. Hsu PI, Lai KH, Liu CP: **Esomeprazole with clopidogrel reduces peptic ulcer recurrence, compared with clopidogrel alone, in patients with atherosclerosis.** *Gastroenterology* 2011, **140**(3):791–798. PubMed PMID: 21144850.

25. Gaglia MA Jr, Torguson R, Hanna N, Gonzalez MA, Collins SD, Syed AI, Syed AI, Ben-Dor I, Maluenda G, Delhaye C, Wakabayashi K, Xue Z, Suddath WO, Kent KM, Satler LF, Pichard AD, Waksman R: **Relation of proton pump inhibitor use after percutaneous coronary intervention with drug-eluting stents to outcomes.** *Am J Cardiol* 2010, **105**(6):833–888. PubMed PMID: 20211327.
26. Hsiao FY, Mullins CD, Wen YW, Huang WF, Chen PF, Tsai YW: **Relationship between cardiovascular outcomes and proton pump inhibitor use in patients receiving dual antiplatelet therapy after acute coronary syndrome.** *Pharmacoepidemiol Drug Saf* 2011, **20**(10):1043–1049. PubMed PMID: 21823195.
27. Ahsberg K, Hoglund P, Stael von Holstein C: **Mortality from peptic ulcer bleeding: the impact of comorbidity and the use of drugs that promote bleeding.** *Aliment Pharmacol Therapeut Symp* 2010, **32**(6):801–810. PubMed PMID: 20653635.
28. Jepsen P, Vilstrup H, Lash TL: **Development and Validation of a Comorbidity Scoring System for Patients With Cirrhosis.** *Gastroenterology* 2014, **146**(1):147–156. quiz e15-6.
29. Bratanic A, Puljiz Z, Ljubicicz N, Caric T, Jelicic I, Puljiz M, Puljiz M, Perko Z: **Predictive factors of rebleeding and mortality following endoscopic hemostasis in bleeding peptic ulcers.** *Hepatogastroenterology* 2013, **60** (121):112–117. PubMed PMID: 22709912.
30. Lau JY, Barkun A, Fan DM, Kuipers EJ, Yang YS, Chan FK: **Challenges in the management of acute peptic ulcer bleeding.** *Lancet* 2013, **381** (9882):2033–2043. PubMed PMID: 23746903.
31. Kwok CS, Jeevanantham V, Dawn B, Loke YK: **No consistent evidence of differential cardiovascular risk amongst proton-pump inhibitors when used with clopidogrel: meta-analysis.** *Int J Cardiol* 2013, **167**(3):965–974. PubMed PMID: 22464478.
32. Focks JJ, Brouwer MA, van Oijen MG, Lanas A, Bhatt DL, Verheugt FW: **Concomitant use of clopidogrel and proton pump inhibitors: impact on platelet function and clinical outcome- a systematic review.** *Heart* 2013, **99**(8):520–527. PubMed PMID: 22851683.
33. Kwok CS, Nijjar RS, Loke YK: **Effects of proton pump inhibitors on adverse gastrointestinal events in patients receiving clopidogrel: systematic review and meta-analysis.** *Drug Saf* 2010, **34**(1):47–57. PubMed PMID: 21047145. Epub 2010/11/05. eng.
34. Hulot JS, Collet JP, Silvain J, Pena A, Bellemain-Appaix A, Barthelemy O, Cayla G, Beygui F, Montalescot G: **Cardiovascular risk in clopidogrel-treated patients according to cytochrome P450 2C19*2 loss-of-function allele or proton pump inhibitor coadministration: a systematic meta-analysis.** *J Am Coll Cardiol* 2010, **56**(2):134–143. PubMed PMID: 20620727.
35. Kwok CS, Loke YK: **Meta-analysis: the effects of proton pump inhibitors on cardiovascular events and mortality in patients receiving clopidogrel.** *Aliment Pharmacol Therapeut Symp* 2010, **31**(8):810–823. PubMed PMID: 20102352.
36. Siller-Matula JM, Jilma B, Schror K, Christ G, Huber K: **Effect of proton pump inhibitors on clinical outcome in patients treated with clopidogrel: a systematic review and meta-analysis.** *J Thromb Haemostasis* 2010, **8**(12):2624–2641. PubMed PMID: 20831618.
37. Siller-Matula JM, Spiel AO, Lang IM, Kreiner G, Christ G, Christ G, Jilma B: **Effects of pantoprazole and esomeprazole on platelet inhibition by clopidogrel.** *Am Heart J* 2009, **157**(1):148 e1-5. PubMed PMID: 19081411. Epub 2008/12/17. eng.
38. Bhurke SM, Martin BC, Li C, Franks AM, Bursac Z, Said Q: **Effect of the clopidogrel-proton pump inhibitor drug interaction on adverse cardiovascular events in patients with acute coronary syndrome.** *Pharmacotherapy* 2012, **32**(9):809–818. PubMed PMID: 22744772. Pubmed Central PMCID: 3531962.
39. Leontiadis GI, Howden CW: **PPI co-therapy did not adversely affect outcomes in clopidogrel users.** *Aliment Pharmacol Therapeut Symp* 2012, **35**(2):313–314. PubMed PMID: 22172084.
40. Schmidt M, Johansen MB, Robertson DJ, Maeng M, Kaltoft A, Jensen LO, Tilsted HH, Bøtker HE, Sørensen HT, Baron JA: **Concomitant use of clopidogrel and proton pump inhibitors is not associated with major adverse cardiovascular events following coronary stent implantation.** *Alimentary pharmacology & therapeutics* 2012, **35**(1):165–174. PubMed PMID: 22050009.
41. Valkhoff VE, t Jong GW, Van Soest EM, Kuipers EJ, Sturkenboom MC: **Risk of recurrent myocardial infarction with the concomitant use of clopidogrel and proton pump inhibitors.** *Aliment Pharmacol Therapeut Symp* 2011, **33**(1):77–88. PubMed PMID: 21083580.

CNX-011-67, a novel GPR40 agonist, enhances glucose responsiveness, insulin secretion and islet insulin content in n-STZ rats and in islets from type 2 diabetic patients

Venkategowda Sunil†, Mahesh Kumar Verma†, Anup M Oommen†, Manojkumar Sadasivuni, Jaideep Singh, Dasarahalli N Vijayraghav, Bhawna Chandravanshi, Jayalaxmi Shetty, Sanghamitra Biswas, Anilkumar Dandu, Yoganand Moolemath, Marikunte V Venkataranganna, Baggavalli P Somesh and Madanahalli R Jagannath*

Abstract

Background: GPR40 is a G-protein coupled receptor regulating free fatty acid induced and also glucose induced insulin secretion. We generated neonatally-streptozotocin-treated female rats (n-STZ) and treated them with CNX-011-67, a GPR40 agonist to examine the role of GPR40 in modulation of glucose metabolism, insulin secretion and content.

Methods: Female n-STZ animals were orally administered with CNX-011-67 (15 mg/kg body weight, twice daily) or with vehicle for 8 weeks ($n = 8$ per group). Glucose tolerance in treated animals and insulin secretion, islet insulin content and gene expression in isolated islets were determined. Islets from type 2 diabetic mellitus (T2DM) patients were treated with different concentrations of glucose in presence or absence of CNX-011-67 and insulin secretion was measured.

Results: Treatment of n-STZ rats with GPR40 agonist CNX-011-67 enhanced insulin secretion in response to oral glucose load on day 0 and this response persisted during the treatment period. The treatment also produced a 'memory effect' during which insulin secretion in response to oral glucose load remained enhanced, for a week, even in absence of the agonist. Activation of GPR40 enhanced responsiveness of islets to glucose and increased glucose induced insulin secretion and islet insulin content. An increase in islet mRNA expression of GCK, PDX1, insulin and PC was also observed. Acute treatment of islets from n-STZ rats with GPR40 agonist enhanced cellular ATP content. Activation of GPR40 enhanced mitochondrial calcium level in NIT-1 insulinoma cells. CNX-011-67 increased insulin secretion in islets from T2DM patients which were non-responsive to increased glucose concentration

Conclusions: Our data provide evidence that activation of GPR40 with CNX-011-67 stimulates glucose metabolism, enhances glucose responsiveness, increases insulin secretion and content and that pharmacological activation of GPR40 will prove beneficial for treatment of T2DM.

Keywords: β-cells, CNX-011-67, Glucose stimulated insulin secretion, GPR40, Neonatal streptozotocin, Type 2 Diabetes mellitus, Islet insulin content

* Correspondence: m.r.jagannath@connexios.com
†Equal contributors
Connexios Life Sciences Pvt Ltd, #49, "SHILPA VIDYA" 1st Main, 3rd Phase, JP Nagar, Bangalore 560078, India

Background

Type 2 Diabetes Mellitus (T2DM) is growing in epidemic proportions both in the developed and developing countries and is estimated to affect 438 million humans world-wide by the year 2030 (World Diabetes Foundation). Normally the β-cell responds to an increment in glucose with an increase in insulin to maintain normoglycemia [1,2]. In response to oral glucose an 'early phase' insulin secretion is observed within the first 30 min of ingestion which is reduced in subjects with impaired glucose tolerance suggesting that an impaired first phase is perhaps the earliest detectable abnormality in individuals destined to develop T2DM [3,4]. With onset of β-cells failure there is first a steady increase in postprandial and fasting glucose concentrations leading finally to the development of overt diabetes [1,5-7].

Several therapeutic approaches have been adopted to prevent and/or delay the defects in β-cell function [8,9]. Of relevance to this study is the role of the G protein coupled receptor 40 (GPR40), also known as Free Fatty Acid Receptor 1 in the regulation of β-cell function. GPR40 is highly expressed in human β-cells, brain and endocrine cells of the gastrointestinal tract and is activated by medium and long chain saturated and unsaturated fatty acids and enhance insulin secretion by activating cytosolic calcium flux [10-12]. Over-expression of GPR40 increases whereas its knockout decreases insulin secretion [13,14] indicating its important role for insulin secretion and glucose tolerance. Similarly, its expression is reduced in T2DM islets and is positively correlated with insulin secretion [15]. Hence, GPR40 is an important therapeutic target to treat T2DM. In fact a number of small molecule agonists have been shown to modulate glucose stimulated insulin secretion. Different GPR40 agonists such as GW9508, TAK-875, AS2575959, AMG837 and phenyl propanoic acid derivatives have shown increased insulin secretion in both insulinoma cells and/or in animal models [16-20]. Among these agonists, TAK-875 has been shown to prevent β-cells dysfunction [21] in animal model of diabetes and improves glycemic control in T2DM patients [22,23]. However, none of these abovementioned molecules have been reported to increase insulin secretion in n-STZ model which has high β-cell stress.

While the precise primary defects that trigger β-cell defects are not fully understood, islets from patients with T2DM have been reported to display reduced glucose oxidation [24,25], reduced ATP content in response to an acute glucose stimulation [26] and reduced glucose stimulated insulin secretion (GSIS) [24,25,27]. These changes are associated with a decrease in expression of glucokinase (GCK), glucose transporter 1 and 2 (GLUT1 and 2), and alterations in genes involved in insulin granule exocytosis [24,28,29]. β-cell population in diabetics is reduced by 30% when accompanied by deposition of islet amyloid [30,31] and a 50% decline in β-cell volume is observed in patients with impaired fasting glucose [32]. The similar pathology was reported in neonatal streptozotocin (n-STZ) rats [33-36]. Also stress in β-cell of this model is very high which is similar to the stress seen in T2DM patient's islets.

We have reported previously that chronic treatment of male ZDF rats (insulin resistant model with elevated blood glucose and free fatty acid levels) with CNX-011-67 increased insulin secretion, decreased blood glucose and reduced β-cells apoptosis without affecting body weight [37]. We have shown that chronic β-cell stress mediated by glucolipotoxic conditions reduces GSIS, islet insulin content, ATP levels and expression of genes such as GCK, PDX1 and insulin [38]. Chronic treatment of CNX-011-67 was able to overcome these defects in β-cells functions [37]. In the present study we were interested to evaluate chronic activation of GPR40 in the neonatal streptozotocin (n-STZ) rats which manifests reduced β-cell number, decreased GSIS and severe β-cell stress as seen in T2DM patient islets [33-36]. Chronic treatment with CNX-011-67 resulted in improved glucose responsiveness, phasic glucose stimulated insulin secretion and increased islet insulin content. CNX-011-67 also increased glucose stimulated insulin secretion in human islets from T2DM patient. These results suggest that activation of GPR40 by CNX-011-67 will provide a novel therapeutic approach to improve long-term glycemic control in T2DM patients by regulating β-cell biology.

Methods

Reagents

Glucose was estimated using Accu-check glucometer (Roche Diagnostics, Germany). Ultra-sensitive insulin ELISA kit (Crystal Chem Inc, USA) was used to determine plasma insulin levels. Insulin was estimated in *in-vitro* studies using "ultra-sensitive insulin assay kit" (Mercodia, Sweden) according to the manufacturer's instructions.

Animals

In-bred Wistar rats were provided commercial pelleted food (Provimi, India) and water *ad libitum* and maintained on a 12 h light and 12 h dark cycle during the studies. All animal experiment procedures were approved by the Institutional Animal Ethics Committee of Connexios Life Sciences and were in accordance with the guidelines of Committee For The Purpose Of Control And Supervision On Experiments On Animals (CPCSEA) Govt. of India.

Oral glucose tolerance test (OGTT)

After a 16 h fast, CNX-011-67 (5 mg/kg or 15 mg/kg body weight) or vehicle was administered 30 min or

45 min prior to administration of glucose (2 g/kg b.wt) by oral gavage (n = 8 per group). Blood samples were collected from the tail vein 30 min or 45 min before treatment and at 0, 10, 20, 30, 60 and 120 min after glucose load for estimating glucose and insulin.

Generation and treatment of n-STZ rats

Following breeding, pups were administered 50 mg/kg, i.p of STZ (Sigma-Aldrich, St. Louis, USA) or vehicle on day 2 and 3 of birth and allowed to be with their mothers until weaning at 21 days of age. Subsequently, only animals that were confirmed as glucose intolerant in an oral glucose tolerance test (at the age of 17 weeks) were included in the study. More than 95% of the animals that were administered with STZ were glucose intolerant at 17 week and the rest of the animals developed glucose intolerance 2 weeks later.

Three experimental groups were studied, namely, sham control, n-STZ control and n-STZ + CNX-011-67 (15 mg/kg b.wt.). CNX-011-67 was dissolved in water and administered twice daily by oral gavage (15 mg/kg b. wt.). The n-STZ control animals were administered vehicle (water). Four protocols were followed:

Protocol 1: n-STZ animals were treated with CNX-011-67 (twice daily, 15 mg/kg body weight) or vehicle for 12 weeks (n = 8 per group) and oral glucose tolerance test was performed on day 0 and week 8.

Protocol 2: n-STZ animals were treated with CNX-011-67 (twice daily, 15 mg/kg body weight) or vehicle for 8 weeks (n = 8 per group) and islet mRNA was isolated for RT-PCR based analysis of gene expression.

Protocol 3: n-STZ animals were treated with CNX-011-67 (twice daily, 15 mg/kg body weight) or vehicle for 8 weeks (n = 8 per group) and treatment was withdrawn for 1-week (ninth week of the study). OGTT was performed after week 8 and again after one week of drug withdrawal (9th week). Agonist treatment was reintroduced and continued for a further 3 weeks after which glucose stimulated insulin secretion and insulin content were determined in islets isolated from the animals.

Protocol 4: Islets isolated from n-STZ rats were acutely treated with CNX-011-67 and ATP content was measured.

Daily food intake and body weight were recorded for all the animals in the above protocols

Islet isolation, gluose stimulated insulin secretion and islet insulin content measurement

Animals were killed under anesthesia (due to ethical considerations; all groups of animals were similarly treated) and pancreata were digested with collagenase-II (Sigma-Aldrich, St. Louis, USA) followed by islet separation in a density gradient centrifugation using Histopaque (Sigma diagnostics, St. Louis, MO, USA) as described ear lier [39]. Size-matched islets were handpicked under a stereomicroscope (Nikon) and used for GSIS assay. Briefly, islets were seeded in 24-well culture plates in 1 ml of Krebs-Ringer bicarbonate HEPES (KRBH) buffer with 2.8 mM glucose and incubated at 37°C for 1 h. Islets were then treated with 1 μM of CNX-011-67 in the presence of low (5.6 mM) or high (16.7 mM) glucose for 2 h. The culture supernatant was collected and stored at −70°C for measurement of insulin. Islets were then lysed in lysis buffer and islet insulin content was measured. Both secreted insulin and islet insulin content were normalized with total protein measured using Bradford's reagent (Bio-Rad). Amount of secreted insulin was also normalized with islet insulin content and represented as % of islet insulin content.

Human islets from cadevar T2DM donars were procured from Prodo lab, USA. Size matched islets were hand picked and incubated in KRBH containing 2.8 mM glucose for 1 h. Islets were then incubated with different concentrations of glucose with or without CNX-011-67 (1 μM) for 2 h. The supernatent was collected and used for insulin measurement. Four islets were used in each replicate for the GSIS.

Measurement of mitochondrial and cytosolic calcium flux in N1T1 cells.

NIT1 cells (ATCC) were cultured in Ham's F12 medium (Sigma-Aldrich) supplemented with 15% FBS, 2 mM L-glutamine, 100 U/ml penicillin and 100 μg/ml of streptomycin (All reagents from GIBCO, USA). For experiments, NIT-1 cells were seeded at a density of 40,000 cells/well in 96-well plates and incubated for 72 h. Cells were loaded with Fluo-3 AM (Invitrogen, 2.5 μM) dye for cytosolic calcium measurement or Rhod-2 AM dye (Invitrogen, 4 μM) for mitochondrial calcium measurement for 60 min and washed twice with HEPES buffered saline solution (HBSS) to remove unbound dye. Following a basal measurement, cells were treated with low glucose (2.8 mM), high glucose (16.7 mM) or high glucose with 1 μM of CNX-011-67 and Ca^{2+} levels were measured for 4 min at 6-s intervals using a Biotek Synergy 2 fluorimeter with resulting flux being represented as arbitrary fluorescence units (AFU) [40]. Calcium levels represented refer to net response with background fluorescence corrections. There were no oscillations observed and the response was sustained for nearly 12 minutes.

Quantitative Real-time PCR (qPCR)

Total RNA was extracted from islets using Tri-reagent (Sigma, St. Louis, MO, USA), followed by chloroform extraction and isopropyl alcohol precipitation. This total RNA (500 ng) was used for cDNA synthesis by reverse transcription (ABI, Foster City, CA, USA). mRNA levels were quantified using SYBR Green PCR Master Mix (Eurogenetic, Belgium) using 5 ng of cDNA. Genes analyzed in the present study were GCK, PC, PDX1 and insulin. For quantification of gene expression, β-actin was used as internal control (primer sequences are available upon request).

Measurement of β-cell ATP and inositol-tri-phosphate (IP3) content

After preincubation at 2.8 mM glucose for 60 min, groups of ten islets were incubated in tubes containing 0.5 ml KRBH buffer supplemented with 2.8 or 11 mM glucose with or without 300 nM CNX-011-67 for 60 min for ATP and 5 min for IP3 measurement. The islets were then washed twice with 1X cold PBS and lysed in lysing buffer provided by the manufacturer. ATP and IP3 concentrations were measured using ATP determination kit (Molecular Probes, USA) or Rat IP3 ELISA Kit (CUSABIO biotech, China) in a Multi-Mode Micro plate Reader (SpectraMax M5e, Molecular Devices, USA).

Histology and immunohistochemistry of β-cells

Pancreata were dissected out from the animals and fixed in 10% buffered neutral formalin for 48 h. The entire pancreas was collected, weighed, processed and paraffin-embedded. Each block was serially sectioned (4 μm) throughout its length to avoid any bias from regional changes in islet distribution and islet cell composition, and sections were mounted on clean glass slides. Three serial sections were obtained every 100 microns. One was used for hematoxylin and eosin staining, and the remaining for immunofluorescence staining for insulin and PDX1.

Immunofluorescence staining for insulin and PDX1 was carried out using a goat anti-mouse FITC conjugated and goat anti-rabbit Alexafluor conjugated secondary antibody direct labeling technique, respectively. Sections were incubated for 1 h with anti-insulin (Abexome, India) and anti-PDX1 (Abcam, UK) antibodies. Thereafter, FITC- and Alexafluor-conjugated secondary antibodies were applied for 30 min. After staining, sections were mounted in fluromount (Sigma). All hematoxylin and eosin sections were taken for histological evaluation under light microscope.

Images were captured using Zeiss fluorescence microscope using progres® capture pro 2.1 camera. Quantitative evaluation of total β-cell mass was performed using a computer-assisted image analysis (progres®capturepro) software. The relative volume of β-cells was determined by a stereological morphometric method, calculating the ratio between the area occupied by immunoreactive cells and that occupied by total pancreatic cells. Total β-cell mass per pancreas was derived by multiplying this ratio by the total pancreatic weight. The total β-cell nuclei from all stained section were counted, to derive number of β-cells per islet.

Electron microscopy studies

Pancreatic tissue was fixed in 3% gluteraldehyde for 24 h, washed with phosphate buffer twice and post-fixed with 1% Osmium tetroxide. Tissues were then washed with phosphate buffer twice and processed in different grades of alcohol for dehydration and propylene oxide for clearing. Tissues were infiltrated with a mixture of propylene oxide: araldite (1:1) and incubated on a rotator overnight at room temperature. Tissues were transferred to fresh and pure araldite, incubated and then embedded. Blocks were allowed to polymerize for 48 h at 60°C. Ultra thin sections were stained with uranyl acetate and lead citrate and scanned in a Transmission Electron Microscope.

Statistical Analysis

Data values are expressed as mean ± S.E.M. Significance of differences among groups was determined using One-way analysis of variance followed by Dunnett's post-test or by Students unpaired t-test. P value summary: (*) <0.05, (**) <0.01 and (***) <0.001 respectively, when compared with vehicle control.

Results

Phenotypic characterization of n-STZ rats prior to the start of treatment

Table 1 gives body weight, fasting glucose and insulin levels in the neonatally STZ treated adult (n-STZ) rats and sham control rats at week 17 of age, 1 week before commencement of treatment with CNX-011-67. There was no significant difference in body weight and fasting glucose between the sham control and n-STZ groups but the n-STZ animals displayed decreased insulin area under curve (AUC) and severe glucose intolerance during 'Oral Glucose Tolerance Test' (OGTT). Fasting insulin levels in n-STZ animals had declined to 0.174 ± 0.04 ng/ml as compared to 0.31 ± 0.05 ng/ml recorded in the sham control animals.

Table 1 Phenotypic characterization of n-STZ rats (prior to treatment commencement)

	Body weight (g)	Fasting glucose (mg/dl)	Fasting insulin (ng/ml)	Glucose AUC (OGTT) (mg/dl)*min	Insulin AUC (GSIS) (ng/ml)*min
Sham (n = 32)	202 ± 6	83 ± 3	0.31 ± 0.05	14791 ± 255	98 ± 8.6
n-STZ (n = 55)	203 ± 3	80 ± 1.7	0.17 ± 0.04*	31617 ± 931***	79 ± 5.14

Statistical comparison between sham and n-STZ group was conducted by Students t-test (Two-way, unpaired: *p < 0.05 and ***p < 0.001).

Effect of GPR40 agonist treatment on insulin secretion and glucose levels with and without glucose load in Wistar rats

In normal Wistar rats, oral administration of 2 g/kg glucose resulted in a significant increase in insulin secretion (0–30 min AUC 12.45 ± 1.55 vs 4.85 ± 0.63) when compared to control animals while treatment with CNX-011-67 (5 mg/kg body weight) significantly enhanced insulin secretion (0–30" AUC 16.23 ± 2.05 vs 12.45 ± 1.55, 31% increase, $P < 0.05$) in response to oral glucose (Figure 1A lower panel and D) when compared with glucose control. There was a significant decrease in glucose AUC in CNX-011-67 treated animals when compared to untreated animals (0–120 min AUC 14716 ± 360 vs 17400 ± 535, 39% decrease, $P < 0.001$) (Figure 1A upper panel and C). In absence of oral glucose challenge, treatment with CNX-011-67 (15 mg/kg body weight) did not either increase insulin secretion (0–30 min AUC 10.18 ± 1.7 vs 11.73 ± 1.9) (Figure 1B lower panel and E) or decrease blood glucose levels (0–120 min AUC 11049 ± 362 vs 11272 ± 176) (Figure 1B upper panel and F).

Effect of GPR40 agonist treatment on early phase insulin secretion and glucose tolerance in n-STZ rats

The n-STZ group of animals showed loss of insulin secretion capacity in response to an oral glucose challenge (Figure 2A, lower panel). Insulin secretion in response to oral glucose load increased (1.8 fold) in the n-STZ-CNX-011-67 treated animals after administration of the first dose itself (day 0) leading to a significant improvement in glucose tolerance when compared to the (untreated) n-STZ animals (AUCglucose 20057 ± 885 vs 30433 ± 865 respectively, n = 8; $P < 0.01$; Figure 2A upper panel). The improvement in glucose tolerance was almost similar to the glucose tolerance observed in the sham control animals (AUCglucose 17900 ± 217). Chronic administration of CNX-011-67 to n-STZ animals showed no impact on body weight and feed consumption. Histological analysis did not show any organ related toxicity (data not shown). After 8 weeks of treatment with CNX-011-67 agonist, a similar increase in insulin secretion (2-fold, Figure 2B lower panel) in response to oral glucose load and improvement in glucose tolerance was observed in the n-STZ-CNX-011-67 animals compared to the untreated n-STZ animals (17225 ± 786 vs 32480 ± 1697 respectively, n = 8; $P < 0.01$; Figure 2B upper panel) and this improved glucose tolerance was again similar to the glucose tolerance observed in the sham control animals group (18094 ± 501). Similarly, the increase in insulin secretion in first 30 min, on day 0, led to a significant improvement in glucose tolerance in the n-STZ-CNX-011-67 animals when compared to the untreated n-STZ animals (area under the 0–30 min glucose curve: 4232 ± 182 vs 5725 ± 358, respectively, n = 8; $P < 0.01$; Figure 2A upper panel) and was similar to the glucose tolerance observed in the vehicle treated sham control animals (AUCglucose 4221 ± 102). A similar increase in insulin secretion and improvement in glucose tolerance at 30 min post oral glucose load was also observed after 8 weeks of treatment with the n-STZ-CNX-011-67 agonist. A significant aspect of the n-STZ-CNX-011-67 agonist action is the steep increase in the early phase insulin secretion (~1.8–2 fold increase) at 15 min and the significant glucose clearance within 30 min of the oral glucose load. These data indicate that treatment of n-STZ animals with the CNX-011-67 enhanced glucose sensitivity of β-cells and almost normalized insulin secretion in response to oral glucose load.

Effect of withdrawal of CNX-011-67 treatment on insulin secretion in response to oral glucose load

To understand if the chronic effects induced by CNX-011-67 agonist were maintained in the long term n-STZ-CNX-011-67 animals were administered the agonist for 8 weeks and then the treatment was withdrawn for a period of 1 week. Oral glucose tolerance test was performed at end of 8 weeks and again after one week of agonist withdrawal. Since the half life of CNX-011-67 agonist is 6 h in Wistar rats (data not shown), it is unlikely that the compound administered a week earlier remained in circulation in the n-STZ-CNX-011-67 animals. The similar profiles of the oral glucose tolerance tests performed prior to (increase in 27% insulin AUC in n-STZ-CNX-011-67 in 8th week, $P < 0.001$, Figure 2C lower panel) and 1 week after agonist withdrawal (35% increase in insulin AUC in the 9th week, $P < 0.05$, Figure 2D lower panel) respectively indicates that the β-cells in the n-STZ-CNX-011-67 animals remained responsive to glucose even in the absence of the agonist. It appears that the CNX-011-67 induced β-cell population in the n-STZ-CNX-011-67 remains functional and sensitive to stimulatory glucose concentrations even in absence of the agonist.

Effect of CNX-011-67 on GSIS, insulin content of islets, β-cell mass and number

Freshly isolated size-matched islets from sham control, n-STZ and n-STZ-CNX-011-67 animals (8 weeks treatment) were tested *in vitro* in a static glucose stimulated insulin secretion (GSIS) assay. Islets from sham control animals displayed the expected steep increase in insulin secretion upon high glucose stimulation while islets from the n-STZ animals, in sharp contrast, displayed a weak insulin secretory response (60% decrease compared to sham control, $P < 0.001$) indicating a significant loss of β-cell sensitivity to glucose (Figure 3A). However, islets from the n-STZ-CNX-011-67 animals displayed a 55% increase ($P < 0.05$) in insulin secretory (Figure 3A) response that was significantly greater than that observed in islets from n-STZ animals indicating a robust

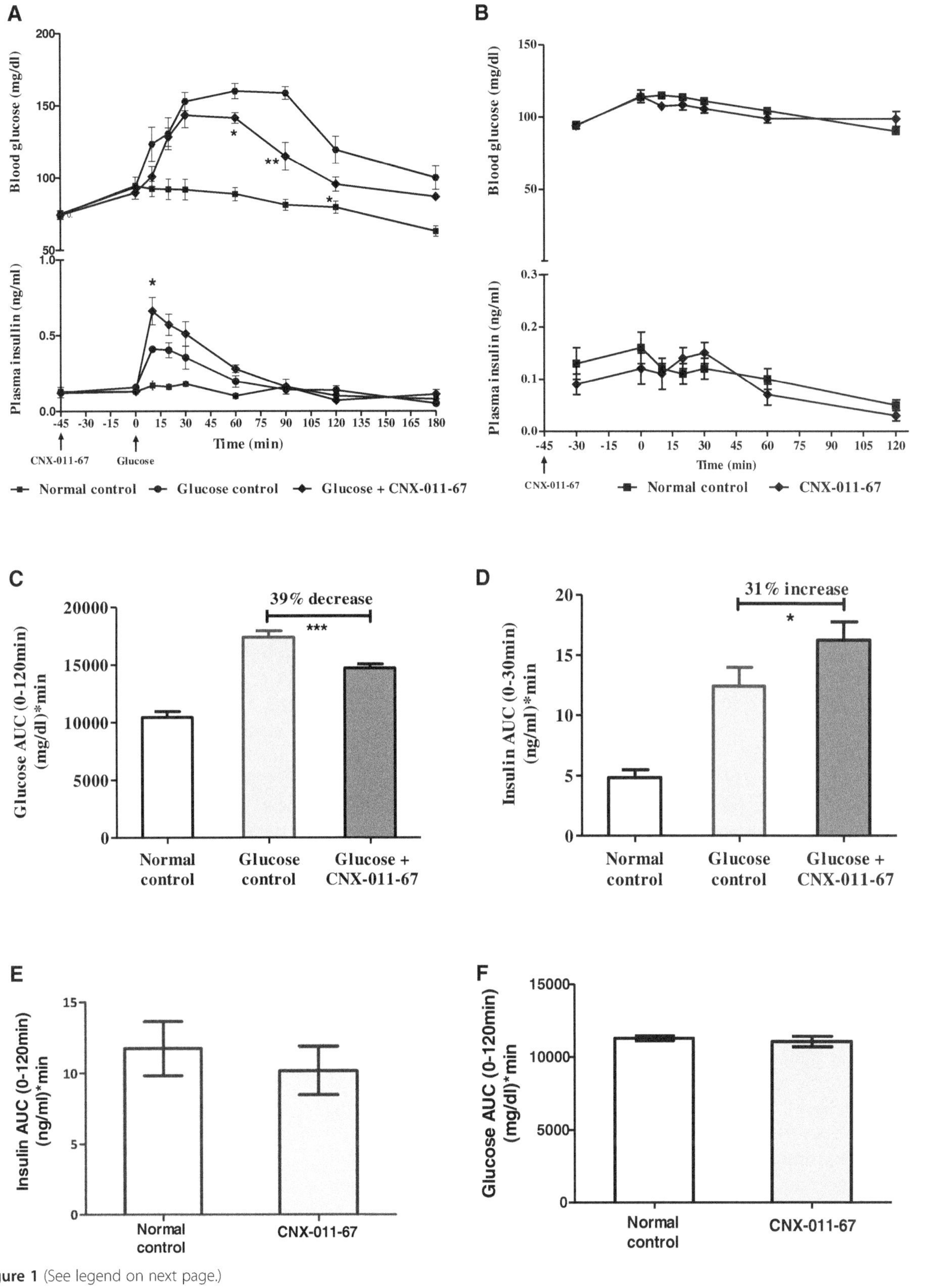

Figure 1 (See legend on next page.)

(See figure on previous page.)
Figure 1 Effect of CNX-011-67 in normal wistar rats and rat islets- OGTT glucose, insulin and GSIS. Effects of CNX-011-67 on blood glucose and insulin levels in normal Wistar rats with **(A)** and without glucose load **(B)**. The rats were dosed with vehicle or CNX-011-67 by oral gavage at −45 min, blood samples obtained at the time intervals indicated in the graphs for glucose and insulin estimation. Effects of CNX-011-67 on total blood glucose **(C)** & insulin **(D)** AUC during the OGTT in Wistar rats. Effects of CNX-011-67 on total insulin **(E)** & blood glucose **(F)** AUC during the OGTT without glucose load in Wistar rats. The percent inhibition of glucose levels was calculated based on the glucose AUC during the 0-120 min OGTT for each group after subtracting the values from those of the normal (no drug and no glucose) control group. Data in all panels are mean ± SEM (n = 8/group). Statistical comparison between control and treatment group was conducted by one-way ANOVA followed by Dunnett's post test correction. (*P < 0.05 and ** P < 0.01).

improvement in β-cell sensitivity to glucose upon CNX-011-67 treatment. Analyses of islet insulin content from the three groups showed a similar trend (Figure 3B). Insulin content in the islets from n-STZ animals was reduced (48% decrease compared to sham control, P < 0.001) indicating a potential reduction in insulin biosynthesis. In contrast, islets from n-STZ-CNX-011-67 animals exhibited a 41% increase (P < 0.05) in insulin content compared to the n-STZ group and more importantly, an increase in insulin biosynthesis was observed upon exposure to 16.7 mM glucose (Figure 3B) indicating increased response to glucose stimulation. When expressed as percent of islet insulin content, insulin secretion from islets prepared from n-STZ animals displayed a 22% decrease (P < 0.05, Figure 3C) while islets from n-STZ-CNX-011-67 animals displayed only a 4% decrease when compared with sham controls. However, the islets from n-STZ-CNX-011-67 animals displayed a 20% increase, though non-significant (P < 0.08), when compared with islets from n-STZ animals (Figure 3C).

Since pancreatic islets from n-STZ animals resemble T2DM human islets in terms of increased stress and reduced insulin secretion, we sought to measure insulin secretion in human islets obtained from T2DM cadaver donors and studied impacts on CNX-011-67 treatment. As shown in Figure 3D, T2DM human islets did not secrete elevated levels of insulin in response to physiological stimulatory glucose concentration (8 mM). Insulin secretion was increased to some extent only at 11 mM glucose concentration and further increase in glucose level showed no further insulin secretion. Treatment of T2DM human islets with CNX-011-67 increased insulin secretion only at stimulatory glucose concentration (8 mM) and had no impact at lower glucose levels (upto 5 mM) (Figure 3D). These data thus further indicate that activation of GPR40 by CNX-011-67 can increase insulin secretion in a glucose dependent manner.

Immunohistochemical analysis of islet sections from sham control, n-STZ and n-STZ-CNX-011-67 animals revealed a modest increase in insulin (Figure 4A) and PDX-1 (Figure 4B) immunofluorescence while electron microscopic studies indicated presence of higher number of electron-dense insulin granules in n-STZ-CNX-011-67 animals (Figure 4C). However, the effect of treatment with CNX-011-67 on β-cell number and β-cell mass was statistically non-significant (Figure 4D & E). Hematoxylin and eosin staining of pancreas showed no detectable change in morphology or structure (data not shown).

Effect of CNX-011-67 on mitochondrial and cytosolic calcium content

As GPR40 is coupled to Gα-q/11 protein and specific ligands like oleic acid induce an increase in cytosolic calcium, we explored whether CNX-011-67 increased cytosolic Ca^{2+} levels. While exposure to stimulatory glucose concentration in NIT-1 cells led to a 43% increase in cytosolic [Ca^{2+}] consistent with earlier reports [41-44], the presence of CNX-011-67 resulted in a further increase by 24% in cytosolic [Ca^{2+}] (Figure 5A). GPR40 agonism by CNX-011-67 thus led to a significant augmentation of cytosolic [Ca^{2+}] over that induced by stimulatory glucose concentrations. CNX-011-67-mediated increase in cytosolic [Ca^{2+}] levels were however dependent on presence of calcium in extracellular medium as inhibition of voltage dependent calcium channels by nitrendipine abrogated increase in cytosolic [Ca^{2+}] levels (data not shown). As GPR40 activation enhanced endoplasmic reticulum Ca^{2+} release, we next examined if this could lead to an increase in mitochondrial [Ca^{2+}]. In NIT-1 cells, while exposure to stimulatory glucose concentrations led to a 20% increase in mitochondrial [Ca^{2+}], presence of CNX-011-67 caused a further increase by 13% in mitochondrial Ca^{2+} levels (Figure 5B).

Effect of treatment with CNX-011-67 on islet ATP and inositol-tri-phosphate (IP3) content in n-STZ islets

Freshly isolated islets from sham control animals displayed enhanced ATP synthesis when exposed to stimulatory glucose concentration and this was enhanced further in the presence of CNX-011-67 (P < 0.01, Figure 5C). On the contrary, ATP synthesis in islets freshly isolated from n-STZ animals was already high, as previously reported [45], even at low glucose concentrations when compared to sham control, and exposure to stimulatory glucose levels induced only a marginal increase in ATP synthesis as expected. However, the presence of CNX-011-67 restored ATP synthesis in the islets from n-STZ animals in response to stimulatory glucose concentrations to almost

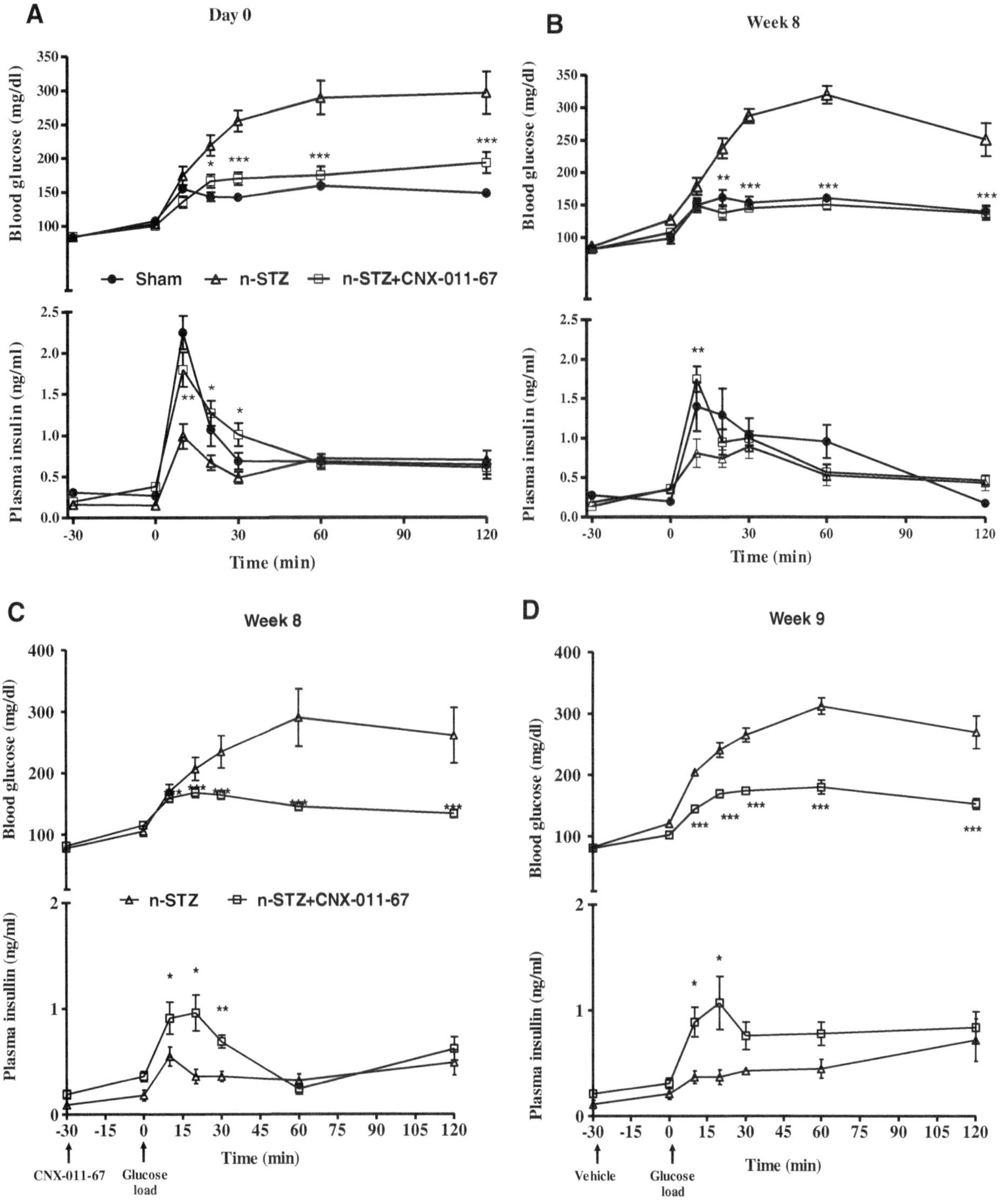

Figure 2 Effect of CNX-011-67 on OGTT glucose and insulin levels in n-STZ rats. On day 1 **(A)** and week 8 **(B)**. Blood samples were collected from the tail vein at the intervals indicated in the graph for estimating insulin and glucose levels. The lower panel represents the OGTT glucose and insulin levels at the end of the study in n-STZ-CNX-011-67 rats on week 8 **(C)** and week 9 **(D)** which is one week after agonist withdrawal. In all the experiments, animals were fasted for 16 h and oral glucose administered at 2 g/kg load. On week 8, CNX-011-67 was administered 30 min before oral glucose load. Blood samples were collected from the tail vein at the intervals indicated in the graph for estimating insulin and glucose levels. Open triangle: n-STZ; Closed circle: Sham control; Open square: n-STZ-CNX-011-67. Data in all panels are mean ± SEM (n = 8/group). Statistical comparison between control and treatment group was conducted by one-way ANOVA followed by Dunnett's post test correction. (*P < 0.05, ** P < 0.01 and *** P < 0.001).

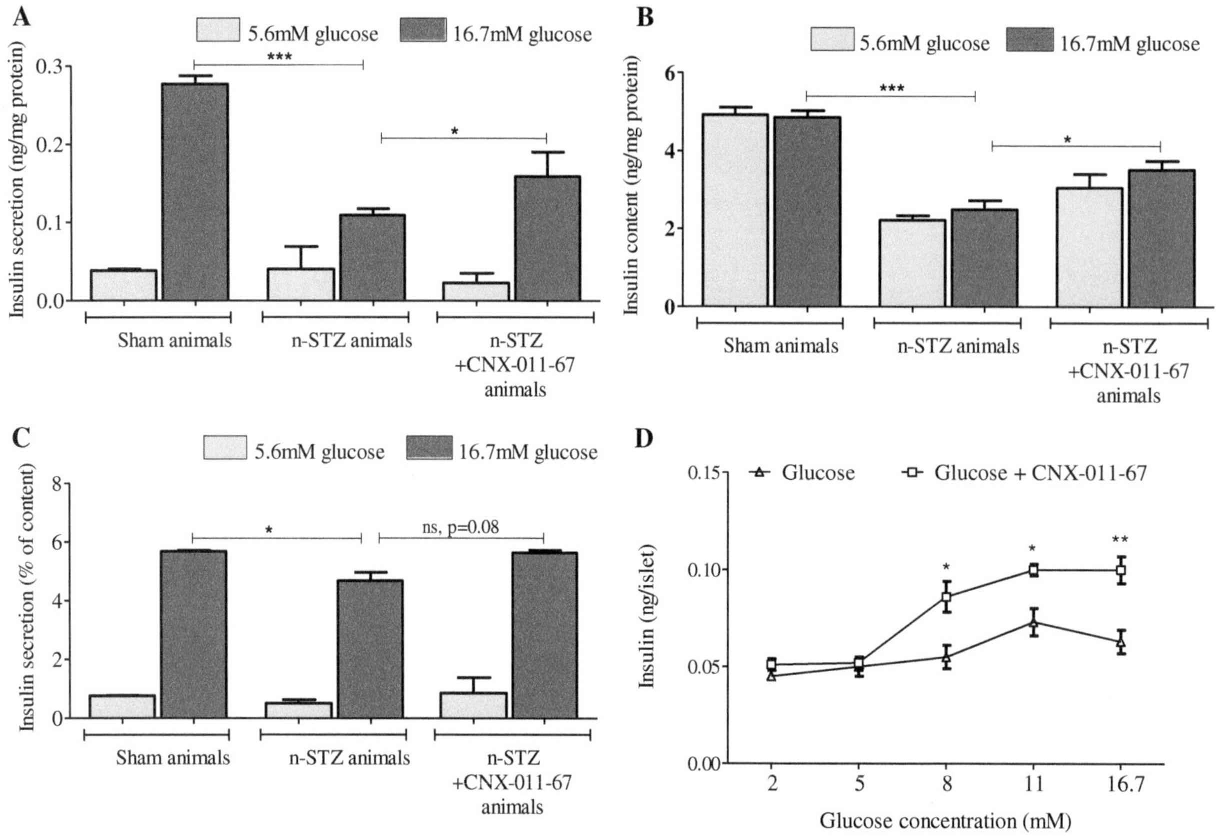

Figure 3 CNX-011-67 increases islet insulin secretion and content. Insulin secretion **(A)**, islet insulin content **(B)**, ratio of secreted insulin to insulin content represented as percentage **(C)** of islets from sham control, n-STZ and n-STZ-CNX-011-67 animals after treatment with CNX-011-67 for 8 weeks. Freshly isolated rat islets were preincubated with 2.8 mM glucose for 30 min and later incubated with 5.6 mM and 16.7 mM glucose for 120 min. Both insulin secretion and islet insulin content were measured. Secreted insulin and islet insulin content are presented as ng of insulin/mg protein. **(D)** CNX-011-67 increases insulin secretion in human islets from T2DM patients. The islets from T2DM did not show glucose responsiveness as elevated glucose concentration (8 mM) could not increase insulin secretion. CNX-011-67 treatment resulted in increased glucose responsiveness as CNX-011-67 facilitated insulin secretion only at higher glucose concentration. Values represent mean ± S.E.M ($n = 4$). Statistical analysis was performed by Students t-test (Two-way, unpaired: *$P < 0.05$, **$P < 0.01$ and ***$P < 0.001$).

control levels suggesting enhanced glucose metabolism ($P < 0.01$, Figure 5C). IP3 content in islets was also significantly enhanced by addition of CNX-011-67 in agreement with earlier observations [46] that the signal transduction of GPR40 involves phospholipase C activation, and elevation of intracellular IP3 leading to intracellular calcium release (Figure 5D).

Treatment with CNX-011-67 enhances expression of factors regulating glucose metabolism and insulin synthesis

To investigate the molecular mechanisms underlying CNX-011-67 mediated increase in insulin secretion and insulin content, we examined the expression of factors regulating glucose metabolism and insulin synthesis in islets isolated from sham control, n-STZ and n-STZ-CNX-011-67 rats (Figure 6). In n-STZ animals while expression of PDX-1 was decreased ($P < 0.05$, Figure 6A), expression of pyruvate carboxylase (PC, Figure 6D) was significantly increased and that of glucokinase (GCK, Figure 6B) and insulin genes (Figure 6C) remained unchanged when compared with sham controls. Expression of all these four factors showed a significant increase in the islets from n-STZ-CNX-011-67 rats indicating that chronic treatment with CNX-011-67 has a beneficial effect on expression of genes that are critical for regulating glucose metabolism and insulin synthesis.

Discussion

The objective of this study was to investigate the therapeutic effects of CNX-011-67, a specific GPR40 agonist, in ameliorating the defects in glucose responsiveness of β-cells and insulin secretion in the neonatally STZ-treated adult Wistar rat model. Female rats were selected for the present study as loss in insulin secretion capacity in neonatally STZ treated adult animals remain uniform irrespective of the sex of the animals [47]. The n-STZ model represents a model having reduced β-cell

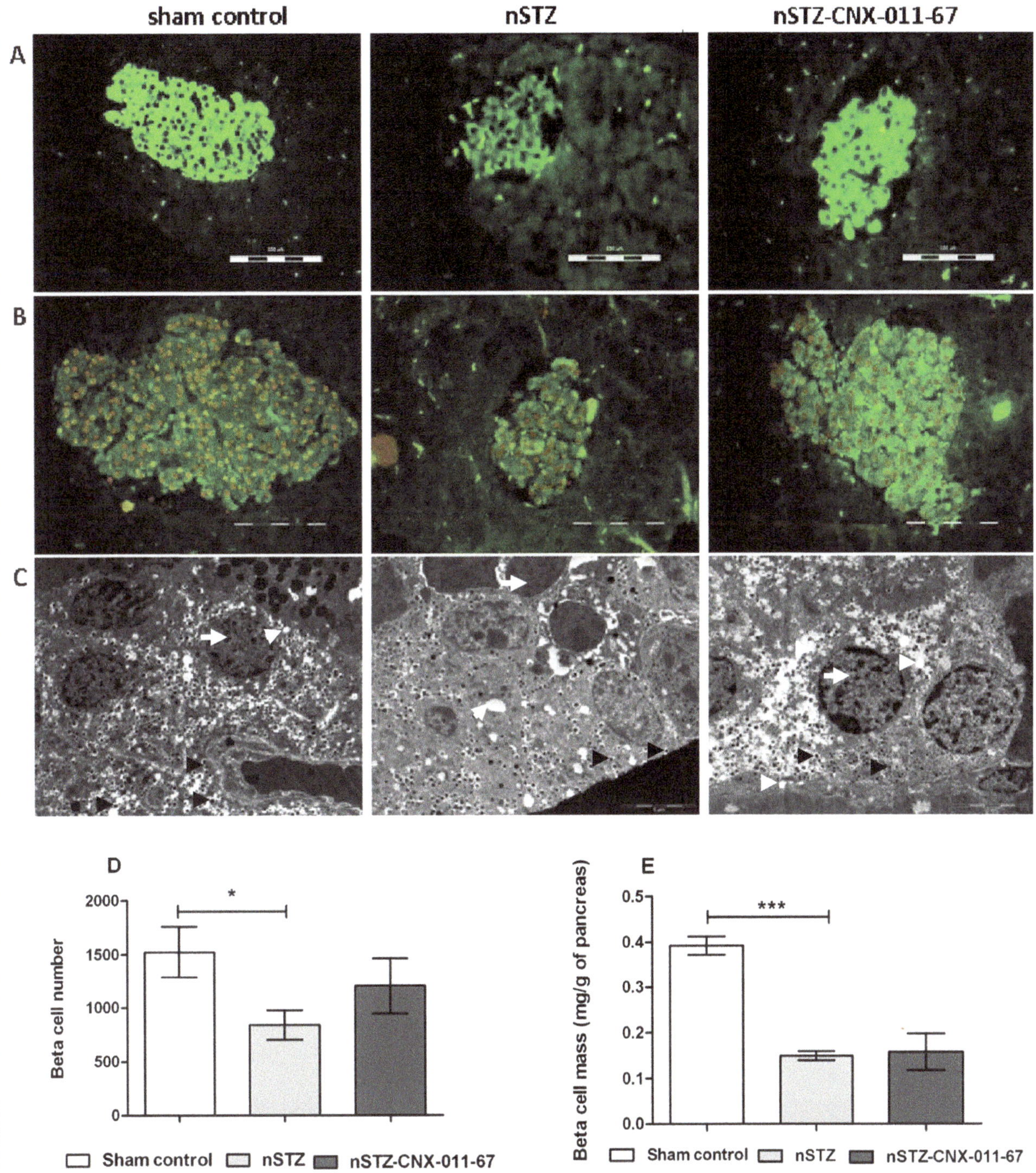

Figure 4 CNX-011-67 improves islet insulin content, β-cell mass and number-immuno fluorescence staining and elctron microscope studies of CNX-011-67 treatment in islets and β-cell. Sections from sham control, n-STZ and n-STZ-CNX-011-67 Islets stained for insulin content using Immuno fluorescent staining (FITC; green) **(A)**. Double immuno fluorescence staining for PDX1 (red; alexafluor 555) and insulin (green; FITC) representing all groups **(B)**. Electron microscope images of β-cells from sham control, n-STZ and n-STZ-CNX-011-67 animals, treated animals showed improvement and increased number of dense-core insulin granules when compared with n-STZ animals. Mitochondria and endoplasmic reticulum health have restored in treatment **(C)**. White arrow: nucleus, white arrowheads: mitochondria, black arrowheads: insulin vesicles. The n-STZ animals showed decreased β-cell number and mass when compared with normal control animals. The treated animals exhibited non significant increase in the β-cell number and β-cell mass **(D & E)**. Images were taken at 40× magnification for immunohistochemical analysis and 4800× magnification for electron micrographs. Scale bar: 5 μm. Data in all panels are mean ± S.E.M (n = 6). Statistical analysis was performed by Students t-test (two-way, unpaired: *P < 0.05 and ***P < 0.001).

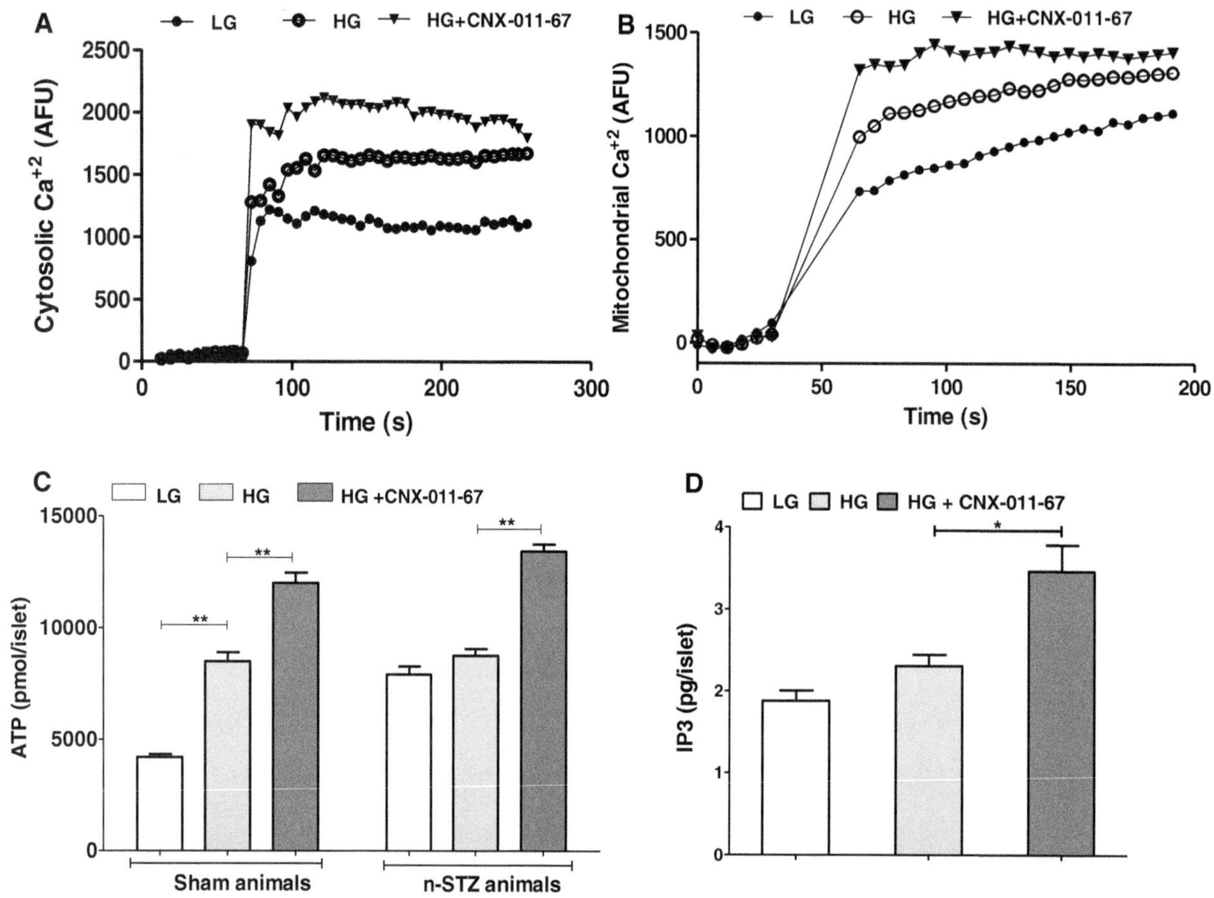

Figure 5 CNX-011-67 increases both cytosolic and mitochondrial calcium in NIT1 cells and ATP levels in rat islets. Cultured NIT1 cells were loaded with Fluo-3 AM dye for cytosolic calcium measurement **(A)** and Rhod-2 AM dye for mitochondrial calcium measurement **(B)** for 60 min. Following a basal measurement, cells were treated with low glucose (2.8 mM), high glucose (16.7 mM) or high glucose (16.7 mM) with 1 μM of CNX-011-67 followed by measurement of Ca^{2+} levels for 4 min at 6-s intervals. The resulting flux was represented as arbitrary fluorescent units (n = 3). **(C)** Islet ATP content from sham control and n-STZ animals. **(D)** Islet IP3 content in normal Wistar rat islets. Islets were preincubated with 2.8 mM glucose for 1 h and later incubated with low glucose (LG, 2.8 mM), high glucose (HG, 11 mM) or high glucose (11 mM) with 1 μM of CNX-011-67 for 60 min for ATP and 5 min for IP3 measurement. ATP (pmol) and IP3 (pg) content are presented per islet. Values represent mean ± S.E.M (n = 4). Statistical analysis was performed by Students t-test (Two-way, unpaired: * $P < 0.05$ and ** $P < 0.01$).

number and increased β-cells stress indicating thus the β-cells pathology in this model is similar to what seen in human diabetic patients [30-32]. Acute treatment with CNX-011-67 induced a significant increase in insulin secretion in response to oral glucose stimulation and chronic treatment for eight weeks induced significant changes in expression of genes involved in glucose metabolism and insulin synthesis leading to enhanced insulin content in islets.

A number of small molecules such as GW9508, TAK-875, AS2575959 and AMG837 have been synthesized to activate GPR40 to induce insulin secretion [16-20] in different model systems. However, none of these molecules have shown for their potency to increase insulin secretion in n-STZ animals, a model where β-cell stress is high. Moreover, it is not clear from present literature whether GPR40 activation has any impact on β-cells glucose metabolism which is an important factor for insulin release. Though, Alquier et al. [14] reported that GPR40 knock out did not alter fuel metabolism under normal condition, the same can not be corroborated for GPR40 activation under disease conditions. In this report and in the earlier study [37] we provide evidences, though indirectly, that CNX-011-67 increases glucose metabolism in β-cells.

Since, increased insulin secretion for prolonged period can cause β-cells exhaustion which can instead complicate the pathology, it become important to study whether the increase in insulin secretion by GPR40 activation has any impact on islet insulin content. Interestingly, we have observed that CNX-011-67 can actually increase the islet insulin content despite increasing

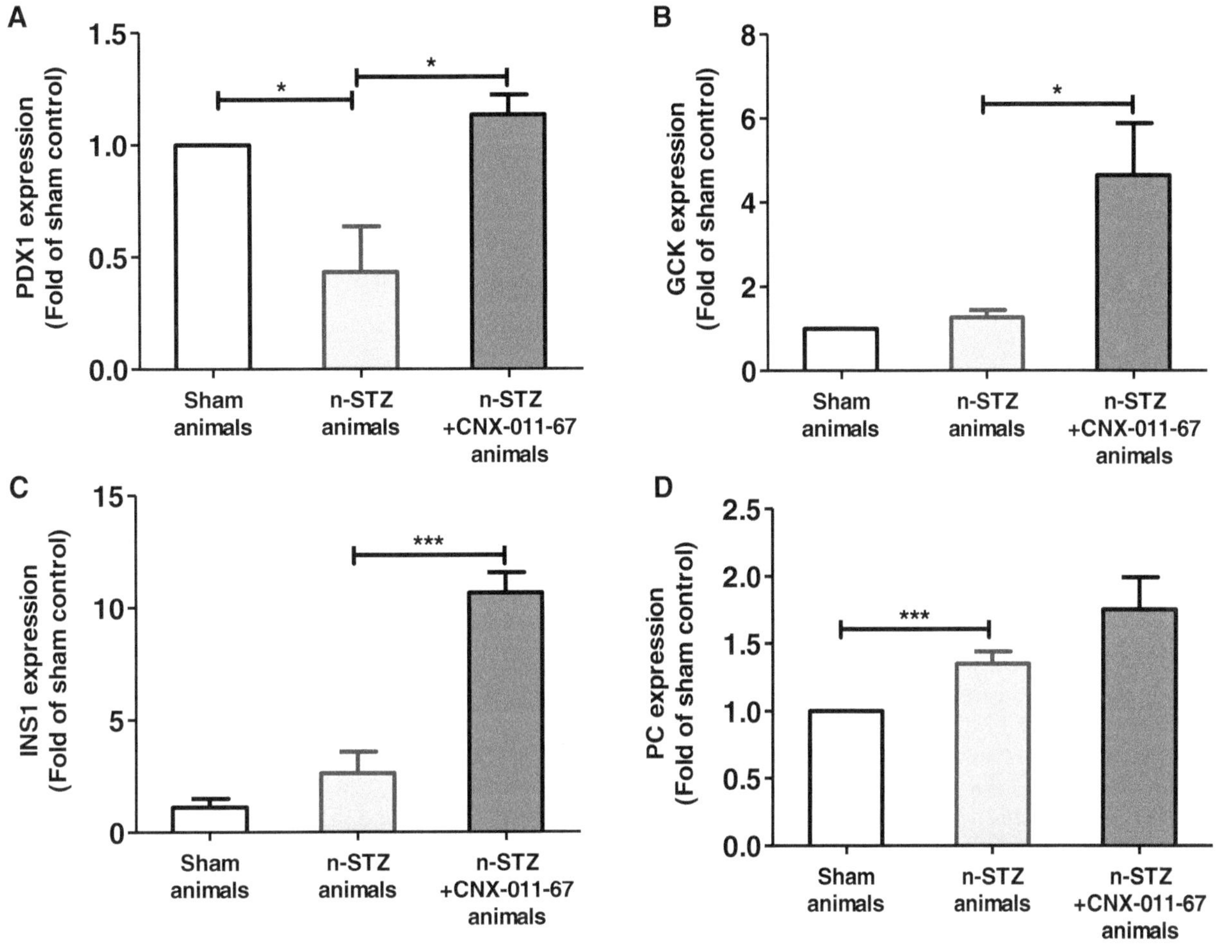

Figure 6 Effect of CNX-011-67 on islet gene expression. mRNA levels of PDX1 **(A)**, GCK **(B)**, INS1 **(C)** and PC **(D)** in islets from sham control, n-STZ and n-STZ-CNX-011-67 rats were measured as mentined in the methods. The mRNA levels of all the genes were expressed relative to β-actin mRNA. Values represent mean ± S.E.M (n = 4). Statistical analysis was performed by Students t-test (Two-way, unpaired: * $P < 0.05$ and *** $P < 0.001$).

insulin secretion thereby indicating that insulin synthesis is improved. This was further substantiated by increased expression of insulin and PDX1.

It is well known that increase in β-cell glucose metabolism and ATP synthesis activates voltage-gated Ca^{2+} channels culminating in influx of extracellular Ca^{2+} and insulin granule exocytosis [48,49]. Acute treatment with CNX-011-67 significantly enhanced cytoplasmic and mitochondrial [Ca^{2+}] in NIT-1 cells and increased IP3 and ATP levels in islets prepared from normal Wistar rats and n-STZ rats, respectively. These observations suggest that acute exposure of n-STZ islets to CNX-011-67 perhaps leads to an increase in islet cytoplasmic and mitochondrial [Ca^{2+}] levels [50,51] leading to activation of the dehydrogenases of the citric acid cycle and enhanced ATP content observed in the n-STZ islets (Figure 5C). The defective Calcium-activated oxidative metabolism and ATP synthesis reported in islets in n-STZ animal models [52] is likely overcome by acute treatment with CNX-011-67 and results in enhanced insulin secretion in response to stimulatory glucose concentrations.

The above sequence of molecular alterations perhaps explains the enhanced insulin secretion observed in the n-STZ-CNX-011-67 rats on day 0 itself, following the first exposure to CNX-011-67 (Figure 2A). The acute phase of insulin release observed in the first 10 min following oral glucose stimulation in the n-STZ-CNX-011-67 rats on day 0 is attributable to mechanisms such as enhanced mitochondrial [Ca^{2+}], glucose metabolism and ATP synthesis, that together trigger exocytosis of a small number of insulin granules from the readily releasable pool in a K_{ATP} channel-dependent manner as described previously [53-55]. Such an effect is also evident in the acute reversal of loss of insulin secretion observed in islets from n-STZ rats after exposure to CNX-011-67 suggesting that the mechanism of action of the agonist ensures glucose responsiveness and enhances hormone secretion. This explains, in part, the acute increase in insulin secretion observed on day 0 of treatment with CNX-011-67. A similar acute effect on glucose stimulated insulin secretion was also evident in normal Wistar rats (Figure 1). The robust insulin secretion observed after eight weeks of treatment with the GPR40 agonist suggested an improvement in β-cell number or function. The enhanced glucose stimulated insulin secretion and insulin content observed in cultured islets prepared from the n-STZ-CNX-011-67 rats when exposed to 16.7 mM glucose (Figure 3A & B) indicates an improvement in glucose responsiveness of the β-cells and is also one reason for the sustained insulin secretion observed in the treated animals.

In the n-STZ animals, the reduced insulin secretion and insulin content can be explained by defective mitochondrial activity leading to reduced ATP synthesis in spite of normal expression levels of mRNA of GCK, insulin and PC genes involved in upstream events of glucose metabolism. The increase in mRNA levels of PDX1, GCK and PC in the n-STZ-CNX-011-67 rats indicates improved glucose metabolism (Figure 6 A, B & D) initiated by the agonist while the increase in insulin mRNA and higher ATP availability support higher insulin synthesis (Figures 6C and 5C).

Even though we have not provided any direct evidence to support that GPR40 activation enhances β-cell glucose oxidation our study provides indirect evidence to link activation of GPR40 with enhanced glucose metabolism in β-cells. Since glucose metabolism and ATP content are directly related in pancreatic β-cells and we observed an increase in ATP content hence we speculate that glucose metabolism is increased. Moreover, GCK expression is reported to be reduced after STZ treatment [56] leading to a reduced glucose metabolism, and with CNX-011-67 treatment we observed an up-regulated expression of GCK further indicating that glucose metabolism in enhanced after CNX-011-67 treatment.

The near-normal insulin secretory response to oral glucose maintained in n-STZ-CNX-011-67 rats even after the withdrawal of the agonist can be explained by the change in expression of multiple genes involved in glucose metabolism and insulin synthesis. For example, it has been previously reported that in Zucker diabetic fatty rats a reduced expression of GLUT2 was associated with reduced insulin response to higher glucose concentrations, and transgenic overexpression of GLUT2 rescued the mice from early death [57,58]. Treatment of n-STZ rats with sodium tungstate enhanced phosphorylation of PDX-1 and increased β-cell replication and insulin producing cells [25].

In the present study, the significant increase in islet insulin content and modest increase in area of insulin positive cells observed after 12 weeks treatment with CNX-011-67 most likely occurs due to a synergy resulting from a coordinated increase in expression of PDX1, and genes (insulin, GCK, and PC) involved in glucose metabolism and ATP synthesis. The electron micrographs not only indicate the preponderance of dense insulin granules in islets from n-STZ-CNX-011-67 rats, almost similar to the islets from sham control rats, but also show that there is an increase in the number of granules docked at the membrane and ready for release upon glucose stimulation. It may be mentioned here that treatment of Wistar rats with CNX-011-67 at 5 and 15 mg/kg did not increase serum GLP1 levels and hence the effects observed in the β-cells in this study are attributable to the direct activation of GPR40 on β-cells by CNX-011-67. We recently reported a similar increase in ATP synthesis, islet insulin content and enhanced early phase insulin secretion in male ZDF rats upon treatment with CNX-011-67 [37].

The decrease in insulin secretion in T2DM patients is attributed both to a loss in β-cell mass and to an increase in number of β-cells that respond poorly to glucose [59]. Pancreatic β-cells from diabetic patients display a decrease in expression of GCK, GLUT 1 and 2, genes involved in insulin granule exocytosis, show reduced glucose oxidation and ATP content resulting in reduced glucose stimulated insulin release. Further, patients with T2DM display a reduced early phase insulin secretion in response to oral glucose stimulation. The incretin glucagon like peptide-1 (GLP-1) has demonstrated trophic effects on β-cells as evidenced by increased differentiation of pancreatic ductal cells, reduced apoptosis and enhanced proliferation of β-cells in animal models [60] and incretin-based therapies have been developed to treat T2DM in humans. On account of its ability to enhance Gαq/11 signaling, GPR40 agonism represents a novel therapeutic approach to ameliorate the defects in insulin secretion observed in patients with T2DM. The phenotype of impaired glucose metabolism, lower content of insulin, lower rate of insulin biosynthesis and content and a persistent impairment of insulin release especially at higher glucose concentration appear to be similar in islets from adult n-STZ rats and from T2DM patients.

Chronic treatment of CNX-011-67 did not show any impact on body weight, feed consumption and pancreata histology and also no toxic effects were observed. Thus, CNX-011-67 is a novel, non-toxic, potent small molecule having insulin secretion ability in a glucose dependent manner. These results are in consistent with our earlier study [37] where we have shown insulin secreting ability of CNX-011-67 in male ZDF animal model without any detectable impact on feed intake or body weight. Taken together, CNX-011-67 is an orally available small molecule capable of enhanced insulin secretion in a glucose dependent manner. Therefore, the CNX-011-67 holds promise as a future therapeutic agent to meet the demand of insulin secretion in T2DM patients whose β-cells are under chronic stress.

Conclusions

This study suggests that β-cells that are non-responsive to glucose, for various reasons, can be pharmacologically revived by CNX-011-67- mediated activation of GPR40 to synthesize and secrete insulin in response to glucose stimulation. The ability of CNX-011-67 to overcome the 'glucose incompetence' of islet β-cells and increase insulin secretion and content in response to stimulatory glucose concentrations has clear implications for treating T2DM.

Abbreviations

GPR40: Gprotein coupled receptor 40; T2DM: Type 2 diabetes mellitus; n-STZ: Neonatelly straptozotocin treated; GSIS: Glucose stimulates insulin secretion; GCK: Glucokinase; GLUT: Glucose transporter; PC: Pyruvate carbozylase; IP3: Inositol-tri-phosphate; AUC: Area under curve; OGTT: Oral glucose tolerance test.

Competing interests

The authors declare that they have no competing interests.

Authors' contributions

VS, JS, DNV, BC, JS, SB carried out the experiments; MKV, MKS, YM, AD designed the study and carried out the analysis. MKV, MOA, MW and BPS interpreted the data and drafted the manuscript. MRJ supervised the progress and critically revised the manuscript. All authors read and approved the final manuscript.

Acknowledgements

We would like to thank all the members of the *in vitro* and *in vivo* experimentation group with specific mention of Nagesh Gowda, Vasuda Kadam, Aparna K, Ashokkumar Reddy, Shilpa PC at Connexios Life Sciences Pvt Ltd. for their assistance in the study. We thank Dr. Rohit N Kulkarni, Department of Cell Biology, Joslin Diabetes Center, Boston, MA for his valuable inputs for composing the manuscript and Dr. B.K. Chandrasekhar Sagar, Dept. of Neuropathology, at National Institute of Mental Health and Neurosciences, Bangalore, India for his valuable contribution in electron microscopy.

References

1. Bergman RN: **Towards physiological understanding of glucose tolerance: minimal-model approach (Lilly Lecture).** *Diabetes* 1989, **38**:1512–1527.
2. Reaven GM, Hollenback CB, Chen YD: **Relationship between glucose tolerance, insulin secretion and insulin action in non-obese individuals with varying degrees of glucose tolerance.** *Diabetologia* 1989, **32**:52–55.
3. Caumo A, Luzi L: **First-phase insulin secretion: does it exist in real life? Considerations on shape and function.** *Am J Physiol Endocrino Metab* 2004, **287**:E372–E385.
4. Gerich JE: **Is reduced first-phase insulin release the earliest detectable abnormality in individuals destined to develop type 2 diabetes?** *Diabetes* 2002, **51**:S117–S121.
5. DeFronzo RA: **From the triumvirate to the ominous octet: A new paradigm for the treatment of Type 2 Diabetes Mellitus.** *Diabetes* 2009, **58**:773–795.
6. Diamond MP, Thornton K, Connolly-Diamond M, Sherwin RS, DeFronzo RA: **Reciprocal variation in insulin stimulates glucose uptake and pancreatic insulin section in women with normal glucose tolerance.** *J Soc Gynecol Invest* 1995, **2**:708–715.
7. Lillioja S, Mott DM, Spraul M, Ferraro R, Foley JE, Ravussin E, Knowler WC, Bennett PH, Bogardus C: **Insulin resistance and insulin secretary dysfunction as precursors of non-insulin-dependent diabetes mellitus. Prospective studies of Pima Indians.** *N Engl J Med* 1992, **329**:1988–1992.
8. Fineman MS, Cirincione BB, Maggs D, Diamant M: **GLP-1 based therapies: differential effects on fasting and postprandial glucose.** *Diabetes Obes Metab* 2012, **14**:675–688.
9. Richter B, Bandeira-Echtler E, Bergerhoff K, Clar C, Ebrahim SH: **Pioglitazone for type 2 diabetes mellitus.** *Cochrane Database Syst Rev* 2006, **18**, CD006060.
10. Briscoe CP, Tadayyon M, Andrews JL, Benson WG, Chambers JK, Eilert MM, Ellis C, Elshourbagy NA, Goetz AS, Minnick DT, Murdock PR, Sauls HR Jr, Shabon U, Spinage LD, Strum JC, Szekeres PG, Tan KB, Way JM, Ignar DM, Wilson S, Muir AI: **The orphan G protein-coupled receptor GPR40 is activated by medium and long chain fatty acids.** *J Biol Chem* 2003, **278**:11303–11311.
11. Shapiro H, Shachar S, Sekler I, Hershfinkel M, Walker MD: **Role of GPR40 in fatty acid action on the beta cell line INS-1E.** *Biochem Biophys Res Commun* 2005, **335**:97–104.
12. Itoh Y, Kawamata Y, Harada M, Kobayashi M, Fujii R, Fukusumi S, Ogi K, Hosoya M, Tanaka Y, Uejima H, Tanaka H, Maruyama M, Satoh R, Okubo S, Kizawa H, Komatsu H, Matsumura F, Noguchi Y, Shinohara T, Hinuma S, Fujisawa Y, Fujino M: **Free fatty acids regulate insulin secretion from pancreatic beta cells through GPR40.** *Nature* 2003, **422**:173–176.
13. Nagasumi K, Esaki R, Iwachidow K, Yasuhara Y, Ogi K, Tanaka H, Nakata M, Yano T, Shimakawa K, Taketomi S, Takeuchi K, Odaka H, Kaisho Y: **Overexpression of GPR40 in pancreatic beta-cells augments glucose-stimulated insulin secretion and improves glucose tolerance in normal and diabetic mice.** *Diabetes* 2009, **58**:1067–1076.
14. Alquier T, Peyot ML, Latour MG, Kebede M, Sorensen CM, Gesta S, Ronald Kahn C, Smith RD, Jetton TL, Metz TO, Prentki M, Poitout V: **Deletion of GPR40 impairs glucose-induced insulin secretion in vivo in mice without affecting intracellular fuel metabolism in islets.** *Diabetes* 2009, **58**:2607–2615.
15. Del Guerra S, Bugliani M, D'Aleo V, Del Prato S, Boggi U, Mosca F, Filipponi F, Lupi R: **G-protein-coupled receptor 40 (GPR40) expression and its regulation in human pancreatic islets: the role of type 2 diabetes and fatty acids.** *Nutr Metab Cardiovasc Dis* 2010, **20**:22–25.
16. Feng XT, Leng J, Xie Z, Li SL, Zhao W, Tang QL: **GPR40: a therapeutic target for mediating insulin secretion.** *Int J Mol Med* 2012, **30**:1261–1266.
17. Yashiro H, Tsujihata Y, Takeuchi K, Hazama M, Johnson PR, Rorsman P: **The effects of TAK-875, a selective G protein-coupled receptor 40/free fatty acid 1 agonist, on insulin and glucagon secretion in isolated rat and human islets.** *J Pharmacol Exp Ther* 2012, **340**:483–489.
18. Briscoe CP, Peat AJ, McKeown SC, Corbett DF, Goetz AS, Littleton TR, McCoy DC, Kenakin TP, Andrews JL, Ammala C, Fornwald JA, Ignar DM, Jenkinson S: **Pharmacological regulation of insulin secretion in MIN6 cells through the fatty acid receptor GPR40: identification of agonist and antagonist small molecules.** *Br J Pharmacol* 2006, **148**:619–628.
19. Tanaka H, Yoshida S, Minoura H, Negoro K, Shimaya A, Shimokawa T, Shibasaki M: **Novel GPR40 agonist AS2575959 exhibits glucose metabolism improvement and synergistic effect with sitagliptin on insulin and incretin secretion.** *Life Sci* 2014, **94**:115–121.
20. Lin DC, Zhang J, Zhuang R, Li F, Nguyen K, Chen M, Tran T, Lopez E, Lu JY, Li XN, Tang L, Tonn GR, Swaminath G, Reagan JD, Chen JL, Tian H, Lin YJ, Houze JB, Luo J: **AMG 837: a novel GPR40/FFA1 agonist that enhances insulin secretion and lowers glucose levels in rodents.** *PLoS One* 2011, **6**:e27270.
21. Ito R, Tsujihata Y, Matsuda-Nagasumi K, Mori I, Negoro N, Takeuchi K: **TAK-875, a GPR40/FFAR1 agonist, in combination with metformin prevents progression of diabetes and β-cell dysfunction in Zucker diabetic fatty rats.** *Br J Pharmacol* 2013, **170**:568–580.
22. Kaku K, Araki T, Yoshinaka R: **Randomized, double-blind, dose-ranging study of TAK-875, a novel GPR40 agonist, in Japanese patients with inadequately controlled type 2 diabetes.** *Diabetes Care* 2013, **36**:245–250.
23. Burant CF, Viswanathan P, Marcinak J, Cao C, Vakilynejad M, Xie B, Leifke E: **TAK-875 versus placebo or glimepiride in type 2 diabetes mellitus: a**

phase 2, randomised, double-blind, placebo-controlled trial. *Lancet* 2012, **379**:1403–1411.
24. Del Guerra S, Lupi R, Marselli L: **Functional and molecular defects of pancreatic islets in human type 2 diabetes.** *Diabetes* 2005, **54**:727–735.
25. Fernández-Alvarez J, Conget I, Rasschaert J, Sener A, Gomis R, Malaisse WJ: **Enzymatic, metabolic and secretory patterns in human islets of Type 2 (non-insulin-dependent) diabetic patients.** *Diabetologia* 1994, **37**:177–181.
26. Anello M, Lupi R, Spampinato D, Piro S, Masini M, Boggi U, Del Prato S, Rabuazzo AM, Purrello F, Marchetti P: **Functional and morphological alterations of mitochondria in pancreatic beta cells from type 2 diabetic patients.** *Diabetologia* 2005, **48**:282–289.
27. Deng S, Vatamaniuk M, Huang X, Doliba N, Lian MM, Frank A, Velidedeoglu E, Desai NM, Koeberlein B, Wolf B, Barker CF, Naji A, Matschinsky FM, Markmann JF: **Structural and function abnormalities in the islets isolated from type 2 diabetic subjects.** *Diabetes* 2004, **53**:624–632.
28. Gunton JE, Kulkarni RN, Yim S, Okada T, Hawthorne WJ, Tseng YH, Roberson RS, Ricordi C, O'Connell PJ, Gonzalez FJ, Kahn CR: **Loss of ARNT/HIF1beta mediates altered gene expression and pancreatic islet dysfunction in human type 2 diabetes.** *Cell* 2005, **122**:337–349.
29. Ostenson CG, Gaisano H, Sheu L, Tibell A, Bartfai T: **Impaired gene and protein expression of exocytotic soluble N-ethylmaleimide attachment protein receptor complex proteins in pancreatic islets of type 2 diabetic patients.** *Diabetes* 2006, **55**:435–440.
30. Clark A, Jones LC, de Koning E, Hansen BC, Mathews DR: **Decreased insulin secretion in Type 2 diabetes: A problem of cellular mass or function.** *Diabetes* 2001, **50**:S169–S171.
31. Rahier J, Goebbels RM, Henquin JC: **Cellular composition of the human diabetic pancreas.** *Diabetologia* 1983, **24**:366–371.
32. Butler AE, Janson J, Bonner-Weir S, Ritzel R, Rizza RA, Butler PC: **β-cell deficit and increased β-cell apoptosis in humans with type 2 diabetes.** *Diabetes* 2003, **52**:102–110.
33. Bonner-Weir S, Trent DE, Honey RN, Weir GC: **Responses of neonatal rat islets to streptozotocin: limited B-cell regeneration and hyperglycemia.** *Diabetes* 1981, **30**:64–69.
34. Junod A, Lambert AE, Stanffacher W, Renold AE: **Diabetogenic action of streptozotocin relationship of the dose to metabolic response.** *J Clin Invest* 1969, **48**:2129–2139.
35. Marathe PA, Parekar RR, Shinde SP, Rege NN: **A split dose regimen of streptozotocin to induce diabetes in a neonatal rat model.** *Ind J Pharmacol* 2008, **38**:432–433.
36. Portha B, Movassat J, Cuzin-Tourrel C, Bailbe D, Giriox P, Serradas P, Dolz M, Kergoat M: **Neonatally Streptozotocin induced (n-STZ) diabetic rats: A family of type 2 diabetes models.** In *Animal Models of Diabetes.* 2nd edition. Edited by Shafrir E. Boca Raton, FLA: CRC Press; 2007:223–250.
37. Gowda N, Dandu A, Singh J, Biswas S, Raghav V, Lakshmi MN, Shilpa PC, Sunil V, Reddy A, Sadasivuni M, Aparna K, Verma MK, Moolemath Y, Anup MO, Venkataranganna MV, Somesh BP, Jagannath MR: **Treatment with CNX-011-67, a novel GPR40 agonist, delays onset and progression of diabetes and improves beta cell preservation and function in male ZDF rats.** *BMC Pharmacol Toxicol* 2013, **14**:28.
38. Somesh BP, Verma MK, Sadasivuni MK, Mammen-Oommen A, Biswas S, Shilpa PC, Reddy AK, Yateesh AN, Pallavi PM, Nethra S, Smitha R, Neelima K, Narayanan U, Jagannath MR: **Chronic glucolipotoxic conditions in pancreatic islets impair insulin secretion due to dysregulated calcium dynamics, glucose responsiveness and mitochondrial activity.** *BMC Cell Biol* 2013, **14**:31.
39. Lacy PE, Kostianovsky M: **Method for the isolation of intact islets of Langerhans from the rat pancreas.** *Diabetes* 1967, **16**:35–39.
40. Antunes CM, Salgado AP, Rosário LM, Santos RM: **Differential patterns of glucose-induced electrical activity and intracellular calcium responses in single mouse and rat pancreatic islets.** *Diabetes* 2000, **49**:2028–2038.
41. Dula SB, Jecmenica M, Wu R, Jahanshahi P, Verrilli GM, Carter JD, Brayman KL, Nunemaker CS: **Evidence that low-grade systemic inflammation can induce islet dysfunction as measured by impaired calcium handling.** *Cell Calcium* 2010, **48**:133–142.
42. Hamakawa N, Yada T: **Interplay of glucose-stimulated Ca^{2+} sequestration and acetylcholine-induced Ca^{2+} release at the endoplasmic reticulum in rat pancreatic beta-cells.** *Cell Calcium* 1995, **17**:21–31.
43. Lenzen S, Lerch M, Peckmann T, Tiedge M: **Differential regulation of $[Ca^{2+}]i$ oscillations in mouse pancreatic islets by glucose, alpha-ketoisocaproic acid, glyceraldehyde and glycolytic intermediates.** *Biochim Biophys Acta* 2000, **1523**:65–72.
44. Nunemaker CS, Bertram R, Sherman A, Tsaneva-Atanasova K, Daniel CR, Satin LS: **Glucose modulates $[Ca^{2+}]_i$ oscillations in pancreatic islets via ionic and glycolytic mechanisms.** *Biophys J* 2006, **15**:2082–2096.
45. Matschinsky FM, Pagliara AS, Stillings SN, Hover BA: **Glucose and ATP Levels in Pancreatic Islet Tissue of Normal and Diabetic Rats.** *J Clin Invest* 1976, **58**:1193–1200.
46. Fujiwara K, Maekawa F, Yada T: **Oleic acid interacts with GPR40 to induce Ca^{2+} signaling in rat islet beta-cells: mediation by PLC and L-type Ca^{2+} channel and link to insulin release.** *Am J Physiol Endocrinol Metab* 2005, **289**:E670–E677.
47. Bacova Z, Najvirtova M, Krizanova O, Hudecova S, Zorad S, Strbak V, Benicky J: **Effect of Neonatal Streptozotocin and Thyrotropin-Releasing Hormone Treatments on Insulin Secretion in Adult Rats.** *Gen Physiol Biophys* 2005, **24**:181–197.
48. Meglasson MD, Matschinsky FM: **Pancreatic islet glucose metabolism and regulation of insulin secretion.** *Diabetes Metab Rev* 1986, **2**:163–214.
49. Newgard CB, McGarry JD: **Metabolic coupling factors in pancreatic beta-cell signal transduction.** *Annu Rev Biochem* 1995, **64**:689–719.
50. Taylor CW, Genazzani AA, Morris SA: **Expression of inositol triphosphate receptors.** *Cell Calcium* 1999, **26**:237–251.
51. Vermassen E, Parys JB, Mauger JP: **Subcellular distribution of the inositol 1,4,5-triphosphate receptors: functional relevance and molecular determinants.** *Biol Cell* 2004, **96**:3–17.
52. Portha B, Blondel O, Serradas P, McEvoy R, Giroix MH, Kergoat M, Bailbe D: **The rat model of non-insulin dependent diabetes induced by neonatal streptozotocin.** *Diabetes Metab* 1989, **15**:61–75.
53. Ashcroft FM, Harrison DE, Ashcroft SJ: **Glucose induces closure of single potassium channels in isolated rat pancreatic beta-cells.** *Nature* 1984, **312**:446–448.
54. Cook DL, Hales CN: **Intracellular ATP directly blocks K^+ channels in pancreatic B-cells.** *Nature* 1984, **311**:271–273.
55. Straub SG, Sharp GW: **Glucose-stimulated signaling pathways in biphasic insulin secretion.** *Diabetes Metab Res Rev* 2002, **18**:451–463.
56. Park C, Kim JR, Shim JK, Kang BS, Park YG, Nam KS, Lee YC, Kim CH: **Inhibitory effects of streptozotocin, tumor necrosis factor-alpha, and interleukin-1beta on glucokinase activity in pancreatic islets and gene expression of GLUT2 and glucokinase.** *Arch Biochem Biophys* 1999, **362**:217–224.
57. Johnson JH, Ogawa A, Chen L, Orci L, Newgard CB, Alam T, Unger RH: **Underexpression of beta cell high Km glucose transporters in noninsulin-dependent diabetes.** *Science* 1990, **250**:546–549.
58. Thorens B, Guillam MT, Beermann F, Burcelin R, Jaquet M: **Transgenic reexpression of GLUT1 or GLUT2 in pancreatic beta cells rescues GLUT2-null mice from early death and restores normal glucose-stimulated insulin secretion.** *J Biol Chem* 2000, **275**:23751–23758.
59. Clark A, Wells CA, Buley ID, Cruickshank JK, Vanhegan RI, Matthews DR, Cooper GJ, Holman RR, Turner RC: **Islet amyloid, increased A-cells, reduced B-cells and exocrine fibrosis: quantitative changes in the pancreas of type 2 diabetes.** *Diabetes Res* 1988, **9**:151–159.
60. Holst JJ, Vilsbøll T, Deacon CF: **The incretin system and its role in type 2 diabetes mellitus.** *Mol Cell Endocrinol* 2009, **297**:127–136.

Diazoxide protects against doxorubicin-induced cardiotoxicity in the rat

Lisa Drange Hole[1*], Terje Hjalmar Larsen[2,3], Kjell Ove Fossan[1], Fredrik Limé[1] and Jan Schjøtt[1,4]

Abstract

Aim: Chemotherapy with doxorubicin is limited by cardiotoxicity. Free radical generation and mitochondrial dysfunction are thought to contribute to doxorubicin-induced cardiac failure. In this study we wanted to investigate if opening of mitochondrial K_{ATP}-channels by diazoxide is protective against doxorubicin cardiotoxicity, and if 5-hydroxydecanoate (5-HD), a selective mitochondrial K_{ATP}-channel antagonist, abolished any protection by this intervention.

Methods: Wistar rats were divided into 7 groups ($n = 6$) and followed for 10 days with 5 intervention groups including the following treatments: (1) Diazoxide and doxorubicin, (2) diazoxide and 5-hydroxydecanoate (5-HD), (3) 5-HD and doxorubicin, (4) diazoxide and saline and (5) 5-HD and saline. On day 1, 3, 5 and 7 the animals received intraperitoneal (i.p.) injections with 10 mg/kg diazoxide and/or 40 mg/kg 5-HD, 30 minutes before i.p. injections with 3.0 mg/kg doxorubicin. One control group received only saline injections and the other control group received saline 30 minutes prior to 3.0 mg/kg doxorubicin. On day 10 the hearts were excised and Langendorff-perfused. Cardiac function was assessed by an intraventricular balloon and biochemical effects by release of hydrogen peroxide (H_2O_2) and troponin-T (TnT) in effluate from the isolated hearts, and by myocardial content of doxorubicin.

Results: Doxorubicin treatment produced a significant loss in left ventricular developed pressure (LVDP) ($p < 0.05$) and an increase in both H_2O_2 and TnT release in effluate ($p < 0.05$). Diazoxide significantly attenuated the decrease in LVDP ($p < 0.05$) and abolished the increased release of H_2O_2 and TnT ($p < 0.05$). 5-HD abolished the effects of pretreatment with diazoxide, and these effects were not associated with reduced myocardial accumulation of doxorubicin.

Conclusions: Pretreatment with diazoxide attenuates doxorubicin-induced cardiac dysfunction in the rat, measured by physiological indices and TnT and H_2O_2 in effluate from isolated hearts. The effect could be mediated by opening of mitochondrial K_{ATP}-channels, reduced doxorubicin-associated free radical generation and decreased cardiomyocyte damage. Diazoxide represents a promising protective intervention against doxorubicin-induced acute cardiotoxicity.

Keywords: Doxorubicin, Troponin T, Hydrogenperoxide, Doxorubicinol, Heart, Rat, 5-hydroxydecanoate, Cardiotoxicity, Ex vivo, Diazoxide

Background

Doxorubicin is a widely used chemotherapy drug, but its application is associated with cardiotoxicity. Free radical generation and mitochondrial dysfunction are thought to contribute to doxorubicin-induced cardiac failure [1,2]. Dose reduction protocols have been proposed to avoid the risk of delayed cardiotoxicity, but this might be at the expense of the anticancer effect [3]. In addition, impaired calcium handling and cellular damage mediated by reactive oxygen species, have been proposed as toxic mechanisms to explain both acute and delayed cardiotoxicity of anthracyclines [4-6].

Diazoxide has been in clinical use since the early 1960's to treat severe non-malignant and malignant hypertension in hospitalized adults and acute severe hypertension in hospitalized children. Diazoxide is also used to treat hypoglycaemia. The mechanisms of diazoxide's clinical action relate predominantly to the opening of pancreatic and smooth muscle K_{ATP}-channels [7].

Mitochondria are the major effectors of cardioprotection by mechanisms that open the mitochondrial K_{ATP}-channel, including ischemic and pharmacological

* Correspondence: lisa.drange.hole@helse-bergen.no
[1]Section of Clinical Pharmacology, Laboratory of Clinical Biochemistry, Haukeland University Hospital, 5021 Bergen, Norway
Full list of author information is available at the end of the article

preconditioning [8]. Pharmacological preconditioning, mimicking ischemic preconditioning, is suggested as an intervention to reduce doxorubicin cardiotoxicity [9]. Morphine has been demonstrated to mimic preconditioning in cardiomyocytes [10,11]. We have previously observed increased mortality in rats pretreated *in vivo* with morphine before doxorubicin (32). In a follow-up study we pretreated rats with morphine, isolated the hearts and exposed them to doxorubicin in a Langendorff perfusion system (unpublished data). We found that pretreatment with morphine *in vivo* was associated with a cardiodepressive effect in isolated hearts before doxorubicin exposure. After exposure to doxorubicin *ex vivo*, isolated hearts from rats pretreated with morphine were associated with increased release of hydrogen peroxide (H_2O_2), increased release of troponin-T (TnT), increased myocardial contracture and increased myocardial content of doxorubicin. These findings were in contrary to results from a comparable study [9] which found that morphine was protective against doxorubicin cardiotoxicity. Based on these opposing results we wanted to investigate further, whether pharmacological preconditioning could reduce doxorubicin cardiotoxicity.

Direct stimulation of myocardial δ_1-opioid receptors leads to opening of mitochondrial K_{ATP}-channels and a resultant increase in intracellular free radical signals *in vitro* [10]. Recently, nicorandil, a mitochondrial K_{ATP}-channel opener, has successfully been administered to counteract the toxic effects of doxorubicin [12,13]. In light of our previous results, we now wanted to bypass the opioid receptors in this experiment, and study how direct opening of mitochondrial K_{ATP}-channels interacts with the cardiotoxic mechanisms of anthracyclines. We used diazoxide, a selective mitochondrial K_{ATP}-channel agonist, known to have protective properties against cardiac ischemia [7,14]. We also used 5-hydroxydecanoate (5-HD), a selective mitochondrial K_{ATP}-channel antagonist. 5-HD inhibits the increase in free radicals seen with δ_1-opioid receptor activation, and abolishes cardioprotection afforded by ischemic preconditioning [7]. Our model combines drug treatment *in vivo* with the study of hearts *ex vivo*, yielding direct physiological information on systolic and diastolic cardiac function combined with biochemical indices like H_2O_2, TnT and measurement of myocardial content of doxorubicin.

Methods

Materials

Doxorubicin was purchased from Meda AS (Slemmestad, Norway), diazoxide, 5-hydroxydecanoate and pentobarbital from Haukeland Hospital Pharmacy (Bergen, Norway), heparin from Leo Pharma A/S (Oslo, Norway), and ingredients for the Krebs-Henseleit bicarbonate buffer from Merck KGaA (Darmstadt, Germany). This study conforms to the Guide for the Care and Use of Laboratory Animals published by the US National Institutes of Health (NIH Publication No. 85–23, revised 1996) and was approved by the Animal Care and User Committee in Norway with document number: ID 1766 FOTS, and certified institution number 066 Vivarium, University of Bergen.

Animals

Male Wistar rats weighing 200 ± 20 grams were purchased from Taconic (Ejby, Denmark). The animals were housed in grid-bottom metal wire cages in a room maintained at a 12 hour light/dark cycle at a temperature of 20–22°C. They were acclimatised for two weeks, housed three per cage and allowed free access to food pellets (Pellets rodent, Special Diets Services, Essex, UK) and tap water until i.p. injection of diazoxide, 5-HD, saline or doxorubicin. The animals were separated in individual cages based on their respective treatment protocols.

Langendorff perfusion model

The perfusion medium was a modified, oxygenated (95% O_2 and 5% CO_2) Krebs-Henseleit bicarbonate buffer (KHBB) (pH 7.4) containing in mM: 118.5 NaCl, 25.0 $NaHCO_3$, 1.2 $MgSO_4$, 4.7 KCl, 1.2 KH_2PO_4, 11.0 D-glucose, and 1.25 $CaCl_2$. Hearts were excised after anaesthesia of the rats with an i.p. injection of pentobarbital 50 mg/kg (0.1 ml/100 g bodyweight) and heparinised i.p. (0.1 ml 500 IU/100 g bodyweight). Anaesthesia was evaluated by the pedal-withdrawal reflex. The heart was rapidly excised and immediately placed in cold (4°C) KHBB to temporarily stop its beating and preserve it from ischemic injury prior to perfusion. The heart was mounted on a steel cannula placed in the aorta and perfused retrogradely in a Langendorff system with the use of thermostated (37°C) reservoirs (Lauda, Lauda-Königshofen, Germany), perfusion lines and heart chamber. Pressure regulated flow was performed at 100 cmH_2O (73 mmHg), while volume regulated flow (12.5 ml/min) was performed by use of an Alitea peristaltic pump (Alitea, Stockholm, Sweden). A water-filled latex balloon was placed in the left ventricle and connected to a pressure transducer (Memscap AS, Skoppum, Norway) for the recording of left ventricular pressure (LVDP) and secondarily derived contractility indices. Left ventricular end-diastolic pressure (LVEDP) was adjusted between 4 and 8 mmHg. A second pressure transducer was connected to a side arm on the aortic cannula for the recording of aortic pressure (AoP), an index of coronary vascular resistance during volume-regulated perfusion. Pressure signals were amplified (Quadbridge, AD Instruments, London, UK) and recorded using a PowerLab data acquisition system (AD Instruments, East Sussex, UK). AoP, LVDP, LVEDP, left ventricular pressure first derivatives maximum (dp/dt_{max}) and minimum (dp/dt_{min}) were continuously displayed and recorded. Pacing (300 beats per minute by electric stimulation of 5 V amplitude of 3 ms duration) was obtained by placing one electrode on the right auricle and one on the steel cannula. Pacing was used to maintain a standard contractile response to the experimental drugs in the model not influenced by changes in heart rate and/or periods of arrhythmia. Coronary flow rate was measured by timed collection of the coronary perfusate that dripped from the heart. At the end of the perfusion protocol, hearts were removed from the Langendorff system and myocardial tissue from the left ventricle was dissected free and immediately frozen in liquid helium and stored at −80°C until analysis of doxorubicin and doxorubicinol was performed, within 14 days of termination of the perfusion protocol. Effluent samples of 1 mL were collected in 1.5 mL polypropylene Eppendorf micro test tubes (Eppendorf Vertrieb, Wesseling-Berzdorf, Germany) from each heart, at the end of the perfusion protocol, and stored at 0°C, until analysis for TnT within 4 days of termination of the perfusion protocol. Effluent samples of 1 mL were collected in Eppendorf tubes from each heart at the end of the perfusion protocol, placed in a thermostated (37°C) Eppendorf rack heated by a Lauda reservoir (Lauda, Königshofen, Germany), and immediately analysed for H_2O_2. All experiments and analysis were carried out between 7 am and 7 pm.

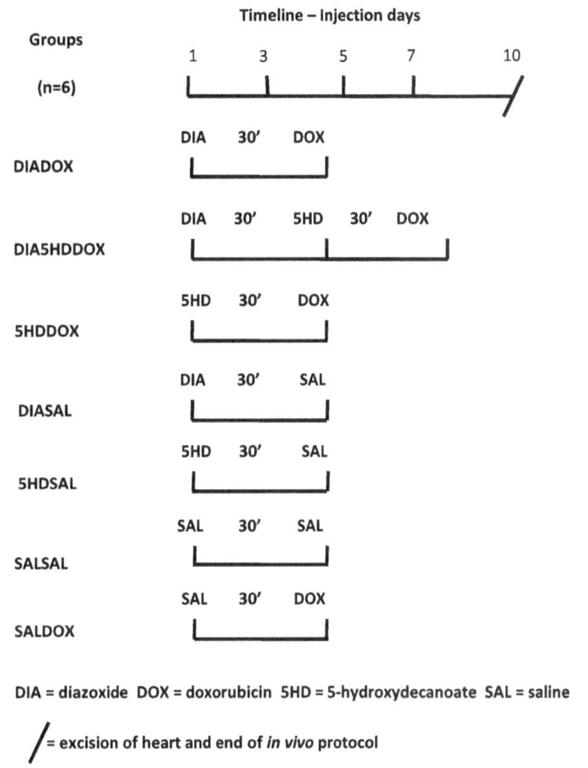

Figure 1 Drug treatment protocols.

Experimental design

DIADOX (n = 6) received pretreatment with an i.p. injection of 10 mg/kg diazoxide 30 minutes before an i.p. injection of 3 mg/kg doxorubicin.
DIA5HDDOX (n = 6) received pretreatment with an i.p. injection of 10 mg/kg diazoxide 30 minutes before an i.p. injection of 40 mg/kg 5-HD, 30 minutes before an i.p. injection of 3 mg/kg doxorubicin.
5HDDOX (n = 6) received pretreatment with an i.p. injection of 40 mg/kg 5-HD 30 minutes before an i.p. injection of 3 mg/kg doxorubicin.
DIASAL (n = 6) received pretreatment with an i.p. injection of 10 mg/kg diazoxide 30 minutes before an i.p. injection of 0.9% saline.
5HDSAL (n = 6) received pretreatment with an i.p. injection of 40 mg/kg 5-HD 30 minutes before an i.p. injection of 0.9% saline.
SALSAL (n = 6) received pretreatment with an i.p. injection of 0.9% saline 30 minutes before another i.p. injection of 0.9% saline.
SALDOX (n = 6) received pretreatment with an i.p. injection of 0.9% saline 30 minutes before an i.p. injection of 3 mg/kg doxorubicin.

Injections were given on day 1, 3, 5 and 7 and protocols are illustrated in Figure 1. On day 10 hearts were excised and Langedorff-perfused with the following protocol: 15 minutes stabilisation period with pressure-regulated flow, followed by 5 minutes with pressure-regulated flow and 5 minutes with volume-regulated flow. During the latter 10 minutes physiological data were recorded, and cardiac effluent samples collected for the evaluation of biochemical and pharmacological parameters. The perfusion protocol is illustrated in Figure 2.

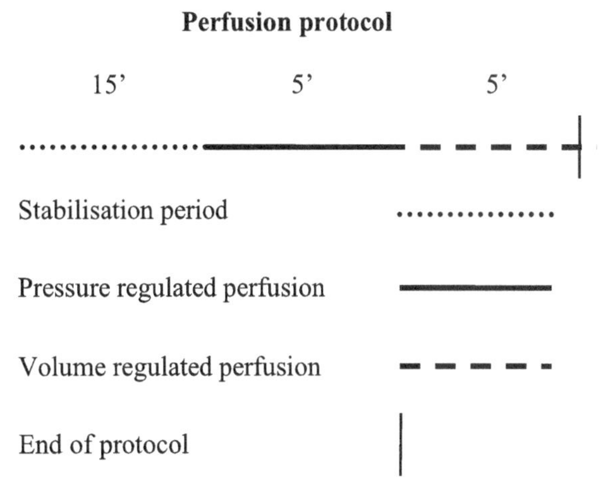

Figure 2 Perfusion protocol.

Quantification of doxorubicin and doxorubicinol

Doxorubicin and doxorubicinol were quantified by high performance liquid chromatography (HPLC-MS/MS) (1200 series RRLC, Agilent Technologies, USA) coupled to an Agilent 6410 triple quadrupole mass spectrometer using positive electrospray ionisation (Agilent Technologies, USA). Frozen left ventricular tissue was minced and weighted out in a glass tube with a screw cap and homogenized in physiological saline (2 ml/100 mg tissue) with a tissue homogenizer (Ultra Turrax, Sigma Aldrich, Germany). 1000 µl of sample was added 100 µl of daunorubicin as internal standard (IS), and 200 µl of buffer (1 M TRIZMA, pH 11.1) and mixed well before extraction with 4 ml ethylacetate/heptane (80/20 vol/vol). The samples were mixed using a rotary blender for 15 minutes and then centrifuged at 3500 rpm for 10 minutes at 10°C. The organic phase was evaporated to dryness at 50°C under nitrogen then dissolved in 100 µl of methanol followed by 100 µl of distilled water. The extract was mixed thoroughly and transferred to silanized vials before analysis. 25 µl of extract was injected and separated on a Zorbax SB-Aq (2.1 x 50 mm, 1.8 µm particles, Agilent Technologies, USA) column using gradient elution with acetonitrile and 0.1% formic acid in water. Quantification was performed using multiple reaction monitoring (MRM) mode at m/z 546.1 → 363.1 for doxorubicinol, m/z 544.1 → 361.1 for doxorubicin and m/z 528.1 → 321.1 for daunorubicin (IS).

Effluent content of H_2O_2

H_2O_2 in cardiac effluent was measured using an Apollo 4000 electrochemical detection system (World Precision Instruments, Sarasota, Florida, USA). The electrode was calibrated using 9 serial dilutions of H_2O_2 in phosphate buffered saline with added aniline. The current recorded from the effluent was then calculated as µM H_2O_2. Samples were kept at 37°C during measurement. The electrode was allowed 3 minutes of stabilisation and 1 minute of recording.

Effluent content of TnT

TnT in cardiac effluent was measured using an Elecsys 2010 immunoassay analyzer (Roche Diagnostics Norway AS, Oslo, Norway), based on the sandwich principle. Total duration of assay: 9 minutes. 1st incubation: 50 µL of sample, a biotinylated monoclonal cardiac TnT-specific antibody, and a monoclonal cardiac TnT-specific antibody labeled with a ruthenium complex (Tris(2,2-bipyridyl)ruthenium(II)-complex (Ru(bpy))) reacted to form a sandwich complex. 2nd incubation: After addition of streptavidin-coated microparticles, the complex became bound to the solid phase via interaction of biotin and streptavidin. The reaction mixture was aspirated into the measuring cell where the microparticles were magnetically captured onto the surface of the electrode. Unbound substances were then removed with ProCell. Application of a voltage to the electrode then induced chemiluminescent emission which was measured by a photomultiplier. Results were determined via a calibration curve which was instrument-specifically generated by 2-point calibration and a master curve (5-point calibration) provided via the reagent barcode. Detection limit was 5.0 ng/L.

Statistics

All results are reported as mean values ± standard deviation (SD) in tables. Groups were compared with regards to parameters with a one-way analysis of variance (ANOVA) and subsequently Fisher's protected least-significant difference test. SPSS for Windows version 17.0 was used and $p < 0.05$ was considered statistically significant.

Results

All physiological results from the pressure regulated perfusion are presented in Table 1 and all physiological results from the volume regulated perfusion are presented in Table 2. Biochemical results and doxorubicin analysis are presented in Table 3.

During pressure regulated perfusion LVDP was significantly ($p < 0.05$) higher in DIADOX (136.6 ± 2.9 mmHg) compared to SALDOX (120.4 ± 3.6 mmHg) and LVEDP was significantly ($p < 0.05$) lower in DIADOX (9.3 ± 1.5 mmHg) compared to SALDOX (15.4 ± 2.2 mmHg). There was no significant difference in LVDP, LVEDP or coronary flow in DIA5HDDOX or 5HDDOX versus SALDOX.

During volume regulated perfusion LVDP was significantly ($p < 0.05$) higher in DIADOX (141.5 ± 6.9 mmHg) compared to SALDOX (117.1 ± 9.1 mmHg). LVEDP was significantly ($p < 0.05$) lower in DIADOX (9.6 ± 2.5 mmHg) compared to SALDOX (18.0 ± 13.2 mmHg). AoP was significantly ($p < 0.05$) lower in DIADOX (103.9 ± 2.2 mmHg) compared to SALDOX (133.7 ± 5.0 mmHg). dp/dt_{max} was significantly ($p < 0.05$) higher in DIADOX (3697.4 ± 141.0 mmHg/s) compared to SALDOX (2777.8 ± 386.9 mmHg/s). dp/dt_{min} was not significantly different in DIADOX versus SALDOX, and there was no significant difference in LVDP, LVEDP, AoP, dp/dt_{max} or dp/dt_{min} in DIA5HDDOX or 5HDDOX versus SALDOX. There was no significant difference in dp/dt_{max} or dp/dt_{min} between any of the groups during pressure regulated perfusion.

Coronary flow was significantly higher ($p < 0.05$) in DIADOX (11.3 ± 1.8 ml/min) compared to SALDOX (8.9 ± 1.7 ml/min) during pressure regulated perfusion. There was no significant difference in coronary flow during pressure regulated perfusion in DIA5HDDOX or 5HDDOX versus SALDOX.

Table 1 Physiological results from pressure regulated perfusion

	DIADOX	DIA5HDDOX	5HDDOX	DIASAL	5HDSAL	SALSAL	SALDOX
LVDP (mmHg)	136.6 ± 2.9*	122.9 ± 4.4	117.5 ± 5.2	146.4 ± 6.8*	144.6 ± 5.1*	152.7 ± 11.0*	120.4 ± 3.6
LVEDP (mmHg)	9.3 ± 1.5*	16.1 ± 1.8	14.9 ± 2.7	8.2 ± 1.5*	8.1 ± 1.6*	8.3. ± 1.6*	15.4 ± 2.2
AoP (mmHg)	73.0 ± 0	73.0 ± 0	73.0 ± 0	73.0 ± 0	73.0 ± 0	73.0 ± 0	73.0 ± 0
Heart rate (beats per minute)	300 ± 0	300 ± 0	300 ± 0	300 ± 0	300 ± 0	300 ± 0	300 ± 0
dp/dt_{max} (mmHg/s)	3525.5 ± 949.9	3295.3 ± 895.9	3283.4 ± 621.9	3647.4 ± 563.7	3522.5 ± 120.1	4499.1 ± 887.2	3026.6 ± 150.0
dp/dt_{min} (mmHg/s)	−2176.5 ± 1147.9	−2012.3 ± 282.3	−1952.7 ± 373.9	−2921.9 ± 200.3	−3050.9 ± 277.6	−3060.1 ± 311.3	−2173.0 ± 195.1
Coronary flow (ml/min)	11.3 ± 1.8*	9.5 ± 0.7	8.8 ± 1.2	11.8 ± 1.2*	12.0 ± 1.3*	12.6 ± 0.4*	8.9 ± 1.7

Values presented as mean ± standard deviation (SD). *Significantly different from hearts in SALDOX, $p < 0.05$.

There was no significant difference in doxorubicin or doxorubicinol accumulation in myocard in any of the intervention groups versus SALDOX. TnT was significantly ($p < 0.05$) lower in DIADOX (67.3 ± 7.9 ng/L) compared to SALDOX (121.0 ± 17.2 ng/L). H_2O_2 concentration in effluate was significantly ($p < 0.05$) lower in DIADOX (54.9 ± 2.6 μM) compared to SALDOX (73.5 ± 2.4 μM). There was no significant difference in TnT or H_2O_2 in DIA5HDDOX or 5HDDOX versus SALDOX.

Discussion

Pretreatment with diazoxide attenuated doxorubicin-induced cardiac dysfunction in the rat in the present study. Doxorubicin treatment produced a significant loss in left ventricular developed pressure (LVDP) ($p < 0.05$) both in volume- and pressure regulated perfusion similar to previous reports [15,16]. Diazoxide significantly attenuated this decrease in LVDP ($p < 0.05$) in both perfusion protocols. Diazoxide also improved diastolic dysfunction in doxorubicin treated hearts, by lowering the elevation of LVEDP ($p < 0.05$) in both perfusion protocols, compared to animals that received both diazoxide and 5-HD. The protective effect of diazoxide is equivalent to that of ischemic preconditioning, and diazoxide is often used as a pharmacological means to induce preconditioning [7]. The drug has previously been described as an agent with a unique molecular target by opening of mitochondrial K_{ATP}-channels in cardioprotection. However, more recently a consensus seems to emerge that there are numerous effectors involved in the cardioprotective effects of diazoxide, and these effectors may synergistically contribute to its cardioprotective properties [7].

With volume regulated flow, the effects on doxorubicin-induced coronary vascular resistance, can be studied in parallel with effects on myocardial contractility. During volume regulated perfusion, aortic pressure, an indirect measure of coronary resistance, was increased in hearts that received both diazoxide and 5-HD, or just 5-HD, before doxorubicin. However, diazoxide pretreatment attenuated this effect. The vasodilatory effects of diazoxide in vascular smooth muscle are due to opening of vascular K_{ATP}-channels. K_{ATP}-channels have a pronounced role in controlling coronary blood flow and the coronary reserve, particularly in the resistance arterioles [17]. In some studies diazoxide has been noted to improve coronary flow, which is associated with cardioprotection, in perfused hearts [18], despite the fact that the coronary flow reserve is low in crystalloid-perfused hearts [19]. Coronary flow was significantly higher ($p < 0.05$) in DIADOX compared to SALDOX during pressure regulated perfusion. This effect was abolished with 5-HD. Based on these results, improved cardiac function associated with preserved coronary flow during pressure regulated perfusion, and attenuated increase in aortic pressure during volume regulated perfusion, could account for some of the cardioprotective effects of diazoxide.

Table 2 Physiological results from volume regulated perfusion

	DIADOX	DIA5HDDOX	5HDDOX	DIASAL	5HDSAL	SALSAL	SALDOX
LVDP (mmHg)	141.5 ± 6.9*	127.9 ± 4.3	108.1 ± 9.3	149.5 ± 10.8*	155.6 ± 13.0*	162.9 ± 14.7*	117.1 ± 9.1
LVEDP (mmHg)	9.6 ± 2.5*	16.0 ± 2.2	15.8 ± 2.1	10.6 ± 1.8*	8.2 ± 1.0*	9.3 ± 1.6*	18.0 ± 13.2
AoP (mmHg)	103.9 ± 2.2*	124.2 ± 5.1	130.5 ± 7.3	82.7 ± 6.0*	76.0 ± 3.5*	76.9 ± 3.6*	133.7 ± 5.0
Heart rate (beats per minute)	300 ± 0	300 ± 0	300 ± 0	300 ± 0	300 ± 0	300 ± 0	300 ± 0
dp/dt_{max} (mmHg/s)	3697.4 ± 141.0*	2512.9 ± 302.0	2950.7 ± 237.5	4583.6 ± 546.9*	3935.7 ± 213.6*	3973.6 ± 246.9*	2777.8 ± 386.9
dp/dt_{min} (mmHg/s)	−2380.6 ± 157.0	−2176.4 ± 154.8	−2530.1 ± 251.4	−2940.8 ± 261.6	−3041.6 ± 403.1	2862.0 ± 295.1	−2579.8 ± 329.1
Coronary flow (ml/min)	12.5 ± 0	12.5 ± 0	12.5 ± 0	12.5 ± 0	12.5 ± 0	12.5 ± 0	12.5 ± 0

Values presented as mean ± standard deviation (SD). *Significantly different from hearts in SALDOX, $p < 0.05$.

Table 3 Biochemical results and drug analysis

	DIADOX	DIA5HDDOX	5HDDOX	DIASAL	5HDSAL	SALSAL	SALDOX
Troponin -T effluate concentration ng/L	67.3 ± 7.9*	126.3 ± 20.5	130.0 ± 16.9	27.0 ± 4.9*	26.8 ± 4.9*	28.0 ± 5.3*	121.0 ± 17.2
H_2O_2 effluate concentration (μM)	54.9 ± 2.6*	72.8 ± 9.2	70.6 ± 5.7	24.8 ± 3.0*	26.1 ± 2.5*	22.8 ± 1.7*	73.5 ± 2.4
Doxorubicin tissue concentration nmol/g	1.9 ± 0.3	2.7 ± 0.4	3.3 ± 1.8	0 ± 0	0 ± 0	0 ± 0	2.6 ± 0.5
Doxorubicinol tissue concentration nmol/g	0.4 ± 0	0.7 ± 0.3	0.4 ± 0.1	0 ± 0	0 ± 0	0 ± 0	0.5 ± 0.2

Values presented as mean ± standard deviation (SD). *Significantly different from hearts in SALDOX, $p < 0.05$.

Diazoxide pretreated hearts had lower concentrations of H_2O_2 in cardiac effluate compared to hearts that were pretreated with 5-HD and diazoxide or 5-HD alone. Diazoxide is an inhibitor of the mitochondrial complex II protein, succinate dehydrogenase (SDH). This inhibition also occurs in the heart [20]. The activity of SDH is a site of reactive oxygen species (ROS) generation, and the possibility has been raised that diazoxide and other SDH inhibitors mediate some of their cardioprotective effects via modulation of ROS production. Which ROS signals cardioprotection is mediated through is not fully understood [8]. Opening of mitochondrial K_{ATP}-channels leads to increased ROS, leading to a persistent open state of the channel. The ROS responsible for this is not known [7]. H_2O_2 has been proposed as one candidate for this effect, although one study concludes that H_2O_2 is not the mediator of mitochondrial K_{ATP}-channel-dependent ROS signalling [8]. In our study we found higher levels of H_2O_2 in effluate from hearts that had not undergone diazoxide pretreatment before doxorubicin, or that had received both 5-HD and diazoxide before doxorubicin. The level of H_2O_2 associated with cellular signalling is much lower than the levels associated with cardiotoxicity [21]. The present study was not designed to examine signalling effects, and our observations are thus associated with the reduced cardiotoxicity of doxorubicin. This is supported by our observation of diazoxide improving diastolic dysfunction in doxorubicin treated hearts, by lowering the elevation of LVEDP. Diastolic dysfunction and contracture is proposed to be related to ROS generation [22,23].

Diazoxide pretreated hearts also had lower concentrations of TnT in cardiac effluate compared to hearts that were pretreated with 5-HD and diazoxide or 5-HD alone. Troponins are myocardial regulatory proteins, which regulate the calcium mediated actin and myosin interaction. Troponin-T is widely used as a specific marker to diagnose myocardial infarction. Doxorubicin is associated with increased TnT in serum and in heart effluate [15,24,25].

Finally, pretreatment with diazoxide was not associated with decreased myocardial accumulation of doxorubicin or doxorubicinol which suggest that the protective effects did not involve a change of distribution of the anthracycline to the heart *in vivo*.

Limitations

In this study we wanted to investigate if opening of mitochondrial K_{ATP}-channels by diazoxide is protective against doxorubicin cardiotoxicity. Mitochondrial K_{ATP}-channels have been implicated as important mediators of preconditioning [26,27]. However, the evidence for their role in preconditioning is primarily based on the effects of pharmacological agents, in particular, diazoxide and 5-HD. Diazoxide has been reported to be a specific opener of mitochondrial K_{ATP} channels, but studies have suggested that its mechanism of cardioprotection may be due to other actions, such as inhibition of succinate dehydrogenase [28,29], activation of sarcolemmal K_{ATP} channels [30] or transient opening of the mitochondrial permeability transition pore [31]. In addition, it might be argued that the complex metabolic effects of 5-HD severely limit its usefulness as a 'selective' blocker of mitochondrial K_{ATP} channels [32]. Furthermore, since their identification heavily relies on the use of diazoxide as a specific opener and 5-HD as a specific blocker, the very existence of mitochondrial K_{ATP} channels may be questioned. This skeptical view is supported by a study in which no changes in mitochondrial matrix volume induced by diazoxide or 5-HD could be detected [33]. Hence, one view on 5-HD is that it should no longer be considered a useful tool for studying the role of mitochondrial K_{ATP} channels in preconditioning [32]. Thus, although diazoxide attenuated doxorubicin-induced cardiac dysfunction in our results, our model was not designed to establish the precise protective mechanisms. Furthermore, we cannot exclude that the protective effects involved a change in distribution of doxorubicin to different compartments within the heart.

Conclusion

The main observation in the present results is that pretreatment with diazoxide attenuates doxorubicin-induced cardiac contractile dysfunction, and attenuates release of biomarkers of cardiotoxicity in effluate without decreasing the accumulation of doxorubicin. 5-HD completely abolished this effect of diazoxide in our rat model. A possible mechanism could be opening of mitochondrial K_{ATP}-channels. However, we cannot exclude other effects of the drug, including opening of vascular K_{ATP}-channels. The low specificity of 5-HD, calls for additional studies of mechanisms of a promising protective intervention.

Abbreviations

5-HD: 5-hydroxydecanoate; H_2O_2: Hydrogen peroxide; TnT: Troponin-T; LVDP: Left ventricular developed pressure; KHBB: Krebs-Henseleit bicarbonate buffer; LVEDP: Left ventricular end-diastolic pressure; AoP: Aortic pressure; dp/dt_{max}: Left ventricular pressure first derivatives maximum; dp/dt_{min}: Left ventricular pressure first derivatives minimum; HPLC-MS/MS: High performance liquid chromatography; MRM: Multiple reaction monitoring; SD: Standard deviation; ANOVA: Analysis of variance; ROS: Reactive oxygen species; SDH: Succinate dehydrogenase.

Competing interest

The authors declare that they have no competing interests.

Authors' contributions

LDH and KOF carried out the pharmacological studies, and drafted the manuscript. LDH carried out the immunochemical analysis and the animal experiments. LDH and FL carried out the hydrogen peroxide analysis, and drafted the manuscript. LDH, THL and JS conceived of the study, participated in its design and coordination, performed the statistical analysis, and helped to draft the manuscript. All authors read and approved the final manuscript.

Acknowledgements

This work was supported by Bergen Heart Foundation.

Author details

[1]Section of Clinical Pharmacology, Laboratory of Clinical Biochemistry, Haukeland University Hospital, 5021 Bergen, Norway. [2]Institute of Biomedicine, University of Bergen, 5021 Bergen, Norway. [3]Department of Heart Disease, Haukeland University Hospital, 5021 Bergen, Norway. [4]Institute of Clinical Science, Faculty of Medicine and Dentistry, University of Bergen, 5021 Bergen, Norway.

References

1. Hiona A, Lee AS, Nagendran J, Xie X, Connolly AJ, Robbins RC, Wu JC: **Pretreatment with angiotensin-converting enzyme inhibitor improves doxorubicin-induced cardiomyopathy via preservation of mitochondrial function.** *J Thorac Cardiovasc Surg* 2011, **142**(2):396–403 e393.
2. Minotti G, Menna P, Salvatorelli E, Cairo G, Gianni L: **Anthracyclines: molecular advances and pharmacologic developments in antitumor activity and cardiotoxicity.** *Pharmacol Rev* 2004, **56**(2):185–229.
3. Robert J: **Preclinical assessment of anthracycline cardiotoxicity in laboratory animals: predictiveness and pitfalls.** *Cell Biol Toxicol* 2007, **23**(1):27–37.
4. Ferreira AL, Matsubara LS, Matsubara BB: **Anthracycline-induced cardiotoxicity.** *Cardiovasc Hematol Agents Med Chem* 2008, **6**(4):278–281.
5. Gan XT, Cook MA, Moffat MP, Karmazyn M: **Protective effects against hydrogen peroxide-induced toxicity by activators of the ATP-sensitive potassium channel in isolated rat hearts.** *J Mol Cell Cardiol* 1998, **30**(1):33–41.
6. Li W, Xu B, Xu J, Wu XL: **Procyanidins produce significant attenuation of doxorubicin-induced cardiotoxicity via suppression of oxidative stress.** *Basic Clin Pharmacol Toxicol* 2009, **104**(3):192–197.
7. Coetzee WA: **Multiplicity of effectors of the cardioprotective agent, diazoxide.** *Pharmacol Therapeut* 2013, **140**(2):167–175.
8. Garlid AO, Jaburek M, Jacobs JP, Garlid KD: **Mitochondrial reactive oxygen species: which ROS signals cardioprotection?** *Am J Physiol Heart Circ Physiol* 2013, **305**(7):H960–H968.
9. Kelishomi RB, Ejtemaeemehr S, Tavangar SM, Rahimian R, Mobarakeh JI, Dehpour AR: **Morphine is protective against doxorubicin-induced cardiotoxicity in rat.** *Toxicology* 2008, **243**(1–2):96–104.
10. McPherson BC, Yao Z: **Morphine mimics preconditioning via free radical signals and mitochondrial K(ATP) channels in myocytes.** *Circulation* 2001, **103**(2):290–295.
11. Barrere-Lemaire S, Combes N, Sportouch-Dukhan C, Richard S, Nargeot J, Piot C: **Morphine mimics the antiapoptotic effect of preconditioning via an Ins(1,4,5)P3 signaling pathway in rat ventricular myocytes.** *Am J Physiol Heart Circ Physiol* 2005, **288**(1):H83–H88.
12. Ahmed LA, El-Maraghy SA: **Nicorandil ameliorates mitochondrial dysfunction in doxorubicin-induced heart failure in rats: possible mechanism of cardioprotection.** *Biochem Pharmacol* 2013, **86**(9):1301–1310.
13. Abdel-Raheem IT, Taye A, Abouzied MM: **Cardioprotective effects of nicorandil, a mitochondrial potassium channel opener against doxorubicin-induced cardiotoxicity in rats.** *Basic Clin Pharmacol Toxicol* 2013, **113**(3):158–166.
14. Garlid KD, Paucek P, Yarov-Yarovoy V, Murray HN, Darbenzio RB, D'Alonzo AJ, Lodge NJ, Smith MA, Grover GJ: **Cardioprotective effect of diazoxide and its interaction with mitochondrial ATP-sensitive K+ channels. Possible mechanism of cardioprotection.** *Circ Res* 1997, **81**(6):1072–1082.
15. Hole LD, Larsen TH, Fossan KO, Lime F, Schjott J: **A short-time model to study relevant indices of cardiotoxicity of doxorubicin in the rat.** *Toxicol Mech Meth* 2013, **23**(6):412–418.
16. Gharanei M, Hussain A, Janneh O, Maddock HL: **Doxorubicin induced myocardial injury is exacerbated following ischaemic stress via opening of the mitochondrial permeability transition pore.** *Toxicol Appl Pharmacol* 2013, **268**(2):149–156.
17. Akai K, Wang Y, Sato K, Sekiguchi N, Sugimura A, Kumagai T, Komaru T, Kanatsuka H, Shirato K: **Vasodilatory effect of nicorandil on coronary arterial microvessels: its dependency on vessel size and the involvement of the ATP-sensitive potassium channels.** *J Cardiovasc Pharmacol* 1995, **26**(4):541–547.
18. Feng J, Li H, Rosenkranz ER: **Diazoxide protects the rabbit heart following cardioplegic ischemia.** *Mol Cell Biochem* 2002, **233**(1–2):133–138.
19. Deng Q, Scicli AG, Lawton C, Silverman NA: **Coronary flow reserve after ischemia and reperfusion of the isolated heart. Divergent results with crystalloid versus blood perfusion.** *J Thorac Cardiovasc Surg* 1995, **109**(3):466–472.
20. Hanley PJ, Daut J: **K(ATP) channels and preconditioning: a re-examination of the role of mitochondrial K(ATP) channels and an overview of alternative mechanisms.** *J Mol Cell Cardiol* 2005, **39**(1):17–50.
21. Feng RH, Zhang JC, Li XQ, Sun HL, Liu B, Zhao YZ, Tang XD, Li J: **Attenuation of cardiac ischemia/reperfusion injury by transient low hydroperoxide pretreatment in rat.** *Zhongguo ying yong sheng li xue za zhi = Zhongguo yingyong shenglixue zazhi =Chinese J Appl Physiol* 2013, **29**(3):247–250.
22. Valen G, Starkopf J, Takeshima S, Kullisaar T, Vihalemm T, Kengsepp AT, Lowbeer C, Vaage J, Zilmer M: **Preconditioning with hydrogen peroxide (H2O2) or ischemia in H2O2-induced cardiac dysfunction.** *Free Radic Res* 1998, **29**(3):235–245.
23. Essick EE, Wilson RM, Pimentel DR, Shimano M, Baid S, Ouchi N, Sam F: **Adiponectin modulates oxidative stress-induced autophagy in cardiomyocytes.** *PloS one* 2013, **8**(7):e68697.
24. Chennuru A, Saleem MT: **Antioxidant, lipid lowering, and membrane stabilization effect of sesamol against doxorubicin-induced cardiomyopathy in experimental rats.** *BioMed Res Int* 2013, **2013**:934239.
25. Fouad AA, Albuali WH, Al-Mulhim AS, Jresat I: **Cardioprotective effect of cannabidiol in rats exposed to doxorubicin toxicity.** *Environ Toxicol Pharmacol* 2013, **36**(2):347–357.
26. Garlid KD, Dos Santos P, Xie ZJ, Costa AD, Paucek P: **Mitochondrial potassium transport: the role of the mitochondrial ATP-sensitive K(+) channel in cardiac function and cardioprotection.** *Biochim Biophys Acta* 2003, **1606**(1–3):1–21.
27. Gross GJ, Peart JN: **KATP channels and myocardial preconditioning: an update.** *Am J Physiol Heart Circ Physiol* 2003, **285**(3):H921–H930.
28. Lim KH, Javadov SA, Das M, Clarke SJ, Suleiman MS, Halestrap AP: **The effects of ischaemic preconditioning, diazoxide and 5-hydroxydecanoate on rat heart mitochondrial volume and respiration.** *J Physiol* 2002, **545**(Pt 3):961–974.
29. Hanley PJ, Mickel M, Loffler M, Brandt U, Daut J: **K(ATP) channel-independent targets of diazoxide and 5-hydroxydecanoate in the heart.** *J Physiol* 2002, **542**(Pt 3):735–741.
30. Suzuki M, Saito T, Sato T, Tamagawa M, Miki T, Seino S, Nakaya H: **Cardioprotective effect of diazoxide is mediated by activation of sarcolemmal but not mitochondrial ATP-sensitive potassium channels in mice.** *Circulation* 2003, **107**(5):682–685.
31. Hausenloy D, Wynne A, Duchen M, Yellon D: **Transient mitochondrial permeability transition pore opening mediates preconditioning-induced protection.** *Circulation* 2004, **109**(14):1714–1717.

32. Hanley PJ, Drose S, Brandt U, Lareau RA, Banerjee AL, Srivastava DK, Banaszak LJ, Barycki JJ, Van Veldhoven PP, Daut J: **5-Hydroxydecanoate is metabolised in mitochondria and creates a rate-limiting bottleneck for beta-oxidation of fatty acids.** *J Physiol* 2005, **562**(Pt 2):307–318.
33. Das M, Parker JE, Halestrap AP: **Matrix volume measurements challenge the existence of diazoxide/glibencamide-sensitive KATP channels in rat mitochondria.** *J Physiol* 2003, **547**(Pt 3):893–902.

No changes of cholesterol levels with a commercially available glucosamine product in patients treated with lipid lowering drugs: a controlled, randomised, open cross-over trial

Robert Eggertsen[1*], Åke Andreasson[2] and Lennart Andrén[3]

Abstract

Background: The widespread use of natural health products is also a problem, as they could interact with prescribed drugs in patients. One commonly used product is glucosamine for osteoarthritis and some reports have found increased values of cholesterol and other lipids in patients treated with simvastatin for hypercholesterolemia. The aim of this trial was to investigate the effects of glucosamine on s-cholesterol levels (total s-cholesterol, s-HDL, s-LDL) in primary care patients on treatment with simvastatin or atorvastatin.

Methods: Controlled, randomized, open, crossover pharmacodynamic study in two primary health care centres. Patients were treated with Artrox® (glucosamine) 625 mg twice daily and control (a commercially available multivitamin tablet Vitamineral®). The study started with a run-in period of four weeks followed by control or active treatment with randomization of sealed envelopes. Each treatment period was four weeks and the treatment with simvastatin or atorvastatin was unchanged during the study (12 weeks). 34 patients were treated with a stable dose of simvastatin (n=21) or atorvastatin (n=13) for at least three months. Assessments of total s-cholesterol, s-HDL, S-LDL and s-triglycerides were performed in the morning with the patients in a fasting condition. T-tests for paired samples were used for statistical analyses and a p-value <0.05 was considered significant. Endpoints were the differences in lipid values at week 8 and week 12.

Results: All patients completed the study. No significant changes were seen on any of lipid levels in the simvastatin group.

Conclusion: The actual glucosamine product did not change lipid levels of patients treated with simvastatin. Atorvastatin group was too small for safe calculations but was also without changes.

Trial registration: EUDRACT2006-001458-28

Background

There is a widespread use of natural health products [1,2]. It is also known that some of these products can interact with several prescribed drugs [3], causing increased levels for example of cholesterol and other lipids [4,5] when interacting with the metabolism of simvastatin and atorvastatin [4,5]. One drug that is commonly used of patients suffering from osteoarthritis is glucosamine, which is found naturally in the body and also is used by the body as one of the building blocks of cartilage. Some case reports have found increased values of cholesterol and other lipids in patients treated with simvastatin and glucosamine [6] but no prospective studies have been conducted to confirm these data. One long-term study of glucosamine effects on osteoarthritis found no effects on lipids but this was not made on patients treated with simvastatin [7]. One Danish trial found similar results but these patients were not either treated for hypercholesterolemia [8]. We have found effects on patients

* Correspondence: robert.eggertsen@vgregion.se
[1]Department of Medicine/Primary Health Care, University of Gothenburg, Mölnlycke vårdcentral, Ekdalavägen 2, S 435 30, Mölnlycke, Sweden
Full list of author information is available at the end of the article

treated with simvastatin and atorvastatin of St John´s Wort as a consequence of interaction of the CYP3A4 (4,5). In one trial on healthy subjects, glucosamine was tested together with noskapin where no such effects could be demonstrated for glucosamine [9]. Artrox® is a widely used commercially available product containing 750 mg glucosaminehydrochlorid that is equivalent with 625 mg glucosamine. The recommended daily dose is 625 mg given twice daily. Patients in primary health care often ask their doctor of possibilities to take natural remedies or over-the counter drugs together with prescribed medicines. It is therefore important to investigate possible interactions to prevent negative effects and give right advice to the patients. Simvastatin and atorvastatin are to a large extent metabolized by cytocrom P450 3A4. The hypothesis for our study was that glucosamine could interfere with this major metabolic pathway causing a deterioration in lipid control as was reported for three cases in Denmark (8). Against the background that no trial is carried out on patients on treatment for high levels of lipids, we decided to investigate the influence of the commercially available glucosamine product Artrox® on relevant pharmacodynamic interactions in patients with hypercholesterolemia, treated with simvastatin or atorvastatin in a randomized, controlled crossover study.

Methods

There were totally 21 patients with hypercholesterolemia on treatment with a stable dose of simvastatin (10–40 mg once daily) and 13 patients with atorvastatin (10–20 mg daily) that were included in the study. The 11 males and 10 females in the simvastatin group had a mean age of 66 years, range 57–77 years. Fourteen patients had hypertension, nine type 2 diabetes and five had suffered from cardiac infarction or stroke (Table 1). In the atorvastatin group there were nine men and four women with a mean age of 67 years, range 47–75 years. Eight patients had hypertension, five had diabetes, and four had earlier experienced heart infarction or stroke (Table 1).

The study was approved by the Swedish Medical Products Agency and the Regional Ethical Board in Western Sweden.

The study was performed as a randomised, open, cross-over study, where the approved glucosamine containing product Artrox® was compared with an inactive control (a commercially available vitamin product named Vitamineral®). Patients were recruited from the primary health care centres in Mölnlycke and Landvetter in the Western region of Sweden. Eligible patients on simvastatin or atorvastatin treatment were identified by the routinely used data system at the primary health care centres. Patient characteristics are given in Table 1. Patients were invited by an introductory letter which included information about the study. The information leaflet was approved by the regional ethical board and it was sent home to eligible patients. Those who were willing to participate signed an informed consent and were included in the study. No record was made of those patients who did not respond to the information letter.

Table 1 patients characteristics

Simvastatin treatment n = 21		
		Mean
Dose mg	10-40	21
Age years	57-77	66
Male n	11	
Female n	10	
Weight kg	47-110	83
Length cm	157-185	169
Hypertension n	14	
Diabetes n	9	
Heart disease/stroke n	5	
Systolic blood pressure mm Hg	110-178	169
Diastolic blood pressure mm Hg	60-90	78
Heart rate b/min	46-80	62
Atorvastatin treatment n = 13		
		Mean
Dose mg	10-20	15
Age years	47-75	67
Male n	9	
Female n	4	
Weight kg	60-105	87
Length cm	162-181	170
Hypertension n	8	
Diabetes n	5	
Heart disease/stroke n	4	
Systolic blood pressure mm Hg	109-165	142
Diastolic blood pressure mm Hg	64-100	82
Heart rate b/min	50-76	63

Exclusion criteria were; unstable angina pectoris, recent myocardial infarction (within a year), recent stroke (within a year), cardiac failure, HIV and dementia. There have not been shown any significant interactions involving glucosamine except case reports to warfarin treated patients. However, we excluded same drugs as in our earlier trials with St John´s Wort as our hypothesis was a stimulation of CYP3A4. Thus, treatment with birth control pills, warfarin, theofylline, cyclosporine, amitryptilin, nortriptilin, digoxin or sertraline was not allowed.

The study started with a four week run-in period. At the initial visit (week 0), the patients were informed about the study, inclusion and exclusion criteria were verified and a physical examination was performed. All blood samples were obtained in the fasting condition and analysed at the accredited central laboratory at Sahlgrenska University Hospital in Gothenburg (total s-cholesterol, s-HDL-cholesterol, s-LDL-cholesterol and s-triglycerides). The laboratory was unaware of patient treatment. Patients were then to return after 4 weeks (week 4) and another physical examination was performed and blood samples as described at week 0 above were collected. At this visit, the treating physician randomised (using sealed envelopes performed by a person not involved with patients), the order of treatment with active (Artrox®) and control (Vitamineral®). Thus, 50% started with active treatment and the other 50% started with control treatment and all were crossed- over to the other treatment modality after another 4 weeks (week 8). We considered that the treatment period o four weeks was adequate for possible glucosamine effects to vanish and thus no further wash out period was mandatory. Assessment of total s-cholesterol, s-HDL and s-LDL-cholesterol and s-triglycerides were then performed at the end of each treatment period (week 8 and 12). Compliance was verified by pill counting at each visit. The patients were on their regular dose of simvastatin or atorvastatin and the dose of simvastatin and atorvastatin was kept unchanged during the whole study period until all patients completed the study. The mean dose of simvastatin was 21 mg (range 10 mg – 40 mg) and of atorvastatin 14.6 mg (range 10–20 mg).

Glucosamine could have an effect on glucose metabolism as stated in the SPC of the product. In order to exclude negative effects on this variable, HbA1c was followed as a safety measure,

Statistics

T- test for paired samples was used for statistical analyses and a p-value <0.05 was considered significant. The primary efficacy endpoint was the difference in LDL-cholesterol at week 8 and 12 between active treatment and control. Secondary endpoints were the corresponding difference in total cholesterol, HDL-cholesterol and in triglycerides. The study was powered to detect a difference of 0.48 mmol/L with a power of 81.2 % with a significance level of 0.05 (two sided) and a standard deviation within the groups of 0.52. Power calculations showed that participation of 20 subjects would give statistical significance. Randomization procedure was performed by a person not involved with the patients.

Results

Simvastatin group

Basal measurements were made after four weeks of run-in. There were no significant effects on s-LDL, s-HDL, total s-cholesterol, or s-triglycerides after four weeks treatment with glucosamine. Neither were there any significant changes of p-glucose and HbA1c Table 2.

Atorvastatin group

This group (n=13) was too small for safe calculations but also in this group there were no effects on the different lipids that could be demonstrated when compared with run-in determinations and after four weeks of active treatment. Values of p-glucose and HbA1c were also unchanged Table 2.

Table 2 Effects on lipid and glucose values

	Vitamineral mean and SD	Simvastatin mean and SD	P-value
s-LDL mmol/L	2.27+0.61	2.30+0.51	0.81 ns
s-HDL mmol/L	1.62+0.55	1.63+0.60	0.86 ns
s-total cholesterol mmol/L	4.69+0.99	4.76+0.96	0.53 ns
s-triglyceridesmmol/L	1.77+0.76	1.83+0.79	0.63 ns
p-glucose mmol/L	6.77+1.90	6.90+1.62	0.70 ns
HbA1c mmol/mol	5.13+1.10	5.09+0.97	0.57 ns
		Atorvastatin	
s-LDL mmol/L	2.36+0.65	2.36+0.64	1.00 ns
s-HDL mmol/L	1.55+0.40	1.48+0.40	0.10 ns
s-total cholesterol mmol/L	4.51+0.65	4.40+0.89	0.42 ns
s-triglyceridesmmol/L	1.74+1.05	1.59+0.70	0.39 ns
p-glucose mmol/L	7.39+2.08	7.53+2.16	0.38 ns
HbA1c mmol/mol	5.20+1.13	5.18+1.40	0.90 ns

All patients completed the study and no significant side effects were reported.

Discussion

The main finding in our study was that we could not demonstrate any significant effect on total s-cholesterol, s-LDL, S-HDL or s-triglycerides after treatment with the glucosamine product Artrox® on patients treated with neither simvastatin nor atorvastatin for increased levels of lipids. However, the atorvastatin group comprised of 13 patients why safe conclusions could not be drawn from these patients. This is valuable knowledge as the use of glucosamine is widespread and a considerable amount of people is now also treated with lipid lowering drugs.

Many patients are not aware of possibilities for interaction with increasing lipid values and different natural health products that you can buy on the counter [4,5]. We have used one commercial product in our trial but results may be similar with other glucosamine products Also positive effects are described of natural health products as for pomegranate preparations where reductions in LDL-cholesterol have been demonstrated [10,11]. Such products are as a rule not tested for influence on different metabolic interactions, why it is important to make investigations in that field. There are made meta-analysis of the effects of glucosamine but reports of interactions and effects of lipids are missing [12,13]. Reports of glucose rising and induction of insulin resistance of glucosamine have been discussed but not been confirmed in clinical studies [14]. The Swedish Medical Products Agency (MPA) points out that interaction studies are lacking and precaution is important even if the risks of interactions is estimated as low [14]. In our material we could not find any disturbances in the glucose metabolism, however the active treatment period was only four weeks.

A limitation in our study is that it was not double-blind, why we cannot exclude carry-over effects in the cross-over regimen. However, the half life for glucosamine is about two hours why this seems unlikely in treatment periods of four weeks. Furthermore, the study was randomized, and assessment of the lipids was performed by an accredited central laboratory, blinded to the treatment regimen. We can not with used sample sizes definitely exclude that there may be a type 2 error because our study was dimensioned to detect differences between the groups. Further studies with larger materials could be necessary. The metabolism of glucosamine is not known. This was an explanatory study to investigate if there was a signal that could verify clinical observations of possible interactions. If a signal had been detected further studies on possible mechanism had been justified.

Conclusions

We conclude that no increased levels of lipids were seen in patients on lipid lowering drugs as simvastatin if they simultaneously take glucosamine for articulation problems.

Competing interests

None of the authors have any relevant conflicts of interest.

Authors' contributions

All authors planned and managed the study, performed the analysis and wrote the main results and final manuscript. All authors read and approved the final manuscript.

Acknowledgements

The study was funded by the Health and Medical Care Executive Board of the Region Västra Götaland, Sweden.

Author details

[1]Department of Medicine/Primary Health Care, University of Gothenburg, Mölnlycke vårdcentral, Ekdalavägen 2, S 435 30, Mölnlycke, Sweden.
[2]Landvetter vårdcentral, Centrumhuset, S 438 32, Landvetter, Sweden.
[3]Department of Clinical Pharmacology, University of Gothenburg, Sahlgrenska University Hospital, S 413 45, Göteborg, Sweden.

References

1. Thomas KJ, Nicholl JP, Coleman P: **Use and expenditure on complementary medicine in England: a population based survey.** *Complement Ther Med* 2001, **9:**2–11.
2. Hansen B, Grimsgaard S, Launsö L, Fönnebo V, Falkenberg T, Rasmussen N: **Use of complimentary and alternative medicine in the Scandinavian countries.** *Scand J Prim Health Care* 2005, **23:**57–62.
3. Stjernberg L, Berglund J, Halling A: **Age and gender on the use of herbal medicine products and food supplements among the elderly.** *Scand J Prim Health Care* 2006, **24:**50–55.
4. Eggertsen R, Andreasson Å, Andrén L: **Effects of treatment with a commercially available St John´s Wort product (Movina) on cholesterol levels in patients with hypercholesterolemia treated with simvastatin.** *Scand J Prim Health Care* 2007, **25:**154–159.
5. Andrén L, Andreasson Å, Eggertsen R: **Interaction between a commercially available St John´s Wort product (Movina) and atorvastatin in patients with hypercholesterolemia.** *Eur J Clin Pharmacol* 2007, **63:**913–916.
6. Odder EL: **Glucosamine/cholesterol possible interaction.** *Ugeskr Leger* 2004, **166:**3895.
7. Reginster J, Deroisy R, Rovati L, Lee R, Lejeune E, Bruyere O, Giacovelli G, Henrotin Y, Dacre J, Gosett C: **Long-term effects of glucosamine sulphate on osteoarthritis progression: a randomized, placebo controlled trial.** *Lancet* 2001, **357:**251–256.
8. Östergaard K, Hvid T, Hyllested-Winge J: **The effect of glucosamine sulphate on the blood levels of cholesterol of triglycerides-a clinical study.** *Ugeskr Leger* 2007, **169:**407–410.
9. Rosenborg S, Stenberg M, Otto S, Östervall J, Masquelier M, Yue Q-Y, Bertilsson L, Eliasson E: **Clinically significant CYP2C inhibition by noskapine but not by glucosamine.** *Clin Pharmacol Ther* 2010, **88:**343–346.
10. Aviram M, Rosenblad M, Gaitini D, Nitecki S, Hoffman A, Dornfeld L, Volkova N, Presser D, Attias J, Liker H, Hayek T: **Pomegranate juice consumption for 3 years by patients with carotid artery stenosis reduces common carotid intima.media thickness, blood pressure and LDL oxidation.** *Clin Nutr* 2004, **23:**423–433.
11. Esmaillzadeh A, Tahbaz F, Gaieni I, Alavi-Majd H, Azadbakht L: **Concentrated pomegranate juice improves lipid profiles in diabetic patients with hyperlipidemia.** *J Med Food* 2004, **7:**305–308.
12. Wandel S, Juni P, Tendal B, Nuesch E, Villiger P, Welton N, Reichenbach S, Trelle S: **Effects of glucosamine, chondroitin, or placebo in patients with osteoarthritis of hip or knee: network meta-analysis.** *BMJ* 2010, **341:**c4675.

13. Towheed T, Maxwell L, Anastassiades TP, Shea B, Houpt JB, Welch V, Hochberg MC, Wells GA: **Glucosamine therapy for treating osteoarthritis (Review).** *Cochrane Database of Syst Rev* 2005, CD002946.pub2. issue 2 Art No: CD002946.
14. Swedish Medical Products Agency: **Monography. Artrox (glucosamine).** *Information from the MPA* 2002, **13**(6).

17

Bioenergetic study of murine hepatic tissue treated *in vitro* with atorvastatin

Ali S Alfazari[1*], Bayan Al-Dabbagh[1], Saeeda Almarzooqi[2], Alia Albawardi[2] and Abdul-Kader Souid[3]

Abstract

Atorvastatin (a 3-hydroxy-3-methylglutaryl coenzyme-A reductase inhibitor) is a widely used cholesterol-lowering drug, which is recognized for its potential hepatotoxicity. This study investigated *in vitro* effects of this agent on hepatic tissue respiration, ATP content, caspase activity, urea synthesis and histology. Liver fragments from Taylor Outbred and C57Bl/6 mice were incubated at 37°C in Krebs-Henseleit buffer continuously gassed with 95% O_2: 5% CO_2 in the presence and absence of atorvastatin. Phosphorescence O_2 analyzer that measured dissolved [O_2] as a function of time was used to monitor cellular mitochondrial O_2 consumption. The caspase-3 substrate *N*-acetyl-asp-glu-val-asp-7-amino-4-methylcoumarin was used to monitor caspase activity. The rates of hepatocyte respiration (μM O_2 min^{-1} mg^{-1}) in untreated samples were 0.15 ± 0.07 (n = 31). The corresponding rates for samples treated with 50 nM (therapeutic concentration), 150 nM or 1.0 μM atorvastatin for ≤13 h were 0.13 ± 0.05 (n = 19), $p = 0.521$. The contents of hepatocyte ATP ($pmol^{-1}$ mg^{-1}) in untreated samples were 40.3 ± 14.0 and in samples treated with 1.0 μM atorvastatin for ≤4.5 h were 48.7 ± 23.9 ($p = 0.7754$). The concentrations of urea (mg/dL mg^{-1}, produced over 50 min) for untreated samples were 0.061 ± 0.020 (n = 6) and for samples treated with 1.0 μM atorvastatin for ≤6 h were 0.072 ± 0.022 (n = 6), $p = 0.3866$. Steadily, hepatocyte caspase activity and histology were unaffected by treatments with up to 1.0 μM atorvastatin for ≤6 h. Thus, the studied murine model showed preserved hepatocyte function and structure in the presence of high concentrations of atorvastatin.

Keywords: Statins, Mitochondria, Respiration, Caspases, Apoptosis

Background

Statins, 3-hydroxy-3-methylglutaryl coenzyme-A reductase inhibitors, are the most effective class of drugs that treat hypercholesterolemia. These agents reduce hepatocyte cholesterol, which results in up-regulation of the low-density lipoprotein (LDL) receptors and increased clearance of LDL-cholesterol from the plasma. Atorvastatin, (3*R*,5*R*)-7-[2-(4-fluorophenyl)-3-phenyl-4-(phenylcarbamoyl)-5-propan-2-ylpyrrol-1-yl]-3,5-dihydroxyheptanoic acid, is considered "best-in-class" for meeting the recommended treatment guidelines [1].

Elevations of liver alanine and aspartate aminotransferases (ALT and AST) are well-recognized adverse events of atorvastatin [2-4], occurring in about 0.5% of patients, usually in the first few months of therapy [5,6]. Since other lipid-lowering compounds also increase liver aminotransferases, it has been debated whether statin-associated elevated transaminases are due to hepatotoxicity or a reaction to reduced cholesterol [7]. More recent studies have shown statins are well tolerated by patients with primary biliary cirrhosis, hepatitis C and non-alcoholic steatohepatitis [8-10]. Furthermore, a few short-term studies showed statins improved hepatic inflammation in patients with non-alcoholic fatty liver disease [11]. In a prospective, double blind trial of 326 patients with chronic liver disease, fewer patients in the pravastatin group had elevations in ALT compared to placebo (7.5% *vs.* 12.5%, $p = 0.13$) [12]. The recent *post hoc* analysis of safety of atorvastatin in the Greek Atorvastatin and Coronary Heart Disease Evaluation (GREACE) study showed atorvastatin significantly ameliorated elevations of AST and ALT [13]. Other reports in humans and animals showed hepatotoxicities of statins [14], including caspase activation (apoptosis) and induction of mitochondrial disturbances [15]. These toxicities could stem from confounding factors, such

* Correspondence: a.almelaih@uaeu.ac.ae
[1]Department of Internal Medicine, United Arab Emirates University, Al Ain, Abu Dhabi, United Arab Emirates
Full list of author information is available at the end of the article

idiosyncratic reactions, hypercholesterolemia, concomitant medications and co-morbidities (e.g., diabetes mellitus).

The term "cellular bioenergetics" implies the biochemical processes involved in energy metabolism (energy conversion or transformation), and the term "cellular respiration" (mitochondrial O_2 consumption) describes the delivery of metabolites and O_2 to the mitochondria, the oxidation of reduced metabolic fuels with passage of electrons to O_2, and the synthesis of ATP. Impaired bioenergetics or respiration entails interferences with any of these processes.

Apoptosis describes the highly regulated mechanisms responsible for cellular responses to injuries and adverse biological signals. This process produces deleterious morphological and biochemical changes, including mitochondrial disturbances that may lead to cell death [16]. Caspases, cysteine aspartate-directed proteases and members of the interleukin-1β-converting enzyme (ICE), are key executers of apoptosis. Intracellular caspase activity can be monitored using the caspase-3 synthetic substrate *N*-cetyl-asp-glu-val-asp-7-amino-(4-methyl- coumaryl-7-amide) (Ac-DEVD-AMC). Caspase-3 is involved in proteolysis of proteins, including poly(ADP ribose) polymerase. The enzyme cleaves at the C-terminal to Asp^{216} in the asp-glu-val-asp sequence. This 4-amino-acid motif has been utilized for the highly specific caspase-3 substrate Ac-DEVD-AMC. Caspase-3 cleaves the tetrapeptide between D and AMC, releasing the fluorogenic moiety 7-amino-4-methylcoumarin (AMC). The latter can be separated on HPLC and detected by fluorescence with a great accuracy [17].

The primary aim of the study here was to investigate the effects of atorvastatin on hepatocyte bioenergetics and caspase activity. The described *in vitro* murine system allowed accurate assessment of multiple hepatic biomarkers as a function of time using murine liver tissue. The results show liver tissue function and structure are well preserved in the presence of high concentrations of atorvastatin.

Materials and methods

Reagents

Atorvastatin was purchased from Selleck Chemicals (Houston, TX, USA). Pd(II) complex of *meso*-tetra-(4-sulfonatophenyl)-tetrabenzoporphyrin (Pd phosphor) was purchased from Porphyrin Products (Logan, UT). A lyophilized powder of caspase inhibitor I [*N*-benzyloxycarbonyl-val-ala-asp(O-methyl)-fluoromethylketone, zVAD-fmk, *m.w.* = 467.5, a pan-caspase inhibitor] was purchased from Calbiochem (La Jolla, CA). Ac-DEVD-AMC (*N*-acetyl-asp-glu-val-asp-7- amino-4-methylcoumarin; *m. w.* = 675.64; caspase-3 substrate) was purchased from Axxora LLC (San Diego, CA). Complete® protease inhibitor cocktail was purchased from Roche Applied Science (Indianapolis, IN). Glucose (anhydrous), endotoxin- and fatty acid-free bovine serum albumin and remaining reagents were bought from Sigma-Aldrich (St. Louis, MO).

The pan-caspase inhibitor (zVAD-fmk) solution (2.14 mM) was made by dissolving 1.0 mg in 1.0 mL dimethyl sulfoxide and stored at -20°C. Ac-DEVD-AMC solution (7.4 mM) was made by dissolving 5.0 mg in 1.0 mL dimethyl sulfoxide and stored at -20°C. Pd phosphor solution (2.5 mg/mL = 2 mM) was prepared in dH_2O and stored in aliquots at -20°C. NaCN solution (1.0 M) was prepared in dH_2O; the pH was adjusted to ~7.0 with 12 N HCl and stored at -20°C. Glucose oxidase, 10 mg/mL in dH_2O, was stored at -20°C. One tablet of Complete® protease inhibitor cocktail was dissolved in 1.0 mL Water-For-Injection and stored at -20°C.

Mice

Male Taylor Outbred (TO, age: 9-10 weeks, weight: 30-35 g) and C57Bl/6 (age: 9-10 weeks, weight: 20-22 g) mice were maintained at an animal facility that was in compliance with NIH guidelines (http://grants.nih.gov/grants/olaw/references/phspol.htm). The mice were purchased from the Jackson Laboratory (Bar Harbor, ME). All mice were housed in rooms maintained at 22°C with ~60% relative humidity and a 12-hr light/dark cycle. All mice had *ad libitum* access to standard rodent chow and filtered water. All protocols here received approval from the Animal Ethics Committee-United Arab Emirates University-College of Medicine and Health Sciences.

Liver tissue

Mice were anesthetized by sevoflurane inhalation (100 μL per 10 g body weight). Liver specimens (~20 to 30 mg) were collected using a 4-mm human skin biopsy punch (Miltex GmbH, Germany) and *immediately* immersed in 50 mL ice-cold *modified* Krebs-Henseleit (KH) buffer (115 mM NaCl, 25 mM $NaHCO_3$, 1.23 mM NaH_2PO_4, 1.2 mM Na_2SO_4, 5.9 mM KCl, 1.0 mM EDTA, 1.18 mM $MgCl_2$, 10 mM glucose, and 0.5 μL/mL Complete® protease inhibitor cocktail, pH 7.5) continuously gassed with 95% O_2: 5% CO_2 [18].

The samples were then incubated *in vitro* at 37°C in 50 mL in KH buffer (115 mM NaCl, 25 mM $NaHCO_3$, 1.23 mM NaH_2PO_4, 1.2 mM Na_2SO_4, 5.9 mM KCl, 1.25 mM $CaCl_2$, 1.18 mM $MgCl_2$, and 10 mM glucose, pH 7.5) supplemented with 0.5 μL/mL Complete® protease inhibitor cocktail and continuously gassed with 95% O_2: 5% CO_2. For the O_2 measurement, specimens were placed in 1.0 mL KH buffer (air-saturated) containing 0.5% fatty acids-free bovine albumin and 3 μM Pd phosphor. Specimens were also processed for measuring caspase activity, urea synthesis and histology as described below.

Oxygen measurement

Phosphorescence oxygen analyzer was used to monitor O_2 consumption by liver specimens [18,19]. O_2 detection was performed with the aid of Pd phosphor that had absorption maximum at 625 nm and phosphorescence maximum at 800 nm. Samples were exposed to light flashes (600 per min) from a pulsed light-emitting diode array with peak output at 625 nm (OTL630A-5-10-66-E, Opto Technology, Inc., Wheeling, IL). Emitted phosphorescent light was detected by a Hamamatsu photomultiplier tube (928) after first passing it through a wide-band interference filter centered at 800 nm. The amplified phosphorescence decay was digitized at 1.0 MHz by a 20-MHz A/D converter (Computer Boards, Inc., Mansfield, MA).

A program was developed using Microsoft Visual Basic 6, Microsoft Access Database 2007, and Universal Library components (Universal Library for Measurements Computing Devices; http://www.mccdaq.com/daq-software/universal-library.aspx). It allowed direct reading from the PCI-DAS 4020/12 I/O Board (PCI-DAS 4020/12 I/O Board; http://www.mccdaq.com/pci-data-acquisition/PCI-DAS4020-12.aspx). The pulse detection was accomplished by searching for 10 phosphorescence intensities >1.0 volt (by default). Peak detection was accomplished by searching for the highest 10 data points of a pulse and choosing the data point closest to the pulse decay curve [20].

The phosphorescence decay rate ($1/\tau$) was characterized by a single exponential; $I = Ae^{-t/\tau}$, where I = Pd phosphor phosphorescence intensity. The values of $1/\tau$ were linear with dissolved O_2: $1/\tau = 1/\tau^o + k_q[O_2]$, where $1/\tau$ = the phosphorescence decay rate in the presence of O_2, $1/\tau^o$ = the phosphorescence decay rate in the absence of O_2, and k_q = the second-order O_2 quenching rate constant in $s^{-1} \bullet \mu M^{-1}$.

Respiration was measured at 37°C in 1-mL sealed vials. Mixing was with the aid of parylene-coated stirring bars. In vials sealed from air, $[O_2]$ decreased linearly with time, indicating the kinetics of mitochondrial O_2 consumption was zero-order. The rate of respiration (k, in $\mu M\ O_2\ min^{-1}$) was thus the negative of the slope $d[O_2]/dt$. NaCN inhibited respiration, confirming O_2 was consumed in the mitochondrial respiratory chain.

The calibration reaction contained PBS with 3 μM Pd phosphor, 0.5% fat-free albumin, 50 μg/mL glucose oxidase and various concentrations of β-glucose. $[O_2]$ was calculated using, $1/\tau = 1/\tau^o + k_q[O_2]$ [21]. Rates of cellular respiration were normalized per mg of liver tissue (i.e., expressed as μM O_2 consumed per min per mg liver tissue).

ATP content

Liver fragments were homogenized in ice-cold 2% trichloroacetic acid for 2 min and neutralized with 100 mM Tris-acetate, 2 mM EDTA, pH 7.75. The supernatant was collected by centrifugation (1000 × *g* at 4°C for 5 min) and stored at -20°C until analysis. The pH of samples was adjusted to 7.75 immediately before ATP determination. ATP concentration was measured using the Enliten ATP Assay System (Bioluminescence Detection Kit, Promega, Madison, WI). Briefly, 2.5 μL of the acid-soluble supernatant was added to 25 μL of the luciferin/luciferase reagent. The luminescence intensity was measured at 25°C using Glomax Luminometer (Promega, Madison, WI). The ATP standard curve was linear from 10 pM to 100 nM (R^2 >0.9999).

Intracellular caspase activity

Liver specimens were incubated at 37°C in oxygenated KH buffer containing 37 μM Ac-DEVD-AMC with and without 32 μM zVAD-fmk (final volume, 0.5 mL). The tissue was then disrupted by vigorous homogenization and 10 passages through a 27-G needle. The Ac-DEVD-AMC cleavage reaction was quenched with tissue disruption, mainly because caspases became inactive due to dilution. The supernatant was collected by centrifugation (16,300 *g* for 90 min) through a Microcentrifuge Filter (nominal molecular weight limit = 10,000 Dalton, Sigma©), separated on HPLC, and analyzed for the free fluorogenic AMC moiety. The elution time for AMC was about 5.0 min.

HPLC

The analysis was performed on a Waters 1525 reversed-phase HPLC system (Spectra Lab Scientific Inc, Alexandria, VA) that consisted of manual injector, pump and fluorescence detector. The excitation wavelength used was 380 nm and the emission wavelength 460 nm. Solvents A and B were HPLC-grade CH_3OH: dH_2O (1:1; isocratic). The Ultrasphere IP column (4.6 × 250 mm, Beckman) was operated at 25°C at 1.0 mL/min. The run time was 20 min. The injection volume was 50 μL.

Urea synthesis

Liver specimens were incubated at 37°C in 50 mL KH buffer (continuously gassed with 95% O_2: 5% CO_2) with and without 1.0 μM atorvastatin for up to 6 h. Specimens were then removed from the incubation solution every 60 min and placed in 1.0 mL KH buffer supplemented with 10 mM NH_4Cl and 2.5 mM ornithine. The reactions were allowed to continue at 37°C for 50 min with continuous gassing as above. At the end of the incubation period, the solutions were analyzed for urea as described [22]. Blood urea nitrogen (BUN, mmol/L) was measured using standard laboratory methods with an LX20 multiple automated analyzer (Beckman Coulter, CA, USA). For conversion, BUN (mg/dL) = BUN (mmol/L) ÷ 0.357; Urea (mg/dL) = BUN (mg/dL) × 2.14.

Histology

Liver samples were fixed in 10% neutral formalin, dehydrated in increasing concentrations of ethanol, cleared with xylene and embedded in paraffin. Four-micrometer sections were prepared from paraffin blocks and stained with hematoxylin and eosin.

Statistical analysis

Data were analyzed using SPSS statistical package (version 19). The nonparametric test (2 independent variables) Mann-Whitney was used to compare treated and untreated samples. Respiration rates (k_c, in μM O_2 min^{-1} mg^{-1}), cellular ATP content (pmol mg^{-1}), AMC peak areas (arbitrary unit mg^{-1}) and urea (mg/dL per mg liver tissue) for untreated samples were compared with those for treated samples.

Results

Bioenergetics of liver tissue treated with atorvastatin

To assess the effects of atorvastatin on liver tissue bioenergetics, specimens from ten Taylor Outbred (TO) mice and three C57Bl/6 mice were incubated at 37°C with 50 nM (therapeutic concentration; Maier et al. [23]), 150 nM or 1.0 μM atorvastatin and analyzed for cellular O_2 consumption and ATP content as a function of time. Results of representative experiments are shown in Figure 1.

In Figure 1A-B, liver specimens from TO mice were incubated at 37°C in 50 mL KH buffer (continuously gassed with 95% O_2: 5% CO_2) with and without 150 nM atorvastatin for up to 6 h. Samples were alternatively removed from the incubation mixture and processed for O_2 measurement at 37°C. The rate of respiration (k, μM O_2 min^{-1}) was set as the negative of the slope of $[O_2]$ *vs. t*. The values of k_c (μM O_2 min^{-1} mg^{-1}; mean ± SD) for untreated samples were 0.18 ± 0.06 (n = 5, for t from 1.8 to 5.3 h) and for treated samples 0.18 ± 0.05 (n = 3, for t from 1.1 to 3.7 h), $p = 0.9737$.

Liver samples were also incubated as above with and without 50 nM atorvastatin. The value of k_c for untreated tissue was 0.15 μM O_2 min^{-1} mg^{-1} ($t = 1.4$ h) and for treated tissue 0.15 μM O_2 min^{-1} mg^{-1} ($t = 2.2$ h). In 10 independent experiments involving incubations with 50 nM, 150 nM or 1.0 μM atorvastatin for up to 13 h, the rates of respiration for untreated specimens were 0.15 ± 0.07 (n = 31 runs) and for treated specimens 0.13 ± 0.05 (n = 19 runs), $p = 0.521$.

In C57Bl/6 strain, the value of k_c for untreated tissue was 0.10 ± 0.03 ($1.8 < t < 5.3$ h, n = 5) and for tissue treated with 1.0 μM atorvastatin 0.11 ± 0.04 (for t from 1.1 to 3.7 h, n = 4). In another experiment, the value of k_c for untreated tissue was 0.12 ± 0.05 (for t from 1.3 to 5.9 h, n = 4) and treated tissue 0.12 ± 0.04 (for t from 0.5 to 4.4 h, n = 3). Thus, hepatocyte respiration was preserved in the presence of high doses of atorvastatin for up to 13 h.

In Figure 1C-D, liver samples were incubated as above with and without 1.0 μM atorvastatin for up to 6.5 h and processed for measurements of cellular respiration and ATP content. The results are plotted as a function of incubation time in Panel D. The values of k_c for untreated samples (for t from 0 to 5.3 h) were 0.17 ± 0.03 μM O_2 min^{-1} mg^{-1} and for treated samples (for t from 0 to 4.5 h) 0.16 ± 0.02 μM O_2 min^{-1} mg^{-1} ($p = 0.3954$). Cellular ATP at $t = 0$ h was 181.1 ± 8.0 pmol mg^{-1}. For untreated specimens, cellular ATP (in pmol mg^{-1}, measured in triplicates) at $t = 1.3$ h was 33.9 ± 1.7, at $t = 2.0$ h was 61.2 ± 1.4, at $t = 3.5$ h was 32.6 ± 1.4, and at $t = 5.3$ h was 33.4 ± 6.8. For treated specimens, cellular ATP at $t = 0.3$ h was 66.5 ± 3.9, at $t = 3.0$ h was 58.0 ± 7.4 and at $t = 4.5$ h was 21.6 ± 6.1. Thus, the overall ATP contents for untreated samples (for t from 1.3 to 5.3 h) were 40.3 ± 14.0 and for treated samples (for t from 0.3 to 4.5 h) 48.7 ± 23.9 ($p = 0.7754$). In another experiment, ATP contents at 6 h for untreated tissue were 10.5 ± 1.0 (n = 4) and for treated tissue 16.6 ± 0.9 (n = 4). Thus, hepatocyte ATP was highest immediately after tissue collection (*in vivo* levels of hepatocyte bioenergetics) and declined equally in the presence and absence of atorvastatin (*in vitro* levels of hepatocyte bioenergetics).

Hepatocyte caspases in liver tissue treated with atorvastatin

Representative experiments for hepatocyte caspase activity in TO (Panels A-B) and C57BL/6 (Panels C-D) strains are shown in Figure 2. The samples were incubated at 37°C with and without 1.0 μM atorvastatin for 6 h. The specimens were then incubated at 37°C with 37 μM Ac-DEVD-AMC in the presence and absence of zVAD-fmk (32 μM). In untreated samples from the TO strain (Panel A), the AMC peak area (arbitrary unit, reflecting caspase activity) without zVAD was 1,627,780 mg^{-1} and with zVAD was 121,952 mg^{-1} (93% inhibition). In treated samples (Panel B), the AMC peak area without zVAD was 963,346 mg^{-1} and with zVAD was 152,144 mg^{-1} (84% inhibition). In untreated samples from the C57BL/6 strain (Panel C), the AMC peak area without zVAD was 1,988,712 mg^{-1} and with zVAD 125,667 mg^{-1} (94% inhibition). In treated samples (Panel D), the AMC peak area without zVAD was 2,068,736 mg^{-1} and with zVAD 119,295 mg^{-1} (94% inhibition). Thus, hepatocyte caspase activity at 6 h was similar in untreated and treated samples.

Urea synthesis by liver tissue treated with atorvastatin

Liver specimens were incubated at 37°C in 50 ml KH buffer (continuously gassed as above) with and without 1.0 μM atorvastatin for 6 hr. Every 60 min, specimens (sum sample weight = 86.9 ± 5.9 mg) were removed from the incubation solutions and placed in 1.0 mL KH buffer supplemented with 10 mM NH_4Cl and 2.5 mM ornithine. The solutions were then analyzed for urea at min

50. The concentrations of urea (mg/dL per mg liver tissue) for untreated and treated samples were not significantly different (Table 1).

Histology

Representative micrographs of hematoxylin and eosin stained sections of untreated tissue at 0 and 6 hr and tissue treated with 1.0 μM atorvastatin at 6 hr are shown in Figure 3. The incubation conditions were as above. Liver architecture and cytology were preserved in treated and untreated specimens. Inflammation and cholestasis were absent.

Discussion

Asymptomatic increase in hepatic transaminases is most common adverse event of atorvastatin, occurring in

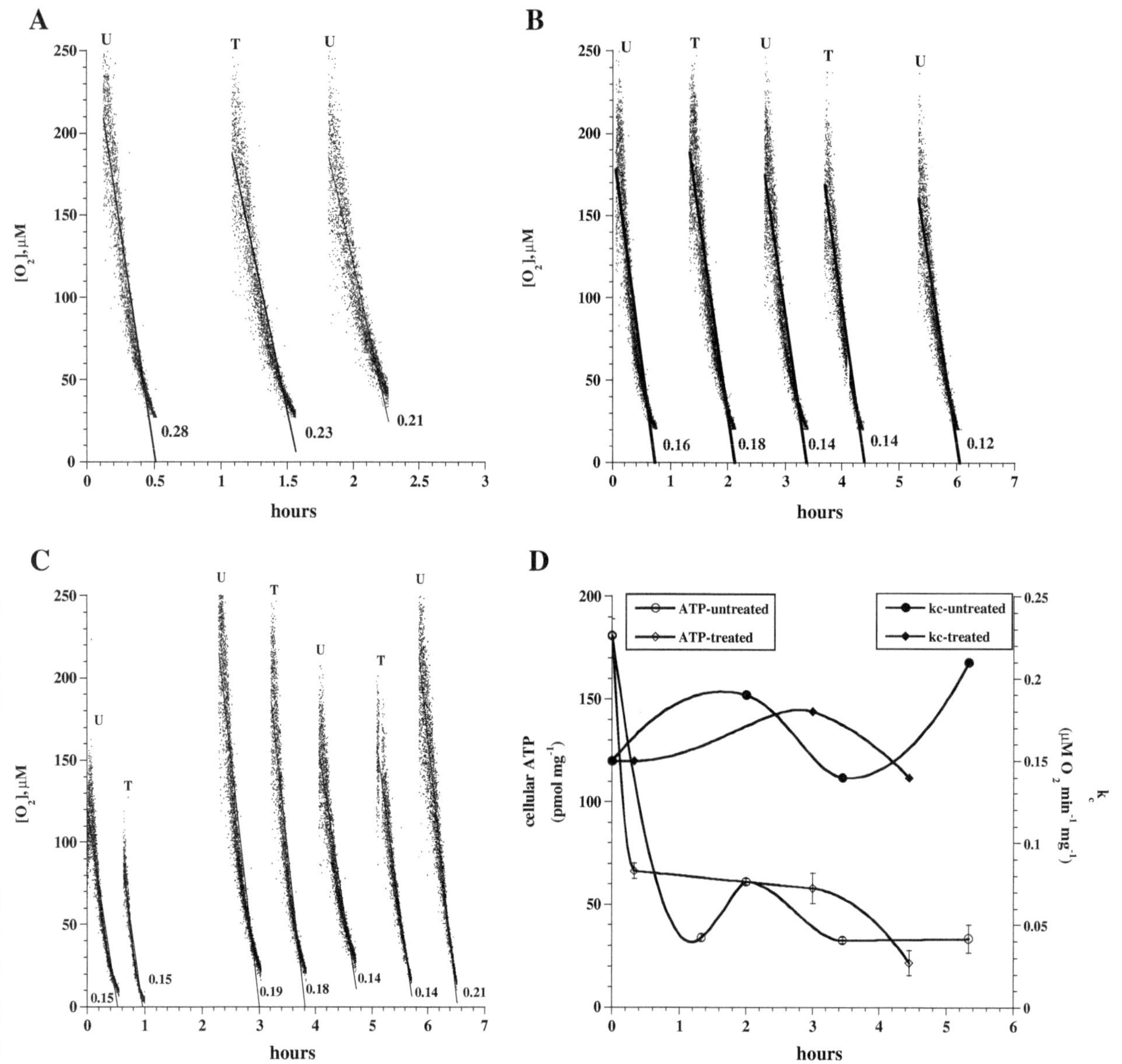

Figure 1 Atorvastatin neither alters hepatocyte respiration nor hepatocyte ATP content. Panels **A-C**: Cellular mitochondrial O_2 consumption with and without atorvastatin. Panels **A-B**, O_2 runs with and without 150 nM atorvastatin. Panel **C**, O_2 runs with and without 1.0 μM atorvastatin. Panel **D**: Cellular ATP content and values of k_c as a function of incubation time. Liver specimens from TO mice were incubated *in vitro* at 37°C in 50 mL KH buffer (continuously gassed with 95% O_2: 5% CO_2) with and without 150 nM (**A-B**) or 1.0 μM (**C-D**) atorvastatin. Cellular O_2 consumption and ATP content were determined as a function of time; $t = 0$ corresponded to tissue collection. The lines in Panels **A-C** are linear fits ($0.873 < R^2 < 0.955$). The rate of respiration (k, μM O_2 min^{-1}) was set as the negative of the slope of $[O_2]$ *vs. t*. The values of k_c (μM O_2 min^{-1} mg^{-1}) are shown at the bottom of each run. The values of k_c in Panel **C** and the cellular ATP content of the same experiment are plotted in Panel **D**. Eleven independent experiments were done with the TO mice and 4 independent experiments were done with the C57Bl/6 mice. U, untreated; T, treated.

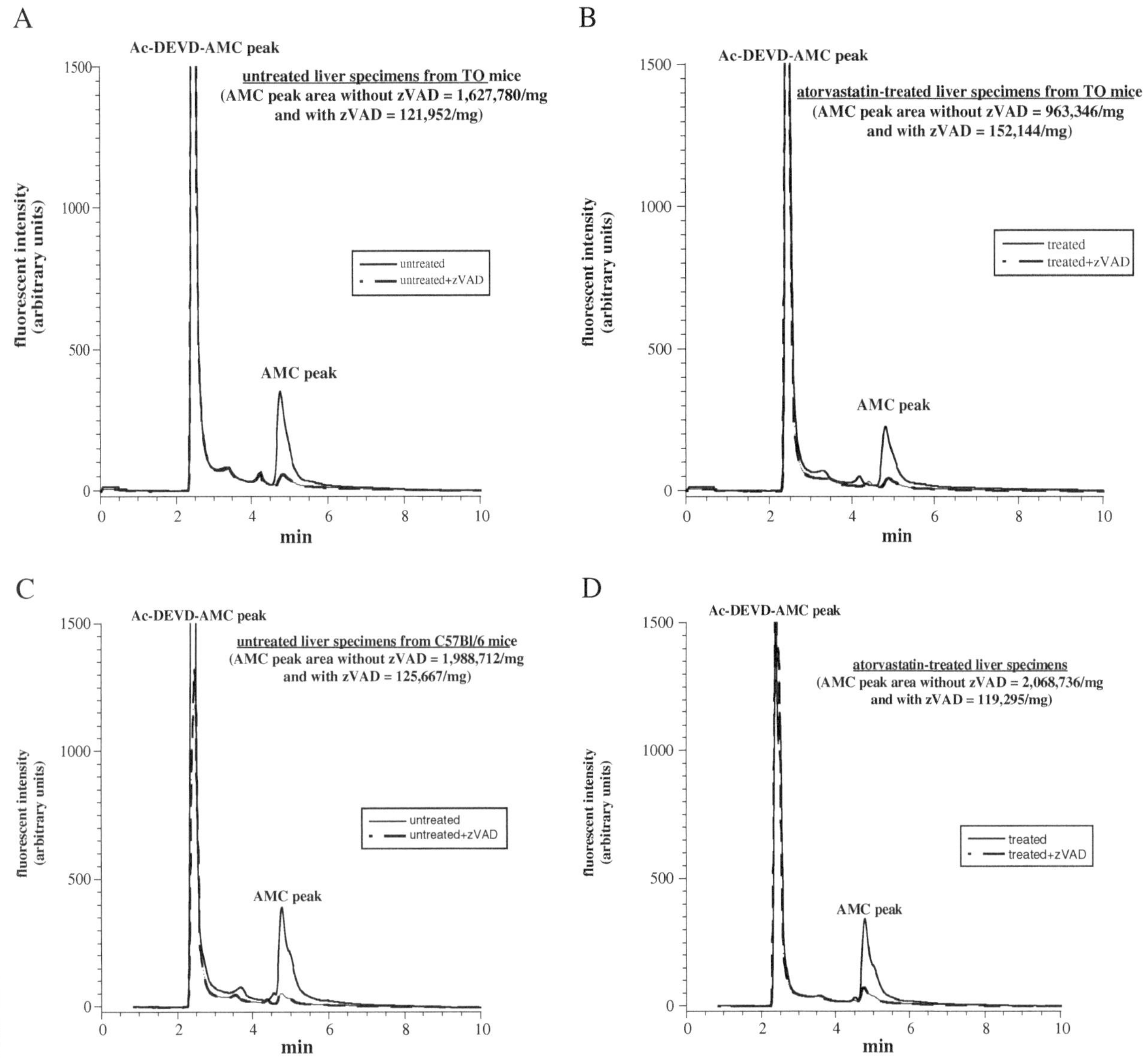

Figure 2 Atorvastatin does not induce hepatocyte caspases. Panel **A**, untreated liver specimens from TO mice. Panel **B**, atorvastatin-treated liver specimens from TO mice. Panel **C**, untreated liver specimens from C57Bl/6 mice. Panel **D**, atorvastatin-treated liver specimens from C57Bl/6 mice. Representative experiments of liver specimens incubated *in vitro* at 37°C with (B and D) and without (A and C) 1.0 μM atorvastatin for 6 hr are shown. At the end of incubation period, the samples (24.7 to 35.1 mg) were rinsed and incubated at 37°C in 1.0 mL oxygenated KH buffer with and without 32 μM zVAD-fmk for 10 min. Ac-DEVD-AMC (37 μM) was then added and the incubation continued for 20 min. The tissues were vigorously disrupted and the supernatants were separated on HPLC and analyzed for the AMC (R_t, ~5.0 min) and Ac-DEVD-AMC peaks (R_t, ~2.5 min). Eleven independent experiments were done with the TO mice and 4 independent experiments were done with the C57Bl/6 mice.

Table 1 Urea synthesis (mg/dL mg^{-1}, produced over 50 min) by liver tissue treated with atorvastatin

Untreated (n =6)	Treated (n =6)	*P*-value
0.061 ± 0.020	0.072 ± 0.022	0.3866

Liver specimens were incubated at 37°C in KH buffer with and without 1.0 μM atorvastatin for 6 hr. Every 60 min, specimens were removed from the incubation solutions and placed in 1.0 mL KH buffer supplemented with 10 mM NH_4Cl and 2.5 mM ornithine. The solutions were then analyzed for urea at min 50. The values are mean ± SD for hr 1 to 6.

about 0.5% of patients [1]. Other hepatocellular injuries, such as cholestasis, immune hepatitis and fulminant liver failure are also possibly linked to atorvastatin use (Bhardwaj and Chalasani [7]; see also atorvastatin product insert). The duration between exposure and onset of toxicity varies, ranging from 12 hours to 52 - weeks. The transaminase elevations, however, are frequently dose-dependent and occur in the first 16 weeks of therapy [3,24].

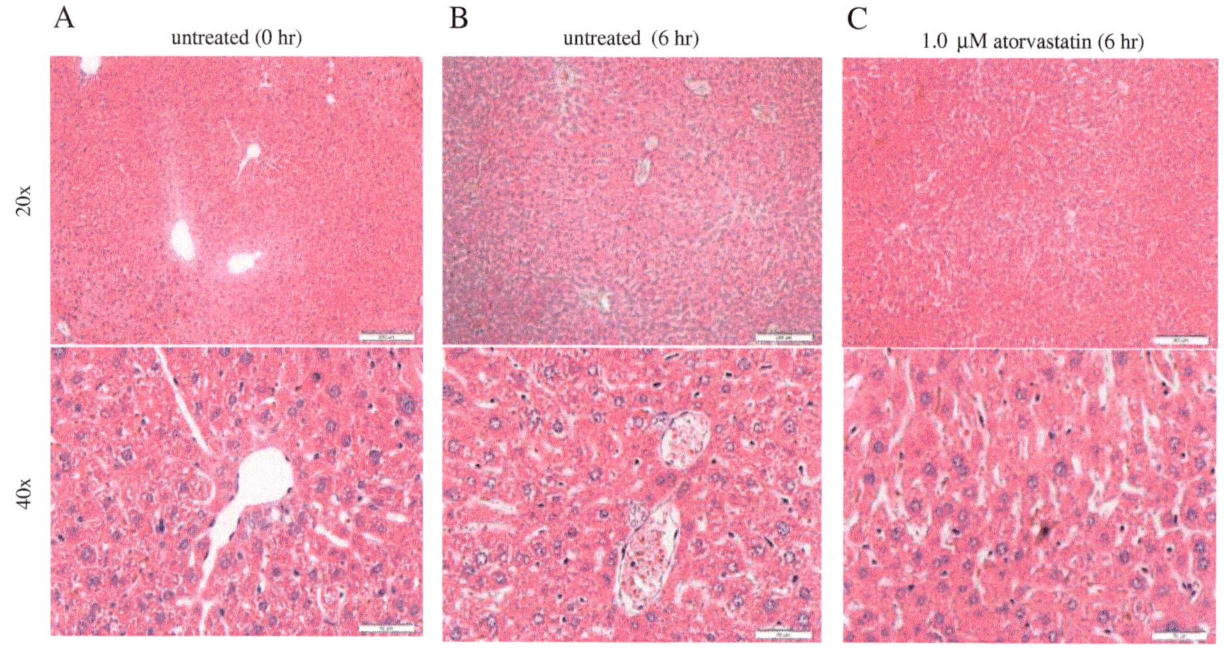

Figure 3 Micrographs of hematoxylin and eosin-stained liver sections from untreated and atorvastatin-treated TO mouse. Results of representative experiment of liver specimens incubated *in vitro* at 37°C with and without 1.0 μM atorvastatin for 6 hr is shown. A liver specimen at 0 hr is also shown. Liver structure and cytology are preserved in treated and untreated specimens. Inflammation and cholestasis are absent. (Hematoxylin and eosin, 10× and 40×).

Oxygen consumption is sensitive to reduced cellular metabolic fuels, as well as to mitochondrial derangements. Cellular respiration is reduced in the presence of nutrient depletion or electron transport chain deficits. The rate of respiration, on the other hand, is enhanced in the presence of proton leak (uncoupling oxidative phosphorylation). As shown previously, measurements of cellular mitochondrial oxygen consumption by the phosphorescence oxygen analyzer are highly sensitive to these cellular insults [17]. Moreover, liver architecture and urea synthesis are typical biomarkers for assessing hepatocyte injury [25].

Hepatotoxicities were evident in diabetic and hypercholesterolemic rats treated with oral atorvastatin (5 mg/kg daily) for two months [14]. Several reports also described statin-induced mitochondrial toxicities (see Dykens and Will [26]). More recently, impaired mitochondrial oxidative phosphorylation, membrane fluidity and coenzyme Q (ubiquinone, a component of the mitochondrial respiratory chain) content were reported in rats treated with 80 mg/kg atorvastatin for 4 weeks. The authors suggested that impaired hepatocyte bioenergetics may play a role in the development of statin-induced hepatotoxicities [15].

Atorvastatin also exerts cytotoxic effects on human hematopoietic tumors by promoting apoptosis through the mitochondrial cell death pathway. Other potential mechanisms involve altering the membrane localization of small GTPases. Treatment with statin resulted in reduction of mitochondrial membrane potential and cytosolic release of the activator of caspases Smac/DIABLO. As a result, caspases 9, 3 and 8 were efficiently activated [27].

This study investigated whether atorvastatin impairs hepatocyte cellular bioenergetics (respiration and ATP content). Strain-specific drug toxicities have been described [28]. Therefore, our animal model always tests different murine strains or a murine strain and a rat strain. The results clearly show preserved murine hepatocyte respiration and ATP content following *in vitro* exposure to 1.0 μM atorvastatin for several hours (Figure 1). This concentration is about 20-fold higher than therapeutic plasma levels. Consistently, hepatocyte caspase activity (Figure 2) and liver architecture (Figure 3) are preserved in the presence of 1.0 μM atorvastatin and indeed inflammation and cholestasis were absent. Thus, in the studied murine hepatic model, atorvastatin was not toxic. It is unknown, however, whether a much longer exposure produces cytotoxicity and will definitely be a venture for future research.

Cellular ATP was highest *immediately* after tissue collection (reflecting *in vivo* levels of bioenergetics) and declined subsequently to a new steady state (reflecting *in vitro* levels of bioenergetics), Figure 1D. This assumption is consistent with the preserved hepatocyte structure (Figure 3) and ultrastructure (data not shown) following tissue collection. Along the same lines, about 50% decline in cortical ATP levels was noted in rat brain

15 min following cortical surgery [29]. The *in vitro* levels of ATP shown in Figure 1D, however, are much higher than those reported for cultured rat hepatocytes at the steady state level (2.44 ± 0.09 pmol mg^{-1}) [25].

Urea synthesis is a sensitive biomarker for hepatocellular functions. As shown in Table 1, the presence of atorvastatin for up to 6 hr had no significant effect on the rate of hepatocyte urea synthesis. Consistently, hepatocyte structure was preserved in the presence of atorvastatin (Figure 3).

Statins inhibit the rate-limiting step of cholesterol biosynthesis catalyzed by HMG-CoA reductase. This inhibition leads to decreased hepatic cholesterol synthesis, up-regulation of low-density lipoprotein (LDL) receptor, and increased clearance of plasma LDL-cholesterol. As a result of inhibiting HMG-CoA reductase, statins could also inhibit the synthesis of important isoprenoids, such as farnesylpyrophosphate (FPP) and geranylgeranylpyrophosphate (GGPP). These intermediates serve as lipid attachments for the post-translational modification of intracellular proteins, such as nuclear lamins, Ras, Rho, Rac and Rap [30]. Hence, the pleiotropic effects of statins may arise from combined cholesterol lowering effects and inhibition of intracellular isoprenoid-dependent proteins.

Conclusion

In conclusion, this *in vitro* study shows that murine hepatocyte bioenergetics, caspase activity and histology are preserved in the presence of high concentrations of atorvastatin for at least 6 hours. These observations are consistent with the fact that long term atorvastatin therapy is well tolerated clinically [8-10].

In pre-clinical drug development, *in vitro* studies are routinely performed prior to *in vivo* testing. Due to potential pharmacodynamic differences, *in vitro* pharmacological studies should be followed by *in vivo* testing. The biomarkers (hepatocyte bioenergetics and caspase activity) described in this study, however, can be easily adapted for *in vivo* studies. Moreover, due to potential species differences in response to atorvastatin, liver tissue from small and large animals (e.g., rats and monkeys) are needed for better prediction of organ toxicity.

Competing interests

The authors declare that they have no competing interests.

Authors' contributions

ASA and BA designed the study, carried out the analysis, interpreted the data and drafted the manuscript. SA and AA performed the histology. AKS supervised the progress and critically revised the manuscript. All authors read and approved the final manuscript.

Acknowledgements

This work was supported by a research grant from Sheikh Hamdan Bin Rashid Al Maktoum Award for Medical Sciences.

Author details

[1]Department of Internal Medicine, United Arab Emirates University, Al Ain, Abu Dhabi, United Arab Emirates. [2]Department of Pathology, United Arab Emirates University, Al Ain, Abu Dhabi, United Arab Emirates. [3]Department of Pediatrics, United Arab Emirates University, Al Ain, Abu Dhabi, United Arab Emirates.

References

1. Newman CB, Palmer G, Silbershatz H, *et al*: **Safety of atorvastatin derived from analysis of 44 completed trials in 9,416 patients.** *Am J Cardiol* 2003, **92**:670–676.
2. Armitage J: **The safety of statins in clinical practice.** *Lancet* 2007, **370**:1781–1790.
3. Liu Y, Cheng Z, Ding L, Fang F, Cheng KA, Fang Q, Shi GP: **Atorvastatin-induced acute elevation of hepatic enzymes and the absence of cross-toxicity of pravastatin.** *Int J Clin Pharmacol Ther* 2010, **48**:798–802.
4. Gillett RC, Norrell A: **Considerations for safe use of statins: liver enzyme abnormalities and muscle toxicity.** *Am Fam Physician* 2011, **83**:711–716.
5. Law M, Rudnicka AR: **Statin safety: a systematic review.** *Am J Cardiol* 2006, **97**:52C–60C.
6. Brown WV: **Safety of statins.** *Curr Opin Lipidol* 2008, **19**:558–562.
7. Bhardwaj SS, Chalasani N: **Lipid lowering agents that cause drug-induced hepatotoxicity.** *Clin Liver Dis* 2007, **11**:597–613.
8. Musso G, Cassader M, Gambino R: **Cholesterol-lowering therapy for the treatment of nonalcoholic fatty liver disease: an update.** *Curr Opin Lipidol* 2011, **22**:489–496.
9. Tandra S, Vuppalanchi R: **Use of statins in patients with liver disease.** *Curr Treat Options Cardiovasc Med* 2009, **11**:272–278.
10. Zamor PJ, Russo MW: **Liver function tests and statins.** *Curr Opin Cardiol* 2011, **26**:338–341.
11. Argo CK, Loria P, Caldwell SH, Lonardo A: **Statins in liver disease: a molehill, an iceberg, or neither?** *Hepatology* 2008, **48**:662–669.
12. Lewis JH, Mortensen ME, Zweig S, Fusco MJ, Medoff JR, Belder R: **Efficacy and safety of high-dose pravastatin in hypercholesterolemic patients with well-compensated chronic liver disease: Results of a prospective, randomized, double-blind, placebo-controlled, multicenter trial.** *Hepatology* 2007, **46**:1453–1463.
13. Athyros VG, Tziomalos K, Gossios TD, *et al*: **Safety and efficacy of long-term statin treatment for cardiovascular events in patients with coronary heart disease and abnormal liver function tests in the GREACE study: a post-hoc analysis.** *Lancet* 2010, **376**:1916–1922.
14. El-Hossary GG, El-Shazly AHM, Mohamed AS, Mansour SM: **Evaluation of therapeutic potential of atorvastatin against diabetic retinopathy: A biochemical histopathological study.** *J Appl Sci Res* 2011, **7**:1527–1535.
15. Ulicna O, Vancova O, Waczulikova I, Bozek P, Sikurova L, Bada V, Kucharska J: **Liver mitochondrial respiratory function and coenzyme Q content in rats on a hypercholesterolemic diet treated with atorvastatin.** *Physiol Res* 2012, **61**:185–193.
16. Ricci JE, Muñoz-Pinedo C, Fitzgerald P, Bailly-Maitre B, Perkins GA, Yadava N, Scheffler IE, Ellisman MH, Green DR: **Disruption of mitochondrial function during apoptosis is mediated by caspase cleavage of the p75 subunit of complex i of the electron transport chain.** *Cell* 2004, **117**:773–786.
17. Tao Z, Penefsky HS, Goodisman J, Souid AK: **Caspase activation by cytotoxic drugs (the caspase storm).** *Mol Pharm* 2007, **4**:583–585.
18. Alsamri MT, Alshamsi M, Al-Salam S, Marzouqi F, Al Mansouri A, Alhammadi S, Balhaj G, Al Dawaar SK, Al Hanjeri RS, Benedict S, Sudhadevi M, Conca W, Penefsky HS, Souid AK: **Measurement of oxygen consumption by murine tissues *in vitro*.** *J Pharmacol Toxicol Meth* 2011, **63**:196–204.
19. Alshamsi M, Alsamri M, Al-Salam S, Conca W, Benedict S, Sudhadevi M, Biradar A, Asefa T, Souid AK: **Biocompatibility study of mesoporous silicate particles with cellular bioenergetics in murine tissues.** *Chem Res Toxicol* 2010, **11**:1796–1805.
20. Shaban S, Marzouqi F, Almansouri A, Penefsky H, Souid AK: **Oxygen measurements via phosphorescence.** *Comput Meth Programs Biomed* 2010, **100**:265–268.
21. Lo LW, Koch CJ, Wilson DF: **Calibration of oxygen-dependent quenching of the phosphorescence of Pd-meso-tetra (4-carboxyphenyl) porphine: A phosphor with general application for measuring oxygen concentration in biological systems.** *Anal Biochem* 1996, **236**:153–160.
22. Takeyori S, Nobuhiko K: **Analysis of regulatory factors for urea synthesis by isolated perfused rat liver.** *J Biochem* 1975, **77**:659–669.

23. Maier K, Hofmann U, Bauer A, Niebel A, Vacun G, Reuss M, Mauch K: **Quantification of statin effects on hepatic cholesterol synthesis by transient (13)C-flux analysis.** *Metab Eng* 2009, **11**:292–309.
24. Clarke AT, Mills PR: **Atorvastatin associated liver disease.** *Digestive and liver disease official journal of the Italian Society of Gastroenterology and the Italian Association for the Study of the Liver* 2006: Retrieved from http://www.ncbi.nlm.nih.gov/pubmed/16777499.
25. Berry MN: **Metabolic properties of cells isolated from adult mouse liver.** *J Cell Biol* 1962, **15**:1–8.
26. Dykens JA, Will Y: **The significance of mitochondrial toxicity testing in drug development.** *Drug Discov Today* 2007, **12**:777–785.
27. Cafforio P, Dammacco F, Gernone A, Silvestris F: **Statins activate the mitochondrial pathway of apoptosis in human lymphoblasts and myeloma cells.** *Carcinogenesis* 2005, **26**:883–891.
28. Lee GH, Nomura K, Kanda H, Kusakabe M, Yoshiki A, Sakakura T, Kitagawa T: **Strain specific sensitivity to diethylnitrosamine-induced carcinogenesis is maintained in hepatocytes of C3H/HeN in equilibrium with C57BL/6 N chimeric mice.** *Cancer Res* 1991, **15**:3257–3260.
29. Marklund N, Salci K, Ronquist G, Hillered L: **Energy metabolic changes in the early post-injury period following traumatic brain injury in rats.** *Neurochem Res* 2006, **31**:1085–1093.
30. Van Aelst L, D'Souza-Schorey C: **Rho GTPases and signaling networks.** *Genes Dev* 1997, **11**:2295–2322.

18

Treatment with CNX-011-67, a novel GPR40 agonist, delays onset and progression of diabetes and improves beta cell preservation and function in male ZDF rats

Nagesh Gowda, Anilkumar Dandu, Jaideep Singh, Sanghamitra Biswas, Vijaya Raghav, Mudigere N Lakshmi, Pavagada C Shilpa, Venkategowda Sunil, Ashokkumar Reddy, Manojkumar Sadasivuni, Kumaraswamy Aparna, Mahesh Kumar Verma, Yoganand Moolemath, Mammen O Anup, Marikunte V Venkataranganna, Baggavalli P Somesh and Madanahalli R Jagannath*

Abstract

Background: The role of G protein-coupled receptor (GPR40), which is highly expressed in pancreatic beta cells, has been studied extensively in the amelioration of beta cell dysfunction in T2D using rat and mouse islets, beta cell lines and in animal models of diabetes. But its potential as a therapeutic target has not been fully explored. This aim of the study is to evaluate the therapeutic potential of CNX-011-67, a highly selective, potent and orally bioavailable GPR40 agonist, in controlling diabetes and other metabolic parameters.

Methods: Seven week old male ZDF rats were treated with either vehicle or CNX-011-67, 5 mg/kg twice daily, for seven weeks. The animals were subjected to oral glucose tolerance and insulin tolerance tests. Plasma glucose, insulin, triglyceride, HbA1c, fructosamine and free fatty acids were measured at selected time points. Pancreas from control and treated animals were subjected to insulin and pancreatic and duodenal homeobox 1 (PDX1) immunohistochemistry and were also evaluated by electron microscopy. Also the potential impact of CNX-011-67 on islet insulin secretion, content, ATP levels and markers of both glucose oxidation, beta cell health in rat islets under chronic glucolipotoxic conditions was evaluated.

Results: Treatment of male ZDF rats with CNX-011-67 for 7 weeks significantly enhanced insulin secretion in response to oral glucose load, delayed the onset of fasting hyperglycemia by 3 weeks, reduced nonfasting glucose excursions, fasting free fatty acids and triglyceride levels. A significant increase in PDX1 expression and insulin content and reduction in plasma fructosamine, HOMA-IR, and beta cell apoptosis were observed. CNX-011-67 improves glucose mediated insulin secretion, insulin gene transcription and islet insulin content in cultured rat islets under chronic glucolipotoxic condition. Also enhanced glucose oxidation in the form of increased islet ATP content and overall improvement in beta cell health in the form of reduced expression of stress markers (TXNIP and CHOP mRNA) were observed.

Conclusions: These findings, suggest that long-term oral therapy with CNX-011-67 could be of clinical value to provide good glycemic control and improve islet beta cell function.

Keywords: GPR40, Zucker diabetic fatty rats, PDX1, GSIS, Type 2 diabetes, Rat islets, Glucolipotoxicity, Insulin content

* Correspondence: m.r.jagannath@connexios.com
Connexios Life Sciences Pvt Ltd, #49, "SHILPA VIDYA" 1st Main, 3rd Phase, JP Nagar, Bangalore 560078, India

Background

Progressive insulin resistance and loss of beta cell function and mass are primary characteristics of type 2 diabetes mellitus. There is thus a need for a robust anti-diabetic therapy that not only provides good glycemic control but also enhances beta cell preservation and thus delays progression of the disease. Several therapeutic approaches have been adopted to prevent the onset and progression of defects in beta-cell function [1-3].

GPR40, Free Fatty Acid Receptor 1, highly expressed in human pancreatic beta cells, brain and endocrine cells of the gastrointestinal tract is activated by medium and long chain saturated and unsaturated fatty acids [4,5]. GPR40 is coupled to Gαq/11 and specific ligands like oleic acid induce an increase in cytosolic [Ca^{2+}] and consequent insulin secretion at stimulatory glucose concentration in a Phospholipase C (PLC) and L-type Ca^{2+} channel dependent manner [6]. Several small-molecule agonists of GPR40 have been reported to enhance glucose-dependent insulin secretion and reduce blood glucose in mice and rodents [7-10] and also in humans [11,12].

Male ZDF rats become hyperlipidemic, hyperinsulinemic and insulin resistant by 7–8 weeks of age and subsequently hyperglycemia sets in the presence of marked hyperinsulinemia. As these animals are initially euglycemic they can be employed to investigate the delay in onset and subsequent control of progression of diabetes by therapeutic agents [13,14].

CNX-011-67 is a highly potent and selective small molecule agonist with an EC50 of 0.24 nM towards human GPR40 (Additional file 1: Figure S1). The objective of the present study was to assess the therapeutic potential of CNX-011-67 on onset and control of hyperglycemia, as well as on beta cell preservation in male ZDF rats.

Methods

Reagents

Glucose was estimated using Accu-check glucometer (Roche Diagnostics, Germany), HbA1c using DCA Vantage™ Analyzer (Siemens Healthcare, USA) and fructosamine using a FAR kit (FAR Diagnostics, Italy). Ultra-sensitive insulin ELISA kit (Crystal Chem Inc, USA) was used to determine plasma insulin levels. Circulating serum TG and plasma FFA were estimated using TAG estimation kit (Diasys Diagnostics system, Germany) and Randox kit (Randox Laboratories, UK) respectively. Triton-X and Fluromount were procured from Sigma-Aldrich.

Animals

Six week old male ZDF rats (Charles River Indianapolis, IN) were housed 4 per cage under a 12-h light/dark cycle with free access to feed (rodent diet DI2450B, Research diets, US) and water, acclimatized for one week, randomized into vehicle and treatment groups and then administered vehicle (water) or CNX-011-67 (5 mg/kg, b.wt, dissolved in water, p.o. twice daily), respectively, for seven weeks. The dose was selected based on a PK/PD study in Wistar rats in which ED50 was achieved at 5 mg/kg b.wt. Body weight, and fed and fasting blood glucose were measured at weekly intervals while feed intake was monitored daily and reported weekly average as g/animal/day. All animal experiment protocols were approved by Institutional Animal Ethics Committee of Connexios Life Sciences Pvt. Ltd.

Oral glucose tolerance test (OGTT)

After 6 weeks of treatment OGTT was performed in 6 h fasted rats by orally administering CNX-011-67 (5 mg/kg) 30 min prior to 2 g/kg oral glucose load and blood samples collected from the tail vein −30 min before molecule administration and 0, 10, 20, 30, 60, 90 and 120 minutes after glucose load for glucose and insulin estimation. HOMA-beta and HOMA-IR were calculated to assess β-cell function and insulin action respectively.

Prolonged post-prandial glucose profile

On day 42 of treatment, glucose in fed state was monitored at 2 h time intervals for a period of 8 h following the OGTT.

Insulin tolerance test (ITT)

ITT was performed on day 48 in 6 h fasted rats. Blood samples, for glucose estimation, were collected prior to and at 2.5, 5, 10, 20, 30 and 60 min after administration of 2 IU/kg (i.p) insulin (Humulin R Insulin, Eli Lilly).

Rat islet isolation

For in vitro experiments reported islets were isolated from male Wistar rats (8 weeks, 180-240 gm body weight; Charles River Lab, USA) as per previously reported [15] and size-matched purified islets were handpicked under a stereo-zoom microscope (Nikon, Japan).

Insulin secretion and islet insulin content measurement

Stock fatty acid solutions were prepared by conjugating Palmitate with fatty acid free-BSA. In brief, Sodium palmitate was dissolved in 50% ethanol and heated at 60°C. The 500 mM stock thus prepared was conjugated with 10% BSA by stirring for 90 min to give a solution with a palmitate:BSA ratio of 3.6:1, filtered and used for experiments. Islets were cultured in growth medium (as control) or glucolipotoxic medium (16.7 mM glucose and 500 μM palmitate) either alone or with CNX-011-67 for 72 h and then transferred into 24-well plates containing 1 ml KRBH (2.5 mM glucose)/well, pre-incubated for 1 h and then induced with indicated glucose concentration alone or with 1 μM CNX-011-67 for 2 h. Secreted insulin was measured using an ELISA kit (Mercodia AB, Sweden) following the manufacturer's protocol. Later, islet lysates were prepared in lysis buffer and used for measuring intracellular islet insulin content. Both secreted insulin and content were expressed as amount of insulin per islet.

Measurement of ATP level

Rat islets were cultured in glucolipotoxic medium for 72 hrs, then incubated in KRBH buffer containing 2.5 mM glucose for 1 h and then induced with either 11 mM glucose (HG) alone or with 11 mM glucose and CNX-011-67 for 1 h. Islets were then lysed and ATP levels were estimated using ATP determination kit (Invitrogen) following the manufacturer's protocol.

RNA isolation, reverse transcription and quantitative real time polymerase chain reaction (qPCR)

Post 72 h of incubation, RNA was isolated, converted to cDNA (ABI, USA) and gene expression was measured using SYBR Green PCR Master Mix (Eurogenetic, Belgium). Gene primers were based on mRNA sequences from the GenBank nucleotide database and designed in-house. Genes analyzed in the present study were GCK, PDX1, Insulin, PPARa, TXNIP and CHOP. For quantification of gene expression, ?-actin was used as internal control (primer sequences are available upon request).

Pancreas histology

Pancreas was fixed in 10% buffered neutral formalin for 48 h and paraffin-embedded, sectioned and stained with H&E or immunofluorescence stain for microscopic examination [16,17]. The pancreas section at the 25th, 26th, 27th , and 28th levels were taken for H&E, insulin immunofluorescence staining, Terminal deoxynucleotide transferase-mediated dUTP Nick end Labeling TUNEL) [18,19] and PDX1 and insulin double immunofluorescence labeling, respectively.

Double immunofluorescence for insulin and PDX-1

Pancreatic sections were de-paraffinized and blocked in 1% BSA in PBS for 30 min at RT and incubated with a mixture of primary antibodies against insulin (Abexome, India) and PDX1 (Abcam USA) for 60 min at RT, followed by washing with PBS. Sections were then incubated with a mixture of secondary antibody (goat anti-mouse FITC conjugated secondary antibody for Insulin, Molecular Probes, Invitrogen and goat anti-rabbit conjugated with Alexafluor555, BioServices, India) for 30 min at RT and mounted using fluromount. Localization and distribution of insulin (green fluorescence) and PDX-1 (orange fluorescence) were assessed and the images were captured at 400X magnification. The number of PDX1-positive nuclei was counted in all islets (12 per animal) in the entire tissue section and values expressed as mean ± SEM.

Assessment of islet apoptosis

To detect apoptosis, TUNEL staining was performed using ApopTag Peroxidase in situ Apoptosis detection kit (S7100) (Chemicon® International, Inc), according to the manufacturer's instructions. The entire pancreas section was evaluated under light microscope at 400X magnification. Apoptosis-positive nuclei were counted within the islets on the whole pancreatic section area [19-21].

Electron microscopy

Pancreas tissues were fixed in 3% glutaraldehyde for 24 h and processed for electron microscopy as described previously [17,22]. Three sections per group were scanned and images were captured using a Transmission electron microscope, Technai-G2 (Biotwin, FEI, Netherlands) at magnifications of 4800X, 11000X and 23000X. All photographs were analyzed manually. Insulin granules were assessed as mature granules (with an electron-dense core, tetrahedral or hexagonal in shape, surrounded by a peripheral halo) or as immature granules (with a less electron-dense core and a reduced or even absent halo) [23,24].

Assessment of insulin signaling by AKT phosphorylation

Lean control, ZDF control and ZDF rats treated with CNX-011-67 for 7 weeks were sacrificed by cervical dislocation. 10 mg of tissue samples were collected from adipose (subcutaneous), muscle (soleus) and liver from each animal. Lysates were prepared by homogenization. Lysates (50 µg each from liver, muscle and adipose) were subjected to SDS-PAGE, transferred onto nitrocellulose membranes and probed with primary antibody against p-AKT and total AKT (Cell signaling, USA) and developed by enhanced chemiluminescence (West Pico, Thermo Scientific, USA). The relative levels of p-AKT compared to Total AKT were quantified using Image J Ver. 4.2, NIH, Bethesda.

Statistical analysis

Statistical analyses were performed using Unpaired Student's t-test or with One-Way ANOVA with Dunnett's Post test correction, as appropriate. P value summary: (*) <0.05, (**) <0.01 and (***) <0.001 respectively, when compared with vehicle control.

Results

CNX-011-67 delays onset of fasting hyperglycemia in ZDF rats

In lean control animals fasting glucose was 94 ± 4.3 mg/dl on day 0 and was 87 ± 1.7 mg/dl by end of the 7 week study. In the ZDF control animals fasting glucose reached 119 ± 5.14 mg/dl after 4 weeks treatment, kept increasing and reached 204 ± 32 mg/dl at end of 7 weeks. In contrast in the CNX-011-67 treated animals fasting glucose was 98 ± 2.7 mg/dl at start of the study and crossed the 100 mg/dl mark only after 6 weeks of treatment and reached 133 ± 12 at end of the study. Treatment with CNX-011-67 attenuated increase in fasting glucose and resulted in a 3 week delay in onset of hyperglycemia (Figure 1A).

CNX-011-67 provides good control of hyperglycemia in ZDF rats

In the control ZDF animals fed glucose levels increased from 155 ± 13 mg/dl on day 0 to 403 ± 31 mg/dl at end of 7 weeks study while in the CNX- 011–67 treated animals the corresponding levels for the study period were 152 ± 9.6 mg/dl to 305 ± 41 mg/dl respectively (Figure 1B). In the control ZDF animals blood glucose levels increased significantly upon restoration of access to food from 213 ± 23.79 mg/dl at the end of OGTT on week 6 to 414 ± 32.24 mg/dl at the end of 8 h follow up while in the CNX-011-67 treated animals the corresponding glucose levels were 162 ± 13 mg/dl and 303 ± 31.92 mg/dl respectively resulting in an 18% reduction in glucose AUC (Figure 2A). The food intake during the 8 h follow up period was however not quantified in either group.

CNX-011-67 improves insulin secretion in ZDF rats

During the course of the study there was no difference in fasting and fed insulin levels between the ZDF control

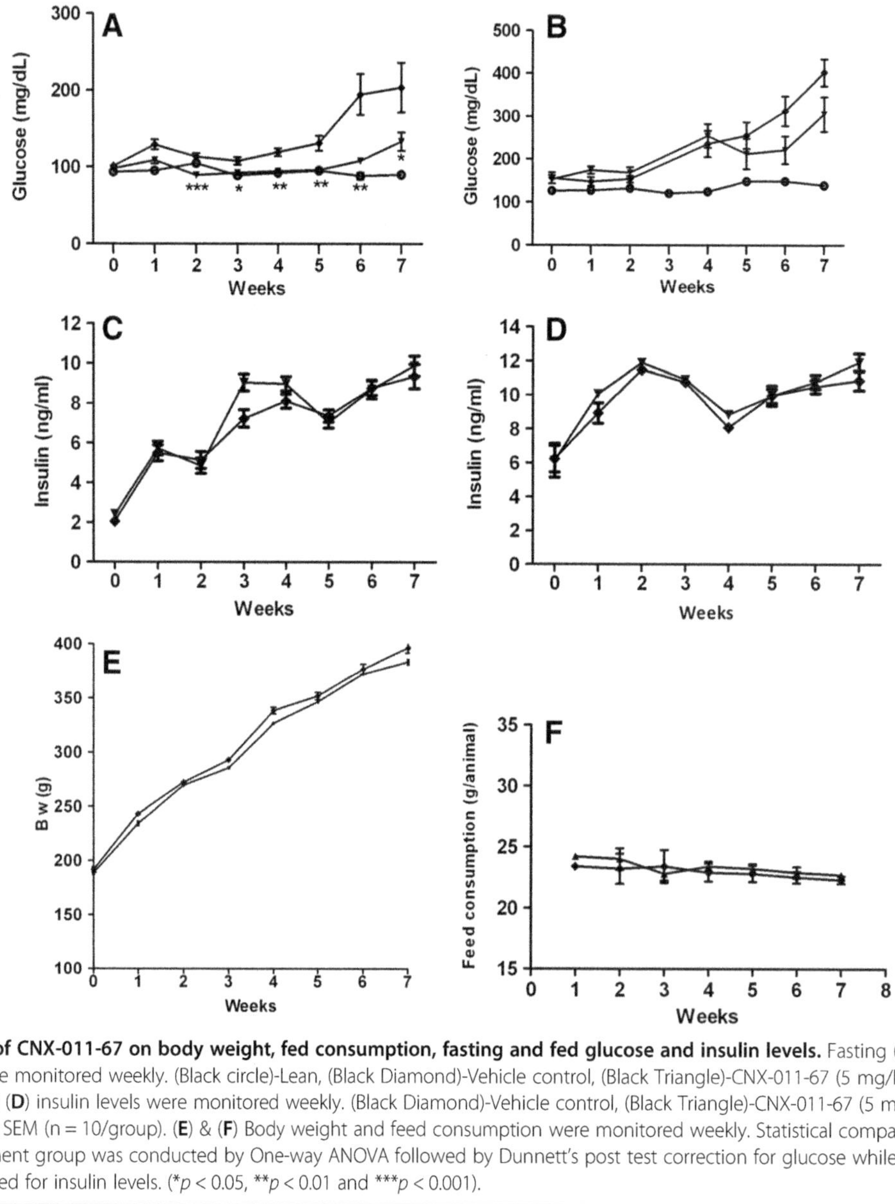

Figure 1 Effects of CNX-011-67 on body weight, fed consumption, fasting and fed glucose and insulin levels. Fasting (**A**) and fed (**B**) Glucose levels were monitored weekly. (Black circle)-Lean, (Black Diamond)-Vehicle control, (Black Triangle)-CNX-011-67 (5 mg/kg). Similarly, fasting (**C**) and fed (**D**) insulin levels were monitored weekly. (Black Diamond)-Vehicle control, (Black Triangle)-CNX-011-67 (5 mg/kg) Data in all panels are mean ± SEM (n = 10/group). (**E**) & (**F**) Body weight and feed consumption were monitored weekly. Statistical comparison between control and treatment group was conducted by One-way ANOVA followed by Dunnett's post test correction for glucose while unpaired Student's t test was performed for insulin levels. (*$p < 0.05$, **$p < 0.01$ and ***$p < 0.001$).

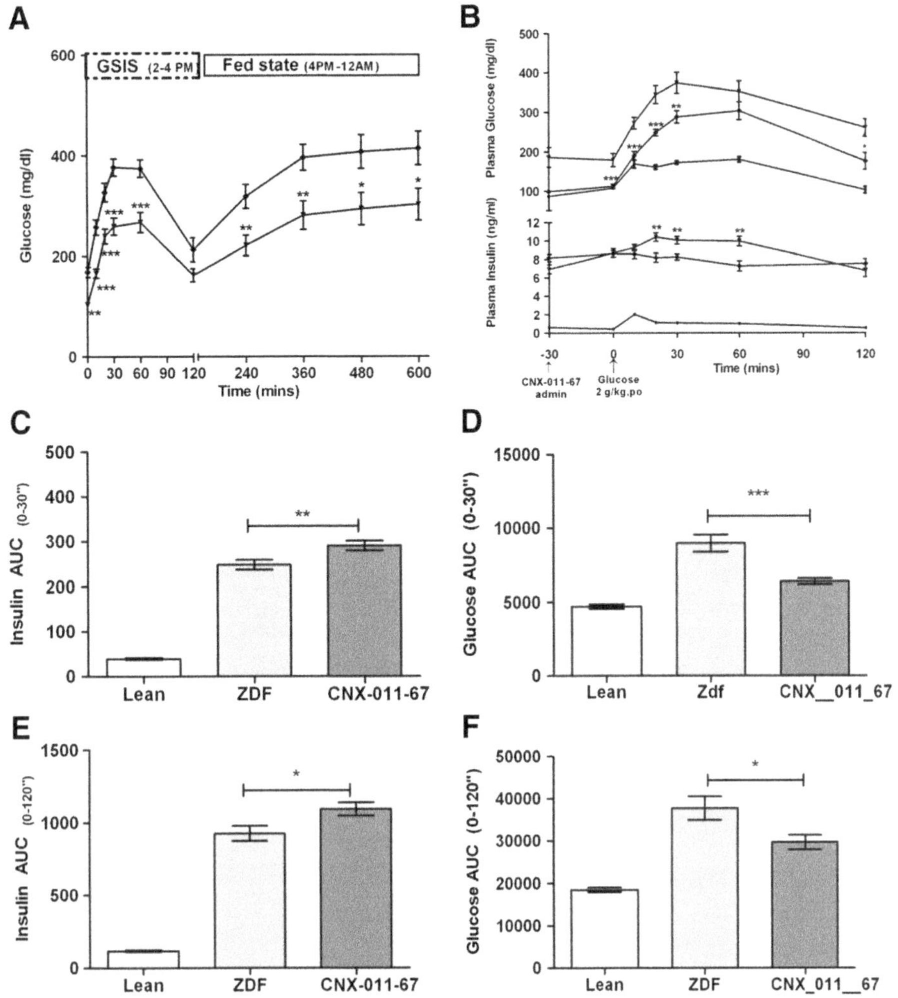

Figure 2 Effects of CNX-011-67 treatment on blood glucose and insulin levels during glucose stimulated insulin secretion. (**A**) A total of 8 h glucose profile was measured in fed state and Glucose AUC was calculated. (**B**) After oral administration of glucose (2 g/kg), plasma glucose and insulin were measured. Also Glucose (**D** & **F**) and Insulin (**C** & **E**) AUC were calculated. (Black circle)-Lean control, (Black Diamond)-Vehicle control and (Black Triangle)-CNX-011-67 (5 mg/kg)). Data in all panels are mean ± SEM. Data in all panels are mean ± SEM (n = 10/group). Statistical comparison was conducted by One-way ANOVA with Dunnett's post test correction to arrive at the significance level when compared with ZDF control. (*$p < 0.05$, ** p <0.01 and *** $p < 0.001$).

and CNX-011-67 treated animals (Figures 1C, D). However in an OGTT performed on day 42 of the study the 0–30' insulin AUC was significantly higher ($p < 0.05$) (291 ± 11 vs. 249 ± 11) (Figure 2C) and the corresponding 0–30' glucose AUC significantly lower ($p < 0.01$) (6389 ± 207 vs. 8964 ± 576) in the CNX-011-67 treated animals when compared to the ZDF control animals (Figure 2D). Similarly the 0–120' insulin AUC was significantly higher ($p < 0.05$) (1093 ± 46 vs. 926 ± 52) (Figure 2E) and the corresponding 0–120' glucose AUC significantly lower ($p < 0.05$) (29641 ± 1712 vs. 37716 ± 2767) in the CNX-011-67 treated animals (Figure 2F) when compared to the ZDF control animals indicating development of severe glucose intolerance in the control ZDF animals. In treated animals the increase in insulin levels from 6.95 ± 0.49 ng/ml at 0 min to 10.42 ± 0.47 ng/ml at 20 min and to 10.04 ± 0.42 ng/ml at 30 min post glucose load was highly significant ($p < 0.01$) (Figure 2B).

The significant difference in glucose tolerance in the OGTT observed with CNX-011-67 appears to be lost when the AUC Glucose is calculated above the basal values. This difference in the basal values between CNX-011-67 treated and control ZDF animals persists even after the onset of feeding upon switching off of the lights by 6 pm. Even though insulin levels at the various time points were not measured it appears that the difference in blood glucose levels could be due to enhanced insulin secretion in response to incremental glucose ingestion induced by CNX-011-67.

CNX-011-67 improves insulin signaling in peripheral tissues and enhances glucose clearance

In ZDF control animals, an average decrease of 14, 22 and 34% in p-AKT to total-AKT levels was observed in adipose, skeletal muscle and liver respectively when compared to lean control group, indicating relatively higher insulin resistance. In contrast, the tissues from CNX-011-67 treated ZDF rats showed enhanced p-AKT to total-AKT levels (an average of 2.7, 3.7 and 3.3 fold increase in adipose, skeletal muscle and liver, respectively) over those from ZDF control animals (Figure 3B) indicating an improvement in insulin signaling in the periphery. The representative blot from one animal in each group has been presented in Figure 3A.

In insulin tolerance test the decrease in blood glucose levels in the CNX-011-67 treated animals, non-significant in the first 10 min, became significant ($p < 0.05$) at 20 and 30 min post insulin administration when compared with control ZDF animals (Figure 3C). This agrees with the significant difference observed in HOMA-IR between ZDF control animals (64 ± 6.17) and CNX-011-67 treated animals (42 ± 6) indicating a reduction in insulin resistance in the treated animals (Table 1).

CNX-011-67 decreases serum FFA and triglyceride levels in ZDF rats

At the end of 3rd week there was a significant ($p < 0.01$) decrease in both plasma FFAs (0.97 ± 0.05 mmol/l vs. 1.27 ± 0.02 mmol/l) and triglyceride levels (263 ± 20 mg/dl vs. 370 ± 16 mg/dl) in the CNX-011-67 treated animals when compared to the ZDF control animals. Similar differences

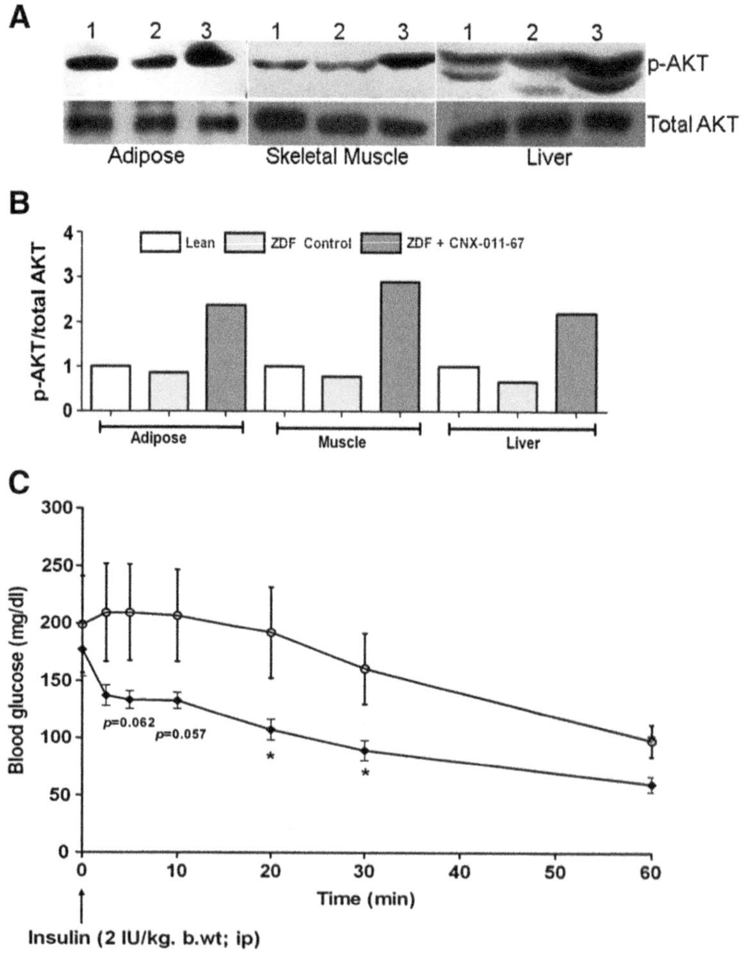

Figure 3 Effects of CNX-011-67 treatment on insulin signaling in peripheral tissues. (**A** and **B**) At the end of treatment, adipose, muscle and liver samples from lean (1), ZDF Control (2) and ZDF rats treated with CNX-011-67 (3) were subjected to western blots for p-AKT and total AKT. Blot in figure **A** is the data from one animal in each group (quantification was represented as fold change across all animals in each group, n = 5). (**C**) ITT was performed in male ZDF rats to determine the effect of CNX-011-67 on insulin induced glucose clearance. Glucose levels were monitored for a period of 60 minutes after insulin challenge. (Open circle)-Vehicle control (Black diamonds)-CNX- 011-67 (5 mg/kg). Data in all panels are mean ± SEM (n = 7 in control group / n = 8 in treated group). Statistical comparison between control and treatment group was conducted by unpaired Student's t test for comparison with baseline values within groups (*$p < 0.05$, ** $p < 0.01$ and *** $p < 0.001$).

Table 1 Effects of CNX-011-67 on blood HbA1c, Fructosamine, PDX1 and apoptotic positive cells

Parameters	Groupings		
	Lean control	**ZDF control**	**CNX-011-67 (5 mg/kg)**
HbA1c	3.84 ± 0.08	5.50 ± 0.30	5.18 ± 0.11
Fructosamine	92.47 ± 10.68	236.36 ± 19.08	111.25 ± 10.61**
HOMA-IR	2.16 ± 0.74	64.26 ± 6.18	41.82 ± 2.59*
HOMA-beta	117.34 ± 39.35	1520.20 ± 227.30	2206.79 ± 418.69
PDX1 positive cells	650 ± 49	461 ± 47.50	589 ± 43
Apoptotic cells	00 ± 00	47 ± 8.7	29 ± 4.6

Data in all panels are mean ± SEM (n = 10/group). Statistical comparison was conducted by One-way ANOVA with Dunnett's post test correction to arrive at the significance level when compared with ZDF control. (*$p < 0.05$ and **$p < 0.01$).

were observed even at end of the study between ZDF control and treated animals (Figures 4A, B).

CNX-011-67 decreases HbA1c and fructosamine

After 7 weeks of treatment HbA1c level was 5.18% in CNX-011-67 compared to 5.5% in the control ZDF group and the difference was not statistically significant. However plasma fructosamine levels of 111 ± 26 μmol/l in CNX-011-67 treated animals was significantly ($p < 0.01$) lesser than 237 ± 17 μmol/l in the control ZDF animals (Table 1).

CNX-011-67 significantly improves insulin secretion in rat pancreatic islets

Exposure of islets to chronic glucolipotoxic conditions significantly ($p < 0.05$) reduced glucose stimulated insulin secretion. However, treatment with CNX-011-67 during exposure to glucolipotoxicity significantly ($p < 0.01$) restored GSIS (Figure 5A). Similarly treatment with CNX-011-67 significantly increased ($p < 0.01$) islet insulin content when compared to that in chronic glucolipotoxic control islets (Figure 5B).

CNX-011-67 enhances glucose metabolism and ATP synthesis

Glucose-mediated increase in ATP levels and mRNA expression of GCK were significantly reduced under glucolipotoxic conditions as compared to control islets. Chronic activation by CNX-011-67 reversed the effect of glucolipotoxicity and significantly enhanced islet ATP content and expression of GCK mRNA (Figures 5C, D).

CNX-011-67 enhances mRNA expression of genes involved in insulin synthesis, and reduces expression of genes involved in stress and apoptosis

Chronic glucolipotoxicity reduced islet mRNA expression of PDX1, INS1 and PPARa whereas increased TXNIP and CHOP significantly when compared to control islets. Exposure of islets to CNX-011-67 under chronic glucolipotoxic conditions, significantly restored expression of these same genes to wild type levels (Figures 6A, B, C, D, E).

CNX-011-67 improves PDX1 expression in islets

Beta cells in the ZDF lean controls displayed good immuno-reactivity to PDX1 antibody and high staining intensity. Male ZDF animals with distorted islet

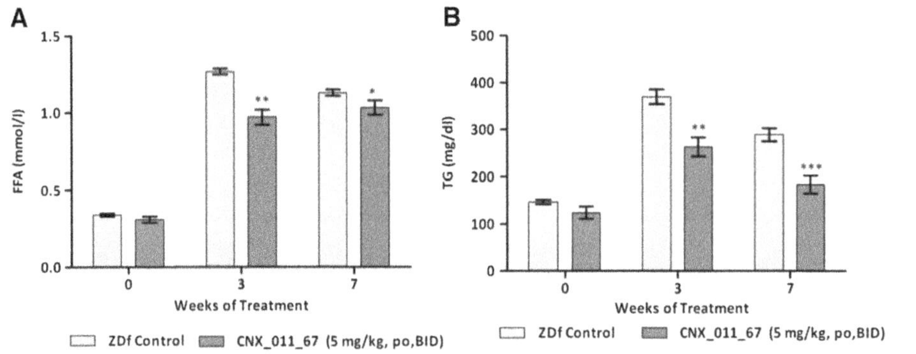

Figure 4 Effects of CNX-011-67 on FFA and TG levels in male ZDF rats. CNX-011-67 reduced both serum FFA (**A**) and serum TG (**B**) in ZDF rats when compared with vehicle control rats. Data in all panels are mean ± SEM (n = 10/group). Statistical comparison between control and treatment group was conducted by unpaired Student's t test for comparison with baseline values within groups (*$p < 0.05$, ** $p < 0.01$ and ***$p < 0.001$).

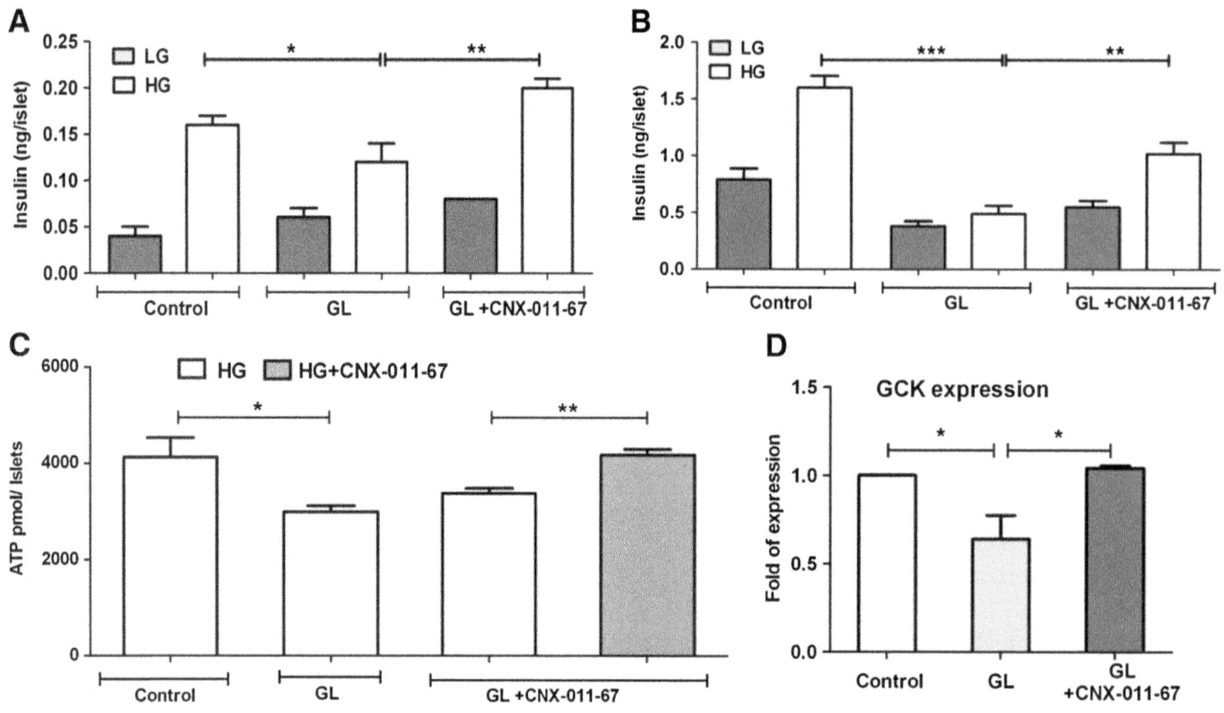

Figure 5 Effect of CNX-011-67 on insulin secretion, content, ATP and GCK expression. Rat islets were cultured under normal condition (control) or with high glucose and palmitate (glucolipotoxic condition; GL) or with CNX-011-67 under GL condition for 72 h. Post 72 h, islets was treated with 2 mM glucose (LG) or 11 mM glucose (HG) for 2 h and secreted insulin was measured (**A**). Islets were then lysed and lysate was used for intracellular insulin content measurement (**B**). Data (A) and (B) are representative of ten independent experiments (N = 10, *n* = 4). For ATP measurements, post 72 h of glucolipotoxicity in the presence or absence of CNX-011-67, islets were incubated with either 11 mM glucose (HG) alone or with HG + CNX-011-67 for 1 h. Islets were then lysed and ATP levels were estimated (N = 1, *n* = 3) (**C**). For GCK expression studies (**D**), RNA was isolated post 72 h of treatment and expression of GCK mRNA was measured as described under Methods (N = 2, *n* = 4). Statistical analysis was performed by Students t-test (Two-way, unpaired) or One-Way ANOVA with Dunnett's post test correction, as appropriate (*$p < 0.05$, ** $p < 0.01$ and ***$p < 0.001$).

architecture showed uneven immunoreactivity to PDX1 antibody and staining intensity was either low or completely absent. CNX-011-67 treated animals showed a marked improvement in islet morphology and displayed intense PDX1 immunostaining in comparison with ZDF control animals. A reduction in PDX1-positive nuclei number was observed in ZDF animals (461 ± 48 ZDF vs. 650 ± 49, lean control), whereas a marked improvement was observed in CNX-011-67 treated animals (589 ± 43 vs. 461 ± 48, ZDF control) (Figures 7G, I). The values, though not statistically significant, suggest enhanced PDX-1 expression in CNX-011-67 treated animals.

CNX-011-67 decreases β-Cell apoptosis

Morphological features of apoptosis, including pyknotic nuclei, were readily detectable in all pancreatic sections. The number of TUNEL-positive apoptotic beta cells was markedly increased in ZDF control animals compared with lean control. There were no fragmented nuclear apoptotic cells localized within the islets in lean control animals. The number of TUNEL positive apoptotic cells were significantly reduced in CNX-011-67 treated animals (47 ± 9 vs. 29 ± 5). A reduction of ~35% in apoptosis-positive nuclei was observed upon treatment with CNX-011-67 (Table 1).

Electron microscopy

Islets from ZDF control animals were either without or with a decreased number of insulin granules with electron-dense cores with many situated away from the plasma membrane indicating low number of docked granules ready for release (Figure 8). These islets also had large number of vacuoles. Islets from CNX-011-67 treated animals displayed an appreciable improvement in number of insulin granules with electron-dense cores surrounded by peripheral halo, tetrahedral or hexagonal in shape well distributed within the cytoplasm and also arrayed close to the plasma membrane indicating much improved docking of vesicles.

CNX-011-67 improves islet insulin content and morphology

Immunohistochemical analysis showed improvement in insulin stained area (morphological assessment) and a

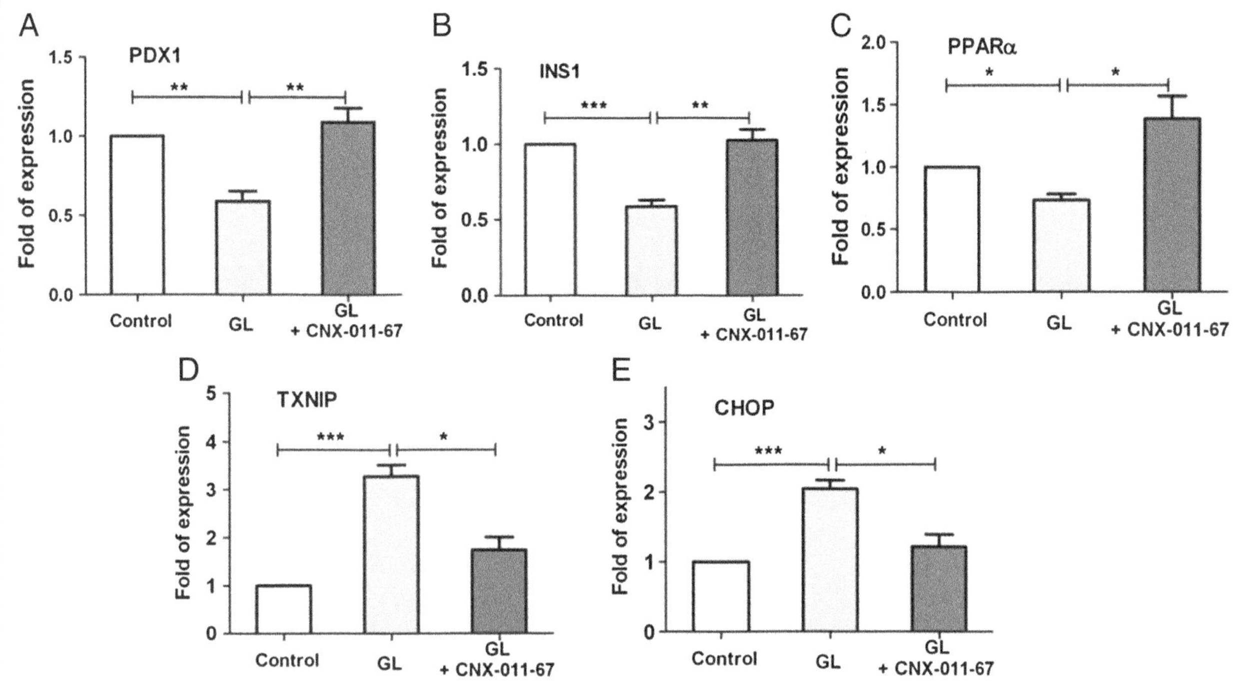

Figure 6 Impact of CNX-011-67 on islet insulin synthesis and β-cell stress. Post 72 h of treatments, RNA was isolated and expression of (**A**) PDX1, (**B**) INS1, (**C**) PPARα, (**D**) TXNIP and (**E**) CHOP mRNA expression were measured as described under Methods (N = 2, $n = 4$). Statistical analysis was performed by One-Way ANOVA with Dunnett's post test correction (*$p < 0.05$, **$p < 0.01$ and ***$p < 0.001$).

larger number of insulin stained cells in CNX-011-67 treated animals (694 ± 114 vs. 526 ± 26, ZDF control) indicating improved insulin content when compared to control ZDF animals (Figures 7D, E, F). Islets from ZDF lean control animals were compact and had a typical organized architecture while islets from control ZDF animals appeared enlarged and disorganized indicating loss of architecture. H&E staining of islets from ZDF control animals indicated a distorted architecture of islets which was distinctly improved upon CNX-011-67 treatment (Figures 7A, B, C). Enlarged and disorganized islets with extensions into the surrounding exocrine tissue were observed in ZDF control islets and a marked improvement was observed in animals treated with CNX-011-67 for seven weeks.

Discussion

A significant finding of the study has been the robust control of both the onset and progress of hyperglycemia by CNX-011-67. Considering that fed and fasting insulin levels did not vary between the animals in the treated and the control groups during the study period it appears that the enhanced first and second phase insulin secretion induced by the agonist (Figure 2B) is responsible for the robust glycemic control achieved in the treated animals. It is well documented in literature that an enhanced early phase insulin secretion has a direct effect on shutting off hepatic glucose output [25,26] and insulin is known to suppress lipolysis in adipocytes [27].

CNX-011-67 does not display any off target effect on lipolysis in 3 T3-L1 cells (data not shown) nor does the molecule activate PPARγ at concentrations below 10 μM. Though data on lipolysis in adipocytes derived from control and CNX-011-67 treated animals from this study is not available the enhanced level of p-Akt in the adipocytes from CNX-011-67 treated animals (Figures 3A & B) seems to indicate enhanced insulin signalling even at the end of the study period. We therefore suggest that the reduction in serum free fatty acids level in the treated rats is a direct effect of the enhanced insulin delivery and action in the adipocytes that reduces lipolysis. We are aware that additional studies are necessary to establish the direct effect of CNX-011-67 mediated increase in first phase insulin secretion in controlling lipolysis in adipocytes. The enhanced first phase insulin secretion (Figure 2B), reduction in free fatty acids (Figure 4A) and the increased insulin signaling in liver observed in CNX-011-67 treated animals (Figure 3A) perhaps explain the significant control over fasting glucose achieved in the study.

Even though there was no reduction in food intake or in body weight all through the treatment period the significant attenuation of the increase in blood glucose levels in the initial phase of the feeding period (6 pm – 12 pm; Figure 2A) is indicative of reduction in

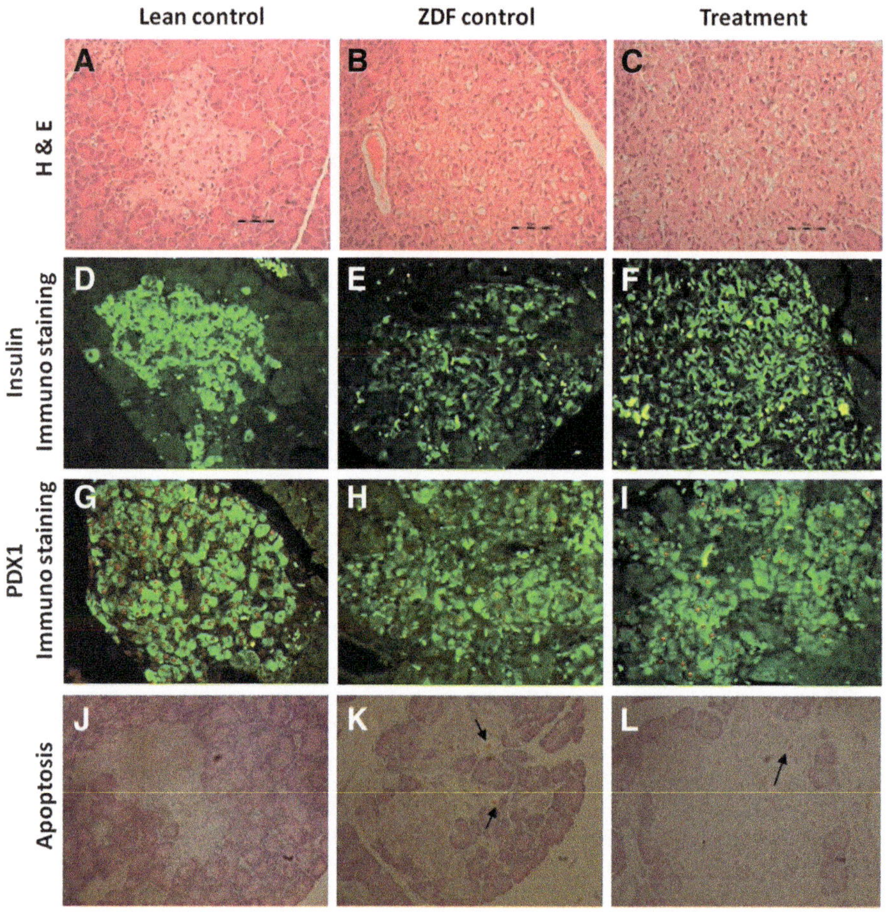

Figure 7 Histology, Immunohistochemistry of Pancreas and metabolic parameters in male ZDF rats. A-C: **H** and **E** stained pancreatic Islets sections from Lean control, ZDF control and CNX-011-67 treatment group. Magnifications at 400X. Islets with normal architecture from Lean control (**A**,**B**) and with distorted architecture in ZDF animals **D-F**: Immunofluorescent staining for insulin in consecutive sections of Pancreas. Immunostaining intensity of B-cells for Insulin is good in Lean control, poor in ZDF control and improved in Treatment group. **G-I**: Double immuno fluorescence staining for PDX1 (red) and insulin (green) of rat pancreatic islets. Compared to ZDF control the number of PDX1 positive nucleus (red) in the treatment appears to be increased. **J-L**: Brown colored apoptotic beta cells (arrow) in a pancreatic islet. Compared to ZDF control, apoptotic beta cells in treatment are found to be reduced.

peripheral insulin resistance in CNX-011-67 treated animals. The reduction in insulin resistance assumes importance as CNX-011-67 does not impact GLP1 levels in vivo (14 ± 0.58 vs. 15.98 ± 0.32 ZDF control active GLP1).

A reduction in circulating free fatty acid levels is reported to impact functioning of various organs and can thus affect multiple physiological parameters. Increased flux of free fatty acid into muscle reduces glucose uptake, into liver enhances gluconeogenesis and into pancreas can reduce insulin secretion and increase apoptosis [28]. The enhanced insulin secretion in response to glucose load (Figure 2B) and the significant reduction in free fatty acid levels early in treatment (Figure 4A) could have facilitated increased insulin signaling in liver, adipose and muscle (Figure 3A) thereby resulting in good control of fed glucose levels (Figure 2A). It is tempting to speculate (in absence of any supporting data) that the significant reduction in serum triglycerides could be due to a reduction in lipolysis in adipocytes (and consequent reduction in flux of free fatty acids into liver) and an improved glucose uptake in muscle.

In the present study it can perhaps be assumed that the significant control on serum free fatty acids levels achieved during the initial weeks of treatment has to a significant extent reduced insulin resistance in the periphery and thus improved glycemic control. In fact there is a significant reduction in HOMA-IR at end of the study (Table 1) and a significant increase in insulin secretion in response to glucose on day 42 of treatment when compared to control ZDF rats (Figure 2A). The insulin tolerance test (Figure 4) indicates overall reduction in insulin resistance in CNX-011-67 treated rats.

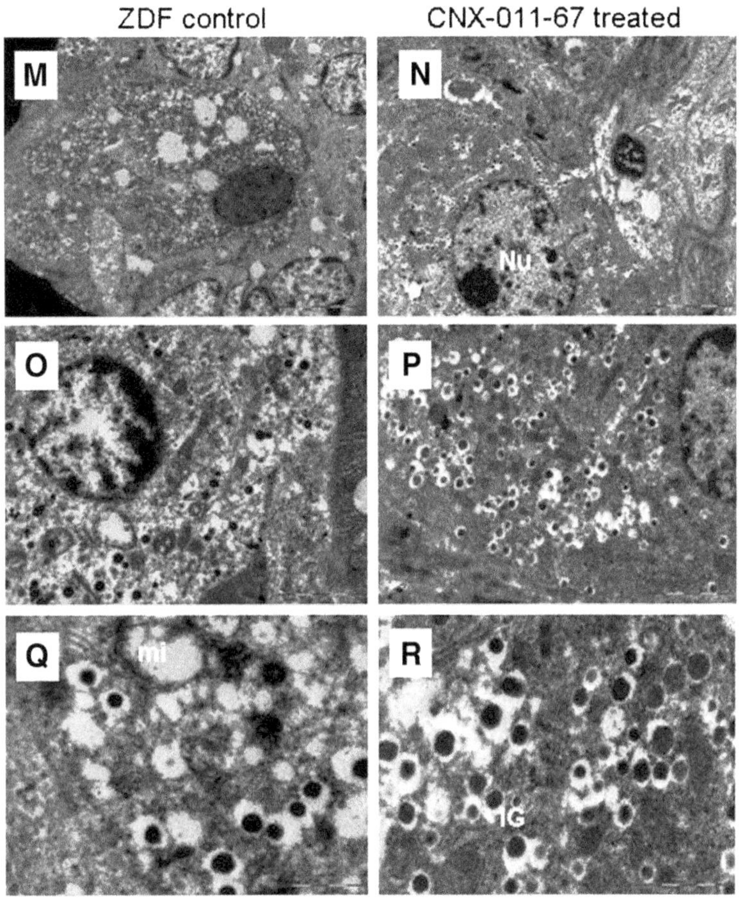

Figure 8 Electron microscope images of Beta cells from male ZDF and CNX-011-67 treated rats. Magnification at 4800 X (**M** and **N**), 11000 X (**O** and **P**), 23000X (**Q** and **R**). NU- Nucleus, mi-Mitochondria, IG- Insulin granules.

Multiple genes are involved in maintaining beta cell function. We restricted our study to a few select genes namely PDX1, INS1, GCK, PPARα, CHOP and TXNIP known to have significant impact on beta cell glucose metabolism, insulin synthesis, secretion and apoptosis.

Peroxisome proliferator-activated receptor alpha (PPA Ralpha) is known to modulate insulin secretion [29] and is reported to protect against fatty acid induced dysfunction by preserving carbohydrate metabolism [30] and can also increase insulin gene transcription. TXNIP serves as a critical link between glucose toxicity and beta-cell apoptosis [31], mediates ER stress [32] and glucocorticoid mediated [33] cell death and lack of TXNIP protects against mitochondria-mediated apoptosis [34].

We consider the enhanced insulin-stained area in islets to be probably due to CNX-011-67 mediated activation of GPR40 that can potentially stimulate ATP synthesis and modulate expression of genes mentioned above under the prevailing conditions of FFAs and glucose levels in the animals. Data from OGTT (Figure 2B), immunohistochemistry (Figures 7A, B, C), TUNEL assay (Figures 7J, K, L) and the increase in number of insulin granules with electron dense cores (Figure 8) seem to strongly support the above assumption.

Significant differences between control ZDF and CNX-011-67 treated animals in fed glucose levels (255 ± 31 vs. 212 ± 35 mg/dl) developed only by week 5 and continued to widen till end of study (406 ± 31 vs. 305 ± 41 mg/dl) while moderate differences in fasting glucose levels (119 ± 5.1 vs. 94.3 ± 4 mg/dl) that developed by week 4 of treatment sharply increased by week 6 (195 ± 26 vs. 108.3 ± 3.7 mg/dl) and week 7 (204 ± 32 vs. 133 ± 12 mg/dl). The HbA1c reduction of 0.32% reflects the control on glucose exercised by CNX-011-67 mainly during this period. The half-lives of glycosylated Hb being 30, 16 and 15 days in man, mouse and rat, respectively [35] the difference in HbA1c levels of 0.32%, between control ZDF and CNX-011-67 treated animals is achieved in a time period that covers two half-life of rat glycosylated Hb. The significant difference in fructosamine levels indicates effective control of glucose levels by CNX-011-67. Inspite of an improvement in first phase insulin secretion and reduction in fasting glucose levels beta cell function as assessed by HOMA-B displayed non-significant improvement. It is reported that estimates of cell function using HOMA have been shown to correlate well with estimates using hyperglycemic clamps and with the acute insulin response from the IVGTT [36]. In this study we have not employed either hyperglycemic clamps or performed IVGTT and hence the HOMA-B arrived at may not reflect the actual improvement in beta cell function achieved in this study.

In male ZDF rats a combination of lipotoxicity and hyperglycemia increase loss of β-cells through apoptosis [37,38] and peripheral acting agents like Rosiglitazone, Metformin, Troglitazone or even the DPP-IV inhibitor FE 999011 that provided significant control over free fatty acids, glucose and triglycerides, improved beta cell function and delayed the progression to diabetes [3,39,40]. Some of the pharmacological effects shown by CNX-011-67 in the present study are similar to the effects observed earlier in preclinical studies with other GPR40 agonists [7,8].

Conclusions

The delay in the onset and robust control of hyperglycemia observed in this study appear to be mediated by the combined effects of enhanced phasic insulin secretion, improvement in glucose sensitivity of beta cells, increased insulin content and reduction in beta cell apoptosis. Though we have not determined the changes in gene expression in the beta cells of treated rats in this study the increase in expression of PDX1 protein and increase in insulin stained area (Figure 7) and a reduction in beta cell apoptosis suggest that CNX-011-67 treatment could have modulated expression of many of the critical genes involved in insulin synthesis, insulin secretion and beta cell apoptosis in the male ZDF rats. From the foregoing data it appears that CNX-011-67 has the potential to provide good and durable glycemic control in type 2 diabetes patients.

Additional file

Additional file 1: Figure S1. CNX-011-67 is highly specific to GPR40.

Competing interests

The authors declare that they have no competing interests.

Authors' contributions

NG, JS, SB, DNVR, MNL, PCS, VS, AR carried out all the experiments; AD, MKS, KA, MKV, YM designed the study, carried out the analysis. MOA, MW and BPS interpreted the data and drafted the manuscript. MRJ supervised the progress and critically revised the manuscript. All authors read and approved the final manuscript.

Acknowledgements

We thank Dr. B.K. Chandrasekhar Sagar, Dept. of Neuropathology, at National Institute of Mental Health and Neurosciences, Bangalore, India for his valuable contribution in electron microscopy. We also thank Dr. T.S. Sridhar, Division of Molecular Medicine, St. John's Research Institute, Bangalore, for the review of the article. These studies were supported by Connexios Life Sciences PVT LTD, a Nadathur Holdings Company.

References

1. Fineman MS, Cirincione BB, Maggs D, Diamant M: **GLP-1 based therapies: differential effects on fasting and postprandial glucose.** *Diabetes Obes Metab* 2012, **14:**675–688.
2. Richter B, Bandeira-Echtler E, Bergerhoff K, Clar C, Ebrahim SH: **Pioglitazone for type 2 diabetes mellitus.** *Cochrane Database Syst Rev* 2006, **18**, CD006060.
3. Sreenan S, Sturis J, Pugh W, Burant CF, Polonsky KS: **Prevention of hyperglycemia in the Zucker diabetic fatty rat by treatment with metformin or troglitazone.** *Am J Physiol* 1996, **271:**742–747.
4. Briscoe CP, Peat AJ, McKeown SC, Corbett DF, Goetz AS, Littleton TR, McCoy DC, Kenakin TP, Andrews JL, Ammala C, Fornwald JA, Ignar DM, Jenkinson S: **Pharmacological regulation of insulin secretion in MIN6 cells through the fatty acid receptor GPR40: identification of agonist and antagonist small molecules.** *Br J Pharmacol* 2009, **148:**619–628.
5. Shapiro H, Shachar S, Sekler I, Hershfinkel M, Walker MD: **Role of GPR40 in fatty acid action on the beta cell line INS-1E.** *Biochem Biophys Res Commun* 2005, **335:**97–104.
6. Fujiwara K, Maekawa F, Yada T: **Oleic acid interacts with GPR40 to induce Ca2+ signaling in rat islet beta-cells: mediation by PLC and L-type Ca2+ channel and link to insulin release.** *Am J Physiol Endocrinol Metab* 2005, **289:**670–677.
7. Tan CP, Feng Y, Zhou YP, Eiermann GJ, Petrov A, Zhou C, Lin S, Salituro G, Meinke P, Mosley R, Akiyama TE, Einstein M, Kumar S, Berger JP, Mills SG, Thornberry NA, Yang L, Howard AD: **Selective small-molecule agonists of G protein-coupled receptor 40 promote glucose-dependent insulin secretion and reduce blood glucose in mice.** *Diabetes* 2008, **57:**2211–2219.
8. Tsujihata Y, Ito R, Suzuki M, Harada A, Negoro N, Yasuma T, Momose Y, Takeuchi K: **TAK-875, an orally available G protein-coupled receptor 40/free fatty acid receptor 1 agonist, enhances glucose-dependent insulin secretion and improves both postprandial and fasting hyperglycemia in type 2 diabetic rats.** *J Pharmacol Exp Ther* 2011, **339:**228–327.
9. Lin DC, Zhang J, Zhuang R, Li F, Nguyen K, Chen M, Tran T, Lopez E, Lu JY, Li XN, Tang L, Tonn GR, Swaminath G, Reagan JD, Chen JL, Tian H, Lin YJ, Houze JB, Luo J: **AMG 837: a novel GPR40/FFA1 agonist that enhances insulin secretion and lowers glucose levels in rodents.** *PLoS One* 2011, **6:**e27270.
10. Luo J, Swaminath G, Brown SP, Zhang J, Guo Q, Chen M, Nguyen K, Tran T, Miao L, Dransfield PJ, Vimolratana M, Houze JB, Wong S, Toteva M, Shan B, Li F, Zhuang R, Lin DC: **A Potent class of GPR40 full agonists engages the enteroinsular axis to promote glucose control in rodents.** *PLoS One* 2012, **7:**e46300.
11. Burant CF, Viswanathan P, Marcinak J, Cao C, Vakilynejad M, Xie B, Leifke E: **TAK-875 versus placebo or glimepiride in type 2 diabetes mellitus: a phase 2, randomised, double-blind, placebo-controlled trial.** *Lancet* 2012, **379:**1403–1411.
12. Kaku K, Araki T, Yoshinaka R: **Randomized, Double-Blind, Dose-Ranging Study of TAK-875, a Novel GPR40 Agonist, in Japanese Patients With Inadequately Controlled Type 2 Diabetes.** *Diabetes Care* 2013, **36:**245–250.
13. Tokuyama Y, Sturis J, DePaoli AM, Takeda J, Stoffel M, Tang J, Sun X, Polonsky KS, Bell GI: **Evolution of beta cell dysfunction in the male Zucker diabetic fatty rat.** *Diabetes* 1995, **44:**1447–1457.
14. Yuen VG, Vera E, Battell ML, Li WM, McNeill JH: **Acute and chronic oral administration of bis(maltolato) oxovanadium (IV) in Zucker diabetic fatty (ZDF) rats.** *Diabetes Res Clin Pract* 1999, **43:**9–19.
15. Carter JD, Dula SB, Corbin KL, Wu R, Nunemaker CS: **A practical guide to rodent islet isolation and assessment.** *Biol Proced Online* 2009, **11:**3–31.
16. Luna L: *AFIP Manual of Histological Staining Methods.* New York: McGraw Hill; 1968.
17. Culling CFA, Allison RT, Bair WT: *Cellular pathology technique.* London: Butterworths; 1985.
18. Kerr JFR, Wyllie AH, Currie AR: **Apoptosis: a basic biological phenomenon with wideranging implications in tissue kinetics.** *Br J Cancer* 1972, **26:**239–257.
19. Wyllie AH, Kerr JFR, Currie AR: **Cell death: the significance of apoptosis.** *Int Rev Cytol* 1980, **68:**251–306.
20. Garrity MM, Burgart LJ, Riehle DL, Hill EM, Sebo TJ, Witzig T: **Identifying and Quantifying Apoptosis: Navigating Technical Pitfalls.** *Mod Pathol* 2003, **16:**389–394.

21. Bruin JE, Gerstein HC, Morrison KM, Holloway AC: **Increased pancreatic beta cell apoptosis following fetal and neonatal exposure to nicotine is mediated via the mitochondria.** *Toxicol Sci* 2008, **103**:362–370.
22. Watari N, Tsukagoshi N, Honma Y: **The correlative light and electron microscopy of the islets of Langerhans in some lower vertebrates.** *Arch Histol* 1970, **31**:371–392.
23. Mihail N, Craciun C: **An ultrastructural description of the cell types in the endocrine pancreas of the pigeon.** *Anat Anz Jena* 1982, **152**:229–237.
24. Misawa E, Tanaka M, Nomaguchi K, Nomaguchia K, Yamada M, Toida T, Takase M, Iwatsuki K, Kawada T: **Administration of phytosterols isolated from aloe vera gel reduce visceral fat mass and improve hyperglycemia in Zucker diabetic fatty (zdf) rats.** *Obes Res Clin Pract* 2008, **2**:239–245.
25. Del Prato S: **Loss of early insulin secretion leads to postprandial hyperglycaemia.** *Diabetologia* 2003, **46**:2–8.
26. Rebrin K, Steil GM, Getty L, Bergman RN: **Free fatty acid as a link in the regulation of hepatic glucose output by peripheral insulin.** *Diabetes* 1995, **44**:1038–1045.
27. Koopmans SJ, Sips HC, Bosman J, Radder JK, Krans HM: **Antilipolytic action of insulin in adipocytes from starved and diabetic rats during adenosine-controlled incubations.** *Endocrinology* 1989, **125**:3044–3050.
28. Bajaj M, Suraamornkul S, Romanelli A, Cline GW, Mandarino LJ, Shulman GI, DeFronzo RA: **Effect of a sustained reduction in plasma free fatty acid concentration on intramuscular long-chain fatty Acyl-CoAs and insulin action in type 2 diabetic patients.** *Diabetes* 2005, **54**:3148–3153.
29. Sugden MC, Holness MJ: **Potential role of peroxisome proliferator-activated receptor-alpha in the modulation of glucose-stimulated insulin secretion.** *Diabetes* 2004, **53**(Suppl 1):S71–S81.
30. Frigerio F, Brun T, Bartley C, Usardi A, Bosco D, Ravnskjaer K, Mandrup S, Maechler P: **Peroxisome proliferator-activated receptor alpha (PPARalpha) protects against oleate-induced INS-1E beta cell dysfunction by preserving carbohydrate metabolism.** *Diabetologia* 2010, **53**:331–340.
31. Chen J, Saxena G, Mungrue IN, Lusis AJ, Shalev A: **Thioredoxin-interacting protein: a critical link between glucose toxicity and beta-cell apoptosis.** *Diabetes* 2008, **57**:938–944.
32. Oslowski CM, Hara T, O'Sullivan-Murphy B, Kanekura K, Lu S, Hara M, Ishigaki S, Zhu LJ, Hayashi E, Hui ST, Greiner D, Kaufman RJ, Bortell R, Urano F: **Thioredoxin-interacting protein mediates ER stress-induced β cell death through initiation of the inflammasome.** *Cell Metab* 2012, **16**:265–273.
33. Reich E, Tamary A, Sionov RV, Melloul D: **Involvement of thioredoxin-interacting protein (TXNIP) in glucocorticoid-mediated beta cell death.** *Diabetologia* 2012, **55**:1048–1057.
34. Chen J, Fontes G, Saxena G, Poitout V, Shalev A: **Lack of TXNIP protects against mitochondria-mediated apoptosis but not against fatty acid-induced ER stress-mediated beta-cell death.** *Diabetes* 2010, **59**:440–447.
35. Rendell M, Stephen PM, Paulsen R, Valentine JL, Rasbold K, Hestorff T, Eastberg S, Shint DC: **An interspecies comparison of normal levels of glycosylated hemoglobin and glycosylated albumin.** *Comp Biochem Physiol B* 1985, **81**:819–822.
36. Wallace TM, Levy JC, Matthews DR: **Use and abuse of HOMA modeling.** *Diabetes Care* 2004, **27**:1487–1495.
37. Lee Y, Hirose H, Ohneda M, Johnson JH, McGarry JD: **Beta-cell lipotoxicity in the pathogenesis of non-insulin-dependent diabetes mellitus of obese rats: impairment in adipocyte-beta-cell relationships.** *Proc Natl Acad Sci USA* 1994, **91**:10878–10882.
38. Pick A, Clark J, Kubstrup C, Levisetti M, Pugh W: **Role of apoptosis in failure of beta-cell mass compensation for insulin resistance and beta-cell defects in the male Zucker diabetic fatty rat.** *Diabetes* 1998, **47**:358–364.
39. Smith SA, Lister CA, Toseland CD, Buckingham RE: **Rosiglitazone prevents the onset of hyperglycaemia and proteinuria in the Zucker diabetic fatty rat.** *Diabetes Obes Metab* 2000, **2**:363–372.
40. Sudre B, Broqua P, White RB, Ashworth D, Evans DM, Haigh R, Junien JL, Aubert ML: **Chronic inhibition of circulating dipeptidyl peptidase IV by FE 999011 delays the occurrence of diabetes in male zucker diabetic fatty rats.** *Diabetes* 2002, **51**:1461–1469.

A randomized, placebo-controlled trial to determine the course of aminotransferase elevation during prolonged acetaminophen administration

Kennon Heard[1,2*], Jody L Green[1,3], Victoria Anderson[1], Becki Bucher-Bartelson[1,4] and Richard C Dart[1,2]

Abstract

Background: Acetaminophen administration for more than 4 days causes aminotransferase elevation in some subjects. The objective of this randomized, placebo-controlled trial is to describe the course of alanine aminotransferase (ALT) elevation in subjects administered 4 g/day of acetaminophen for at least 16 days.

Methods: A randomized, placebo controlled trial of acetaminophen (4 g/day) vs placebo. Subjects were healthy volunteers with normal liver enzymes. The primary outcome was the course of ALT during acetaminophen administration. All subjects were treated for a minimum of 16 days. Subjects with ALT elevation at day 16 were continued on treatment until these elevations resolved up to a maximum of 40 days. Subjects were also evaluated for elevation of INR or serum bilirubin as evidence of hepatic dysfunction.

Results: 157/205 (77%) completed acetaminophen subjects had no ALT elevation or transient elevations that resolved by day 16. Of the 48 subjects who had ALT elevations at study day 16, 47 continued on acetaminophen and had resolution by study day 40. One acetaminophen subject did not have resolution by study day 40, and the course of aminotransferase elevation suggests an alternative cause. One placebo subject had an ALT elevation at day 16 that resolved by day 22. The highest observed ALT among all acetaminophen subjects was 191 IU/L. The mean ALT at day 16 was 4.4 IU/L higher for the acetaminophen than for the placebo group. No subject developed liver dysfunction.

Conclusions: A minority of subjects treated with 4 g/day of acetaminophen for 16 days will have low-grade aminotransferase elevations that are not accompanied by liver dysfunction and resolve if administration is continued.

Trials registration: Clintrials.gov NCT00743093 registered August 26, 2008

Keywords: Alanine aminotransferase, Drug-induced liver injury, Hepatotoxicity

Background

Acetaminophen (paracetamol) is a commonly used analgesic and antipyretic that has an excellent safety profile when taken in doses of 4 g/day or less [1]. However, several studies have found that a significant percentage of subjects who ingest 2–4 g of acetaminophen per day for more than 4 consecutive days develop asymptomatic elevation of serum alanine aminotransferase (ALT) activity [2-6]. These studies generally stopped dosing before the ALT elevations resolved. Multiple clinical studies have not identified any cases of liver failure with long-term acetaminophen use [7-11]. In contrast to prospective studies that found no cases of liver failure, there are anecdotal reports of patients who develop liver failure while allegedly taking therapeutic doses [12]. Given the widespread use of acetaminophen, if asymptomatic elevations of aminotransferase activity with therapeutic doses can progress to liver failure, even rarely, there is a substantial risk to public health.

* Correspondence: Kennon.Heard@rmpdc.org
[1]Rocky Mountain Poison and Drug Center, Denver Health, Denver, CO, USA
[2]University of Colorado Department of Emergency Medicine, Aurora, CO, USA
Full list of author information is available at the end of the article

The course of these aminotransferase activity elevations when acetaminophen is administered longer than 4 consecutive days is not well characterized. Anecdotally, patients take acetaminophen for years (as single ingredient and in combination with opioids) without symptomatic liver injury. In a small, placebo controlled 4-week study measuring the effect of acetaminophen on warfarin-induced anticoagulation, Parra reported a dose-dependent elevation in mean serum aminotransferase activity in subjects at two weeks during treatment with 2 or 4 g/day of acetaminophen [5]. Unlike other studies, acetaminophen was continued despite the mild increases in aminotransferase activity. These elevations resolved by week 4 of treatment and no subject had evidence of liver dysfunction. However, this study only included 15 acetaminophen-treated subjects and serum aminotransferase activity was only measured at baseline, 2 and 4 weeks. While this study suggests that the aminotransferase elevations resolve if therapy is continued, the course is not fully characterized.

The objective of this study is to describe the changes in serum aminotransferase activity in healthy subjects taking 4 g/day of acetaminophen for a minimum of 16 days and continued until any observed ALT elevations resolve. Our secondary aims were to determine if subjects who had aminotransferase elevations developed liver dysfunction and finally to determine if subjects who develop these elevations share any obvious demographic or clinical characteristics.

Methods

Trial design

This was a randomized, placebo controlled trial. Subjects were randomized 4:1 acetaminophen to placebo. This randomization plan was intended to increase the power of the study to detect infrequent adverse events in the acetaminophen group. This study was registered with clinicaltrials.gov (NCT00743093) and approved by The Colorado Multiple Institutional Review Board.

Participants

This was an outpatient study; subjects were evaluated at one of two clinical research sites. Subjects were recruited from a research listserv, posters, classified advertisement website (Craigslist) postings and media advertising. All subjects provided informed consent.

We included male and female subjects who were age 18 years or older and who did not have any of the following exclusion criteria: History of acetaminophen ingestion on any of the four days preceding study enrollment or a measurable serum acetaminophen concentration at time of enrollment; laboratory testing suggesting active viral hepatitis A,B or C infection; any of the following tests greater than the upper limit of normal at screening: serum aminotransferase or total bilirubin, International Normalized Ratio (INR) or alkaline phosphatase activity; platelet count less than 125,000/mL; positive pregnancy test; history of cholelithiasis (without cholecystectomy); history of heavy ethanol use defined as consuming more than an average of 3 alcohol containing drinks daily or 3 or more alcohol containing drinks on any given day over the preceding 2 weeks prior to study enrollment [13]; new prescription medication started within the previous 30 days; taking isoniazid or warfarin; currently has anorexia nervosa or reports a fasting type diet; clinically intoxicated, psychiatrically impaired or unable to give informed consent for any reason; known hypersensitivity or allergy to acetaminophen.

Interventions

Subjects were administered acetaminophen 4 g/day or placebo. Subjects were instructed to take 2 × 500 mg tablets every 4 hours for 4 doses each day (the exact timing varied but subjects were asked to take the doses every 4 hours after the first dose each day). The subjects noted the time of ingestion for each dose in a study diary. They also recorded other medications and alcohol consumption. Compliance was verified by study diary and pill counts at each study visit.

We included a placebo group for two reasons. First we recognized that there is day-to-day variation in aminotransferase activity and we felt it was important to be able to account for this variation as we quantified the effect of acetaminophen. Second, we have planned secondary studies to identify potential characteristics and biomarkers that may suggest a mechanism for these elevations.

The following tests were performed at each visit: serum aminotransferase (alanine aminotransferase-ALT and aspartate aminotransferase-AST), total bilirubin (TBL) and International Normalized Ratio (INR). Additional testing at the screening visit (study day −7 to −1) included a complete blood count, hepatitis A and C antibodies, hepatitis B antigen, serum acetaminophen and serum pregnancy (females only). Serum acetaminophen concentrations were also measured at day 10 and 16 for safety purposes but were not reported to study personnel unless they were above the critical concentration for our laboratory (>40 mcg/mL or 264 micromol/L) to maintain blinding. Adverse events were recorded using a structured interview at each visit. Subjects were specifically asked if they had nausea, vomiting, abdominal pain or jaundice and asked if they had any other symptoms.

Patients were evaluated (including laboratory testing as described above) on study days 0 (baseline), 4, 7, 10, 13 and 16. At day 16, subjects were assessed for resolution (as defined in the outcome section below). Subjects who did not meet resolution criteria by day 16 went into the extended dosing period. In the extended study period, subjects continued treatment as assigned and continued to be evaluated every 3 days until study day 40. If the subject did not have resolution by study day 40, the study drug administration was stopped and the subject was monitored every 3 days until day 49. If the subject did not have resolution by that point, they were referred to a hepatologist for further evaluation and monitoring (Figure 1).

Outcomes

As ALT is considered a more specific biomarker for the liver than AST, the primary outcome of this study was resolution of ALT elevation. Resolution criteria were defined at day 16 as an ALT that was less than 47 IU/L (the upper limit of the reference range for our laboratory) and within 10 IU/L of the subject's baseline value. Subjects who did not meet resolution criteria were continued on the study protocol.

The resolution criteria after day 16 were dependent on the day 16 ALT values.

If the subject had a day 16 ALT >47 IU/L, we required 2 consecutive ALT values less than or equal to 47 IU/L for resolution. If the day 16 ALT was <47 IU/L but >10 IU/L above baseline, resolution occurred when they had 2 consecutive non-increasing ALT measurements less than or equal to 47 IU/L (however they could have a final ALT more than 10 IU/L above their baseline, Figure 1). Our secondary outcome was the proportion of subjects who developed liver dysfunction defined by elevation of the INR above 1.4 or serum bilirubin >2× baseline [14].

As the primary study objective was to document the course of ALT while taking 4 gram per day of acetaminophen, our a-priori analysis plan was to restrict outcome analysis to subjects who completed the full protocol (i.e. met resolution criteria or reached study day 40). For safety reasons, subjects who withdrew from the study were required to have at least one measurement of ALT off study drug.

To assure subject safety, subjects were withdrawn if they developed drug induced liver injury as defined by the United States Food and Drug Administration Drug-Induced Liver Injury Premarketing Clinical Evaluation Guidelines [14]: ALT or AST >8× the upper limit of normal (ULN); ALT or AST >5× ULN for more than 2 weeks, ALT or AST >3× ULN and (total bilirubin >2× ULN or INR >1.5); ALT or AST >3× ULN with the appearance of worsening of fatigue, nausea, vomiting, right upper quadrant pain or tenderness, fever, rash, or eosinophilia.

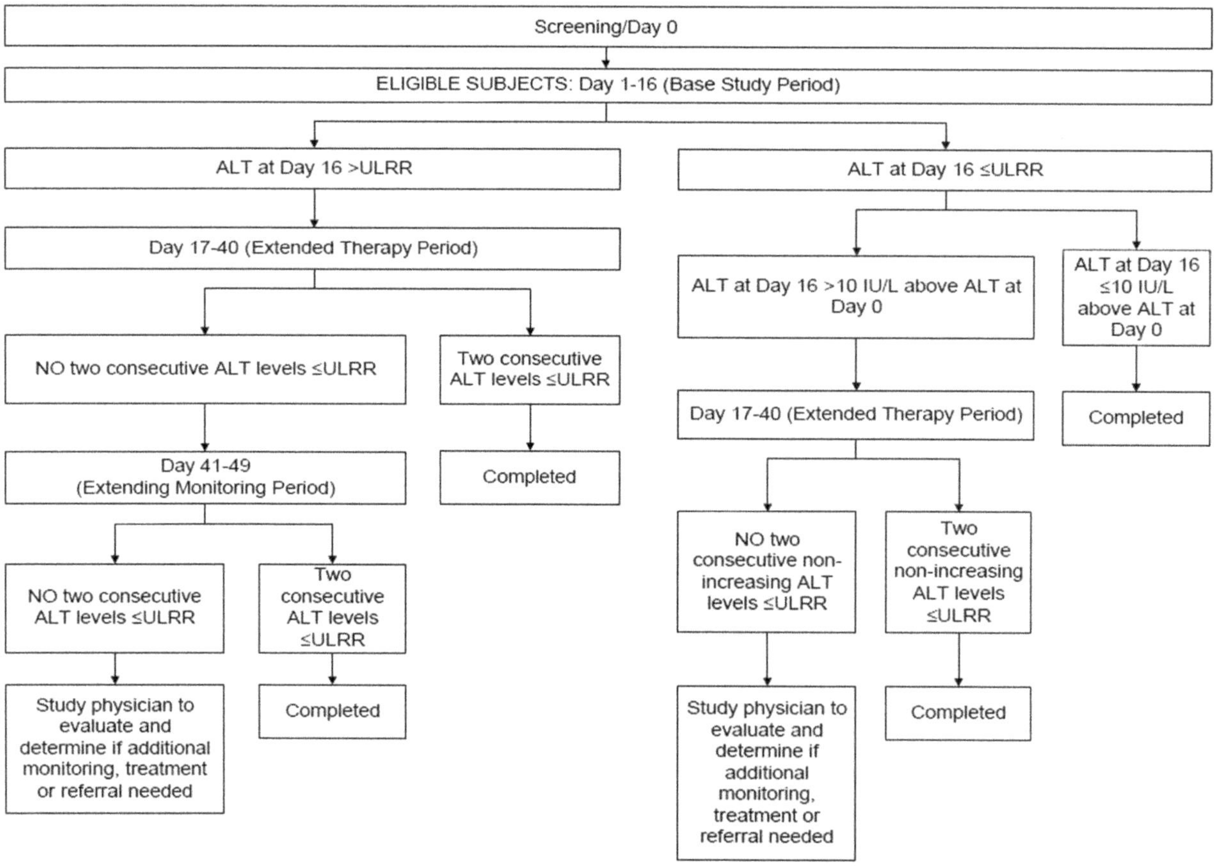

Figure 1 Subject flow and study decision points.

Sample size

As our primary purpose was to describe the course of ALT changes there was no obvious endpoint to use for power calculations. Therefore, we elected to power our study to measure the proportion of patients who did not meet resolution criteria by study day 40. We selected 40 days as a small previous study had suggested that many patients resolve by day 28 [5]. We determined that a sample size of 300 completed subjects (240 acetaminophen: 60 placebo) was appropriate for our endpoint. This assumes that no subjects in the acetaminophen group would have ALT elevations that did not resolve by day 40. Zero out of 240 subjects would result in an upper 95% confidence limit for probability that the true incidence of non-resolution would be less than 0.015 (less than 1.5% of subjects would not resolve by day 40). We assumed a 15% screen failure and a 15% dropout rate.

Randomization

Sequence generation was performed using pre-numbered packages dispensed according to a computer generated randomization list. We used block randomization within the following strata: Hispanic females, Hispanic males, non-Hispanic females, and non-Hispanic males. A separate randomized list of assignments was created for each site based on these strata. We stratified by Hispanic ethnicity as a previous study has suggested that the response to acetaminophen differs between Hispanic and non-Hispanic subjects [6].

Allocation concealment mechanism

Placebo and acetaminophen tablets were provided by McNeil Consumer Healthcare and were identical in appearance. Study medications were packaged into 1-week supplies by a researcher not involved in subject management or data collection.

Implementation

Tablets were dispensed during a study visit as a 1-week supply and the doses for each day were provided in a labeled packet.

Blinding

Participants, investigators and statisticians were all blinded to the treatment groups during the main treatment period (days 0–16). We did not assess the success of blinding. When a subject met the criteria to stop at day 16, the treatment group assignment was unblinded to allow recruitment of acetaminophen-treated subjects into a follow-up study. This occurred after completion of the final study visit (including adverse event recording). The physician assessing relatedness of adverse events and the statistician performing the analysis remained blinded to subject treatment group until the study database was locked.

Statistical methods

Demographic characteristics are presented as medians and interquartile ranges for continuous variables and proportions for categorical variables.

For our primary outcome analysis, we calculated a 95% confidence interval on the proportion of subjects in the active treatment arm with unresolved, persistent elevation of ALT. To determine if ALT elevations were accompanied by changes in liver function (secondary analysis), we calculated a 95% confidence interval on the proportion of subjects in the active treatment arm with elevations of bilirubin or INR.

In a pre-planned exploratory analysis, we analyzed potential associations between aminotransferase elevations and demographic and clinical characteristics. We used logistic regression (PROC LOGISTIC) to determine if any of the following characteristics were associated with our 3 secondary outcomes: age, sex, race/ethnicity (Caucasian, Black, Hispanic, other), baseline ALT, body mass index (BMI) and average daily alcohol consumption (number of 14 gm servings of ethanol per day averaged over the study duration). The 3 outcomes of interest (defined above) were having an ALT elevation more than 1.5 times baseline, having an ALT elevation more than 10 IU/L above baseline, or meeting extension criteria at study day 16.

Results

A total of 398 subjects were screened for the study, 122 were excluded at baseline, 276 were randomized and 252 completed the study. Of the 122 excluded patients, 109 (89.3%) did not meet eligibility criteria at screening and baseline and 13 withdrew participation prior to confirming full eligibility (5 withdrew consent, 5 did not return for baseline eligibility assessments, and 3 withdrew because they could not tolerate the venipuncture). The most common reasons for screen failure (subjects could fail more than 1 criteria) were elevated bilirubin (n = 47), elevated INR (n = 22), elevated ALT or AST (n = 28), elevated alkaline phosphatase (n = 4), positive viral hepatitis markers (n = 17), history of excessive alcohol consumption (n = 9), starting a new prescription in the preceding month (n = 4) and history of acetaminophen ingestion in the 3 days prior to enrollment (n = 3). The study was started on August 20, 2008 and stopped on August 16, 2011 at less than the planned number of subjects due to a higher than expected (31%) screen failure rate. Figure 2 is a CONSORT diagram showing the disposition of study subjects. Placebo and acetaminophen-treated subjects had similar baseline characteristics (Table 1).

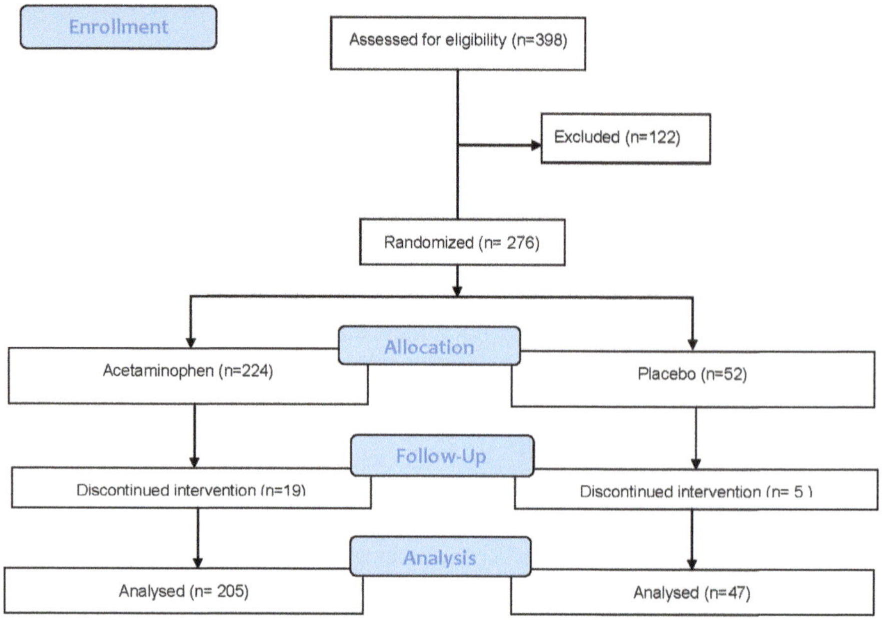

Figure 2 Consort diagram for study subjects.

The median ALT in the acetaminophen group (Figure 3 panels A-D) was unchanged from baseline at study day 4, but increased by 6 IU/L to 26 IU/L on study day 7. The highest median ALT was observed on study day 10 (26.5 IU/L) and the median ALT decreased to 23.5 IU/L by study day 16. Changes in AST followed a slightly more accelerated course of elevation with the median increasing from 21 IU/L at baseline to 27 IU/L on day 7 and decreasing back to 23 IU/L on day 16 (Figure 4 panels A-D). While there was some day-to-day variation in subject measurements, the median ALT and AST in the placebo group was stable throughout the study period (Figures 3 and 4 panel E). The changes in ALT over time in the acetaminophen group were significant ($p < 0.001$ repeated measure ANOVA) and the day 16 ALT was higher for the acetaminophen than the placebo group ($p < 0.001$).

Table 1 Baseline characeteristics of study patients

	Placebo (n = 47)	Acetaminophen (n = 205)
Age (years)	32 (19.0, 64.0)	34 (18.0 to 74.0)
Male	12 (25.5%)	57 (27.8%)
Race		
White	35 (74.5%)	142 (69.3%)
Hispanic	4 (8.5%)	33 (16.1%)
Black	4 (8.5%)	13 (6.3%)
Other/Mixed	4 (8.5%)	17 (8.3%)
Body Mass Index	23.8 (17.3, 48.8)	25.8 (16.5, 53.5)
Self-reported ethanol use	35 (74.5%)	167 (81.5%)
Baseline ALT	17.0 (11.0, 47.0)	19.0(9.0, 44.0)

Note: median (range) were provided for Age, BMI and Baseline ALT.

Of the 205 acetaminophen subjects who completed the study, 157 (77%) did not have ALT elevations or had transient elevations that met resolution criteria by study day 16. Forty-eight completed subjects (23%) in the acetaminophen group and 1 subject (2%) in the placebo group had ALT elevation that met criteria at day 16 to enter the extended treatment phase. Of these 49 subjects, the majority ($n = 31$) entered the extended treatment phase because they had an ALT greater than10 IU/L above their baseline but less than or equal to the upper resolution criteria limit of 47 IU/L (including the one placebo subject) at study day 16. One subject had an ALT less than10 IU/L above their baseline but greater than 47 IU/L while 17 subjects had an ALT that was both greater than10 IU/L above their baseline and greater than 47 IU/L. Among the 49 subjects who entered the extended treatment period, 19 had a final ALT value at least 10 IU above the baseline ALT value.

Overall, 204/205 (99.5%; 95% confidence interval 97.0 to 99.9%) acetaminophen subjects and 47/47 (100%, 95% confidence interval 91.0 to 100%) placebo subjects met criteria for resolution of ALT elevation by study day 40 or less while on continued study dosing regimen (acetaminophen or placebo). The median INR was 1.0 for the acetaminophen group at all time points through study day 36. The two subjects who had an INR measured at study day 40 had a median INR of 1.1. No patient in either group had liver dysfunction defined as elevation

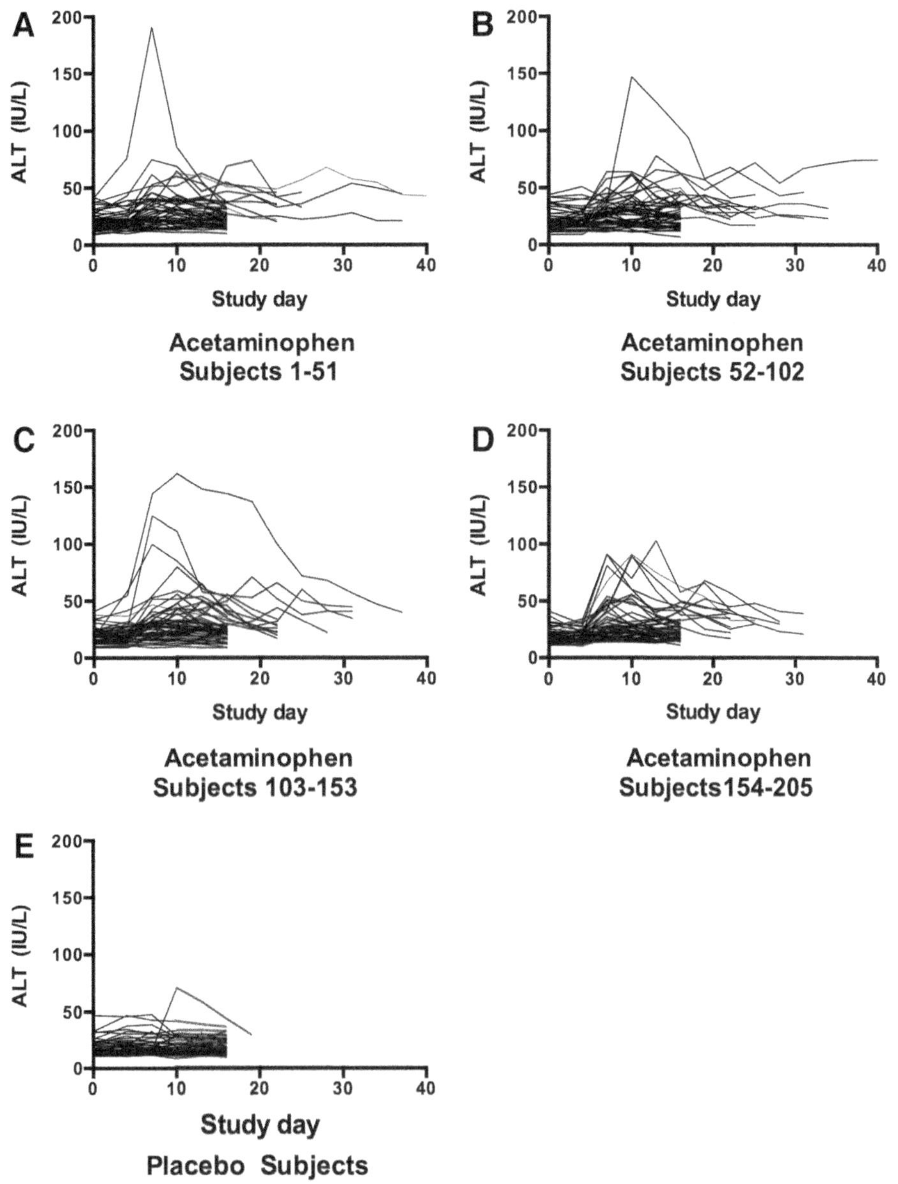

Figure 3 Course of ALT for subjects administered acetaminophen (Panels A-D) and placebo (Panel E). Acetaminophen subjects were split into 4 groups to allow better resolution of subject values.

in INR above 1.4 or bilirubin greater than 2 times their baseline measurement. No subject had a serum acetaminophen concentration greater than 40 mcg/mL (264 micromol/L).

The subject in the acetaminophen group who had an ALT elevation that did not resolve by day 40 was monitored for an additional three weeks after ending acetaminophen administration. After stopping study medication, her ALT continued to trend upward to a maximum of 105 IU/L on study Day 63 (Figure 5) and her INR and bilirubin remained normal. She had no symptoms of liver injury. She was referred for evaluation by a hepatologist but did not follow-up.

Among the completed subjects, 110 (54%) of acetaminophen subjects and 40 placebo subjects (85%) had a peak ALT less than 1.5 times their baseline while 95 acetaminophen subjects (46%) and 7 placebo subjects (15%) had an ALT greater than 1.5 times their baseline. Among the completed subjects, 115 (56%) acetaminophen subjects and 40 (85%) placebo subjects had a peak ALT < 10 U/L above baseline while 90 acetaminophen subjects (44%) and 7 placebo subjects (15%) had an ALT > 10 IU/L above their baseline. For each of these outcomes a logistic model was constructed to identify clinical or demographic characteristics associated with the outcome in the acetaminophen group. The independent factors in the model

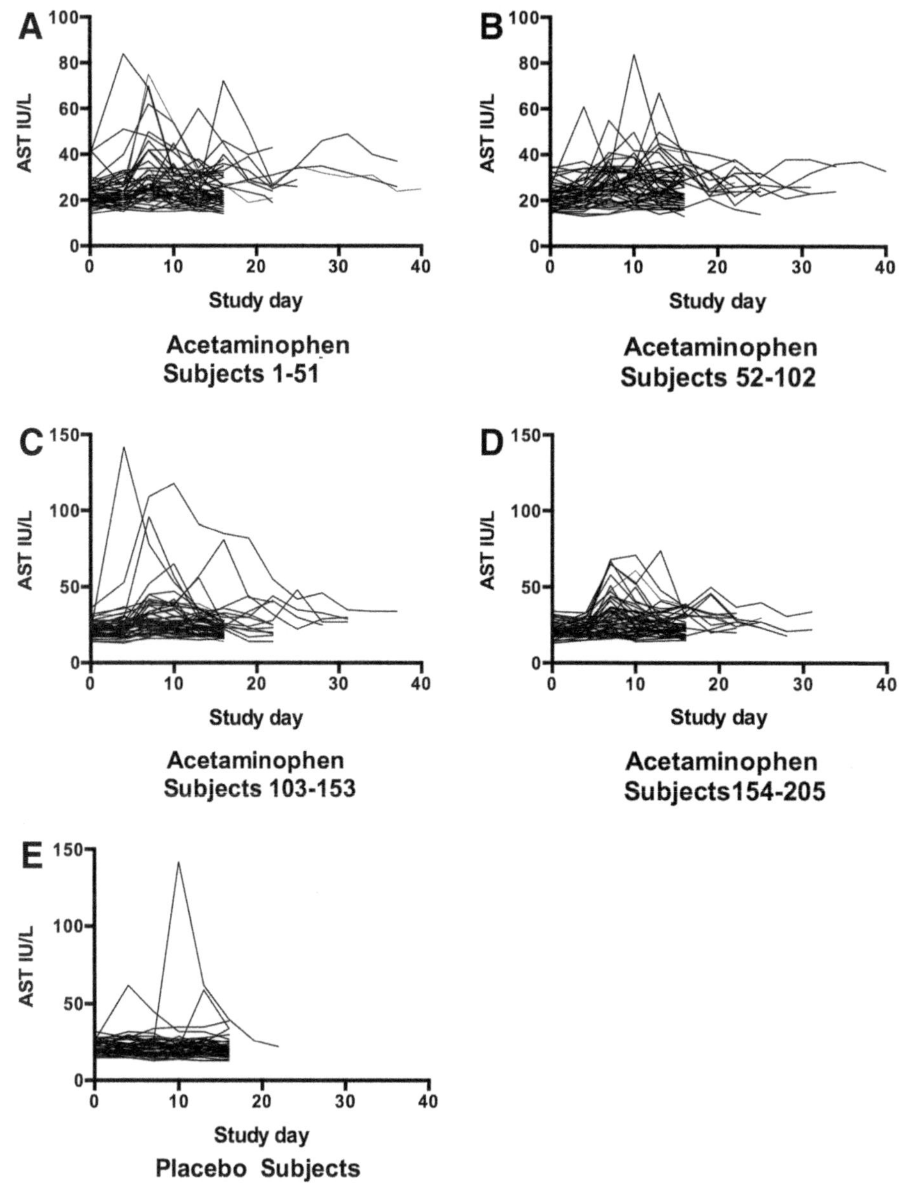

Figure 4 Course of AST for subjects administered acetaminophen (Panels A-D) and placebo (Panel E). Acetaminophen subjects were split into 4 groups to allow better resolution of subject values.

included demographics and baseline variables (age, sex ethnicity, baseline ALT, alcohol user, BMI) and study group. Age, sex, baseline ALT, alcohol use and BMI were not related to any outcome (Table 2). Ethnicity was not associated with entering the extended dosing outcome group. African American subjects were at increased risk for having an ALT increase more than 10 IU/L and there was an overall trend that non-Caucasian subjects had higher rates of all outcomes.

A total of 19 acetaminophen subjects and 5 placebo subjects were withdrawn from the study after receiving at least one dose of study medication. Reasons for withdrawal included non-compliance (5 acetaminophen, 2 placebo), adverse event other than stopping criteria (4 acetaminophen, 1 placebo), day 0 ALT > 47 IU/L (4 acetaminophen) and subject request (6 acetaminophen, 2 placebo). The reasons subjects gave for requesting to be removed from the trial were: inconvenience/too much time required to participate (4 acetaminophen); no transportation (1 acetaminophen, 1 placebo); moved out of state (1 acetaminophen); and no reason given (1 placebo). No subject who requested withdrawal had any symptoms of liver injury. At the time of withdrawal, the median (range) ALT for acetaminophen subjects was 19.5 IU/L (17.0, 26.0 IU/L) for those withdrawn for non-compliance, 19 IU/L (15.0 to 28.0 IU/L) for those withdrawn after adverse events and

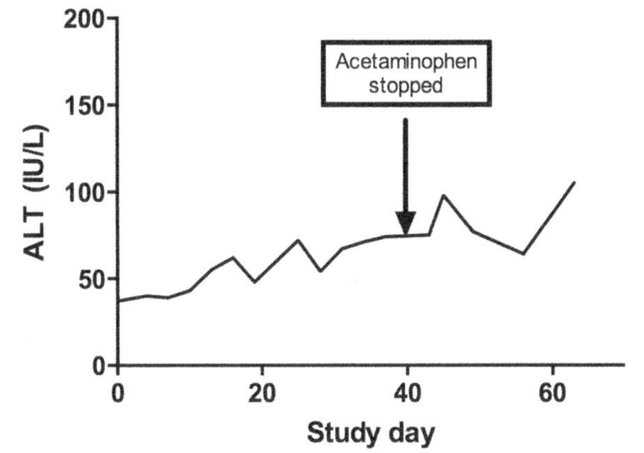

Figure 5 Course of ALT for the one subject who did not have resolution of ALT elevation by study day 40. Acetaminophen was stopped at study day 40 and ALT continued to elevate.

40.0 IU/L (13 to 120 IU/L) for those requesting withdrawal. Two subjects requesting withdrawal had an ALT above the reference range. One subject had a peak ALT of 120 on study day 10 that had decreased to 67 IU/L on day 28 when the subject stopped taking acetaminophen and withdrew. A follow-up ALT off medication on study day 30 was 54 IU/L. A second subject had an ALT of 36 on study day 16, stopped taking study medication on study day 18 and had an ALT of 119 IU/L on study day 21. His ALT decreased to 46 IU/L on study day 24 while not taking acetaminophen. For the placebo subjects requesting withdrawal, the ALT values at withdrawal were both 15 IU/L, for those removed for non-compliance the ALTs at the time of withdrawal were 11 and 21 IU/L and the subject removed for an adverse event had an ALT of 15 IU/L at the time of withdrawal. All subjects withdrawn had decreasing ALT documented on follow-up testing.

Self-reported medication compliance, as measured by the diary was similar for both groups. The median (interquartile range) percent of days where subjects took all 4 doses was 100% (86.7 to 100%) for the acetaminophen group and 86.5% (81.1 to 100%) for the placebo group.

Adverse events

The overall proportion of subjects reporting any adverse event was 62.3%; 65.6% of the acetaminophen subjects and 48.1% of the placebo subjects. The characteristics of the adverse events are listed in the online supplement (Additional file 1: Table S3.pdf Adverse Events). The most commonly reported adverse events were gastrointestinal. The majority of adverse events were rated as unrelated or possibly related to study drug. Nausea was the most frequent adverse event rated as probably related or related to study drug. No serious adverse events were reported. The proportion of acetaminophen-treated subjects suffering adverse events was similar for those who had an ALT elevation >10 IU/L: nausea 15/90 (16.7%) in those with elevation and 19/115 (16.5%) in those without; vomiting 2/90 (2.2%) in those with elevation and 2/115 (1.7%) in those without and abdominal pain 6/90 (6.7%) in those with elevation and 6/115 (5.2%) in those without.

Discussion

We found that ingestion of 4 grams per day of acetaminophen for a minimum of 16 days caused no significant change in ALT in approximately half of subjects, and a transient elevation that resolved by day 16 in approximately a quarter of patients. The remaining quarter of patients had modest ALT elevations that resolved when administration was continued over the next 24 days in all but one subject. The maximum observed ALT was 191 IU/L. No patient experienced drug-induced liver injury as defined by a Food and Drug Administration

Table 2 Adjusted risk for secondary outcomes for subjects treated with 4 g/acetaminiophen/day

	Extended dosing		ALT increase > 10 IU/L		ALT increase >50% above baseline	
Variable	Odds ratio	95% Confidence interval	Odds ratio	95% Confidence interval	Odds ratio	95% Confidence interval
Female (vs Male)	1.47	0.64 to 3.73	1.03	0.53 to 2.03	1.21	0.61 to 2.39
Race						
Caucasian	1.0	Ref	1.0	Ref	1.0	Ref
Black	1.71	0.47 to 6.26	3.56	1.02 to 12.45	1.80	0.54 to 5.99
Hispanic	1.86	0.79 to 4.40	1.45	0.66 to 3.2	1.67	0.75 to 3.69
Other	1.85	0.58 to 5.91	1.40	0.50 to 3.96	1.81	0.63 to 5.24
Age (per yr)	1.01	0.98 to 1.04	1.02	0.99 to 1.04	1.02	1.00 to 1.05
Baseline ALT (Per IU/L)	1.03	0.98 to 1.08	1.01	0.97 to 1.05	0.96	0.92 to1.00
BMI	0.98	0.93 to 1.04	0.98	0.93 to 1.03	0.99	0.94 to 1.04
No ethanol use	1.81	0.81 to 4.1	0.90	0.42 to 1.92	0.89	0.42 to 1.88

guideline despite continued therapy with acetaminophen while their aminotransferase activity was elevated. The proportion of acetaminophen subjects experiencing gastrointestinal symptoms was similar for those with and without ALT elevations.

Only one patient's ALT elevation failed to resolve during continued administration of acetaminophen. The subject had no changes in INR or bilirubin, suggesting there was no liver dysfunction. Furthermore, this subject's aminotransferase elevation continued to increase for 3 weeks after acetaminophen was stopped. As with any single case observation, it is not possible to determine causality, even within a clinical trial. However, this pattern of slowly progressive ALT elevation weeks after exposure is not consistent with acetaminophen-induced liver injury [15] and data from other randomized trials suggests that ALT elevations suspected to be related to acetaminophen resolve once acetaminophen is stopped [2,4,6,8]. This pattern of ALT increase suggests an alternative cause of aminotransferase elevation such as infection [16] or a change in diet [17]. Unfortunately, the subject declined a comprehensive hepatology evaluation (as planned in the study protocol). This limited our ability to identify potential causes for her ALT elevation.

As noted in previous studies [3,6], we found no association between aminotransferase elevation (using either of two definitions) and age or gender. While a previous study suggested an increased risk of elevation for Hispanic subjects [6], our study found no difference between Hispanic and Caucasian subjects. We also found no association between ethanol use and aminotransferase elevation. While there have been no previous trials that directly compare the effect of acetaminophen between drinkers and non-drinkers, separate studies have reported the effect sizes in these two groups. A study of moderate ethanol users administered 4 g/day of acetaminophen for 10 days reported a median ALT elevation of 8 IU/L [3] while a similar study in non-drinkers (using a more frequent sampling pattern) reported a median ALT elevation of 15 IU/L [4]. The current study suggests that the aminotransferase elevations do not differ between drinkers and non-drinkers and suggests that the differences in the previous trials are due to different sampling methods.

The degree of aminotransferase elevation caused by repeated therapeutic doses of acetaminophen has varied greatly among prior studies. Studies of ambulatory subjects have consistently reported that the highest observed elevation is less than 3 times the upper limit of normal [3-5,18], while studies of subjects confined to a clinical research facility reported elevations more than 8 times the upper limit of normal [2,6]. While the exact reason for these differences is not clear, there is meta-analytic evidence that subjects on a clinical research unit may increase their aminotransferase activity independent of treatment [19]. This meta-analysis compared the change in ALT for the placebo groups in studies where subjects were admitted to a clinical research unit to the change in ALT for the placebo group in studies where subjects were ambulatory. They noted that almost 10% of placebo treated patients on a clinical research unit had an increase in ALT that was at least 50% of the reference range width, while no outpatient subjects had elevations of this degree. It is possible that the marked increases observed in the acetaminophen group within studies using a clinical research unit are due to a potentiation of the acetaminophen effect by confinement. The clinical implications of an interaction between hospitalization and suggested acetaminophen-induced ALT elevations warrant further investigation. In a small observational study of inpatients (surgical and medical patients), acetaminophen users had an increased risk of developing an elevation of ALT compared to non-acetaminophen users [20]. While the elevations observed in this study were minimal, it is possible that acetaminophen-induced ALT elevations could progress to clinical liver injury if potentiated by other factors such as CYP 2E1 induction, malnutrition or oxidative stress. However, analysis of prospective trials that treated adult or pediatric patients with the therapeutic doses for a variety of medical conditions found no cases of acute liver failure [1,21].

Acetaminophen is frequently used in both combination and single ingredient products for prolonged periods. The rarity of alleged cases of hepatic injury from therapeutic doses is strong evidence that these doses are safe even though ALT elevations occur. Until recently, ALT elevations alone during pre-clinical studies were considered a signal that would often lead a company to stop seeking approval for candidate drugs. However, the recent guidelines emphasize the importance of changes in hepatic function (INR and bilirubin) in addition to elevations of aminotransferase activity [22]. These guidelines recognize that a large number of medications cause self-limited ALT elevations that are not a precursor to clinical liver injury and are not an indication to stop therapy.

Other medications that cause self-limited aminotransferase elevations include amiodarone, tacrine, heparin, isoniazid and the statins [23-27]. While liver failure has rarely been linked to isoniazid and amiodarone, there are no cases definitively caused by tacrine or heparin and the cases linked to the statins have been questioned [28]. These observations have led some to postulate that these transient elevations of the serum transaminase reflect hepatic adaptation [22]. While the mechanism is not clear hepatic adaptation may also occur with repeated acetaminophen dosing.

Our study population was limited to healthy volunteers, so it is possible that subjects with underlying liver disease or other medical conditions may have a different course of

ALT activity during prolonged acetaminophen dosing. Our internal validity is limited by the loss of several subjects prior to completing the protocol. It is possible that these subjects would not have resolved prior to completing the study. This would lead us to underestimate the proportion of subjects who did not resolve. We were also limited by not reaching our planned sample size, and this decreased our overall study power. Our study is also limited by the use of two biomarkers (ALT and AST). It is possible that other biomarkers may produce different patterns of change.

Conclusions

It is now clear that therapeutic doses of acetaminophen when administered for consecutive days may cause mild to moderate ALT elevations. These aminotransferase elevations are relatively common, usually less than 10 IU/L, not accompanied by liver dysfunction and resolve even when acetaminophen therapy is continued.

Additional file

Additional file 1: Table S3. Adverse Events by class for all randomized subjects. Subjects were treated with acetaminophen (4 g/day) or placebo).

Abbreviation

AST: Aspartate aminotransferase; ALT: Alanine aminotransferase; BMI: Body mass index; CI: Confidence interval; INR: International Normalized Ratiol; ULN: Upper limit of normal.

Competing interests

This work was funded by an investigator-initiated award from McNeil Consumer Healthcare to Denver Health. The funding sponsor had no role in the conduct or analysis of the research. The manuscript was reviewed by the funding sponsor for proprietary information prior to publication, but the authors had the final decisions on all content. All authors were employees of Denver Health at the time of this study. Denver Health has research, consulting and clinical contracts with McNeil Consumer Healthcare. All authors received only their salary for work on this project. Dr. Heard was supported in part by Award Number K08DA020573 from the National Institute on Drug Abuse. The content is solely the responsibility of the authors and does not necessarily represent the official views of the National Institute on Drug Abuse or the National Institutes of Health.

Authors' contributions

KH, JLG, RCD designed the study, KH, VA and JLG performed the research, BBB analyzed the data, KH drafted the manuscript and all authors contributed substantially to the revisions. KH had full access to the data and assumes responsibility for the manuscript. All authors read and approved the final manuscript.

Acknowledgements

The authors would like to thank the research staff at the Rocky Mountain Poison Center for their work on this project.

Author details

[1]Rocky Mountain Poison and Drug Center, Denver Health, Denver, CO, USA. [2]University of Colorado Department of Emergency Medicine, Aurora, CO, USA. [3]Vanderbilt School of Nursing, Nashville, TN, USA. [4]Colorado School of Public Health, Aurora, CO, USA.

References

1. Dart RC, Bailey E: **Does therapeutic use of acetaminophen cause acute liver failure?** *Pharmacotherapy* 2007, **27**:1219–1230.
2. Harrill AH, Watkins PB, Su S, Ross PK, Harbourt DE, Stylianou IM, Boorman GA, Russo MW, Sackler RS, Harris SC, Smith PC, Tennant R, Bogue M, Paigen K, Harris C, Contractor T, Wiltshire T, Rusyn I, Threadgill DW: **Mouse population-guided resequencing reveals that variants in CD44 contribute to acetaminophen-induced liver injury in humans.** *Genome Res* 2009, **19**:1507–1515.
3. Heard K, Green JL, Bailey JE, Bogdan GM, Dart RC: **A randomized trial to determine the change in alanine aminotransferase during 10 days of paracetamol (acetaminophen) administration in subjects who consume moderate amounts of alcohol.** *Aliment Pharmacol Ther* 2007, **26**:283–290.
4. Heard KJ, Green JL, Dart RC: **Serum alanine aminotransferase elevation during 10 days of acetaminophen use in nondrinkers.** *Pharmacotherapy* 2010, **30**:818–822.
5. Parra D, Beckey NP, Stevens GR: **The effect of acetaminophen on the international normalized ratio in patients stabilized on warfarin therapy.** *Pharmacotherapy* 2007, **27**:675–683.
6. Watkins PB, Kaplowitz N, Slattery JT, Colonese CR, Colucci SV, Stewart PW, Harris SC: **Aminotransferase elevations in healthy adults receiving 4 grams of acetaminophen daily: a randomized controlled trial.** *JAMA* 2006, **296**:87–93.
7. Bradley JD, Brandt KD, Katz BP, Kalasinski LA, Ryan SI: **Comparison of an antiinflammatory dose of ibuprofen, an analgesic dose of ibuprofen, and acetaminophen in the treatment of patients with osteoarthritis of the knee.** *N Engl J Med* 1991, **325**:87–91.
8. Kuffner EK, Temple AR, Cooper KM, Baggish JS, Parenti DL: **Retrospective analysis of transient elevations in alanine aminotransferase during long-term treatment with acetaminophen in osteoarthritis clinical trials.** *Curr Med Res Opin* 2006, **22**:2137–2148.
9. Pincus T, Koch GG, Sokka T, Lefkowith J, Wolfe F, Jordan JM, Luta G, Callahan LF, Wang X, Schwartz T, Abramson SB, Caldwell JR, Harrell RA, Kremer JM, Lautzenheiser RL, Markenson JA, Schnitzer TJ, Weaver A, Cummins P, Wilson A, Morant S, Fort J: **A randomized, double-blind, crossover clinical trial of diclofenac plus misoprostol versus acetaminophen in patients with osteoarthritis of the hip or knee.** *Arthritis Rheum* 2001, **44**:1587–1598.
10. Temple AR, Benson GD, Zinsenheim JR, Schweinle JE: **Multicenter, randomized, double-blind, active-controlled, parallel-group trial of the long-term (6–12 months) safety of acetaminophen in adult patients with osteoarthritis.** *Clin Ther* 2006, **28**:222–235.
11. Altman RD, Zinsenheim JR, Temple AR, Schweinle JE: **Three-month efficacy and safety of acetaminophen extended-release for osteoarthritis pain of the hip or knee: a randomized, double-blind, placebo-controlled study.** *Osteoarthritis Cartilage* 2007, **15**:454–461.
12. Prescott LF: **Therapeutic misadventure with paracetamol: fact or fiction?** *Am J Ther* 2000, **7**:99–114.
13. Gronbaek M, Becker U, Johansen D, Gottschau A, Schnohr P, Hein HO, Jensen G, Sorensen TI: **Type of alcohol consumed and mortality from all causes, coronary heart disease, and cancer.** *Ann Intern Med* 2000, **133**:411–419.
14. **Guidance for Industry Drug-Induced Liver Injury: Premarketing Clinical Evaluation.** http://www.fda.gov/downloads/Drugs/GuidanceComplianceRegulatoryInformation/Guidances/UCM174090.pdf.
15. Singer AJ, Carracio TR, Mofenson HC: **The temporal profile of increased transaminase levels in patients with acetaminophen-induced liver dysfunction.** *Ann Emerg Med* 1995, **26**:49–53.
16. Maheshwari A, Ray S, Thuluvath PJ: **Acute hepatitis C.** *Lancet* 2008, **372**:321–332.
17. Kechagias S, Ernersson A, Dahlqvist O, Lundberg P, Lindstrom T, Nystrom FH: **Fast-food-based hyper-alimentation can induce rapid and profound elevation of serum alanine aminotransferase in healthy subjects.** *Gut* 2008, **57**:649–654.
18. Sudano I, Flammer AJ, Periat D, Enseleit F, Hermann M, Wolfrum M, Hirt A, Kaiser P, Hurlimann D, Neidhart M, Gay S, Holzmeister J, Nussberger J, Mocharla P, Landmesser U, Haile SR, Corti R, Vanhoutte PM, Lüscher TF, Noll G, Ruschitzka F: **Acetaminophen increases blood pressure in patients with coronary artery disease.** *Circulation* 2010, **122**:1789–1796.
19. Narjes H, Nehmiz G: **Effect of hospitalisation on liver enzymes in healthy subjects.** *Eur J Clin Pharmacol* 2000, **56**:329–333.

20. Mitchell SJ, Hilmer SN, Murnion BP, Matthews S: **Hepatotoxicity of therapeutic short-course paracetamol in hospital inpatients: impact of ageing and frailty.** *J Clin Pharm Ther* 2011, **36**:327–335.
21. Lavonas EJ, Reynolds KM, Dart RC: **Therapeutic acetaminophen is not associated with liver injury in children: a systematic review.** *Pediatrics* 2010, **126**:e1430–e1444.
22. Senior JR: **Monitoring for hepatotoxicity: what is the predictive value of liver "function" tests?** *Clin Pharmacol Ther* 2009, **85**:331–334.
23. Chalasani N, Aljadhey H, Kesterson J, Murray MD, Hall SD: **Patients with elevated liver enzymes are not at higher risk for statin hepatotoxicity.** *Gastroenterology* 2004, **126**:1287–1292.
24. Nolan CM, Goldberg SV, Buskin SE: **Hepatotoxicity associated with isoniazid preventive therapy: a 7-year survey from a public health tuberculosis clinic.** *JAMA* 1999, **281**:1014–1018.
25. Pollak PT, Shafer SL: **Use of population modeling to define rational monitoring of amiodarone hepatic effects.** *Clin Pharmacol Ther* 2004, **75**:342–351.
26. Watkins PB, Zimmerman HJ, Knapp MJ, Gracon SI, Lewis KW: **Hepatotoxic effects of tacrine administration in patients with Alzheimer's disease.** *JAMA* 1994, **271**:992–998.
27. Olsson R, Korsan-Bengtsen BM, Korsan-Bengtsen K, Lennartsson J, Waldenstrom J: **Serum aminotransferases after low-dose heparin treatment. Short communication.** *Acta Med Scand* 1978, **204**:229–230.
28. Tolman KG: **The liver and lovastatin.** *Am J Cardiol* 2002, **89**:1374–1380.

Liver and renal safety of tenofovir disoproxil fumarate in combination with emtricitabine among African women in a pre-exposure prophylaxis trial

Justin Mandala[1*], Kavita Nanda[2], Meng Wang[2], Irith De Baetselier[3], Jennifer Deese[2], Johan Lombaard[4], Fredrick Owino[5], Mookho Malahleha[6], Rachel Manongi[7], Douglas Taylor[2] and Lut Van Damme[1,8]

Abstract

Background: Safety of tenofovir disoproxil fumarate/emtricitabine (TDF-FTC) has been studied more extensively among HIV-infected patients than among HIV-uninfected people. Using data from a pre-exposure trial – FEM-PrEP –, we determined the cumulative probabilities of grade 1+ ALT, AST and creatinine and grade 2+ phosphorus toxicities; ALT/AST toxicities by baseline hepatitis B status; and change in mean creatinine, phosphorus, ALT and AST levels controlling for TDF-FTC adherence.

Methods and findings: FEM-PrEP was a randomized, blinded, placebo-controlled trial of daily TDF-FTC among women in Africa. Enrolled women were in general good health, HIV antibody negative, 18 to 35 years old, hepatitis B surface antigen negative, and had normal hepatic and renal function at baseline. AST, ALT, phosphorus and serum creatinine were measured regularly throughout the trial. TDF-FTC concentrations were measured to assess adherence to TDF-FTC. The cumulative probabilities of grade 1+ creatininemia and grade 2+ phosphatemia toxicities were not statistically different between TDF-FTC and placebo arms. The cumulative probabilities of grade 1+ ALT and AST toxicities were higher among participants in the TDF-FTC arm than in the placebo arm ($p = 0.03$ for both). The proportions of grade 1+ and grade 2+ ALT or AST toxicities were significantly higher in participants who were hepatitis B virus surface antibody (HBsAb) positive than in those who were HBsAb-negative. Women with good adherence had higher mean change from baseline to week 4 in their AST levels (2.90 (0.37, 5.42); $p = 0.025$) than women with less than good adherence.

Conclusions: We did not observe a significant relationship between randomization to TDF-FTC and creatinine or phosphorus toxicities. Women randomized to TDF-FTC had higher rates of mild to moderate ALT/AST toxicities, especially women with prior hepatitis B virus exposure. We also observed a significant increase in AST from baseline to week 4 among women who had higher adherence to TDF-FTC during that interval.

Trial register: #NCT00625404, February 19, 2008.

Keywords: Pre-exposure prophylaxis, HIV, Safety, Women, Africa, Tenofovir disoproxil fumarate, Emtricitabine

* Correspondence: JMandala@fhi360.org
[1]FHI 360, 1825 Connecticut Ave, Suite 800, NW, Washington, DC 20009, USA
Full list of author information is available at the end of the article

Background

Decades into HIV prevention research, there is strong evidence that the use of antiretrovirals (ARV) as pre-exposure prophylaxis (PrEP) significantly reduces the risk of acquiring HIV infection in men and women [1-5]. While the safety of tenofovir disoproxil fumarate (300 mg)/emtricitabine (200 mg) (TDF-FTC) has been extensively studied among HIV-infected patients, limited data are available among HIV-uninfected people [6-10]. Here we report on the hepatic and renal safety of TDF-FTC in a pre-exposure prophylaxis clinical trial – FEM-PrEP – among HIV negative women in Africa [11].

FEM-PrEP was a randomized, double-blind, placebo-controlled trial of once-daily oral TDF-FTC in Africa among women at high risk of acquiring HIV via sexual intercourse. The study was stopped early due to futility, likely due to low adherence to the daily oral regimen by study participants [11].

The primary safety endpoints included grade 2+ creatinine toxicities and grade 3+ alanine aminotransferase (ALT), aspartate aminotransferase (AST), and phosphorus based on the U.S. NIH, NIAID Division of AIDS (DAIDS) grading table and on local normal ranges [12]. Secondary safety outcomes included grade 1+ ALT, AST and creatinine toxicities and grade 2+ phosphorus. Due to overall low TDF-FTC exposure in the study population, we also conducted exploratory analyses controlling for actual TDF drug levels [11,13].

We report on the cumulative probabilities of grade 1+ ALT, AST and creatinine toxicities and grade 2+ phosphorus; ALT/AST toxicities by baseline hepatitis B status; and change in means of creatinine, phosphorus, ALT and AST levels controlling for TDF-FTC adherence.

Methods

Ethics statement

The trial and informed consent forms were approved by all applicable ethics and regulatory committees: The Protection of Human Subjects Committee of FHI360, the US Food and Drug Administration, the ethics committee (EC) of the University Hospital of Antwerp, the Institutional Review Board of ITM, the Kenyatta National Hospital/University of Nairobi Ethics and Research Committee, the Republic of Kenya Ministry of Health (MoH- Pharmacy & Poisons Board), Kilimanjaro Christian Medical Center Research EC of Tanzania, National Institute for Medical Research of Tanzania, London School of Hygiene and Tropical Medicine EC, Tanzania Food and Drugs Authority, Medunsa Campus Research and EC of South Africa, University of the Free State EC and Medicines Control Council of South Africa. Written informed consent was obtained from all participants prior to conducting any study procedures.

Context: FEM-PrEP study

The details of the FEM-PrEP study have been described elsewhere [11]. The trial was approved by all applicable ethical and regulatory committees and participants provided written informed consent before any procedures were performed. Women were recruited from Pretoria and Bloemfontein, South Africa; Bondo, Kenya; and Arusha, Tanzania. Eligibility criteria required that women be HIV antibody negative, 18 to 35 years old, in general good health, hepatitis B virus surface antigen (HBsAg) negative and have no evidence of abnormal hepatic or renal function at baseline (i.e., serum creatinine < 1.5 mg/dl, creatinine clearance ≥ 60 ml/min estimated by the Cockcroft-Gault method, ALT and AST <2× local upper limit of normal [ULN] and serum phosphorus levels above the lower limit of the normal range and below DAIDS grade 3). Participants attended study visits at screening, enrollment (2–4 weeks later), and at 4-week intervals thereafter for up to 60 weeks (52 weeks on product followed by eight weeks off product). Plasma and upper layer packed cell (ULPC) aliquots were stored for TDF-FTC concentration testing at monthly visits; hepatic and renal (AST, ALT, creatinine and phosphorus) parameters were evaluated at weeks 4, 12, 24, 36, 52, 56 and when clinically indicated [13].

Laboratory analysis

AST, ALT, phosphorus and serum creatinine assays were performed according to manufacturer procedures. Samples were processed within two hours after collection. The VITROS DT II instrument (Ortho-Clinical Diagnostics, Inc., Johnson & Johnson, Buckinghamshire, UK) was used in Kenya until May 2010, thereafter the VITROS 250 (Ortho-Clinical Diagnostics, Inc., Johnson & Johnson, Buckinghamshire, UK), the CX5 Beckman Chemistry Analyzer (Beckman Coulter, Inc, Fullerton, CA, USA) was used at both South African sites and the Cobas Integra 400 Plus (Roche Diagnostics GmbH, Mannheim, Germany) was used at the Tanzanian site.

Site-specific laboratory normal ranges (LNR) were used due to unknown population similarities/differences and different instrumentation used across sites. Manufacturer recommended, or nationally/regionally established LNRs were used during the first two to three months of the trial while site-specific LNRs were developed. The local LNR was identified and verified, using Sigma Diagnostic guidelines, by the central laboratory (Institute of Tropical Medicine, Antwerp, Belgium) [14]. Details of the verification process will be described in a separate manuscript. Locally verified ranges were used for final grading of all biochemistry toxicities in Kenya and South Africa. In Tanzania, due to the delay in study initiation and early closure of the trial, local LNR were not verified; manufacturer LNRs were used instead.

The central laboratory provided on-site training in good clinical laboratory practice and technical training for all protocol-required laboratory tests, and conducted quality assurance activities including co-development of site standard operating procedures (SOPs) and analytical plans, assay and equipment validation, external quality assessment (EQA) schemes, and equipment calibration and maintenance. In addition, central lab staff conducted, at a minimum, annual site visits to verify proper conduct of laboratory procedures and review source data.

TDF-FTC concentration analysis on stored samples was conducted at the University of North Carolina at Chapel Hill. Tenofovir (TFV) was measured in plasma and tenofovir diphosphate (TFV-DP) in ULPC. Laboratory procedures for TDF-FTC concentration analysis were published previously [11,13]. Adherence was qualitatively classified on a 6-point scale based on drug concentration data, with the top two adherence scores being "good" and "excellent" (good = plasma TFV levels >10 ng/ml and ULPC intracellular TFV-DP between 100,000-1,000,000 femtomoles/million cells, excellent = plasma TFV levels >10 ng/ml and ULPC intracellular TFV-DP between >1,000,000 femtomoles/million cells) [13].

Management of toxicity and study product interruptions

Protocol-defined toxicities were defined and managed according to clinical assessment, grade and relatedness to the study product as assessed by study clinicians [12]. Study product was temporarily or permanently withdrawn as per protocol-described criteria.

Hepatotoxicity grade 2 was defined as 2.6 -5.0 × upper limit of normal (ULN), if determined to be related to the study product, the study product was interrupted and was restarted only if AST/ALT decreased to ≤ grade 1. Hepatotoxicity grade 3 was defined as 5.1 - 10.0 × ULN and study product was interrupted independent of relatedness assessment. Study product was restarted if AST/ALT decreased to ≤ grade 1. Hepatotoxicity grade 4 was defined as > 10.0 × ULN and study product was permanently withdrawn independent of relatedness.

Creatininemia grade 1 was defined as 1.1 -1.3 × ULN and grade 2 as 1.4 -1.8 × ULN; study product was interrupted for both grades regardless of the relatedness to study product use and was restarted if creatininemia decreased to < grade 1 or < 1.3× baseline. Study product was permanently withdrawn for creatininemia grade 2 determined to be related to the study product, and for any creatininemia grade 3 (>1.8 × ULN)

Study product was also permanently withdrawn when there was hypophosphatemia associated with elevated creatininemia, low creatinine clearance or proteinuria. In case of pregnancy, study product was interrupted and resumption allowed after delivery and completion of breastfeeding or with evidence of pregnancy loss/termination). Study product was immediately discontinued in participants who HIV seroconverted.

Sample selection

The analysis population consisted of all women randomized into the trial, excluding participants who never received study product, returned all product unused, or never returned for a follow-up visit. TDF-FTC concentration data were available for a random sub-cohort of 150 participants assigned TDF-FTC, (50 from each of the three sites where HIV infections took place, i.e., Bloemfontein, Pretoria and Bondo).

Statistical analyses

Cumulative probabilities of grade 1+ creatinine, ALT and AST and grade 2+ phosphorus were plotted with data pooled across sites by treatment group over time using Kaplan-Meier methods. In addition, the number and of percentage of women experiencing toxicities by grade were summarized by baseline HBsAg status and treatment group; fisher exact tests were used to compare differences between groups.

For the random sub-cohort of 150 women in the TDF-FTC arm, we further assessed the association between adherence to TDF-FTC and change from baseline to week 4 in creatinine, phosphorus, ALT, and AST levels using generalized linear models, with adjustment for baseline level, age, body mass index, oral contraceptive (OC) use at enrollment and study site. A similar analysis was done for change from last visit on-product and first visit after product use ceased (at study exit or earlier product withdrawal). SAS 9.3 (SAS Institute, Cary, NC) was used for all analyses; statistical significance was defined as $p \leq 0.05$.

Results

Characteristics of enrolled population

The analysis included a total of 2,058 women who were enrolled during June 2009 to April 2011. There were 701 and 707 person-years of follow up in the TDF-FTC and placebo arms respectively. Demographic characteristics, medical history and self-reported sexual behavior at baseline have been reported elsewhere and were generally similar between both groups [11]. At enrolment 20.8% and 21.4% of participants were hepatitis B surface antibody (HBsAb) positive in the TDF-FTC and placebo arms respectively.

Kidney toxicity

The cumulative probabilities of grade 1+ creatinine or grade 2+ phosphatemia toxicities were higher in the TDF-FTC arm, although neither of these differences were statistically significant (Figures 1 and 2).

Six participants developed grade 2+ creatininemia: four (0.4%) in the TDF-FTC arm and two (0.2%) in the

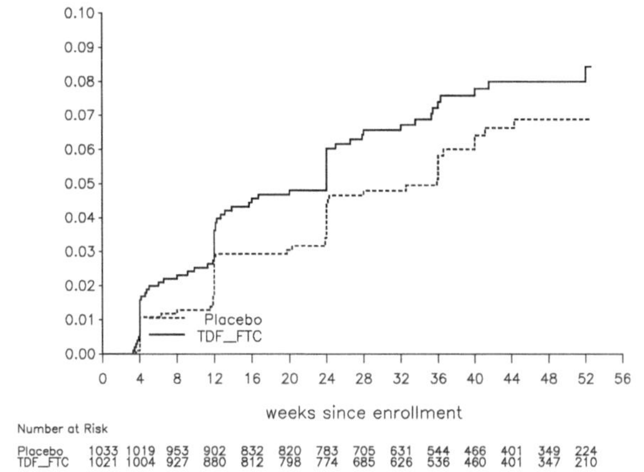

Figure 1 **Cumulative probability of grade 1+ creatinine toxicity, with number of participants at risk at the start of 4-week intervals (log-rank test, stratified on site, p = 0.128).**

placebo arm. Their baseline creatininemia levels were comparable to the average baseline creatininemia at their respective sites. Among the four participants in the TDF-FTC arm, the grade 2+ creatininemia resolved after 1, 2, 16 and 28 weeks respectively; among the two in the placebo arm, one resolved after 6 weeks and decreased to a grade 1 for 10 weeks in the second participant. The latter participant was referred to a nephrologist at the closing of the trial; she later self-reported that her creatinine returned to normal, though results could not be validated by the study team.

None of the six participants with grade 2+ creatininemia reported taking concomitant medication at the time of the event. TDF-FTC drug concentration data were available for the four participants in the TDF-FTC arm: one was classified as having excellent adherence, two as having good adherence, and one as not adherent in the interval prior to the event.

Hepatic toxicity

The cumulative probabilities of grade 1+ ALT and AST toxicities were higher among participants in the TDF-FTC arm than in the placebo arm (p = 0.03 for both) (see Figures 3 and 4).

Sixteen participants developed grade 3+ ALT and/or AST toxicities: eight in the TDF-FTC arm and eight in the placebo arm. Baseline AST/ALT levels among these participants were comparable to the average ALT/AST in their respective sites. In three of these 16 participants, the grade 3+ ALT/AST occurred at the time of HIV seroconversion (one in the TDF-FTC arm and two in the placebo arm), and 11 of the 16 (six in the TDF-FTC arm and five in the placebo arm) events occurred in participants who had received the hepatitis B vaccine. Six participants (two in the TDF-FTC arm and four in the placebo arm) with grade 3+ ALT/AST toxicities reported taking a concomitant medication at the time of the event; medications included acetaminophen, ibuprofen, diclofenac and metronidazole. All grade 3+ ALT/AST toxicities were resolved between two and eight weeks without any difference in time to resolution between TDF-FTC and placebo arms. One participant (in the placebo arm) with grade 3+ ALT at week 12 never returned to the study clinic despite intense tracing efforts. Drug level data were available for seven participants in the TDF-FTC arm with grade 3+ ALT/AST: two were classified as having excellent adherence, one as having good adherence and four as non-adherent in the interval before the event.

At one site – Bondo – the proportion of grade 2+ AST toxicities was significantly higher in the TDF-FTC arm (5.0%) than in the placebo arm (1.9%) (p = 0.02). Also, overall, Bondo observed higher proportions of grade 1+ AST toxicities (43.1% in TDF-FTC arm vs. 36.4% in placebo arm) compared to Bloemfontein (5.7% vs. 3.7%

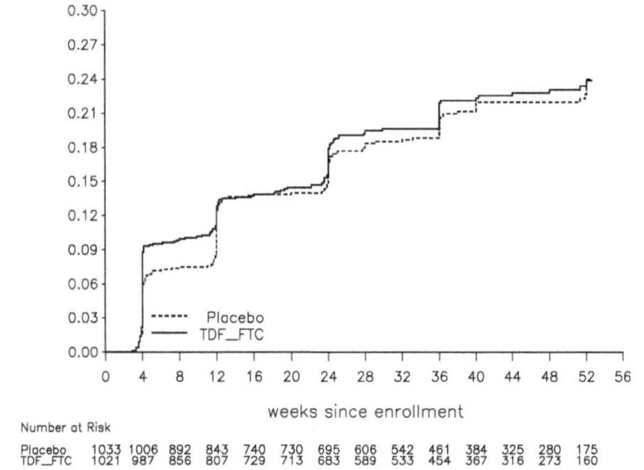

Figure 2 **Cumulative probability of grade 2+ phosphorus toxicity, with number of participants at risk at the start of 4-week intervals (log-rank test, stratified on site, p = 0.621).**

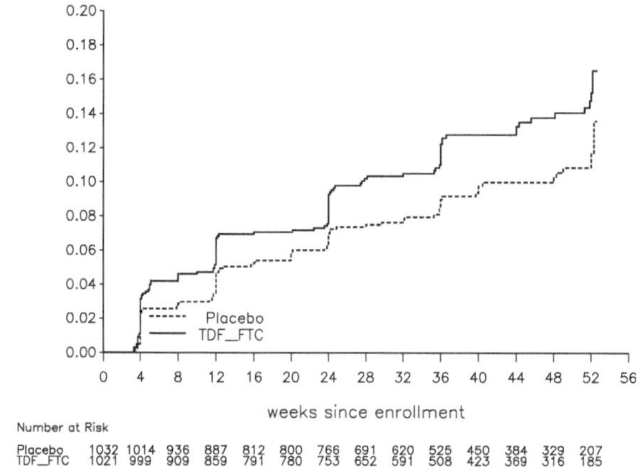

Figure 3 **Cumulative probability of grade 1+ AST toxicity, with number of participants at risk at the start of 4-week intervals (log-rank test, stratified on site, p = 0.025).**

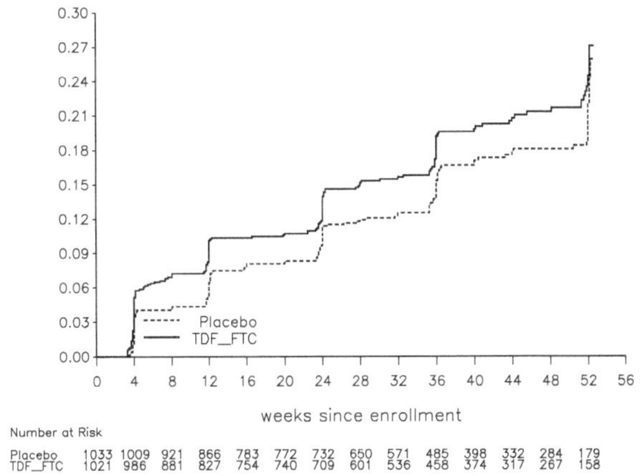

Figure 4 **Cumulative probability of grade 1+ AST toxicity, with number of participants at risk at the start of 4-week intervals (log-rank test, stratified on site, p = 0.025).**

respectively), Pretoria (2.9% vs. 2.4% respectively), and Arusha (0% vs. 3.6% respectively). At baseline, Bondo participants had a higher exposure to hepatitis B.

In the TDF-FTC arm, the proportions of grade 1+ and grade 2+ ALT or AST toxicities were significantly higher in participants who were HBsAb positive than in those who were HBsAb negative; for grade 1+, 31.6 vs. 22.4% respectively, $p < 0.007$ and for grade 2+, 5.6 vs. 2.6% respectively, $p < 0.047$ (Table 1). In the placebo arm, only the proportion of grade1+ ALT or AST toxicities was significantly more frequent in HBsAb positive participants vs. HBsAb negative participants; 29.5 vs. 17.1%, $p < 0.001$ (Table 2).

TDF-FTC concentrations and observed kidney or hepatic toxicities

TDF-FTC concentration data from a sub-cohort of 150 women indicated that very few consistently took the study drug, making it impossible to assess the impact of continuous exposure over longer periods and liver/kidney function. However, the percentage of women with evidence of good adherence in their first four weeks of participation (~40%) was sufficient to assess the impact of short-term drug use. We observed that women with evidence of good adherence had higher mean change from baseline to week 4 in their AST levels (2.90 (0.37, 5.42); $p = 0.025$) as compared to women with less than good adherence. However, corresponding changes in ALT (1.54 (−1.44, 4.52); $p = 0.31$), creatinine (0.19 (−2.60, 2.98); $p = 0.89$) and phosphorus (0.02 (−0.04, 0.08); $p = 0.53$) were not statistically significant. We did not observe an association between adherence to TDF-FTC and change in ALT, AST, creatinine or phosphorus levels between the final drug-use interval and four weeks after product withdrawal.

Discussion

In this article we report on change (grade 1+) in renal and hepatic function among African women who were assigned to the active TDF-FTC arm of a randomized, placebo-controlled clinical trial of HIV pre-exposure prophylaxis. While we did not find significant differences in renal functions, we observed a significant increase in the cumulative probabilities of grade 1+ hepatotoxicity, as measured by ALT and AST, among women assigned TDF-FTC.

Our safety findings are comparable to other PrEP studies which also did not observe more frequent renal toxicity in the active arm than in the placebo one [2,5,15].

With regard to hepatic toxicity, we observed more frequent elevated ALT or AST in participants with previous exposure to hepatitis B virus; which is consistent with the finding in the Bondo site of significantly more grade 2+ AST toxicities and higher population exposure to

Table 1 Laboratory toxicities during scheduled follow-up in the TDF-FTC arm by previous exposure to HBV

	HBsAb negative (N=804)					HBsAb positive (N=215)					
	No. of events	No. of women	% of women	Person years	Rate (per 100) person-years	No. of events	No. of women	% of women	Person years	Rate (per 100) person-years	Difference (P-value)#
ALT or AST											
Grade 1 or higher	238	180	22.4	449.4	40.05	91	68	31.6	123.4	55.09	9.2 (0.007)
Grade 2 or higher	24	21	2.6	525.0	4.00	12	12	5.6	152.0	7.90	3.0 (0.047)
Grade 3 or higher	6	6	0.7	532.6	1.13	2	2	0.9	156.6	1.28	0.2 (0.678)
Grade 4	1	1	0.1	535.8	0.19	1	1	0.5	157.2	0.64	0.3 (0.378)
PHO G2+ and creatininemia											
Grade 1 or higher	11	10	1.2	532.5	1.88	2	2	0.9	156.4	1.28	−0.3 (1.0000)
Grade 2 or higher	0	0	0.0	535.8	0.00	1	1	0.5	156.7	0.64	0.5 (0.2110)
Grade 3 or higher	0	0	0.0	535.8	0.00	1	1	0.5	156.7	0.64	0.5 (0.2110)
Grade 4	0	0	0.0	535.8	0.00	0	0	0.0	157.4	0.00	0 (-)

#Difference in the proportions of participants experiencing toxicities.

Table 2 Laboratory toxicities during scheduled follow-up in the placebo arm by previous exposure to HBV

	HBsAb negative (N=808)					HBsAb positive (N=224)					
	No. of events	No. of women	% of women	Person years	Rate (per 100) person-years	No. of events	No. of women	% of women	Person years	Rate (per 100) person-years	Difference (P-value)#
ALT or AST											
Grade 1 or higher	163	138	17.1	476.1	28.99	79	66	29.5	138.4	47.70	12.4 (0.0001)
Grade 2 or higher	20	19	2.4	527.6	3.60	4	4	1.8	165.0	2.42	−0.6 (0.7996)
Grade 3 or higher	8	8	1.0	531.3	1.51	0	0	0.0	166.4	0.00	−1.0 (0.2126)
Grade 4	2	2	0.2	533.0	0.38	0	0	0.0	166.4	0.00	−0.2 (1.0000)
PHO G2+ and creatininemia											
Grade 1 or higher	3	2	0.2	532.6	0.38	0	0	0.0	166.2	0.00	−0.2 (1.0000)
Grade 2 or higher	0	0	0.0	533.3	0.00	0	0	0.0	166.2	0.00	0 (-)
Grade 3 or higher	0	0	0.0	533.3	0.00	0	0	0.0	166.2	0.00	0 (-)
Grade 4	0	0	0.0	533.3	0.00	0	0	0.0	166.2	0.00	0 (-)

#Difference in the proportions of participants experiencing toxicities.

hepatitis B virus (39% in Bondo vs. 13%, 10% and 32%, in Bloemfontein, Pretoria, and Arusha, respectively). Additional observations are needed to confirm this preliminary finding, particularly in settings where hepatitis B virus prevalence is high and TDF-FTC will be considered for PrEP. Drug-induced liver injury (DILI) is a possible explanation of our findings. DILI has been described in patients with pre-existing hepatic illness like non-alcoholic fatty liver disease (NAFLD), hepatitis C virus related chronic hepatitis [16,17]. Our study was not designed to verify association between our observations and any of these specific pre-existing conditions.

None of the laboratory toxicities observed was accompanied by specific renal or hepatic clinical symptoms. The lack of clinical symptoms is likely due to the relatively moderate level of the toxicities observed, frequent testing and subsequent interruption or withdrawal of the study product.

Although these data indicate that the use of TDF-FTC as PrEP is safe with regard to kidney and hepatic toxicity, the results must be considered in light of overall low adherence to study product. Further, our study used the serum creatinine level and the Cockcroft-Gault formula to assess glomerular filtration and phosphatemia to assess proximal tubular function. Some studies have suggested that more sophisticated formulas – e.g. *four-variable Modification of Diet in Renal Disease formula* (MRDR equation) [18,19] – and multifactor algorithms are more accurate in assessing glomerular filtration and proximal tubular function. In a study comparing tenofovir-containing to tenofovir-sparing HAART in patients living with HIV, Horberg et al., using the MDRD equation, found that the tenofovir-exposed group had a statistically greater percentage of patients with glomerular filtration decline but not creatininemia rising to greater than 2.0 mg/dL [10]. HIV/AIDS patients treated with ARVs can develop kidney and/or liver toxicity for many other reasons than the use of TDF-FTC: HIV infection itself, other ARVs or any other medication to manage their HIV/AIDS condition. In our study, participants were HIV uninfected and healthy at baseline and took limited concomitant medication [20,21].

Our analysis and conclusions are also limited by short overall TDF-FTC exposure (i.e., follow-up was < = 52 weeks); studies and expert opinions suggest that kidney toxicities may increase over time with prolonged exposure to TDF-FTC [10,22].

The main limitation of our study is the limited adherence of participants to the study drug; only about 40% exhibited good adherence during any given test interval, and far fewer exhibited consistently good adherence over the course of their participation [11]. Nonetheless, in the TDF-FTC arm we observed higher cumulative probabilities of grade 1+ of ALT/AST and a higher proportion of participants with grade 2+ ALT/AST when previously exposed to HBV.

Conclusion

In our study population of healthy young African women, we did not observe a significant relationship between randomization to TDF-FTC and creatinine or phosphorus toxicities although we were limited in our ability to adequately assess these relationships due to overall low adherence to the study product. Women randomized to TDF-FTC had higher rates of mild to moderate ALT/AST toxicities, especially women with prior hepatitis B virus exposure. We also observed a significant increase from baseline to week four in AST values among women who were highly adherent to TDF-FTC during that interval.

Competing interests

The authors declare that they have no competing interests.

Authors' contributions

JM contributed to acquisition, analysis and interpretation of data as well as to drafting the manuscript; KN contributed to acquisition and interpretation of data as well as to revising the manuscript; MW contributed to data analysis and revised the manuscript; IdB contributed to laboratory analysis and revised the manuscript; JD contributed to data interpretation and revised the manuscript; JL, FO, MO and RM contributed data acquisition and revised the manuscript; DT contributed data analysis and interpretation as well as to revising the manuscript; LvD conceived the study, contributed to acquisition, analysis and interpretation of data as well as to revising the manuscript. All authors read and approved the final manuscript.

Acknowledgements

The authors are grateful to the women who participated in the FEM-PrEP trial, to the study staff, to the communities who partnered with us to conduct the trial, and to all of our collaborators in Africa, Belgium, and the United States. The views expressed in this publication do not necessarily reflect those of FHI 360, the funding agencies, or Gilead Sciences, Inc. JM, KN, MW, IDB, JD, JL, FO, MM, RM, DT and LVD for the FEM-PrEP Study Group.

Funding

This work was made possible by grants funded by the United States Agency for International Development (USAID): the Contraceptive and Reproductive Health Technologies and Research Utilization Program, and the Preventive Technologies Agreement No. GHO-A-00-09-00016-00. Early support was also provided by the Bill & Melinda Gates Foundation. Gilead Sciences, Inc. donated TDF-FTC and placebo. Views expressed in this publication do not necessarily reflect those of FHI 360 or the agencies that funded the study.

Author details

[1]FHI 360, 1825 Connecticut Ave, Suite 800, NW, Washington, DC 20009, USA. [2]FHI 360, Durham, NC, USA. [3]Institute of Tropical Medicine, Antwerp, Belgium. [4]JOSHA Research, Bloemfontein, South Africa. [5]Impact Research and Development Organization, Kisumu, Kenya. [6]Setshaba Research Centre, Soshanguve, Pretoria, South Africa. [7]Kilimanjaro Christian Medical Center, Kilimanjaro region, Tanzania. [8]The Bill & Melinda Gates Foundation, Seattle, WA, USA.

References

1. Baeten JM, Haberer JE, Liu AY, Sista N: **Preexposure prophylaxis for HIV prevention: where have we been and where are we going?** *J Acquir Immune Defic Syndr* 2013, **63**(Suppl 2):S122–S129.
2. Grant RM, Lama JR, Anderson PL, McMahan V, Liu AY, Vargas L, Goicochea P, Casapia M, Guanira-Carranza JV, Ramirez-Cardich ME, Montoya-Herrera O, Fernandez T, Veloso VG, Buchbinder SP, Chariyalertsak S, Schechter M, Bekker LG, Mayer KH, Kallas EG, Amico KR, Mulligan K, Bushman LR, Hance RJ, Ganoza C, Defechereux P, Postle B, Wang F, McConnell JJ, Zheng JH, Lee J, *et al*: **Preexposure chemoprophylaxis for HIV prevention in men who have sex with men.** *N Engl J Med* 2010, **363**(27):2587–2599.
3. Choopanya K, Martin M, Suntharasamai P, Sangkum U, Mock PA, Leethochawalit M, Chiamwongpaet S, Kitisin P, Natrujirote P, Kittimunkong S, Chuachoowong R, Gvetadze RJ, McNicholl JM, Paxton LA, Curlin ME, Hendrix CW, Vanichseni S: **Antiretroviral prophylaxis for HIV infection in injecting drug users in Bangkok, Thailand (the Bangkok Tenofovir Study): a randomised, double-blind, placebo-controlled phase 3 trial.** *Lancet* 2013, **381**(9883):2083–2090.
4. Celum C, Baeten JM: **Antiretroviral-based HIV-1 prevention: antiretroviral treatment and pre-exposure prophylaxis.** *Antivir Ther* 2012, **17**(8):1483–1493.
5. Thigpen MC, Kebaabetswe PM, Paxton LA, Smith DK, Rose CE, Segolodi TM, Henderson FL, Pathak SR, Soud FA, Chillag KL, Mutanhaurwa R, Chirwa LI, Kasonde M, Abebe D, Buliva E, Gvetadze RJ, Johnson S, Sukalac T, Thomas VT, Hart C, Johnson JA, Malotte CK, Hendrix CW, Brooks JT: **Antiretroviral preexposure prophylaxis for heterosexual HIV transmission in Botswana.** *N Engl J Med* 2012, **367**(5):423–434.
6. Karras A, Lafaurie M, Furco A, Bourgarit A, Droz D, Sereni D, Legendre C, Martinez F, Molina JM: **Tenofovir-related nephrotoxicity in human immunodeficiency virus-infected patients: three cases of renal failure, Fanconi syndrome, and nephrogenic diabetes insipidus.** *Clin Infect Dis* 2003, **36**(8):1070–1073.
7. Peyriere H, Reynes J, Rouanet I, Daniel N, de Boever CM, Mauboussin JM, Leray H, Moachon L, Vincent D, Salmon-Ceron D: **Renal tubular dysfunction associated with tenofovir therapy: report of 7 cases.** *J Acquir Immune Defic Syndr* 2004, **35**(3):269–273.
8. Gaspar G, Monereo A, Garcia-Reyne A, de Guzman M: **Fanconi syndrome and acute renal failure in a patient treated with tenofovir: a call for caution.** *AIDS (London, England)* 2004, **18**(2):351–352.
9. Kinai E, Hanabusa H: **Progressive renal tubular dysfunction associated with long-term use of tenofovir DF.** *AIDS Res Hum Retrovir* 2009, **25**(4):387–394.
10. Horberg M, Tang B, Towner W, Silverberg M, Bersoff-Matcha S, Hurley L, Chang J, Blank J, Quesenberry C Jr, Klein D: **Impact of tenofovir on renal function in HIV-infected, antiretroviral-naive patients.** *J Acquir Immune Defic Syndr* 2010, **53**(1):62–69.
11. Van Damme L, Corneli A, Ahmed K, Agot K, Lombaard J, Kapiga S, Malahleha M, Owino F, Manongi R, Onyango J, Temu L, Monedi MC, Mak'Oketch P, Makanda M, Reblin I, Makatu SE, Saylor L, Kiernan H, Kirkendale S, Wong C, Grant R, Kashuba A, Nanda K, Mandala J, Fransen K, Deese J, Crucitti T, Mastro TD, Taylor D: **Preexposure prophylaxis for HIV infection among African women.** *N Engl J Med* 2012, **367**(5):411–422.
12. NIAID, Division of AIDS: *The Division of AIDS Table for Grading the Severity of Adult and Pediatric Adverse Events.* Bethesda, MD, USA: National Institute of Allergy and Infectious Diseases, Division of AIDS; 2004. December 28.
13. Adams JL, Sykes C, Menezes P, Prince HM, Patterson KB, Fransen K, Crucitti T, De Baetselier I, Van Damme L, Kashuba AD: **Tenofovir diphosphate and emtricitabine triphosphate concentrations in blood cells compared with isolated peripheral blood mononuclear cells: a new measure of antiretroviral adherence?** *J Acquir Immune Defic Syndr* 2013, **62**:260–266.
14. Berger L: **Sigma diagnostics: pioneer of kits for clinical chemistry.** *Clin Chem* 1993, **39**(5):902–903.
15. Baeten JM, Donnell D, Ndase P, Mugo NR, Campbell JD, Wangisi J, Tappero JW, Bukusi EA, Cohen CR, Katabira E, Ronald A, Tumwesigye E, Were E, Fife KH, Kiarie J, Farquhar C, John-Stewart G, Kakia A, Odoyo J, Mucunguzi A, Nakku-Joloba E, Twesigye R, Ngure K, Apaka C, Tamooh H, Gabona F, Mujugira A, Panteleeff D, Thomas KK, Kidoguchi L, *et al*: **Antiretroviral prophylaxis for HIV prevention in heterosexual men and women.** *N Engl J Med* 2012, **367**(5):399–410.
16. Tarantino G, Conca P, Basile V, Gentile A, Capone D, Polichetti G, Leo E: **A prospective study of acute drug-induced liver injury in patients suffering from non-alcoholic fatty liver disease.** *Hepatol Res* 2007, **37**(6):410–415.
17. Tarantino G, Minno MNDD, Capone D: **Durg-induced liver injury: is it somehow foreseeable?** *World J Gastroenterol* 2009, **15**(23):2817–2833.
18. Levey AS, Bosch JP, Lewis JB, Greene T, Rogers N, Roth D: **A more accurate method to estimate glomerular filtration rate from serum creatinine: a new prediction equation. Modification of Diet in Renal Disease Study Group.** *Ann Intern Med* 1999, **130**(6):461–470.
19. Levey AS, Coresh J, Greene T, Stevens LA, Zhang YL, Hendriksen S, Kusek JW, Van Lente F: **Using standardized serum creatinine values in the modification of diet in renal disease study equation for estimating glomerular filtration rate.** *Ann Intern Med* 2006, **145**(4):247–254.
20. Calza L, Vanino E, Magistrelli E, Salvadori C, Cascavilla A, Colangeli V, Di Bari MA, Manfredi R, Viale P: **Prevalence of renal disease within an urban HIV-infected cohort in northern Italy.** *Clin Exp Nephrol* 2013, **18**(1):104–112.
21. Mocroft A, Kirk O, Reiss P, De Wit S, Sedlacek D, Beniowski M, Gatell J, Phillips AN, Ledergerber B, Lundgren JD: **Estimated glomerular filtration rate, chronic kidney disease and antiretroviral drug use in HIV-positive patients.** *AIDS (London, England)* 2010, **24**(11):1667–1678.
22. Rodriguez-Novoa S, Alvarez E, Labarga P, Soriano V: **Renal toxicity associated with tenofovir use.** *Expert Opin Drug Saf* 2010, **9**(4):545–559.

Population pharmacokinetic and pharmacodynamic modeling of transformed binary effect data of triflusal in healthy Korean male volunteers: a randomized, open-label, multiple dose, crossover study

Sung Min Park[1,2,3], Joomi Lee[1,2], Sook Jin Seong[1,2,3], Jong Gwang Park[1], Mi-Ri Gwon[1,2,3], Mi-sun Lim[4], Hae Won Lee[1], Young-Ran Yoon[1,2,3], Dong Heon Yang[5], Kwang-Il Kwon[6*] and Seunghoon Han[7,8*]

Abstract

Background: Triflusal is a drug that inhibits platelet aggregation. In this study we investigated the dose-exposure-response relationship of a triflusal formulation by population pharmacokinetic (PK) and pharmacodynamic (PD) modeling of its main active metabolite, hydroxy-4-(trifluoromethyl) benzoic acid (HTB).

Methods: This study was a randomized, open-label, multiple-dose, two-period, two-treatment, comparative crossover design. All volunteers received a single oral loading dose of 900 mg of triflusal on Day 1, followed by a dose of 600 mg/day from Day 2 to 9. Using data from 34 healthy volunteers, 476 HTB plasma concentration data points and 340 platelet aggregation data points were used to construct PK and PD models respectively using NONMEM (version 6.2). As the PD endpoint was qualitative, we implemented binary analysis of 'inhibition' and 'non-inhibition' rather than using the actual value of the test. The final PK-PD model was evaluated using a visual predictive check (VPC) and bootstrap.

Results: The time-concentration profile of HTB over the entire dosing period was described by a one-compartment model with a first-order formation rate constant for HTB. Weight was selected as a covariate for clearance and volume of triflusal, respectively. The structure and the population estimates for triflusal PK were as follows: oral clearance (CL/F) = $0.2 \cdot (\text{weight}/71.65)^{0.845}$ L/h, oral volume of distribution (V/F) = $8.3 \cdot (\text{weight}/71.65)$ L, and $k_f = 0.341\ h^{-1}$. A sigmoid relationship between triflusal concentration and the probability of significant inhibition with shape factor was chosen as the final PD model. No time delay between concentration and response was identified. The final structure between predicted concentration ($C^{\gamma}_{pred,ij}$) and the probability of inhibition of platelet aggregation (IPA) relationship was as follows: Probability of IPA $= C^{19}_{pred,ij}/(84.9^{19}\mu g/mL + C^{19}_{pred,ij})$. Thus, we concluded this relationship is more like quantal concentration-response relationship. The current dosing regimen was considered to be efficacious based on the EC_{50} estimate of 84.9 μg/mL obtained in this study.

Conclusions: A PK and binary probability PD model of triflusal was successfully developed for Korean healthy volunteers. The model may be used to further prediction inhibition of platelet aggregation by triflusal.

Trial registration: Clinical Research Information Service (CRIS), KCT0001299 (Registered December 5, 2014)

Keywords: HTB, Transformed binary data, Platelet aggregation, Binary probability model, NONMEM, Population pharmacokinetics and pharmacodynamics

* Correspondence: kwon@cnu.ac.kr; waystolove@catholic.ac.kr
[6]College of Pharmacy, Chungnam National University, Daejeon, South Korea
[7]Department of Pharmacology, College of Medicine, The Catholic University of Korea, Seoul, South Korea
Full list of author information is available at the end of the article

Background

Triflusal (2-acetoxy-4-(trifluoromethyl) benzoic acid), which is chemically related to salicylate [1] but is not a derivative of acetylsalicylic acid, is an antiplatelet drug [2,3] that selectively inhibits arachidonic acid (AA) metabolism in platelets by irreversibly inhibiting cyclooxygenase-1 (COX-1) and reduces thromboxane B2 (TXB2) production [4,5]. 2-Hydroxy-4-(trifluoromethyl) benzoic acid (HTB), the main active metabolite of triflusal, is formed by deacetylation upon passage through the liver [5]. Triflusal is less effective in inhibiting COX-1 and reducing TXB2 than aspirin, but more effective than HTB [4]. HTB increases the effects of triflusal on COX-1 inhibition compared with salicylic acid, the main metabolite of aspirin, which competes with the prodrug for the active site on the cyclooxygenase enzyme [5,6].

Several previous reports have described the pharmacokinetic (PK) characteristics of triflusal. After oral administration, triflusal is absorbed rapidly within the small intestine, showing an absolute bioavailability of 83–100% [7]. The plasma half-life ($T_{1/2}$) is 0.5 ± 0.1 h for triflusal and 34.4 ± 0.1 h for HTB [4]. More than 60% of the parent drug is eliminated by the kidney [7] and the values for renal clearance for triflusal and HTB were found to be 0.8 ± 0.2 L/h and 0.18 ± 0.04 L/h, respectively [5,8]. HTB reaches steady-state levels after 8–10 days of treatment [5].

The aim of this study was to quantitatively determine the dose-exposure-response relationship of triflusal in healthy Korean male subjects using a population analysis. Additionally, we suggest a method of binary analysis that might be applied to platelet aggregation data to identify pharmacodynamic (PD) markers.

Methods

Inclusion and exclusion criteria

Volunteers aged 20–55 years and within 20% of their ideal body weight [IBW (kg) = height (cm) – 100) × 0.9] were enrolled in the study. Those who were not suitable on the basis of physical examinations and routine laboratory tests (blood hematology, biochemistry, prothrombin time, bleeding time, urinalysis) were excluded.

Study design and ethical considerations

The analysis was performed using data from a randomized, open-label, multiple-dose, two-period, two-treatment, comparative crossover study involving 38 healthy adult males. The clinical trial was conducted at Kyungpook National University Hospital Clinical Trial Center (KNUH CTC) to determine the bioequivalence and non-inferiority of two different triflusal formulations, as reported previously [4].

The study was conducted in accordance with the guidelines of Good Clinical Practice and the Declaration of Helsinki and its amendments at the KNUH CTC, and was approved by the institutional review board at KNUH. Written informed consent was obtained from all volunteers before their participation.

Study drugs and dosage regimen

Triflusal capsule (Disgren capsule, 300 mg), as the reference formulation, and triflusal EC capsule (Disgren enteric-coated capsule, 300 mg), as the test formulation were manufactured and provided by Myung-In Pharm. Co., Ltd (Seoul, Republic of Korea). The subjects received the test or reference formulation in multiple doses, followed by a 13-day washout period and subsequent administration of the alternative formulation. During each period, each subject received a single 900 mg oral loading dose on Day 1, followed by a 600 mg/day maintenance dose (given as two 300 mg capsules once daily) from Day 2 to 9.

Blood sampling procedures

For measurement of the plasma concentration of HTB (PK), whole blood samples were obtained at time 0 (pre-dose), and 24, 48, 96, 144, 168, 192, 192.5, 193, 194, 196, 199, 202, and 216 h after the first dose (from Day 1 to Day 10). For platelet aggregation measurements (PD), sampling was performed at time 0 (pre-dose), and 24, 48, 96, 144, 168, 192, 196, 202, and 216 h post-dose. The overall sampling schema is presented in Figure 1.

Blood (7 mL) for PK analysis was collected into tubes containing sodium heparin, and blood (3 mL) for PD analysis was collected into tubes containing 0.109 mmol/L sodium citrate. An aliquot (1 mL) of each plasma sample was placed in a microcentrifuge tube containing 0.1 mL 0.1 M HCl to prevent degradation of triflusal in the plasma. The remaining samples were chilled promptly on crushed ice to maintain the distribution ratio between triflusal and HTB [9].

HTB plasma concentration measurements

Concentrations of HTB, rather than triflusal, were measured in this study because the level of triflusal is too low to be detected after 4 h when administered orally, as reported by Lee et al. [4,10]. Blood samples were analyzed by high-performance liquid chromatography coupled with tandem mass spectrometry (HPLC-MS/MS) [7]. Quantification was performed by multiple reaction monitoring (MRM) transitions. A C18 column was used to separate the components of the samples by chromatography. Linear calibration curves were analyzed in the range of 1 to 300 μg/mL HTB (coefficient of correlation, r = 0.999). The lower limit of quantification of HTB was 1 μg/mL. The intra-day and inter-day % CVs for HTB were each less than 15%. Figure 2 shows the plasma concentrations of HTB with respect to time.

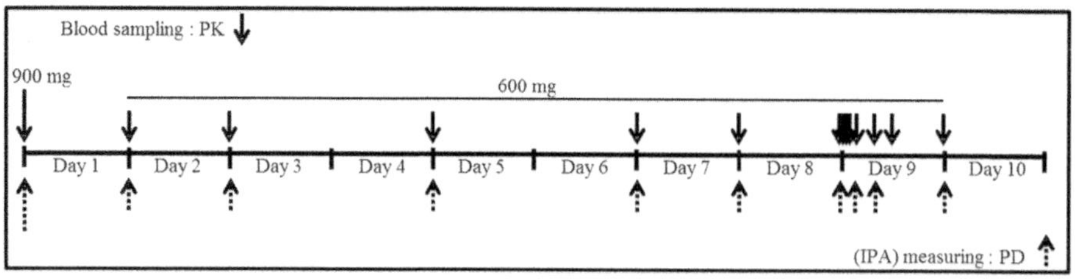

Figure 1 PK and PD study designs. Subjects (n = 34) eligible for this study were given a 900 mg loading dose on day 1, followed by a 600 mg/day maintenance dose on days 2, 3, 5, 7, 8, and 9. For PK assessment, blood samples were obtained at time 0, 24, 48, 96, 144, 168, 192, 192.5, 193, 194, 196, 199, 202 and 216 h. For PD assessment, blood samples were obtained at time 0, 24, 48, 96, 144, 168, 192, 196, 202, and 216 h. PK, pharmacokinetic; PD, pharmacodynamic; IPA, inhibition of platelet aggregation.

Platelet aggregation assessment

The tubes containing sodium citrate were centrifuged (1,000 rpm, 10 min) and 500 μL of platelet-rich plasma (PRP) was collected as the supernatant. The PRP was transferred to microcentrifuge tubes, which were capped to prevent changes in pH upon exposure to air, and the samples were kept on ice. To obtain 500 μL of platelet-poor plasma (PPP), the remaining sample in the original tubes was centrifuged again (3,000 rpm, 10 min) [11]. Platelet aggregation in PRP was assessed using a Chronolog optical aggregometer (Model 490-4D; Chrono-log, Havertown, PA, USA). Cuvettes were lined up along the two rows of the aggregometer, filled with 250 μL of PRP or PPP, and warmed for 5 min at 37°C [12]. To measure the degree of platelet aggregation, 0.5 μL AA was added to the cuvettes as an agonist, and light transmission aggregometry was observed for 5 min. The aggregometer was calibrated with a cuvette containing PRP, equaling 0% light transmission, as the baseline and with a second cuvette containing PPP, equaling 100% light transmission, as the reference [13]. Based on analyses of the blank plasma samples, which were validated in three individuals, the intra-day and inter-day precisions were calculated as (SD/mean) × 100 (%) and ranged from 2.1 to 6.8% and from 2.1 to 7.6%, respectively [4].

Dataset

In the current study, PK and PD data from 34 healthy volunteers who received the reference drug were used for population PK-PD analysis. In total, 476 HTB plasma concentration data points and 340 platelet aggregation (%) data points were included. The latent

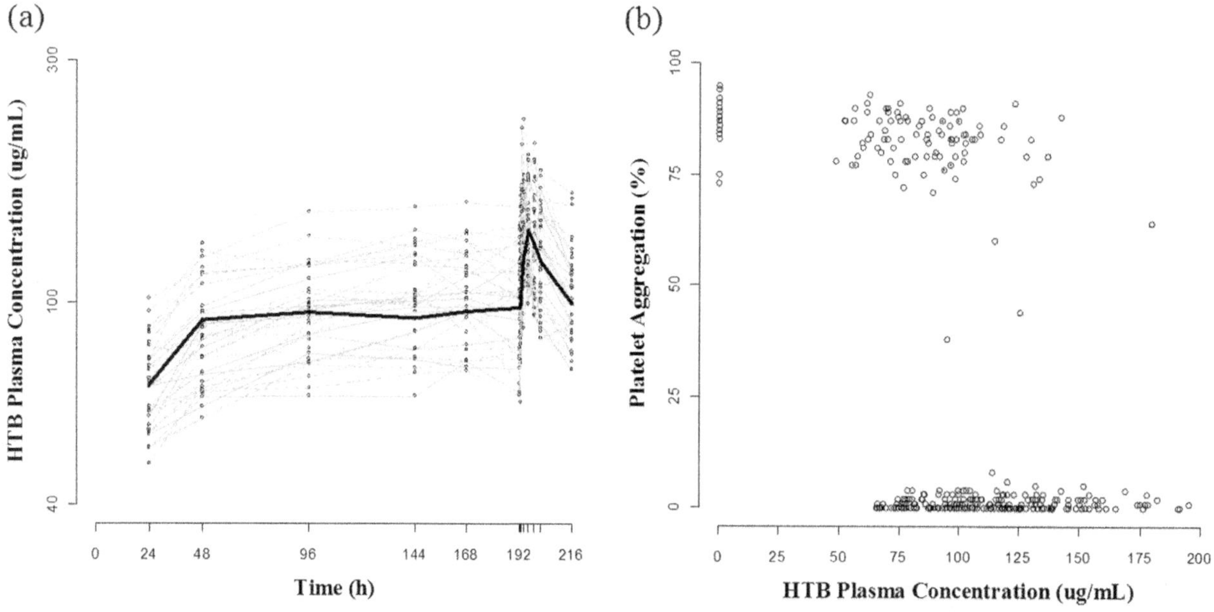

Figure 2 Raw data plot of time-concentration-response profile. (a) Profiles of observed individual and median HTB plasma concentration over time. **(b)** Observed concentration and platelet aggregation at the time of PD sampling.

variables used as candidate covariates were age, height, and weight, and levels of albumin, creatinine, serum aspartate transaminase (*AST*), and alanine transaminase (*ALT*). Creatinine clearance (*CLCR*), calculated using the Cockcroft-Gault equation, was also included.

Population PK-PD model development

The population PK-PD analysis was conducted by nonlinear mixed effects modeling using NONMEM (ver. 6.2; Icon Development Solution, Ellicott City, MD, USA). The estimate and the between-subject variability for PK-PD parameters were investigated. The first-order conditional estimation (FOCE) method with interaction option was used whenever applicable [14]. The between-subject variability of each parameter of the basic model was applied using the exponential model:

$$P_{ij} = \theta_j \times exp\left(\eta_{ij}\right)$$

where P_{ij} is the value of the jth parameter in the ith individual, θ_j is the typical value of the jth population parameter, and η_{ij} is a random variable for the ith individual in the jth parameter. It is assumed that η_{ij} is normally distributed, with a mean of zero and a variance of ω^2, and that $\eta_{ij} \approx N(0, \omega_{ij}^2)$. The residual variability, consisting of intra-individual variability, experimental errors, process noise, and/or model mis-specifications, was modeled using additive ($\varepsilon_{add,ij}$), proportional ($\varepsilon_{pro,ij}$), and combined error structures. The combined additive and proportional error model on the following equation was initially applied to explain the gaps between the observed values and those predicted by individual PK parameters:

$$C_{ij} = C_{pred,ij} \times \left(1 + \varepsilon_{pro,ij}\right) + \varepsilon_{add,ij}$$

where C_{ij} is the jth observed value in the ith individual, and $\varepsilon_{pro,ij}$ and $\varepsilon_{add,ij}$ are the residual intra-individual variability with a mean of zero and variances of σ^2_{pro} and σ^2_{add}, respectively. A similar approach was made to the PD observations. The standard errors, which give information on the precision of the parameter estimates, were explored using NONMEM's "$COVARIANCE" step.

Models were evaluated using diagnostic scatter plots, goodness-of-fit plots, and the log likelihood ratio test (LRT). The results for LRT were considered statistically significant if the objective function value (OFV) decreased by 3.84 ($p = 0.05$); this was used as a cut-off criterion for model improvement.

For PK, various absorption functions and distributional (1-compartment vs. multi-compartment) models were compared. When linking PK-PD relationship, two different models – binary probability and inhibition of build-up – were tried sequentially to find the best description on the PD data. The binary probability model uses a form of relationship similar to the Michaelis-Menten equation, $C^{\gamma}_{pred,ij}/(EC_{50}{}^{\gamma} + C^{\gamma}_{pred,ij})$ to explain instantaneous PK-PD relationship. In this equation, $C_{pred,ij}$ is the estimated concentration over time for individuals, EC_{50} is the plasma concentration corresponding to the half-maximal response, and γ is the shape factor. To implement this approach, the PD data (% platelet aggregation) was transformed to a binary format based upon the finding that the distribution of PD observation (the maximum platelet aggregation observed in each sample) was clearly bimodal (Figure 2). The values above 74% were regarded as no inhibition of platelet aggregation (IPA), and thus as DV = 0, whereas values below 74 were regarded as IPA (DV = 1), according to a guideline presenting the normal ranges for the degree (%) of aggregation in platelet-rich plasma [15]. To find a reliable initial estimate for this model, a logistic regression procedure was performed in advance. For a binary output variable, Y, we can model conditional probability $P(Y = 1 \mid X = x)$ as a function of x [16]. Let $\pi(x)$ be a linear function of x, $\pi(x) = P(Y = 1 \mid X = x)$. The model can be written as $\pi(x) = exp(\beta_0 + \beta_1 x) / exp(\beta_0 + \beta_1 x) + 1$. Equivalently, by a logit transformation, the logistic regression model has a linear relationship, $logit(\pi(x)) = log(\pi(x) / 1 - \pi(x)) = \beta_0 + \beta_1 x$, where β_0 is the intercept coefficient and β_1 is the slope coefficient, for which the sign is positive or negative if $\pi(x)$ is a strictly increasing or decreasing function of x, respectively [17]. Using the frequency of DV = 1 at each time point, the intercept (β_0) and slope (β_1) were estimated using SAS software (ver. 9.2; SAS Institute, Inc., Cary, NC, USA). The inhibition of build-up model was tried to evaluate whether there is a time-delay between concentration and response in the form of continuous variable. The differential equation for platelet aggregation at a certain HTB concentration is as follows [18]:

$$dR/dt = k_{in} \times [1-(I_{max} \cdot C)/(IC_{50} + C)] - k_{out} \times R$$

where dR/dt is the rate of change of the measured response (*R*) over time, k_{in} is the turnover input rate for production of the response, I_{max} is the fraction representing the maximal capacity by which the drug can inhibit platelet aggregation ($0 \le I_{max} \le 1$), *C* is the HTB concentration, IC_{50} is the median inhibition concentration, and k_{out} is the turnover output rate of the response.

Covariate analysis

The parameter-covariate relationship, which explains why PK and PD vary among individuals, was explored using variables in the dataset. In the exploratory analysis, scatter plots of one covariate versus another were used to assess correlations between covariates and of parameters versus covariates. The numerical procedure used generalized additive modeling (GAM), as implemented in the Xpose library (ver. 4.4.0, Department of Pharmaceutical Biosciences of Uppsala University, Uppsala, Sweden) [19] of the 'R' software (ver. 2.15.3; R Foundation for Statistical Computing, Vienna, Austria). In this procedure, a response random variable, Y, is regressed on the individual covariates (X_j) according to the general equation:

$$E\left(Y \,\middle|\, X_1, X_2, \cdots, X_p\right) = s_0 + \sum\nolimits_{j=1}^{p} s_j\left(X_j\right)$$

where the s_0 is an intercept, and $s_1(X_1), \cdots, s_p(X_p)$ are smooth functions that are estimated in a nonparametric fashion. In the equation, candidate covariates with the greatest decrease in the Akaike information criterion were selected as final covariates in the PK model when there was a reduction of at least 3.84 compared with the previous model, and the relationship between the random variable, η, for each parameter and the candidate covariates was improved. Otherwise, they were dropped from the model.

Graphical analyses using goodness-of-fit plots – including observed-versus-population-predicted, observed-versus-individual-predicted, and residual diagnostics – were also conducted to diagnose the degree of model development.

Model evaluation

Bootstrap was recruited to check the robustness of the PK-PD model and parameter estimates. The median value and 95% confidence interval for each parameter were obtained from 1,000 bootstrap dataset. For the PK model, a visual predictive check (VPC) was implemented to further evaluate the accuracy and predictive performance. A total of 1,000 replicate simulation was performed and the 50th (estimated population median), 5th, and 95th percentiles of the created concentrations plotted against time were compared with the overlaid observed concentrations. In addition, predicted concentration-response relationship is plotted with the predicted probability of each concentration data observed at the time of PD sampling.

Sample size determination

We considered the sample size for having an 80% power at a significance level of 0.05 for bioequivalence trials. It was calculated under the condition of the equivalence limit of 22.3%, the true mean difference of 10%, and the standard deviation of 24.2%. The calculation was performed by a formula suggested from Chow et al. [20]. Volunteers were randomly assigned to one of two sequences with simple randomization using SAS software (ver. 9.2; SAS Institute, Inc., Cary, NC, USA).

Statistical analyses

The demographic data were presented using descriptive statistical analysis performed with the standard SPSS package (version 12.0 for Windows, SPSS, College Station, TX, USA). The mean, standard deviation, and range were obtained for each variable.

Results

Study population

Volunteers were recruited from August 2008 to September 2008. In total, thirty-eight volunteers were enrolled in this study. Four subjects dropped out because of severe dental pain, a medication administration error, a missing follow-up urinalysis, or platelet aggregation 1% of baseline in the second period. Data from the remaining 34 subjects were analyzed to construct the PK and PD models. According to the CONSORT flow diagram, Figure 3 shows the subject disposition. The age, height, and weight (means ± SD) of the subjects were 24.1 ± 1.7 years, 176.1 ± 4.9 cm, and 70.8 ± 9.0 kg, respectively (Table 1).

Population PK modeling

The time-concentration profile of HTB over the entire multiple-dosing period was best described by a one-compartment model with first-order formation rate constant of HTB. This model was implemented in the PREDPP library subroutine "ADVAN2 TRANS2" in NONMEM. Residual variability was best described by the proportional error model, which explained the difference between the predicted and observed values for individuals and resulted in a significant decrease in the OFV. Weight was selected as the only covariate candidate after GAM analysis which explains existing knowledge about the PK of the drug. The effect of weight on *CL/F* and *V/F* was explained best with following each equation:

$$CL/F = \theta_1 \times (\text{weight}/71.65)^{\theta 4}$$

$$V/F = \theta_2 \times (\text{weight}/71.65)$$

where θ_1 and θ_2 were the estimated typical values of *CL* and *V* with a median weight (71.65) and θ_4 was the estimated influential factor for weight. Weight produced 30.782 (equivalent to $p < 0.001$, 1 degree of freedom) decrease in the minimized OFV as well as the change in the random BSV for *CL/F* from 18.5% to 14.9% and for *V/F* from 15.6% to 9.5% (as % CV). Because only one demographic variable (weight) was selected as a meaningful covariate, the process of backward covariate exclusion was omitted.

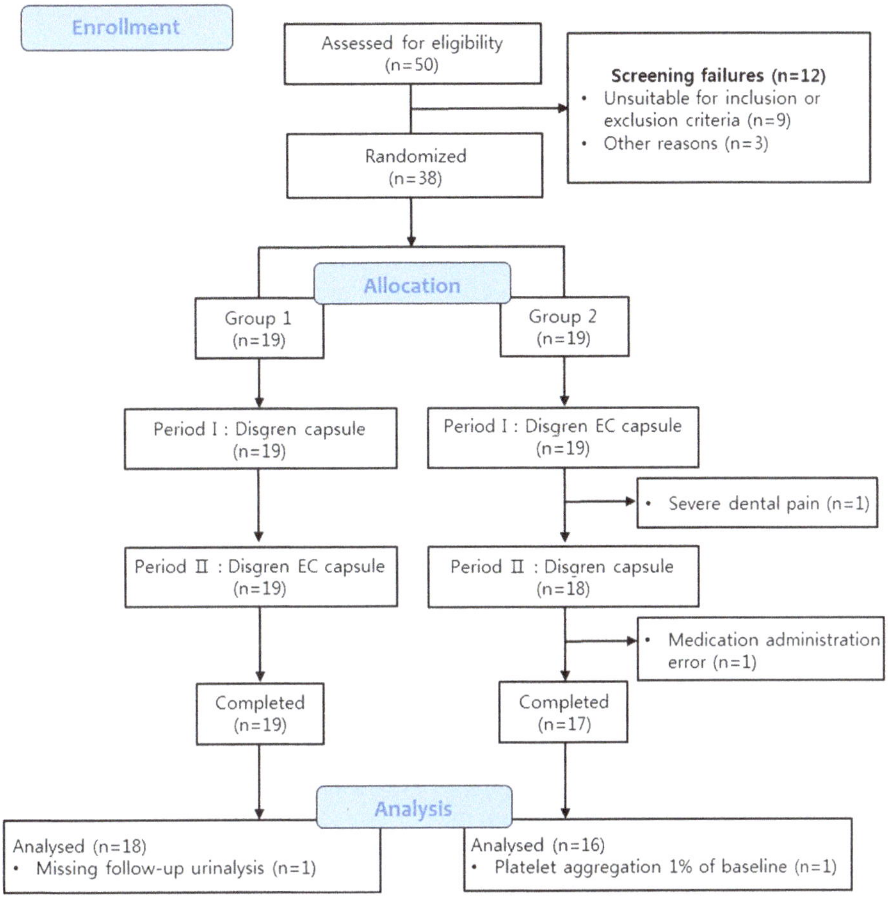

Figure 3 CONSORT flow diagram of subject disposition.

The goodness-of-fit plots for the final PK model are presented in Figure 4. Final estimates from the PK model, explaining the mean value and the between-subject variability, are listed in Table 2. The minimum concentration at steady state ($C_{ss,min}$) was estimated to be 103.5 μg/mL using the values of final population PK parameters; in addition, the estimated value of the accumulation factor was 2.26.

Population PD modeling

The binary probability model was selected as the final PK-PD structure. The results of the estimation from this PD model were as follows: $\gamma = 19$ and $EC_{50} = 84.9$ μg/mL. In addition to these parameter estimates, information such as the observed and predicted number of times that non-aggregation occurred at each time point is shown in Table 3. The between-subject variability was only applied to EC_{50} and was well explained. The values estimated from the PD model are summarized in Table 2.

Table 1 Demographic information of the healthy volunteers

Group	Number of subjects (n = 34) mean ± SD (Min – Max)
Age (years)	24.1 ± 1.7 (21 – 28)
Height (cm)	176.1 ± 4.9 (167.1 – 184.2)
Weight (kg)	70.8 ± 9.0 (53.3 – 89.7)

Model evaluation

The bootstrap results showed acceptable robustness of the model and are presented together with the final estimates in Table 2. The VPC result (Figure 5) showed that the prediction of the simulated data well-matched the observed concentration-time profiles. This graph, representing a visual internal validation of the model, showed that most of the observed data points were overlaid between the 5th and 95th percentiles.

Discussion

The PK and PD characteristics of triflusal were investigated using a non-linear mixed effects analysis. The objective of this study was to develop a population PK and PD model of the triflusal formulation, an established uncoated capsule, in healthy Korean male subjects. Plasma concentrations of the active metabolite, HTB, and the

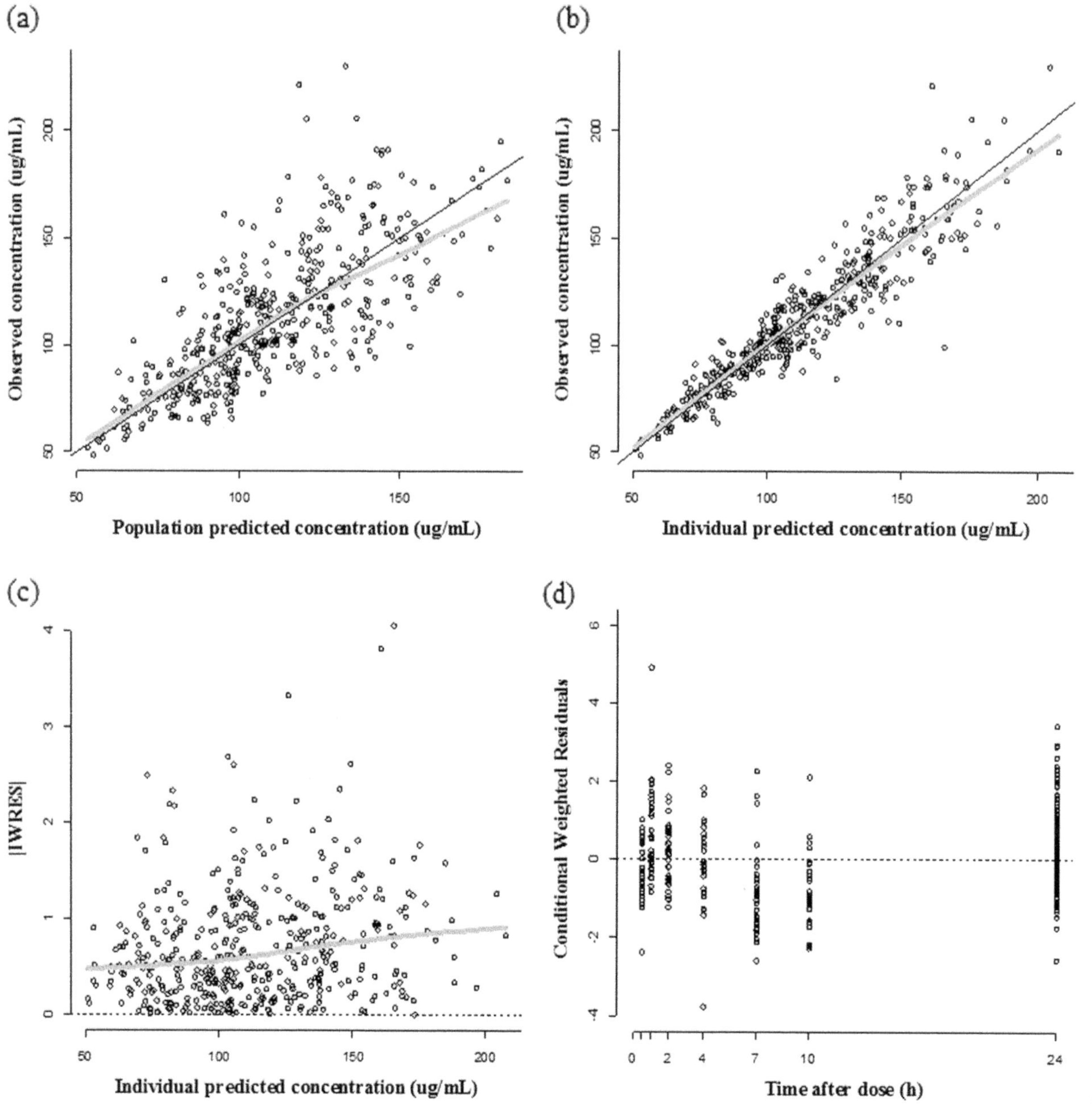

Figure 4 Goodness-of-fit plots of the final population pharmacokinetic model. (a) OBS versus PRED; **(b)** OBS versus IPRED; **(c)** |IWRES| versus IPRED; **(d)** CWRES versus time-after the last dose. Circle: observation; solid black line: line of identity; gray line: loess regression line. OBS, observation; PRED, population prediction; IPRED, individual prediction; |IWRES|, absolute individual weighted residuals; CWRED, conditional weighted residuals.

degree of platelet aggregation inhibition were measured to demonstrate the PK and PD properties. Reasonable estimates for parameters of the PK model were obtained, reflecting the potential for accurately predicting the information sought. The plots of the observed concentrations versus population-predicted or individual-predicted concentrations showed that the PK model was well structured, and the plot of time versus conditional weighted residuals suggested that the errors had homogeneous variances.

Our final HTB PK structure includes first-order formation and 1-compartment disposition. This is plausible judging from the immediate increase in HTB concentration on the day of full-PK study after dosing time and the rate of concentration increase which is the fastest at immediate post-dose and decreases thereafter (Figure 2). This finding is consistent to the model used by Valle et al. [3]. On the contrary, Yun et al. [21] suggested a 2-compartment model for HTB disposition. But we considered this model would behavior like a 1-compartment

Table 2 Final estimates of population PK and PD parameters

Parameter	Description (units)	Estimates from final model		Bootstrap results	Shrinkage (%)
		Estimate	% RSE[a]	Median (95% CI)	
Fixed effect					
Pharmacokinetic					
$CL/F = \theta_1 * (\text{weight}/71.65)^{\theta 4}$					
θ_1	TV of CL/F (L/h) for subject whose weight = 71.65 kg	0.200	2.7	0.1998 (0.1995 – 0.2002)	
θ_4	Exponent of weight proportional to CL/F	0.845	17.4	0.840 (0.830 – 0.850)	
$V_d/F = \theta_2 * (\text{weight}/71.65)$					
θ_2	TV of V_d (L) for subject whose weight = 71.65 kg	8.300	2.7	8.281 (8.267 – 8.295)	
$k_f = \theta_3$	TV of k_f (h^{-1})	0.341	15.1	0.345 (0.341 – 0.348)	
Pharmacodynamic					
θ_5	TV of EC_{50} (μg/mL)	84.9	4.0	85.19 (84.98 – 85.40)	
θ_6	TV of γ	19.2	22.4	20.70 (20.32 – 21.08)	
BSV (%CV)					
Pharmacokinetic					
ω_1^2	BSV for CL/F	14.9	21.0	14.4 (14.3 – 14.5)	0.6
ω_2^2	BSV for V_d	9.5	57.8	8.6 (8.4 – 8.8)	40.2
ω_3^2	BSV for k_f	88.0	26.5	73.5 (72.8 – 74.1)	10.5
Pharmacodynamic					
ω_4^2	BSV for EC_{50}	21.8	28.4	21.4 (21.2 – 21.5)	8.3
ω_5^2	BSV for γ	0 (Fixed)	NE	-	-
Residual error (σ^2)[b]					
Proportional error		0.098	6.5	0.0977 (0.0973 – 0.0981)	11.5

% RSE, % relative standard error; CI, confidence interval; CL/F, oral clearance; TV, typical value at population level; V_d/F, oral volume of distribution; k_f, first-order formation rate constant; EC_{50}, HTB concentration at which the probability of IPA is 50%; γ, shape factor; BSV, between-subject variability; % CV, % coefficient of variation; NE, not estimated.
[a]% RSE is calculated from ω^2.
[b]Additive residual error was not selected.

Table 3 Observed and predicted IPA over time

Time	Number of subjects	Number of observed IPA (%)	Number of predicted IPA (%)
0 h	34	1 (3%)	0 (0%)
24 h	34	2 (6%)	2 (6%)
48 h	34	11 (32%)	11 (32%)
96 h	34	29 (85%)	25 (74%)
144 h	34	25 (74%)	28 (82%)
168 h	34	27 (79%)	30 (88%)
192 h	34	30 (88%)	30 (88%)
196 h	34	34 (100%)	34 (100%)
202 h	34	34 (100%)	34 (100%)
216 h	34	28 (82%)	30 (88%)

IPA, inhibition of platelet aggregation.

model because the distributional rate constant between compartments were much (approximately 60 times) larger than the elimination rate constant and the equilibrium between compartments will be obtained within 1 h after dose. Judging from the time of maximum plasma concentration attainment (postdose 4–5 h), this distributional characteristic might be superimposed by the absorption as well as the elimination.

Covariate model building was established by the relationship between the subjects' body features and parameters in the PK model. Weight accounted for approximately 19 % and 39 % of between-subject variability for CL/F and V/F, respectively, judging from the decrease of ω^2 for corresponding parameters. Particularly, V/F was directly proportional to weight (exponent = 1) and the fact suggested that weight may be used as a scaling factor for triflusal dose. However, definite conclusions could not be made for following reason; 1) this study did not consider the PK of triflusal; thus, weight might be influential to the

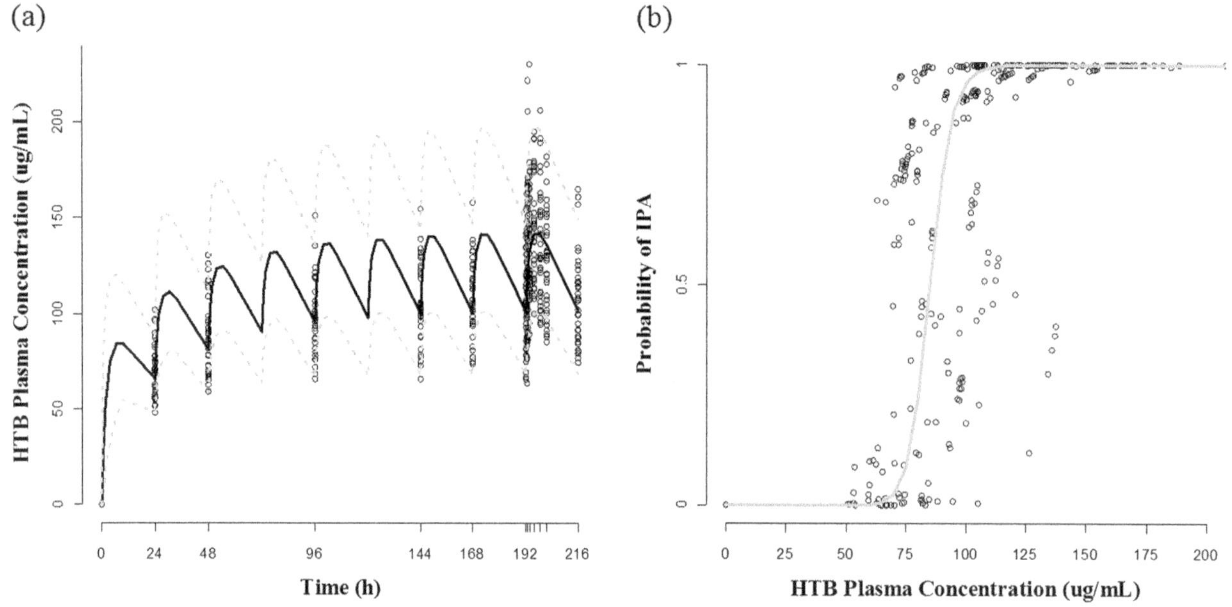

Figure 5 Results of model evaluation. (a) Visual predictive check result. The 5th and 95th percentiles (dashed gray line) and the median value (solid black line) from the simulated data are plotted against the observed concentration data (circle) according to time. **(b)** Predicted HTB concentration-probability of IPA curve; Circle: expected IPA for each HTB concentration measured at the time of PD observation; IPA, inhibition of platelet aggregation.

disposition of triflusal including metabolic fraction to HTB (which was only explained with *F* in this study), 2) the clinical significance of this finding needs further investigations together with its pharmacodynamics variability, therapeutic index and clinical effectiveness. In addition, even though HTB is mainly (>60%) excreted in urine, *CLCR* was not selected as a meaningful covariate for HTB *CL/F*. We consider that the effect of weight superimposed that of *CLCR*. It was expected that studies involving triflusal and HTB PK in patients with various renal function will be essential to elucidate the exact influence of renal function.

Based on the value of EC_{50} (=84.9 μg/mL) estimated in this study, the current dosing regimen was considered to be efficacious judging from the $C_{ss,min}$ value (=103.5 μg/mL) and the concentration-response relationship which showed quantal characteristics ($\gamma = 19$). The saturated value of E_{max} as 1 seemed reasonable, because there was no significant model improvement when the parameter was allowed to be estimated.

Another method, the binary probability model to construct the PD model using transformed binary data, was introduced to show characteristics of the PD data without much information loss. This model resulted in successful explanation of binary data characteristics by the estimates, even though a turnover model was not constructed because of the modified binary data characteristics. To date, this is the first report evaluating quantitative PD data transformed into qualitative binary data possessing one of two values. We recommend this new approach of using probability to estimate parameters that show predictive ability for the presence of platelet aggregation. This model also provided a specific method for potential use with binary data in the case of high intra-individual variability for PD.

This study has some limitations. First, only HTB concentrations were used in our population PK and PD model without measurement of the parent drug. Although triflusal is a prodrug which has no pharmacologic effect, if a study involving the concentration measurement of both triflusal and HTB is conducted, a better description for the HTB formation will be obtained. This approach may enable the identification of influential factors for HTB formation process including first-pass metabolism and hepatic clearance of triflusal. Second, despite the possible loss of information from the data transformation, a PD model using probability (binary data model) was developed to evaluate the extreme values in our PD data, as seen in the scatter diagram. To overcome this problem, more accurate and precise quantitative analytic method to measure the degree of platelet aggregation should be required.

Using the VPC, which is one method of model evaluation, prediction is possible when given not only different dosage- and time-concentrations but also the probability of IPA. Accordingly, optimal dosage regimens could be determined by model-fitted parameter estimates without additional clinical trials. The model may be clinically useful for other similar studies. Finally, this study was conducted in healthy volunteers, rather than in patients. Thus, it is also necessary to construct a model estimating reasonable parameters from patients in a more realistic setting.

Conclusions

A PK and binary probability PD model of triflusal was successfully developed for Korean healthy volunteers. The model may be used to further predict inhibition of platelet aggregation by triflusal.

Competing interests

The authors declare that they have no competing interests.

Authors' contributions

SMP constructed and developed the PK and PD models and drafted the manuscript. JL, SJS, JGP, MRG, MSL, HWL, DHY, and YRY helped prepare datasets, develop the PK and PD models, and interpret the results of the estimated parameters. KIK and SH designed and supervised the clinical study, developed the PK and PD models, and edited the manuscript. All authors read and approved the final manuscript.

Acknowledgements

This research was supported by grants from the National Project for Personalized Genomic Medicine, Ministry of Health & Welfare, Republic of Korea (A111218-PG02); the Bio & Medical Technology Development Program of the National Research Foundation (NRF) funded by the Ministry of Science, ICT & Future Planning, Republic of Korea (NRF-2013M3A9B6046416); the Pfizer Modeling & Simulation Education Center in Korea (PMECK); and the Korea Health 21 R&D Project, Ministry of Health & Welfare, Republic of Korea (A070001).

Author details

[1]Clinical Trial Center, Kyungpook National University Hospital, Daegu, South Korea. [2]Department of Biomedical Science, Kyungpook National University Graduate School, Daegu, South Korea. [3]BK21 Plus KNU Bio-Medical Convergence Program for Creative Talent, Kyungpook National University Graduate School, 680 Gukchaebosang-ro, Jung-gu, Daegu 700-842, South Korea. [4]College of Pharmacy, Yeungnam University, Daegu, South Korea. [5]Department of Internal Medicine, Division of Cardiology, Kyungpook National University School of Medicine, Daegu, South Korea. [6]College of Pharmacy, Chungnam National University, Daejeon, South Korea. [7]Department of Pharmacology, College of Medicine, The Catholic University of Korea, Seoul, South Korea. [8]PIPET (Pharmacometrics Institute for Practical Education and Training), Seoul, South Korea.

References

1. Matias-Guiu J, Ferro JM, Alvarez-Sabin J, Torres F, Jiménez MD, Lago A, Melo T: **Comparison of triflusal and aspirin for prevention of vascular events in patients after cerebral infarction: the TACIP Study: a randomized, double-blind, multicenter trial.** *Stroke* 2003, **34**:840–848.
2. McNeely W, Goa KL: **Triflusal.** *Drugs* 1998, **7**:823–833.
3. Valle M, Barbanoj MJ, Donner A, Izquierdo I, Herranz U, Klein N, Eichler HG, Müller M, Brunner M: **Access of HTB, main metabolite of triflusal, to cerebrospinal fluid in healthy volunteers.** *Eur J Clin Pharmacol* 2005, **61**:103–111.
4. Lee HW, Lim MS, Seong SJ, Lee J, Park J, Seo JJ, Yun HY, Baek IH, Kwon KI, Yoon YR: **A phase I study to characterize the multiple-dose pharmacokinetics, pharmacodynamics and safety of new enteric-coated triflusal formulations in healthy male volunteers.** *Expert Opin Drug Metab Toxicol* 2011, **7**:1471–1479.
5. Anninos H, Andrikopoulos G, Pastromas S, Sakellariou D, Theodorakis G, Vardas P: **Triflusal: an old drug in modern antiplatelet therapy. Review of its action, use, safety and effectiveness.** *Hellenic J Cardiol* 2009, **50**:199–207.
6. Rao GH, Reddy KR, White JG: **Effect of acetaminophen and salicylate on aspirin-induced inhibition of human platelet cyclo-oxygenase.** *Prostaglandins Leukot Med* 1982, **9**:109–115.
7. Murdoch D, Plosker GL: **Triflusal: a review of its use in cerebral infarction and myocardial infarction, and as thromboprophylaxis in atrial fibrillation.** *Drugs* 2006, **66**:671–692.
8. Gonzalez-Correa JA, De La Cruz JP: **Triflusal: an antiplatelet drug with a neuroprotective effect?** *Cardiovasc Drug Rev* 2006, **24**:11–24.
9. Cho HY, Jeong TJ, Lee YB: **Simultaneous determination of triflusal and its major active metabolite, 2-hydroxy-4-trifluoromethyl benzoic acid, in rat and human plasma by high-performance liquid chromatography.** *J Chromatogr B Analyt Technol Biomed Life Sci* 2003, **798**:257–264.
10. Ramis J, Mis R, Forn J, Torrent J, Gorina E, Jane F: **Pharmacokinetics of triflusal and its main metabolite HTB in healthy subjects following a single oral dose.** *Eur J Drug Metab Pharmacokinet* 1991, **16**:269–273.
11. Dong HP, Wu HM, Chen SJ, Chen CY: **The effect of butanolides from Cinnamomum tenuifolium on platelet aggregation.** *Molecules* 2013, **18**:11836–11841.
12. Harrison P, Mackie I, Mumford A, Briggs C, Liesner R, Winter M, Machin S: **Guidelines for the laboratory investigation of heritable disorders of platelet function.** *Br J Haematol* 2011, **155**:30–44.
13. Zhou L, Schmaier AH: **Platelet aggregation testing in platelet-rich plasma: description of procedures with the aim to develop standards in the field.** *Am J Clin Pathol* 2005, **123**:172–183.
14. Beal S, Sheiner L: *NONMEM User's Guide Part I.* San Francisco: University of California at San Francisco; 1992.
15. Chrono-log corporation: *Instruction manual for the chrono-log model 490 optical aggregometers.* Havertown, PA, USA; 2005:31.
16. Agresti A: **Logistic Regression.** In *Categorical Data Analysis.* 2nd edition. New York: Wiley; 2002:166.
17. Casella G, Berger RL: **Regression Models.** In *Statistical Inference.* 2nd edition. California: Wadsworth; 2001:592.
18. Gabrielsson J, Weiner D: **Pharmacodynamic Concepts.** In *Pharmacokinetic and Pharmacodynamic Data Analysis: Concepts and Applications.* 4th edition. Stockholm: Swedish Pharmaceutical Press; 2007:265.
19. Jonsson EN, Karlsson MO: **Xpose–an S-PLUS based population pharmacokinetic/pharmacodynamic model building aid for NONMEM.** *Comput Methods Programs Biomed* 1999, **58**:51–64.
20. Chow SC, Wang H: **On sample size calculation in bioequivalence trials.** *J Pharmacokinet Pharmacodyn* 2001, **28**:155–169.
21. Yun HY, Kang W, Lee BY, Park S, Yoon YR, Yeul Ma J, Kwon KI: **Semi-Mechanistic Modelling and Simulation of Inhibition of Platelet Aggregation by Antiplatelet Agents.** *Basic Clin Pharmacol Toxicol* 2014. in press.

A Swiss real world best practice experience in three different clinical settings of the 6 hour fingolimod first dose observation procedure

Simon P Ramseier[1], Serge Roth[2] and Adam Czaplinski[3*]

Abstract

Background: The Swiss label of oral fingolimod (0.5 mg once daily) requires a 6-hour first dose observation (FDO) including an ECG prior to and 6 hours after the first intake but in comparison to other countries such as Austria, Australia and Canada there are no restrictions regarding the clinical settings of the FDO procedure in Switzerland. We present here our real-world experience of the 6 hour FDO procedure in three different clinical settings, following fingolimod treatment initiation. This is the first report on the FDO of fingolimod in these real-world clinical settings in Swiss patients with multiple sclerosis (MS).

Methods: This was a retrospective, multi-clinic, observational study of 136 patients with relapsing-remitting multiple sclerosis. Summary statistics have been used to present the data.

Results: Only two patients (<1.5% [2/136]) experienced symptoms after the first dose of fingolimod. Atrioventricular conduction abnormalities were reported in 3% (4/136) of patients, which resolved spontaneously within 24 hours of treatment initiation. During the average 6.8 months follow-up, 96% (131/136) of the patients remained on therapy

Conclusions: These findings support the safety and feasibility of FDO and tolerability of fingolimod in real-world clinical settings.

Keywords: Multiple sclerosis, Fingolimod, Cardiovascular function, Heart rate

Background

Fingolimod 0.5 mg once-daily (FTY720; Gilenya™, Novartis Pharma AG, Basel, Switzerland), a sphingosine 1-phosphate (S1P) receptor modulator, is the first oral therapy approved by the Swiss Regulatory Agency for treating patients with relapsing-remitting multiple sclerosis (RRMS) to reduce the frequency of relapses and delay disability progression [1]. Various pharmacodynamics effects of fingolimod are manifested as a consequence of the fingolimod mechanism of action of S1P receptor modulation since these receptors are ubiquitously distributed across different tissues [2]. Fingolimod initiation is associated with a transient reduction in heart rate and possible disturbances in atrioventricular (AV) conduction within the first few hours after first intake [3-5]. Hence, already at the time of market authorization in January 2011, the Swiss label of fingolimod made it a mandate to perform an ECG prior to and after 6 hours of the first dose administration, and recommended regular monitoring of blood pressure and pulse (first dose observation, FDO), which is similar to the current recommendations of other international health authorities. Here, we report for the first time the real-world experience of fingolimod treatment initiation and 6 hours FDO procedure in three different clinical settings outside of University Hospitals (MS centre, day clinic, private practice) since there are no restrictions on location of the FDO procedure in Switzerland.

Methods

Data were collected retrospectively from the charts of RRMS patients treated and monitored as required by the Swiss label for fingolimod between August 2011 and May 2012 at three different locations (i.e. it did not encompass the new recommendations regarding the observation of patients with pre-existing cardiac conditions,

* Correspondence: mc@neurozentrumbellevue.ch
[3]Neurocentre Bellevue, Theaterstrasse 8, Zurich CH-8001, Switzerland
Full list of author information is available at the end of the article

published by the Swiss Regulatory Agency in October 2012 [1]). Site 1 was the MS centre, Cantonal Hospital Aarau, Aarau ($n = 58$), site 2 was the Clinique de Carouge in Carouge (office-based neurologist using a day clinic for FDO, $n = 17$) and site 3 was the Neurocentre Bellevue in Zurich, an office-based neurologist performing the FDO in his practice ($n = 61$). Prior to the FDO appointment all patients received essential information on fingolimod from their treating physician. They were informed about the potential side effects of fingolimod (short and long term), about the FDO procedure, including the reasons for ECG and the 6 h observation. Information was also provided on the required follow-up examinations after FDO over the next few months, including blood analysis and ophthalmological examination required by the Swiss label. Patients received recommendations on taking tablets including explanation of tablet packaging and drug description. The Cantonal Ethics Committee Zurich waived the review of this study as the data were obtained from retrospective chart reviews, and the information was recorded by the investigator in such manner that subjects cannot be identified, directly or through identifiers linked to the subjects.

Results and discussion

Overview of FDO process and associated workload

FDO measurements were performed in the daily clinical setting, which involved an ECG at the beginning and at the end of 6 hours and hourly recording of vital parameters (blood pressure and heart rate) (Figure 1). Between active FDO assessments, performed by the nurse or the physician, patients entertained themselves with activities such as reading, using their personal laptop, lunching together or discussing health related aspects of MS. A nurse took care of up to 2 patients using a single ECG device. She spent two times ten minutes to apply and record the ECG (prior to and 6 hours after the first intake), as well as five times 2 minutes to measure the vital parameters, representing a total workload of 30 minutes for the nurse over the 6 hour period. Interpretation of

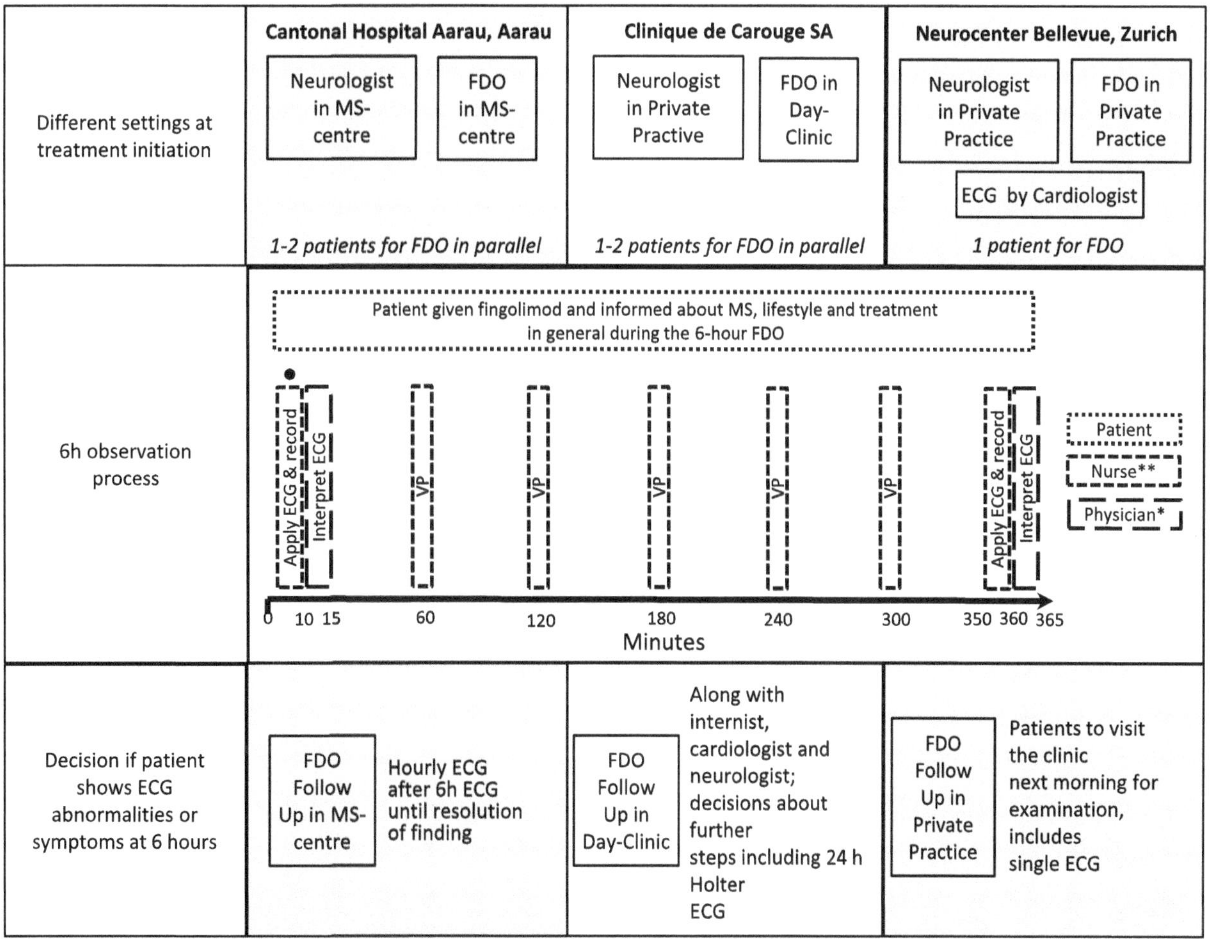

Figure 1 Overview of the FDO process in the three different clinical settings. Not for Neurocentre Bellevue. ECG recording was performed a number of days prior to FDO; *Depends on site, usually internist, cardiologist or neurologist; **Nurse or MS nurse; VP, vital parameters.

Table 1 FDO outcomes in the three centres

	Site 1 Cantonal Hospital, Aarau	Site 2 Clinique de Carouge SA	Site 3 Neurocentre Bellevue	Total
Total number of patients undergoing FDO	58	17	61	136
Patients with no FDO events (n)	57	16	57	130
Patients discharged at 6 hours (n)	57	16	59	132
Patients requiring extended observation after 6 hours (n)	1[a]	0	0	1
Patients requiring observation on 2nd day (n)	0	1[b]	2[c]	3
Symptomatic patients (n)	0	0	2[d]	2
Patients with ECG Abnormalities (n)	1[a]	1[b]	2[c]	4
1st degree AV Block (n)	0	0	2[c]	2
2nd degree AV Block Type I (Wenkebach) (n)	1[a]	1[b]	0	2
2nd degree AV Block Type II (Mobitz Type II) (n)	0	0	0	0
Symptomatic events that resolved by the end of 6 h observation (n)	0	0	2[d]	2
ECG events that had resolved at extended observation or follow-up examination on the 2nd day (n)	1[a]	1[b]	2[c]	4

[a]2nd degree AV block, Wenkebach type: extension of observation by 1 h and repeat of ECG; AV block had resolved.
[b]2nd degree AV block, Wenkebach type: 24 h Holter ECG as a precautionary measure; AV block had resolved and no further finding observed on Holter ECG.
[c]1st degree AV blocks: patients were asked to return to the practice the next day for a single ECG; AV block had resolved.
[d]1 patient with vertigo-like sensation, 1 patient with palpitations (HR in normal range 74 bpm): symptoms had resolved for both patients by the end of the 6 h observation.
AV, atrioventricular; HR, heart rate; bpm, beats per minute.

the ECG was carried out by a physician, representing a workload of 10 minutes altogether (two times five minutes for each ECG). The procedures upon appearance of ECG abnormalities or symptoms after 6 hours varied in the different clinical settings (see Figure 1). If, as stated in the Swiss label, heart rate dropped below 40 bpm during 6 hours FDO, another observation period of 6 hours (including ECG prior to and 6 hours after fingolimod administration) had to be performed on the second day of treatment.

Real-world FDO outcomes in the three centres

Data was collected from 136 RRMS patients. 33 were treatment naïve and 103 were previously treated with interferon beta, glatiramer acetate or natalizumab. In total, 130 (95.5%) patients had uneventful FDO, 6 patients experienced cardiac events associated with the first dose (Table 1). Four patients had an AV block: 2 first-degree AV blocks and 2 second-degree AV blocks of Type Mobitz I. All the AV blocks detected resolved spontaneously within 24 hours. This was ensured either by monitoring with Holter ECG or an on-site ECG the following day. Two patients reported symptomatic events that resolved spontaneously without any pharmacological intervention (1 patient with vertigo-like sensation, 1 patient with palpitations [HR in normal range, 74 bpm]). The average duration of follow up was 6.8 months, and 131 (96%) of patients remained on therapy.

Conclusions

The FDO experience reported here indicates that fingolimod is generally well tolerated upon treatment initiation. The majority of patients had no cardiac events during the FDO. Although symptomatic events were rare, the detection of 1st and 2nd degree Mobitz Type I AV blocks, which in some instances can have clinical implications, highlights the importance of monitoring the patients at treatment initiation and emphasizes the need for comprehensive information beforehand. All 3 participating sites capably facilitated the FDO procedure. Our data, which are in line with the phase 3 trial data [3,4] and other FDO related real-world observational studies [6,7], show that despite strict FDO guidelines in Switzerland, initiation of fingolimod therapy can also take place in clinical settings (MS centre, day clinic, private practice) outside of University Hospitals with a reasonable workload. They also support the safety and feasibility of FDO as well as the good tolerability profile of fingolimod in these real-world clinical settings, as shown by rates of adverse events and drop-outs comparable to those published previously [3,4], supporting the fact that fingolimod can safely be used in MS centres, day clinics and private practices.

Abbreviations

S1P: Sphingosine 1-phosphate; RRMS: Relapsing-remitting multiple sclerosis; AV: Atrioventricular; FDO: First dose observation; ECG: Electrocardiogram.

Competing interests

SPR has participated in advisory boards for Merck Serono (Switzerland), Bayer Schering (Switzerland), Teva Pharma AG (Switzerland), Biogen Idec (Switzerland).
SR has participated in advisory boards for Merck Serono (Switzerland), Bayer Schering (Switzerland), Teva Pharma AG (Switzerland), Biogen Idec (Switzerland), Genzyme (Switzerland) and Novartis (Switzerland).
AC received compensation from Bayer Schering, Biogen Idec, Merck Serono, Novartis, Roche, Teva Pharma AG, Genzyme.

Authors' contribution

AC had primary responsibility for the concept and design. AC, SPR and SR acquired data and performed data analyses. AC drafted and edited the manuscript. AC, SPR and SR made substantial contributions to concept/design and data interpretation, participated in critical review and revision of the manuscript, and take public responsibility for its content. AC, SPR and SR read and approved the final manuscript.

Acknowledgements

The preparation of this article was supported by an independent medical education initiative grant from Novartis Pharma Schweiz AG, which had no influence on the content of the manuscript. No honorarium received for developing this article. We thank Dr. Sandra Gass and Dr. Emilie Jaquiéry of Novartis Pharma Schweiz AG for fruitful discussions with regard to the development of this manuscript. We also thank Dr. Therese Schwender and Shweta Dudeja (Novartis Pharma) for providing editorial support which comprised of checking content and language, formatting, referencing, and incorporating the authors' revisions, all under the direction of the authors. This research received no specific grant from any funding agency in the public, commercial, or not-for-profit sectors.

Author details

[1]Cantonal Hospital Aarau, Aarau, Switzerland. [2]Clinique de Carouge SA, Carouge, Switzerland. [3]Neurocentre Bellevue, Theaterstrasse 8, Zurich CH-8001, Switzerland.

References

1. Swissmedic. Gilenya (Fingolimod) summary of product characteristics. [http://www.swissmedicinfo.ch/]
2. Brinkmann V. FTY720 (fingolimod) in multiple sclerosis: therapeutic effects in the immune and the central nervous system. Br J Pharmacol. 2009;158:1173–82.
3. Kappos L, Radue EW, O'Connor P, Polman C, Hohlfeld R, Calabresi P, et al. A placebo-controlled trial of oral fingolimod in relapsing multiple sclerosis. N Engl J Med. 2010;362:387–401.
4. Cohen JA, Barkhof F, Comi G, Hartung HP, Khatri BO, Montalban X, et al. Oral fingolimod or intramuscular interferon for relapsing multiple sclerosis. N Engl J Med. 2010;362:402–15.
5. DiMarco JP, O'Connor P, Cohen JA, Reder AT, Zhang-Auberson L, Tang D, et al. First-dose effects of fingolimod: pooled safety data from three phase 3 studies. MSARD. 2014;5:629–38.
6. Laroni A, Brogi D, Morra VB, Guidi L, Pozzilli C, Comi G, et al. Safety of the first dose of fingolimod for multiple sclerosis: results of an open-label clinical trial. BMC Neurol. 2014;14:65.
7. Fragoso YD, Arruda CC, Arruda WO, Brooks JB, Damasceno A, Damasceno CA, et al. The real-life experience with cardiovascular complications in the first dose of fingolimod for multiple sclerosis. Arq Neuropsiquiatr. 2014;72:712–4.

Interventions to decrease the risk of adverse cardiac events for patients receiving chemotherapy and serotonin (5-HT3) receptor antagonists: a systematic review

Andrea C Tricco[1], Charlene Soobiah[1], Wing Hui[1], Jesmin Antony[1], Vladi Struchkov[1], Brian Hutton[2], Brenda Hemmelgarn[3], David Moher[2] and Sharon E Straus[1,4*]

Abstract

Background: Patients may experience nausea and vomiting when undergoing chemotherapy or surgery requiring anesthesia. Serotonin 5-hydroxytryptamine 3 (5-HT3) receptor antagonists are effective antiemetics, yet may cause adverse cardiac events, such as arrhythmia. We aimed to identify interventions that mitigate the cardiac risk of 5-HT3 receptor antagonists.

Methods: Electronic databases, trial registries, and references were searched. Studies on patients undergoing chemotherapy or surgery examining interventions to monitor cardiac risk of 5-HT3 receptor antagonists were included. Search results were screened and data from relevant studies were abstracted in duplicate. Risk of bias of included studies was assessed using the Cochrane Effective Practice and Organisation of Care (EPOC) group's risk-of-bias tool. Due to a dearth of included studies, meta-analysis was not conducted.

Results: Two randomized clinical trials (RCT) and 1 non-randomized clinical trial (NRCT) were included after screening 7,637 titles and abstracts and 1,554 full-text articles. Intravenous administration of different dolasetron doses was examined in the NRCT, while dolasetron versus ondansetron and palonosetron versus ondansetron were examined in the RCT. Electrocardiogram (ECG) was the only intervention examined to mitigate cardiac harm. No differences in ECG evaluations were observed between dolasetron or palonosetron versus ondansetron after 15 minutes, 24 hours, and 1 week post-administration in the 2 RCTs. Four deaths were observed in one RCT, which were deemed unrelated to palonosetron or ondansetron administration. Minor increases in PR and QT intervals were observed in the NRCT for dolasetron dosages greater than 1.2 mg/kg 1–2 hours post-administration, but were deemed not clinically relevant.

Conclusions: ECG monitoring of chemotherapy patients administered with 5-HT3 receptor antagonists did not reveal clinically significant differences in arrhythmia between the medications at the examined time periods. The usefulness of ECG to monitor chemotherapy patients administered with 5-HT3 receptor antagonists remains unclear, as all patients received ECG monitoring.

Trial registration: PROSPERO registry number: CRD42013003565

Keywords: Serotonin receptor antagonists, Chemotherapy, Adverse events, Cardiac harm, Systematic review, Electrocardiogram

* Correspondence: sharon.straus@utoronto.ca
[1]Li Ka Shing Knowledge Institute, St. Michael's Hospital, 209 Victoria Street, East Building, Toronto, Ontario M5B 1 W8, Canada
[4]Department of Geriatric Medicine, Faculty of Medicine, University of Toronto, 27 Kings College Circle, Toronto, Ontario M5S 1A1, Canada
Full list of author information is available at the end of the article

Background

Nausea and vomiting are common adverse effects following chemotherapy or surgery requiring anesthesia [1,2]. Serotonin 5-hydroxytryptamine 3 (5-HT3) receptor antagonists can effectively prevent nausea and vomiting for patients undergoing these interventions [1,3-5]. However, a prolonged QT interval has been observed in previous studies of these medications [6,7]. The results of these studies suggest that patients who are administered 5-HT3 receptor antagonists might be at risk of experiencing cardiac harm, yet this has not been confirmed in large-scale studies or systematic reviews.

Diagnostic tests can be used to monitor or mitigate cardiac risk that might be associated with 5-HT3 receptor antagonist administration. For example, electrocardiogram (ECG) provides information on PR and QT prolongation, which may lead to arrhythmia (e.g., torsade de pointes tachycardia) [8], all-cause mortality [9], and sudden death [10]. Cardiac telemetry monitors provide continuous ECG monitoring for 24 hours or longer [11]. Electrolyte imbalances, such as hypocalcemia, hypomagnesemia and hypokalemia can result from persistent vomiting and these abnormalities can cause QT interval prolongation [12]. As such, monitoring might be necessary in patients receiving 5-HT3 antagonists and who are vomiting. However, these diagnostic tests are burdensome to the healthcare system and patients. We aimed to determine whether diagnostic interventions can be implemented to mitigate the risk of adverse cardiac events associated with 5-HT3 receptor antagonists for patients undergoing chemotherapy or surgery through a systematic review.

Methods

We used the Preferred Reporting Items for Systematic Reviews and Meta-analysis (PRISMA) Statement to report the results of our systematic review [13].

Protocol

We developed a protocol that was reviewed by clinicians, systematic review methodologists, pharmacoepidemiologists, and Health Canada. We registered our protocol with the PROSPERO database (CRD42013003565) and published the final version [14].

Eligibility criteria

Studies were included if they examined interventions to monitor cardiac risk associated with 5-HT3 receptor antagonists, such as ECG monitoring, telemetry, adjustment of antiarrhythmics, and electrolyte monitoring and replacement. Studies including patients of all ages receiving 5-HT3 antagonist receptors for nausea and vomiting symptoms post-surgery or after chemotherapy and reporting on arrhythmia (primary outcome), sudden cardiac death, QT prolongation, PR prolongation, and/or all-cause mortality were eligible for inclusion. Experimental studies (randomized clinical trials, quasi-randomized clinical trials, non-randomized clinical trials), quasi-experimental studies (interrupted time series, controlled before and after studies), and cohort studies were included regardless of whether they were unpublished or written in languages other than English.

Information sources and literature search

MEDLINE, EMBASE, and Cochrane Central were searched from inception onwards. The electronic literature search was supplemented by searching trial registers and scanning the reference lists of included studies.

An experienced librarian drafted the search strategies, which were peer reviewed by another expert librarian using the Peer Review of Electronic Search Strategies (PRESS) checklist [15]. The final literature search for MEDLINE has been published previously [14] and is available in the Additional file 1. Literature searches for the other databases can be obtained from the corrsponding author upon request.

Study selection process

The eligibility criteria were calibrated on a random sample of 50 titles and abstracts from the literature search. They were revised to enhance clarity and readability by the team. Subsequently, each title and abstract was screened by two team members, independently. Conflicts were resolved by team discussion. The same process was followed for screening the potentially relevant full-text articles.

Data items and data collection process

Following a similar process to screening, two team members independently abstracted data on study characteristics (e.g., setting, country where the study was conducted, details on the 5-HT3 medications, comparator used, and type of test conducted to assess cardiac risk), patient characteristics (e.g., mean/median age, percent female, type of surgery, type of cancer), and outcome results (e.g., number of patients experiencing arrhythmia, mean and standard deviation for PR prolongation). Companion reports (i.e., duplicate publications reporting the data on the same group of patients) were sorted and authors were contacted for data clarifications.

Methodological quality/risk of bias appraisal

Studies were appraised using the Cochrane Effective Practice and Organisation of Care Risk of Bias Tool [16] and the McHarm tool for reporting adverse events [17].

Synthesis of included studies

We were unable to conduct meta-analysis because none of the studies examined interventions to mitigate harm at the same time point. Furthermore, none of the studies compared an intervention to mitigate harm with a control group. As such, the studies were synthesized descriptively, with a focus on the study characteristics, patient characteristics, and outcome results.

Results

Literature search

Two randomized clinical trials and 1 non-randomized clinical trial [18-20] were included after screening 7,637 titles and abstracts and 1,554 full-text articles (Figure 1).

Study and patient characteristics

The study conduct period was 2000 and 2002 in the randomized clinical trials [19,20] and not reported in the non-randomized clinical trial [18] that was published in 1996 (Table 1). The trials were conducted in the United States [18], multiple European countries [19], and South Korea [20]. One trial examined intravenous dolasetron at 1.2, 1.8, and 2.4 mg/kg administered 30 minutes prior to chemotherapy [18] and another examined intravenous palonosetron 0.25 to 0.75 mg compared to ondansetron 32 mg administered 30 minutes prior to chemotherapy [19]. The third trial examined the effects of intravenous dolasetron 100 mg administered 30 minutes prior to chemotherapy and up to 200 mg orally 2 to 5 days post-chemotherapy compared with another group who received 8 mg of intravenous ondansetron 30 minutes prior to chemotherapy and up to 16 mg intravenously 2–4 hours

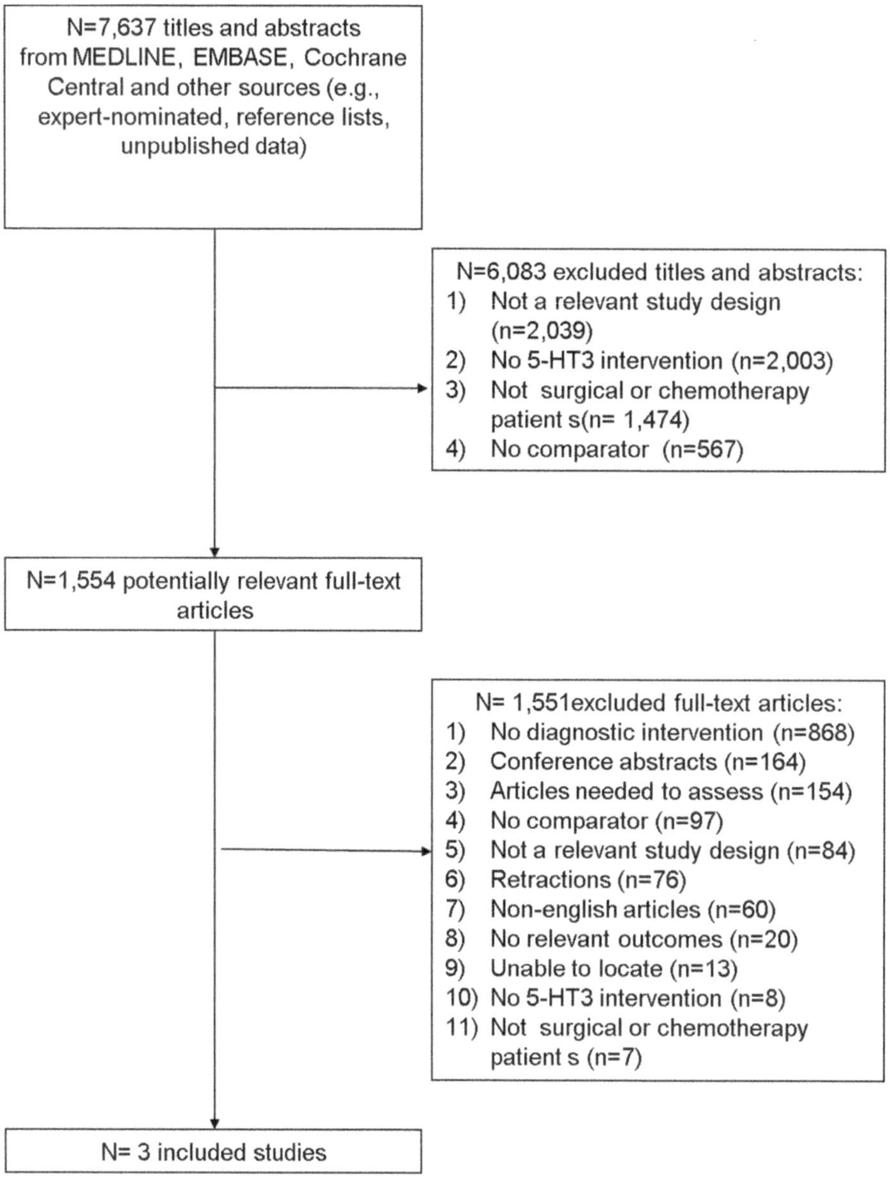

Figure 1 Study flow.

Table 1 Study characteristics

Reference	Study period, country	Study design, # of patients	5-HT3 dose/day	Intervention, examination timing	Outcomes examined
Hesketh [18]	NR, USA	Non-RCT, 44	IV dolasetron 1.2 mg/kg, 1.8 mg/kg, 2.4 mg/kg 30 mins before chemotherapy	ECG, 1–2 hrs and 24–48 hrs	PR, QT
Gralla [19]	August 2000 to October 2001, Germany, Italy, UK, Netherlands, Russia	RCT, 98	IV palonosetron 0.25 mg, IV palonosetron 0.75 mg, IV ondansetron 32 mg 30 mins before chemotherapy	ECG, 15 mins, 24 hrs, 1 wk	Mortality, QT
Kim [20]	April 2002 to October 2002, South Korea	RCT, 114	IV dolasetron 100 mg 30 mins before and 200 mg p.o. 2-5 days after chemotherapy, IV ondansetron 8 mg 30 mins before and IV ondansetron 16 mg 2–4 hrs plus an additional 16 mg/day p.o. 2-5 days after chemotherapy	ECG, 15 mins, 24 hrs, 1 wk	ECG findings unspecified

ECG: electrocardiogram; IV: intravenous; NR: not reported; Non-RCT: non-randomized clinical trial; p.o.: administered orally; RCT: randomized controlled trial.

post-chemotherapy plus an additional 16 mg orally 2–5 days after chemotherapy.

The only intervention identified to mitigate cardiac risk that was examined in the trials was an ECG at various time points. ECG monitoring was not compared with placebo, usual care or another type of diagnostic intervention. The percentage of females included in the trials ranged from 37 to 72% (Table 2). All trials included adult cancer patients with a median (or mean) age ranging from 54 to 56 years. All were receiving a 5-HT3 receptor antagonist for their chemotherapy treatment for various cancer sites. Patients were receiving a variety of chemotherapeutic agents.

Risk of bias assessment

All of the included trials received the same intervention (ECG monitoring) without a comparator group and were assessed for risk of bias (Table 3). The non-randomized clinical trial had the highest risk of bias, with four items assessed as having a high risk of bias [18]. One of the randomized trials had a high risk of bias for allocation concealment and blinding and an unclear risk of bias for random sequence generation and contamination [20]. The other randomized trial had an unclear risk of bias for random sequence generation, contamination, and selective outcome reporting [19]. All of the other risk of bias criteria was assessed as unclear.

Arrhythmia

None of the included trials reported data on arrhythmia, our primary outcome of interest. However, all three trials reported no clinically relevant differences in ECG findings among the patients receiving the 5-HT3 receptor antagonists examined.

Sudden cardiac death and all-cause mortality

Mortality was reported in one of the trials [19]. One withdrawal due to a serious adverse event (pulmonary embolism resulting in death) occurred in the ondansetron group and three other deaths occurred, yet the number of deaths per treatment group was not reported. All deaths were deemed as unlikely or definitely unrelated to the study medications [19]. Although mortality was not specifically reported, no patients dropped out due to mortality in the other two trials [18,20].

QT prolongation

One trial reported no differences between treatment groups in the mean post-dose change from baseline in the QT interval, which was adjusted using the Fridericia correction [19]. The values were 1 ms for palonosetron 0.25 mg, 2 ms for palonosetron 0.75 mg, and 5 ms for ondansetron. Another trial reported median increases in the corrected QT interval as being 11 ms for dolasetron 1.2 mg/kg, 27 ms for dolasetron 1.8 mg/kg, and 39 ms

Table 2 Patient characteristics

Reference	% female	Mean age in years (SD) [range]	Cancer site (%)	Common chemotherapeutic agents* (%)
Hesketh [18]	71	Median 54 (NR) [25–81]	Breast (55), other (45)	Doxorubicin (15), cyclophosphamide (26), 5-FU (43), vincristine (23), methotrexate (14)
Gralla [19]	72	55 (11) [18-NR]	Breast (57), lung (80 < bladder (5), colon (4), rectal (3), small-cell lung (3), gastric (3)	Cyclophosphamide (63), doxorubicin (48), cisplatin (18), methotrexate (16), carboplatin (12)
Kim [20]	37	55.6 (11) [18-NR]	Lung (26), gastric (11), other (29)	5-FU plus cisplatin (27), cisplatin plus the following: taxol, docetaxel, etoposide and ifosfomide, etoposide, gemcitabine, docetaxel plus 5-FU (73)

NR: not reported; SD: standard deviation. *received by >10% of patients.

Table 3 Appraisal of risk of bias, according to Cochrane Effective Practice and Organization of Care risk-of-bias tool [16]

Criterion	Hesketh [18]	Gralla [19]	Kim [20]
Random sequence generation	High	Unclear	Unclear
Allocation concealment	High	Low	High
Similar baseline outcome measures	Unclear	Low	Low
Similar baseline characteristics	Low	Low	Low
Incomplete outcome data	Low	Low	Low
Blinding	High	Low	High
Contamination	Unclear	Unclear	Unclear
Selective outcome reporting	Unclear	Unclear	Unclear
Other bias	High	Low	Low

for dolasetron 2.4 mg/kg [18]. These were considered asymptomatic and not clinically significant. The third trial did not specifically report on this outcome but reported no relevant differences between the treatment groups with respect to ECG findings [20] (Table 4).

PR prolongation

One trial reported median increases in the PR interval as being 1 ms for dolasetron 1.2 mg/kg, 10 ms for dolasetron 1.8 mg/kg, and 22 ms for dolasetron 2.4 mg/kg [18]. A significant dose–response relationship was found between dolasetron and the PR interval at 1–2 hours post-administration. These changes were considered asymptomatic and not clinically significant. The other trials did not specifically report on this outcome but reported no relevant differences between the treatment groups with respect to ECG findings [19,20] (Table 4).

Table 4 QT and PR prolongation

Author, year	Treatment (dose, time of treatment)		
Hesketh [18]			
	Dolasetron (1.2 mg/kg, BC)	Dolasetron (1.8 mg/kg, BC)	Dolasetron (2.4 mg/kg, BC)
QT prolongation*	11 ms	27 ms	39 ms
PR prolongation†	1 ms	10 ms	22 ms
Gralla [19]			
	Palonosetron (0.25 mg, BC)	Palonosetron (0.75 mg, BC)	Ondansetron (32 mg, BC)
QT prolongation*	1 ms	2 ms	5 ms
PR prolongation	NS	NS	NS
Kim [20]			
	Dolasetron (100, BC+ 800 mg, AC)	Ondansetron (8 mg, BC + 80 mg, AC)	
QT prolongation	NS	NS	
PR prolongation	NS	NS	

AC: after chemotherapy treatment; BC: before the start of chemotherapy treatment; NS: not significant. *mean change from baseline; †median change from baseline.

Discussion

In our systematic review, we did not find any clinically relevant changes in the QT interval between different dosages of dolasetron [18] or between palonosetron and ondansetron [19] or dolasetron and ondansetron [20]. Furthermore, we did not find any other significant differences in other ECG changes between these 5-HT3 receptor antagonists at 15 minutes, 1–2 hours, 24 hours, and 1 week post-administration. However, this does not suggest that these agents do not cause cardiac harm. For example, two case series have noted a prolonged QT interval after the administration of 5-HT3 receptor antagonists [6,7]. Both articles were excluded here because they were case series and therefore there was not a comparison group and they did not examine interventions to mitigate the cardiac risk associated with these agents.

We had originally hoped to identify studies in which all patients received a 5-HT3 receptor antagonist and compared an intervention to mitigate cardiac harm (e.g., ECG monitoring) with placebo, usual care or another diagnostic intervention. As we did not identify any such study, the utility of the ECG to monitor adult chemotherapy patients after being administered a 5-HT3 receptor antagonist is currently unclear. Further research is required to recommend ECG monitoring for all adult chemotherapy patients administered a 5-HT3 receptor antagonist, as this would be burdensome to the healthcare system and to patients.

We identified many gaps in the literature in this area. For example, we did not identify studies that tested monitoring cardiac function after the administration of these agents other than the ECG. Similarly, we did not identify studies conducted among children receiving chemotherapy or patients of any age undergoing surgery requiring anesthesia and none of the included studies reported the proportion of patients with prolonged QT or PR intervals. Although unpublished studies were sought, none were identified that examined this research question.

As expected, the non-randomized clinical trial had the greatest risk of bias [18], as random sequence generation, allocation concealment, and blinding was not conducted. The two randomized clinical trials would be improved by adequately reporting random sequence generation, reporting whether contamination was a factor, and providing a protocol so that the potential for outcome reporting bias could be assessed [19,20]. Limitations of our systematic review process include the few studies identified for inclusion. As well, our objective was to compare interventions to mitigate cardiac risk across intervention and comparator groups versus examine cardiac risk after the administration of these agents. As such, we excluded case series, case reports, and cross-sectional studies. We were unable to conduct meta-analysis or assess for publication bias because of the few studies included here.

Conclusions

The utility of the ECG monitoring to mitigate cardiac harm among chemotherapy patients after being administered a 5-HT3 receptor antagonist is unclear; few studies exist that met our eligibility criteria. Future research is necessary to determine whether ECG (or other diagnostic interventions) are beneficial and whether these interventions should be used to monitor other patient populations, including children undergoing chemotherapy and patients of all ages receiving surgery requiring anesthesia.

Additional file

Additional file 1: Literature search for MEDLINE.

Competing interests

The authors declare that they have no competing interests.

Authors' contributions

ACT conceived the study, designed the study, helped obtain funding for the study, generated the tables, interpreted the results, and wrote the manuscript. CS coordinated the study, screened citations for inclusion, abstracted data, and edited the manuscript. WH and VS abstracted data and edited the manuscript. JA helped coordinate the study, screened citations for inclusion, and edited the manuscript. BH, BH, and DM helped conceive the study, interpreted the results, and edited the manuscript. SES conceived the study, designed the study, obtained the funding, interpreted the results, and helped write the manuscript. All authors read and approved the final paper.

Acknowledgments

This systematic review was funded by the Canadian Institutes for Health Research/Drug Safety and Effectiveness Network (CIHR/DSEN). ACT and BH are funded by CIHR/DSEN New Investigator Awards in Knowledge Synthesis. DM is funded by a University of Ottawa Research Chair. SES is funded by a Tier 1 Canada Research Chair in Knowledge Translation.
We thank Laure Perrier for conducting the literature searches and obtaining full-text articles; Erik Blondal for obtaining full-text articles/data abstraction; and Afshin Vafaei, Lisa Strifler, John Ivory, Huda Ashoor, Dr. Paul Khan, Heather McDonald, Emily Reynen, Dr. Roberta Cardoso, Reid Robson, Vera Nincic, Dr. Joanne Ho, Carmen Ng, Christy Johnson, Erin Lillie, Dr. Derek Roberts, and Kelly Mrklas for their assistance with data abstraction/screening for the main project that this review was a part of. We also thank Ana Guzman for formatting our paper.

Author details

[1]Li Ka Shing Knowledge Institute, St. Michael's Hospital, 209 Victoria Street, East Building, Toronto, Ontario M5B 1 W8, Canada. [2]Clinical Epidemiology Program, Centre for Practice-Changing Research, Ottawa Hospital Research Institute, 725 Parkdale Ave., Ottawa, Ontario K1Y 4E9, Canada. [3]Departments of Medicine and Community Health Sciences, University of Calgary, TRW Building, 3rd Floor, 3280 Hospital Drive NW, Calgary, Alberta T2N 4Z6, Canada. [4]Department of Geriatric Medicine, Faculty of Medicine, University of Toronto, 27 Kings College Circle, Toronto, Ontario M5S 1A1, Canada.

References

1. Jin Y, Sun W, Gu D, Yang J, Xu Z, Chen J. Comparative efficacy and safety of palonosetron with the first 5-HT3 receptor antagonists for the chemotherapy-induced nausea and vomiting: a meta-analysis. Eur J Cancer Care (Engl). 2013;22:41–50.
2. Apfel CC, Laara E, Koivuranta M, Greim CA, Roewer N. A simplified risk score for predicting postoperative nausea and vomiting: conclusions from cross-validations between two centers. Anesthesiology. 1999;91:693–700.
3. Rawlinson A, Kitchingham N, Hart C, McMahon G, Ong SL, Khanna A. Mechanisms of reducing postoperative pain, nausea and vomiting: a systematic review of current techniques. Evid Based Med. 2012;17:75–80.
4. Tang DH, Malone DC. A network meta-analysis on the efficacy of serotonin type 3 receptor antagonists used in adults during the first 24 hours for postoperative nausea and vomiting prophylaxis. Clin Ther. 2012;34:282–94.
5. Salvo N, Doble B, Khan L, Amirthevasar G, Dennis K, Pasetka M, et al. Prophylaxis of radiation-induced nausea and vomiting using 5-hydroxytryptamine-3 serotonin receptor antagonists: a systematic review of randomized trials. Int J Radiat Oncol Biol Phys. 2012;82:408–17.
6. Buyukavci M, Olgun H, Ceviz N. The effects of ondansetron and granisetron on electrocardiography in children receiving chemotherapy for acute leukemia. Am J Clin Oncol. 2005;28:201–4.
7. Pinarli FG, Elli M, Dagdemir A, Baysal K, Acar S. Electrocardiographic findings after 5-HT3 receptor antagonists and chemotherapy in children with cancer. Pediatr Blood Cancer. 2006;47:567–71.
8. Malik M, Camm AJ. Evaluation of drug-induced QT interval prolongation: implications for drug approval and labelling. Drug Saf. 2001;24:323–51.
9. Cheng S, Keyes MJ, Larson MG, McCabe EL, Newton-Cheh C, Levy D, et al. Long-term outcomes in individuals with prolonged PR interval or first-degree atrioventricular block. JAMA. 2009;301:2571–7.
10. Ritter JM. Drug-induced long QT syndrome and drug development. Br J Clin Pharmacol. 2008;66:341–4.
11. Tisdale JE, Wroblewski HA, Overholser BR, Kingery JR, Trujillo TN, Kovacs RJ. Prevalence of QT interval prolongation in patients admitted to cardiac care units and frequency of subsequent administration of QT interval-prolonging drugs: a prospective, observational study in a large urban academic medical center in the US. Drug Saf. 2012;35:459–70.
12. Pickham D, Shinn JA, Chan GK, Funk M, Drew BJ. Quasi-experimental study to improve nurses' QT-interval monitoring: results of QTIP study. Am J Crit Care. 2012;21:195–200. quiz 201.
13. Moher D, Liberati A, Tetzlaff J, Altman DG, Group P. Preferred reporting items for systematic reviews and meta-analyses: the PRISMA statement. BMJ. 2009;339:b2535.
14. Tricco AC, Soobiah C, Antony J, Hemmelgarn B, Moher D, Hutton B, et al. Interventions to decrease the risk of adverse cardiac events for post-surgery or chemotherapy patients taking serotonin (5-HT3) receptor antagonists: protocol for a systematic review and network meta-analysis. Syst Rev. 2013;2:45.
15. Sampson M, McGowan J, Cogo E, Grimshaw J, Moher D, Lefebvre C. An evidence-based practice guideline for the peer review of electronic search strategies. J Clin Epidemiol. 2009;62:944–52.
16. Cochrane Effective Practice and Organisation of Care Group Draft Risk of Bias Tool. http://epoccochrane.org/epoc-resources-review-authors.
17. Santaguida P, Raina P, Ismaila A. The development of the McHarm quality assessment scale for adverse events. In: Book The development of the McHarm quality assessment scale for adverse events. 2008.
18. Hesketh PJ, Gandara DR, Hesketh AM, Facada A, Perez EA, Webber LM, et al. Dose-ranging evaluation of the antiemetic efficacy of intravenous dolasetron in patients receiving chemotherapy with doxorubicin or cyclophosphamide. Support Care Cancer. 1996;4:141–6.
19. Gralla R, Lichinitser M, Van Der Vegt S, Sleeboom H, Mezger J, Peschel C, et al. Palonosetron improves prevention of chemotherapy-induced nausea and vomiting following moderately emetogenic chemotherapy: results of a double-blind randomized phase III trial comparing single doses of palonosetron with ondansetron. Ann Oncol. 2003;14:1570–7.
20. Kim JS, Baek JY, Park SR, Choi IS, Kim SI, Kim DW, et al. Open-label, randomized comparison of the efficacy of intravenous dolasetron mesylate and ondansetron in the prevention of acute and delayed cisplatin-induced emesis in cancer patients. Cancer Res Treat. 2004;36:372–6.

Arsenic-induced dyslipidemia in male albino rats: comparison between trivalent and pentavalent inorganic arsenic in drinking water

Olusegun K. Afolabi[1,3], Adedoja D. Wusu[1,4], Olabisi O. Ogunrinola[1,4], Esther O. Abam[1,6], David O. Babayemi[1], Oluwatosin. A. Dosumu[1], Okechukwu. B. Onunkwor[1], Elizabeth. A. Balogun[1,5], Olusegun O. Odukoya[2] and Oladipo Ademuyiwa[1*]

Abstract

Background: Recent epidemiological evidences indicate close association between inorganic arsenic exposure via drinking water and cardiovascular diseases. However, the exact mechanism of this arsenic-mediated increase in cardiovascular risk factors remains enigmatic.

Methods: In order to investigate the effects of inorganic arsenic exposure on lipid metabolism, male albino rats were exposed to 50, 100 and 150 ppm arsenic as sodium arsenite and 100, 150 and 200 ppm arsenic as sodium arsenate respectively in their drinking water for 12 weeks.

Results: Dyslipidemia induced by the two arsenicals exhibited different patterns. Hypocholesterolemia characterised the effect of arsenite at all the doses, but arsenate induced hypercholesterolemia at the 150 ppm As dose. Hypertriglyceridemia was the hallmark of arsenate effect whereas plasma free fatty acids (FFAs) was increased by the two arsenicals. Reverse cholesterol transport was inhibited by the two arsenicals as evidenced by decreased HDL cholesterol concentrations whereas hepatic cholesterol was increased by arsenite (100 ppm As), but decreased by arsenite (150 ppm As) and arsenate (100 ppm As) respectively. Brain cholesterol and triglyceride were decreased by the two arsenicals; arsenate decreased the renal content of cholesterol, but increased renal content of triglyceride. Arsenite, on the other hand, increased the renal contents of the two lipids. The two arsenicals induced phospholipidosis in the spleen. Arsenite (150 ppm As) and arsenate (100 ppm As) inhibited hepatic HMG CoA reductase. At other doses of the two arsenicals, hepatic activity of the enzyme was up-regulated. The two arsenicals however up-regulated the activity of the brain enzyme. We observed positive associations between tissue arsenic levels and plasma FFA and negative associations between tissue arsenic levels and HDL cholesterol.

Conclusion: Our findings indicate that even though sub-chronic exposure to arsenite and arsenate through drinking water produced different patterns of dyslipidemia, our study identified two common denominators of dyslipidemia namely: inhibition of reverse cholesterol transport and increase in plasma FFA. These two denominators (in addition to other individual perturbations of lipid metabolism induced by each arsenical), suggest that in contrast to strengthening a dose-dependent effect phenomenon, the two forms of inorganic arsenic induced lipotoxic and non-lipotoxic dyslipidemia at "low" or "medium" doses and these might be responsible for the cardiovascular and other disease endpoints of inorganic arsenic exposure through drinking water.

Keywords: Trivalent inorganic arsenic, Pentavalent inorganic arsenic, Drinking water, Dyslipidemia

* Correspondence: adelad2@yahoo.com
[1]Department of Biochemistry, Federal University of Agriculture, Abeokuta, Nigeria
Full list of author information is available at the end of the article

Background

Among the plethora of toxicants, arsenic ranks as an environmentally ubiquitous and epidemiologically important metalloid currently poisoning tens of millions of people worldwide [1, 2]. It is found in both inorganic and organic forms and in different valence or oxidation states in the environment.

Chronic exposure to arsenic is associated with a wide range of toxic effects [1, 3]. Cancer of the skin, lung, kidney, liver and urinary bladder are the important cancers associated with these toxic effects [1–3]. Among the non-cancer effects of arsenic, diabetes mellitus, goitre, hepatomegaly, bronchitis, bronchiectasis, cerebrovascular and cardiovascular diseases, are well documented [3–5]. Epidemiological studies have demonstrated that ingestion of arsenic through drinking water might be responsible for these carcinogenic and non-cancer effects of arsenic [3, 4, 6]. In spite of this large body of information about the toxic effects of arsenic, the precise mechanisms of action for the many disease endpoints following acute and chronic arsenic exposure, as well as the threshold for biologic effects and disease risks, remain enigmatic [1].

Over the years, epidemiological studies have identified lipid and lipoprotein abnormalities as independent risk factors in the pathogenesis and progression of atherosclerosis and cardiovascular diseases [7, 8]. There is also increasing evidence that environmental factors/contaminants (most especially heavy metals) contribute to this dyslipidemia [7, 9, 10]. Studies conducted in arsenic-exposed populations revealed a prevalence of nearly a full spectrum of cardiovascular diseases including hypertension, atherosclerosis, blackfoot disease, ischaemic heart diseases, etc. [3, 4]. Therefore, it seems reasonable to hypothesise that the association between arsenicosis and cardiovascular diseases may be mediated through modification of lipid and lipoprotein metabolism. The work reported here explored this hypothesis.

Materials and methods

Chemicals

Sodium arsenite and sodium arsenate were products of Sigma-Aldrich, Missouri, USA.

Animals and treatment

Experimental protocols were conducted in accord with guidelines of the Institutional Animal Care and Use Committee and were approved by the Animal Ethical Committee of the Department of Biochemistry, Federal University of Agriculture, Abeokuta, Nigeria.

Fifty-six male Wistar rats (bred in the College of Veterinary Medicine, Federal University of Agriculture, Abeokuta, Nigeria) with a mean body weight of 130 g were used for the experiments. They were housed in an animal room with normal controlled temperature (22 ± 2 °C) and a regular 12 h light–dark cycle (06:00–18:00 h). They were allowed 14 days to acclimatise before the commencement of arsenic exposure. The animals were maintained on a standard pellet diet.

Animals were divided into 8 groups of 7 animals each. While 2 groups served as control and received distilled water, the remaining groups (3 groups each) were exposed to 50, 100 and 150 ppm arsenic as sodium arsenite and 100, 150 and 200 ppm arsenic as sodium arsenate respectively in their drinking water for 12 weeks. These arsenic concentrations were chosen based on previous studies [11–15]. At the end of arsenic exposure, blood was collected from the animals into heparinised tubes by cardiac puncture under light ether anaesthesia after an overnight fast. Liver, kidney, heart, lung, brain and spleen were also removed from the animals for arsenic and lipid analyses. An aliquot of the blood samples was taken for arsenic determination while the remaining blood samples were centrifuged to separate plasma and red blood cells. All samples were stored at −20 °C until analysed.

Arsenic determination

A portion of the frozen organs (≈200 mg) and whole blood (0.2 ml) were digested in nitric acid. Total arsenic (which would include inorganic and organic forms) was determined using atomic absorption spectrometry. Results are expressed as μg As/ml for blood and μg As/g wet weight for the organs.

Biochemical analyses

Plasma and lipoprotein lipid profiles

Determination of the major lipids (cholesterol, triglycerides, phospholipids and free fatty acids) in plasma and lipoproteins followed established procedures. Details of these have been given in our earlier studies [7, 16–19].

Organ and erythrocyte lipid profiles

Lipids were extracted from the organs (liver, kidney, heart, lung, brain and spleen) as described by Folch et al. (1957) [20] while extraction of erythrocyte lipids followed the procedure described by Rose and Oklander (1965) [21]. After washing with 0.05 M KCl solution, aliquots of the lipid extracts were then used for the determination of lipid profiles. Details of these are given as reported earlier [7, 16–19].

Determination of hepatic and brain HMG-CoA reductase activity

This was determined according to the method of Rao and Ramakrishnan (1975) [22] by measuring the hepatic and brain concentrations of HMG-CoA and mevalonate. The ratio of HMG-CoA to mevalonate is taken as an index of the activity of HMG-CoA reductase. An increase in this ratio indicates inhibition of cholesterogenesis while a decrease indicates enhanced cholesterogenesis.

Statistical analysis

Results are expressed as mean ± SEM. One way analysis of variance (ANOVA) followed by Tukey's test was used to analyze the results with $p < 0.05$ considered significant. Associations among the parameters and their magnitudes were determined using Pearson correlation.

Results

Table 1 depicts the index of arsenic exposure (expressed as weekly arsenic intake/rat) calculated by the formula: water consumption (ml) × arsenic concentration (ppm). Arsenic intake per week was relatively constant in each dose group. For the arsenite-exposed rats, each animal ingested 7.41 ± 0.29 mg As/week in the 50 ppm group, while arsenic ingestion was 13.13 ± 0.69 mg As/week and 17.33 ± 0.60 mg As/week in the 100 ppm and 150 ppm groups respectively. For the 12 weeks of exposure, each animal in the 50 ppm group ingested a total of 88.91 mg of arsenic, while an animal in the 100 ppm group and 150 ppm group had a total arsenic intake of 157.58 mg and 207.90 mg respectively. The arsenate-exposed animals also showed a constant rate of arsenic intake. In the 100 ppm group, an animal consumed on the average, a total of 12.06 ± 0.68 mg As/week, while in the 150 ppm and 200 ppm groups, the intake per week were 16.02 ± 1.07 mg and 22.04 ± 1.87 mg respectively. Total arsenic intake in the groups amounted to 144.75 mg, 192.20 mg and 264.42 mg per rat for the 100 ppm, 150 ppm and 200 ppm doses respectively.

Arsenic levels in some of the tissues in rats administered either arsenite or arsenate in their drinking water are shown in Table 2. Although the administration of the two arsenicals resulted in an accumulation of arsenic in blood, liver, kidney, heart, lung, brain and spleen of the animals, only in the kidney of arsenate-treated and the brain of arsenite-treated animals was the accumulation found to be dose-dependent. In arsenite-treated animals, exposure to an arsenic dose of 50 ppm resulted in arsenic content of 305 μg As/ml of blood. Doubling of the arsenic dose did not result in any further increase in arsenic content. Rather, arsenic content of the blood approached a saturation. At the highest dose of arsenic in the sodium arsenite group (150 ppm), arsenic content of the blood reduced from 301 μg As/ml to 258 μg As/ml. In the arsenate-treated animals, exposure to an arsenic dose of 100 ppm resulted in an arsenic content of 228.44 μg As/ml of blood. Increasing the arsenic dose resulted in a further increase in arsenic content from 228.44 μg As/ml to 267.10 μg As/ml. Increasing the arsenic dose to 200 ppm did not result in any appreciable increase in arsenic content of blood. Rather, arsenic content of blood in this group of animals peaked at 273.23 μg As/ml. In arsenite-exposed animals, the spleen accumulated the highest amount of arsenic, whereas in arsenate-exposed animals, kidney accumulated the highest amount of arsenic.

Dyslipidemia induced by arsenite was characterised by hypocholesterolemia at all the arsenic doses (Fig. 1). At

Table 1 Weekly and total arsenic intakes of each animal on exposure to sodium arsenite and sodium arsenate for 12 weeks through drinking water

Week	Sodium arsenite			Sodium arsenate		
	Arsenic Dose			Arsenic Dose		
	50 ppm	100 ppm	150 ppm	100 ppm	150 ppm	200 ppm
1	9.30	16.00	18.30	16.31	23.27	37.03
2	8.53	16.83	21.30	16.26	21.69	29.94
3	8.57	17.34	19.29	11.80	17.57	26.75
4	8.26	13.54	16.84	12.69	18.56	23.94
5	6.89	13.60	15.43	13.26	15.63	22.06
6	6.84	12.40	16.54	12.49	15.21	19.94
7	6.94	11.77	18.47	10.06	16.67	20.09
8	6.44	10.30	15.60	11.94	13.76	17.73
9	6.49	11.08	15.21	9.86	12.94	17.08
10	6.53	10.97	14.61	9.57	11.91	18.60
11	7.50	11.09	19.59	11.38	12.30	14.67
12	6.63	12.72	16.71	9.14	12.69	16.60
Total intake (mg)	88.91	157.58	207.90	144.75	192.20	264.42
Mean intake/week (mg) (± S.E.M)	7.41 ± 0.29	13.13 ± 0.69	17.33 ± 0.60	12.06 ± 0.68	16.02 ± 1.07	22.04 ± 1.87

Table 2 Arsenic concentrations in the tissues of the animals on exposure to sodium arsenite and sodium arsenate for 12 weeks through drinking water

	Sodium arsenite				Sodium arsenate			
	Arsenic dose				Arsenic dose			
Tissue	Control	50 ppm	100 ppm	150 ppm	Control	100 ppm	150 ppm	200 ppm
Blood (μg/ml)	11.24 ± 2.35a	304.99 ± 15.43b	300.85 ± 18.89b	257.62 ± 12.61c	23.60 ± 2.99a	228.44 ± 31.07b	267.10 ± 13.79c	273.23 ± 14.33c
Liver (μg/g wet weight)	1.73 ± 0.07a	19.92 ± 2.16b	14.85 ± 1.07c	22.44 ± 3.02b	3.54 ± 0.26a	10.03 ± 0.58b	19.32 ± 3.93c	14.19 ± 0.96d
Kidney (μg/g wet weight)	2.06 ± 0.16a	5.56 ± 0.28b	39.54 ± 1.95c	27.36 ± 2.03d	2.06 ± 0.16a	6.31 ± 0.37b	32.84 ± 3.09c	47.90 ± 2.99d
Brain (μg/g wet weight)	0.69 ± 0.05a	3.11 ± 0.24b	24.88 ± 2.57c	35.21 ± 4.33d	1.74 ± 0.15a	18.95 ± 1.81b	31.65 ± 2.15c	22.11 ± 2.10d
Heart (μg/g wet weight)	0.20 ± 0.03a	16.54 ± 1.11b	53.54 ± 5.57c	46.01 ± 2.30c	0.02 ± 0.03a	42.16 ± 2.39c	18.80 ± 3.46b	27.98 ± 2.99b
Lung (μg/g wet weight)	0.71 ± 0.03a	4.97 ± 0.45a	28.73 ± 3.73b	33.20 ± 4.67b	0.75 ± 0.02a	6.64 ± 0.88a	44.80 ± 7.18b	28.39 ± 4.62b
Spleen (μg/g wet weight)	3.37 ± 0.29a	40.35 ± 2.92b	38.08 ± 1.60b	58.32 ± 5.08c	5.88 ± 0.33a	20.66 ± 2.14b	31.41 ± 3.40b	23.12 ± 1.06b

Each value represents the mean ± S.E.M. of 7 rats. Values within a row with different alphabets for each arsenic compound are significantly different at $p < 0.05$

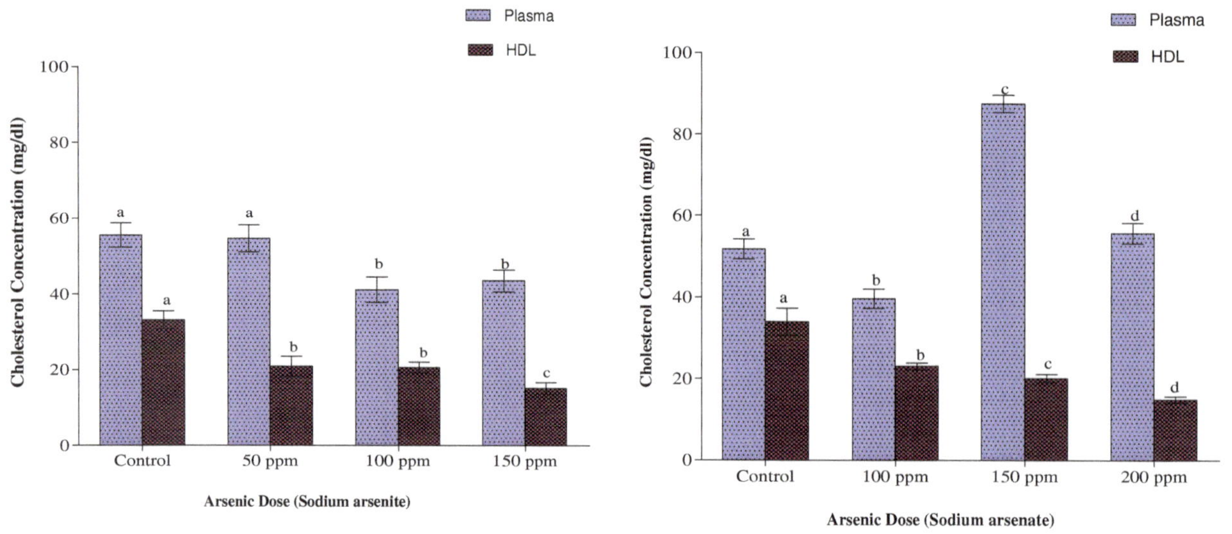

Fig. 1 Effects of arsenite and arsenate on plasma and HDL cholesterol concen-trations. Each bar represents the mean ± S.E.M. of 7 rats. Bars with different alphabets are significantly different at $p < 0.05$

both 100 ppm and 150 ppm doses of arsenic in arsenite-treated animals, cholesterol reduced from 56.48 ± 3.21 mg/dl in control to 41.10 ± 3.35 mg/dl and 43.49 ± 3.87 mg/dl respectively. Arsenate, on the other hand, increased plasma cholesterol by 69 % at the 150 ppm As dose but decreased this lipid by 23 % at 100 ppm As. HDL cholesterol was reduced to the same extent by the two arsenicals. At the highest dose of each arsenical, HDL cholesterol was just about 50 % of control values (Fig. 1).

As indicated in Fig. 2, arsenite elicited a hormetic response in plasma triglyceride concentration in which the 50 ppm As dose up-regulated whereas the 100 ppm As dose down-regulated the plasma triglyceride content. The 50 ppm arsenic dose in arsenite-exposed animals increased the plasma triglyceride content from 46.81 ± 2.25 to 55.32 ± 3.33 mg/dl. Doubling the arsenic dose resulted in a 25 % reduction in triglyceride whereas plasma triglyceride level at highest arsenic dose was not significantly different from the control ($p > 0.05$). Arsenate, on the other hand, induced hypertriglyceridemia at all the doses of arsenic employed. Arsenite exposure at the 50 ppm As dose also caused an elevation of the HDL triglyceride content while, at 150 ppm As dose, the lipid was significantly reduced ($p < 0.05$). With arsenate exposure, however, there was no significant change in HDL triglyceride concentrations except at the 150 ppm As dose where an increase in concentration was observed.

Plasma phospholipid concentrations were significantly reduced in both arsenite- and arsenate-exposed rats at the highest dose ($p < 0.05$) while no significant changes at both the low and medium doses were observed (Fig. 3). Exposure of the animals to either arsenite or arsenate did not result in any significant changes in the HDL phospholipid contents at all the doses employed, although there was a gradual depression of the concentrations as the arsenate doses were increased (Fig. 3).

Cholesterol concentration in the LDL + VLDL fraction was increased on exposure to arsenite and arsenate at all arsenic doses (Fig. 4). The increase in the arsenite-exposed rats amounted to 49 % whereas in arsenate-exposed rats the increases amounted to 30 %, 165 % and 99 % in the 100 ppm, 150 ppm and 200 ppm groups respectively. Triglyceride contents of the LDL + VLDL fraction were not affected by exposure to arsenite but arsenate caused a 2-fold increase in same lipid at 150 ppm and 200 ppm As doses (Fig. 4).

The mean phospholipid concentrations in LDL + VLDL as depicted in Fig. 4 indicate that both arsenite and arsenate exposures resulted in depletion of LDL + VLDL phospholipids. In arsenite-exposed animals, the highest depletion of 52 % was observed at the 100 ppm As dose, but with arsenate, the reduction was maximal in the highest dose group (200 ppm) where 41 % reduction was observed.

The erythrocyte lipid contents of the animals are shown in Fig. 5. Both arsenite and arsenate exposures resulted in significant depression of the cholesterol contents of the red blood cells in the animals ($p < 0.05$). Arsenite-exposure resulted in 35 % and 44 % decreases in cholesterol contents of the erythrocyte of rats with 100 ppm and 150 ppm As respectively. In arsenate-exposed rats, 34, 44 and 39 % reduction resulted from exposure to 100 ppm, 150 ppm and 200 ppm arsenic doses respectively. Arsenite exposure did not affect triglyceride contents of rat erythrocytes as no significant

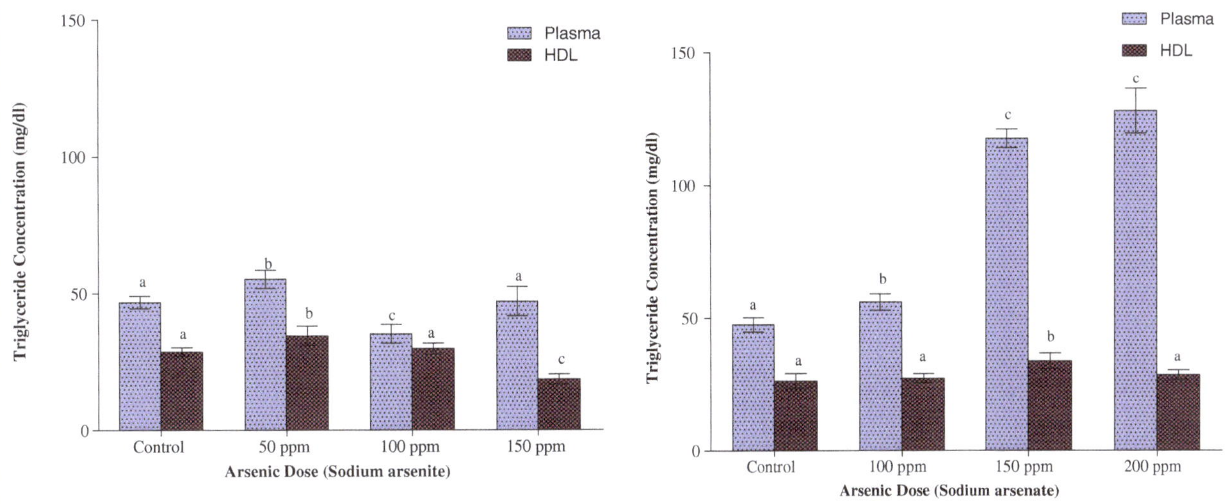

Fig 2 Effects of arsenite and arsenate on plasma and HDL triglyceride concen-trations. Each bar represents the mean ± S.E.M. of 7 rats. Bars with different alphabets are significantly different at $p < 0.05$

change ($p > 0.05$) was observed in the concentrations. Exposure to 100 ppm As in arsenate-exposed animals, however, resulted in a 31 % increase in erythrocyte triglyceride concentration ($p < 0.05$). Increase in the arsenic dose did not result in any further significant increase in the erythrocyte triglyceride.

Phospholipid concentrations in the erythrocyte were markedly lowered on exposure to the two arsenicals, although in both cases, the reduction was not dose-dependent. While the reduction amounted to 51, 29 and 39 % respectively in arsenite-treated animals, it amounted to 32, 16 and 49 % respectively in arsenate-treated animals.

Plasma and erythrocyte FFA concentrations are depicted in Fig. 6. In both arsenite- and arsenate-exposed animals, there was a gradual increase in both plasma and erythrocyte FFA concentrations as the arsenic doses were increased. Comparatively, in the plasma, the increase was more pronounced in arsenate-treated animals whereas in the erythrocytes the increase was more pronounced in arsenite-treated animals.

The effects of the arsenicals on hepatic, renal and brain cholesterol concentrations are depicted in Fig. 7. While arsenite increased hepatic and renal cholesterol by 35 and 82 % respectively, it decreased brain cholesterol by as much as 50 % at the highest dose of arsenic. Arsenate, on the other hand, increased hepatic cholesterol but decreased renal and brain cholesterol concentrations by 50 and 31 % respectively.

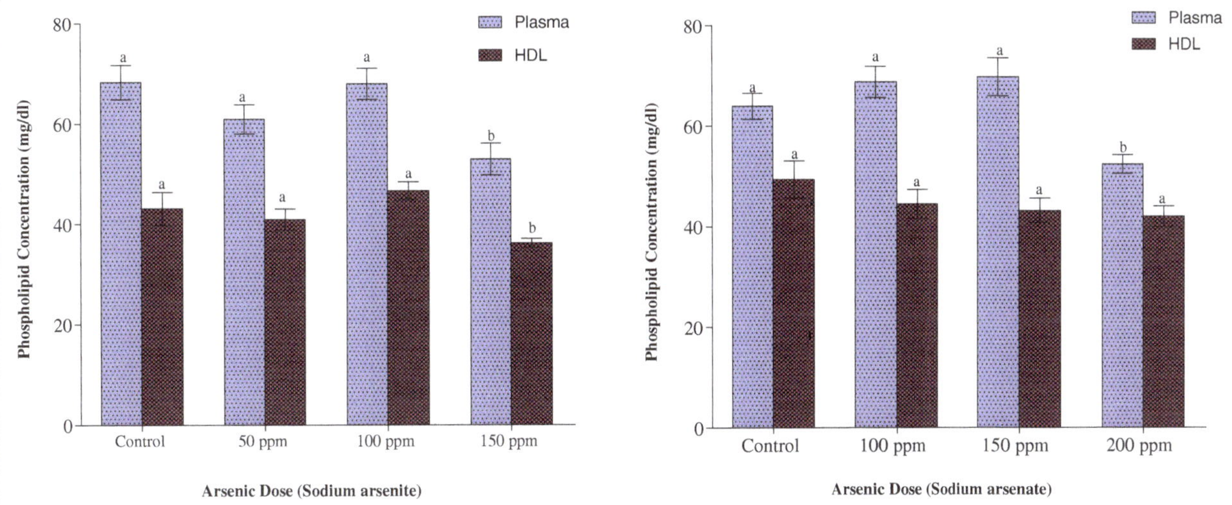

Fig. 3 Effects of arsenite and arsenate on plasma and HDL phospholipid concentrations. Each bar represents the mean ± S.E.M. of 7 rats. Bars with different alphabets are significantly different at $p < 0.05$

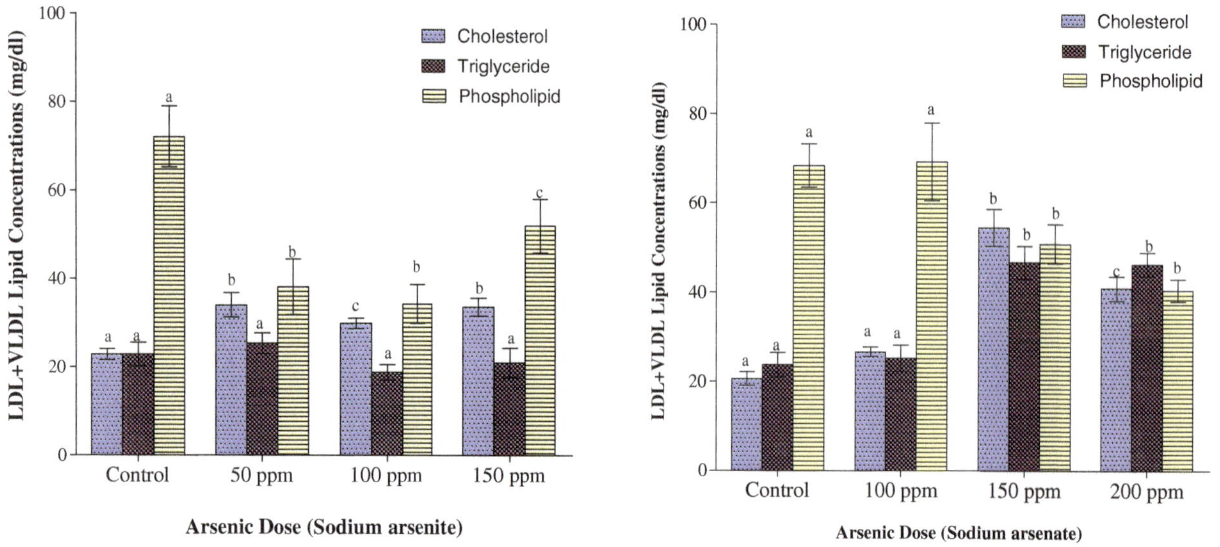

Fig. 4 Effects of arsenite and arsenate on LDL + VLDL cholesterol, triglyceride and phospholipid concentrations. Each bar represents the mean ± S.E.M. of 7 rats. Bars with different alphabets are significantly different at $p < 0.05$

Cardiac, pulmonary and splenic cholesterol contents are shown in Fig. 8. Exposure to the two arsenicals resulted in the depletion of the cardiac cholesterol while increasing pulmonary and splenic cholesterol contents. At the highest dose of each arsenical, cardiac cholesterol was just 23 % (arsenite) and 50 % (arsenate) of control values respectively. In the pulmonary compartment, the pattern of increase was similar for the two arsenicals. In the splenic compartment, however, while the highest increase (42 %) was observed with the highest dose of arsenic in arsenite-exposed animals, it was the 100 ppm As in arsenate-exposed animals that elicited the highest increase (21 %).

Arsenite elicited a hormetic response in hepatic triglyceride concentrations (Fig. 9). While the 50 ppm arsenic dose up-regulated triglyceride concentration by 35 %, the highest dose of arsenic (150 ppm) also caused a 35 % reduction in triglyceride concentration (Fig. 9). Arsenate, on the other hand, increased hepatic triglyceride (11 % and 43 %) at 150 and 200 ppm As doses respectively. Both arsenite and arsenate increased the renal contents of triglyceride. The increase was more pronounced in arsenite-treated animals. The two arsenicals also decreased to the same extent the triglyceride concentration of the brain, although the decrease was not dose-dependent.

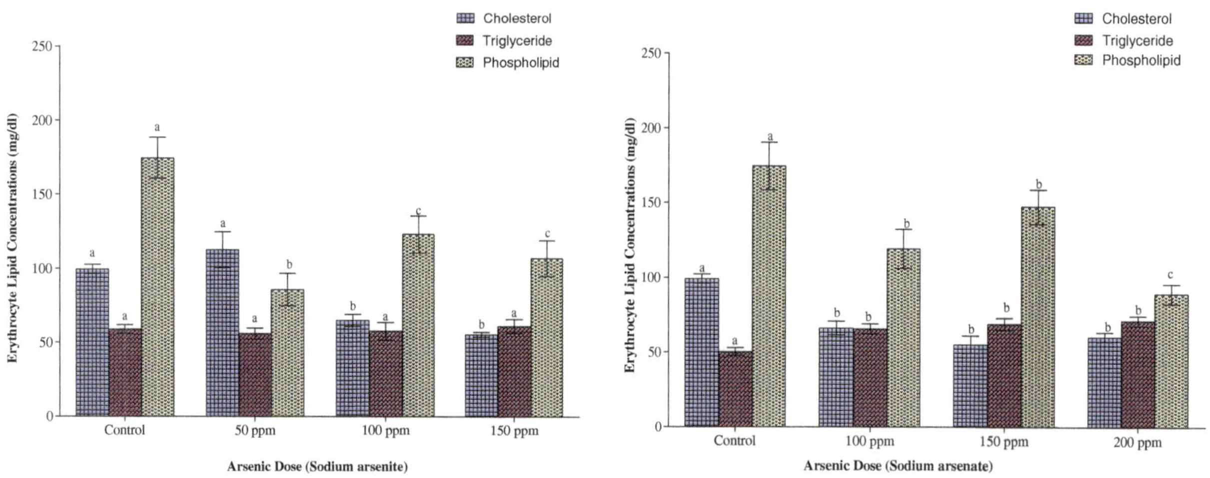

Fig. 5 Effects of arsenite and arsenate on erythrocyte cholesterol, triglyceride and phospholipid concentrations. Each bar represents the mean ± S.E.M. of 7 rats. Bars with different alphabets are significantly different at $p < 0.05$

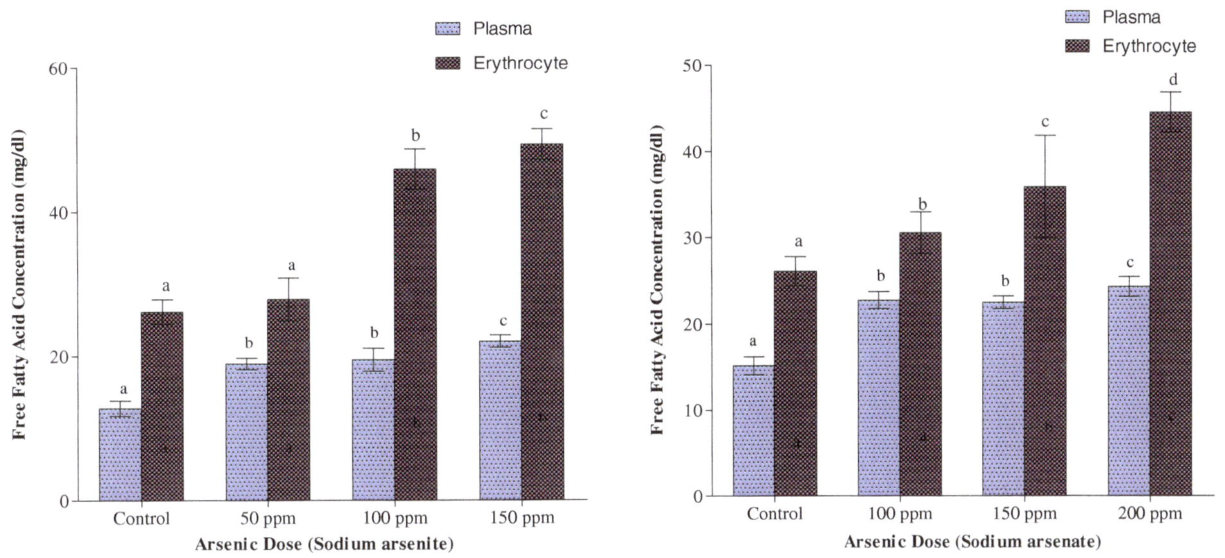

Fig. 6 Effects of arsenite and arsenate on plasma and erythrocyte free fatty acid concentrations. Each bar represents the mean ± S.E.M. of 7 rats. Bars with different alphabets are significantly different at $p < 0.05$

Cardiac, pulmonary and splenic triglyceride contents are shown in Fig. 10. The heart responded to the presence of the two arsenicals in a similar pattern. While the heart responded to the lowest dose of each arsenical with a decrease (64 % in arsenite and 28 % in arsenate), triglyceride contents began to increase with each increasing dose of the arsenicals, although the increase did not reach statistical significance ($p > 0.05$) within the exposed groups. In contrast to the heart, there was a dose-dependent decrease in the triglyceride contents in the lungs in arsenate exposure. Although arsenite also increased pulmonary triglycerides, the increase was not dose-dependent. Exposure to the two arsenicals did not result in any significant change in splenic triglyceride.

The mean phospholipid concentrations in the tissues of the animals as depicted in Figs. 11 and 12 indicate that exposure to both arsenicals resulted in splenic phospholipidosis. Arsenite exposure alone resulted in brain phospholipidosis while arsenate exposure at the highest dose (200 ppm As) resulted in hepatic phospholipidosis. In contrast however, arsenate caused a significant reduction in phospholipid concentrations in the brain, heart and lung of the animals (Fig. 11) whereas it was only in the heart, liver and lung that phospholipid was reduced on exposure to arsenite (Figs. 11 and 12). Renal phospholipids were not affected by any of the arsenicals irrespective of the dose (Fig. 11).

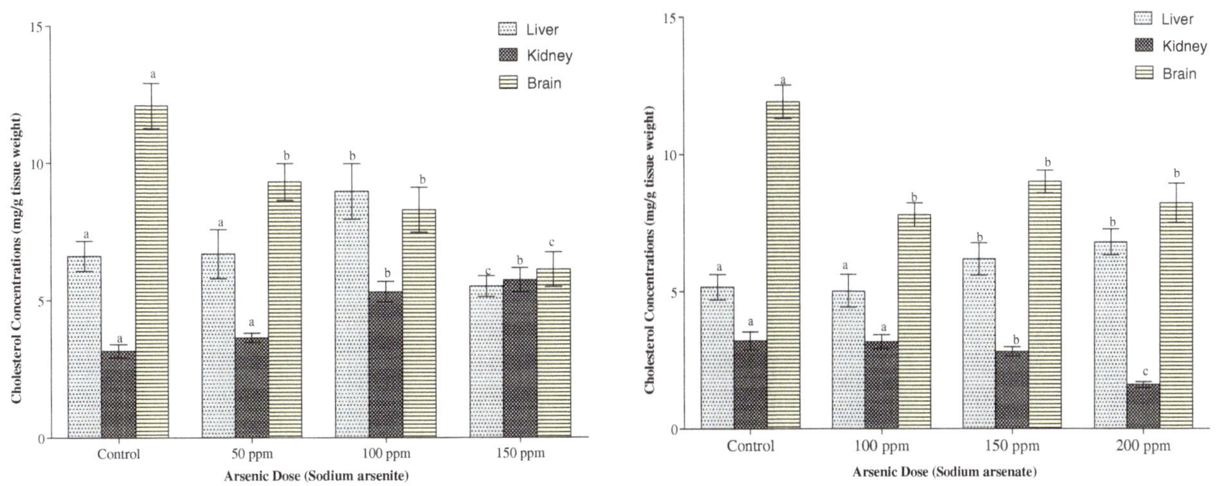

Fig. 7 Effects of arsenite and arsenate on hepatic, renal and brain cholesterol concentrations. Each bar represents the mean ± S.E.M. of 7 rats. Bars with different alphabets are significantly different at $p < 0.05$

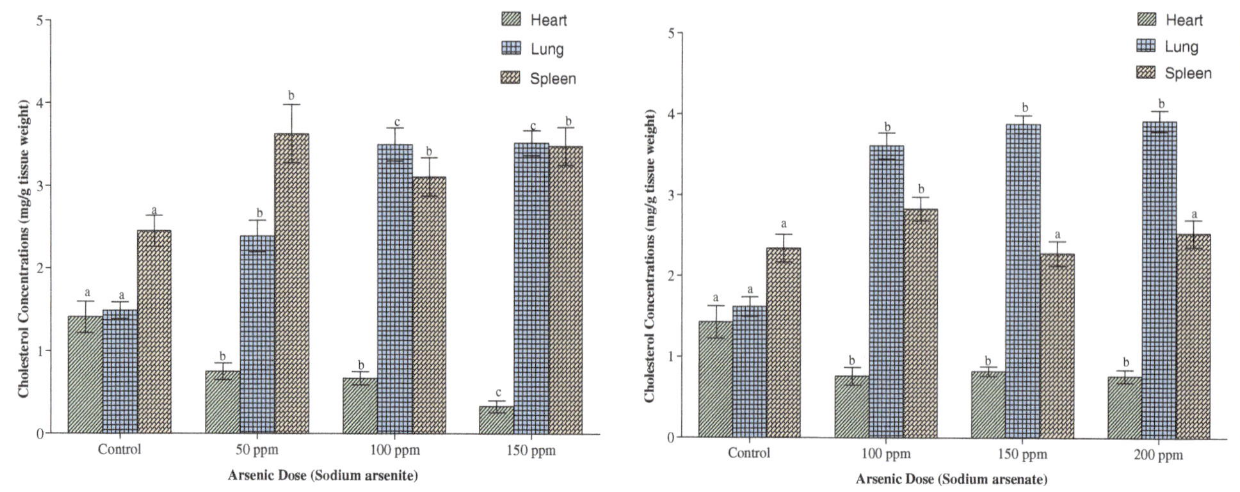

Fig. 8 Effects of arsenite and arsenate on heart, lung and spleen cholesterol concentrations. Each bar represents the mean ± S.E.M. of 7 rats. Bars with different alphabets are significantly different at $p < 0.05$

As indicated in Fig. 13, arsenite (150 ppm As) and arsenate (100 ppm As), inhibited hepatic HMG CoA reductase activity. At other doses of the arsenicals, hepatic HMG CoA reductase was up-regulated by 17 % by the two arsenicals respectively. The activity of the brain enzyme was also up-regulated by the two arsenicals (arsenite 56 % and arsenate 54 %).

The associations between tissue arsenic levels and some lipid parameters are depicted in Table 3. While tissue arsenic levels correlated positively with plasma FFA, reverse cholesterol transport was negatively correlated with tissue arsenic levels. Tissue arsenic levels (with the exception of hepatic arsenic vs. hepatic HMG CoA reductase and brain arsenic vs. hepatic HMG CoA reductase), also correlated positively with hepatic and brain HMG CoA reductase.

Discussion

Arsenic accumulated in all the organs investigated irrespective of the chemical species administered with concentrations raised by many folds compared to control. The rather high level of arsenic in the blood of the exposed rats has been reported by others [13, 23] and is mainly contributed by the erythrocytes which are responsible for the distribution of arsenic throughout the body.

Following exposure to inorganic arsenic, As V is sequentially reduced to As III. The As III produced by this reduction or from direct ingestion is then oxidatively methylated to give pentavalent organic arsenicals, monomethylarsonic acid (MMA) and dimethylarsinic acid (DMA) [24]. This in turn is a function of cellular uptake of the inorganic arsenic in various tissues [25]. Uptake of substances in a cell is a function of the cell membranes.

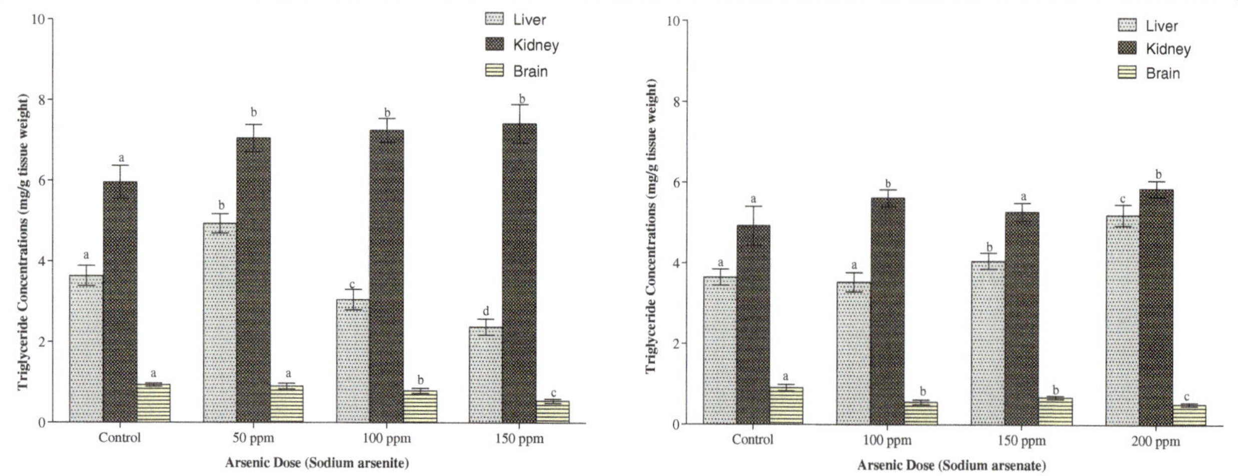

Fig. 9 Effects of arsenite and arsenate on hepatic, renal and brain triglyceride concentrations. Each bar represents the mean ± S.E.M. of 7 rats. Bars with different alphabets are significantly different at $p < 0.05$

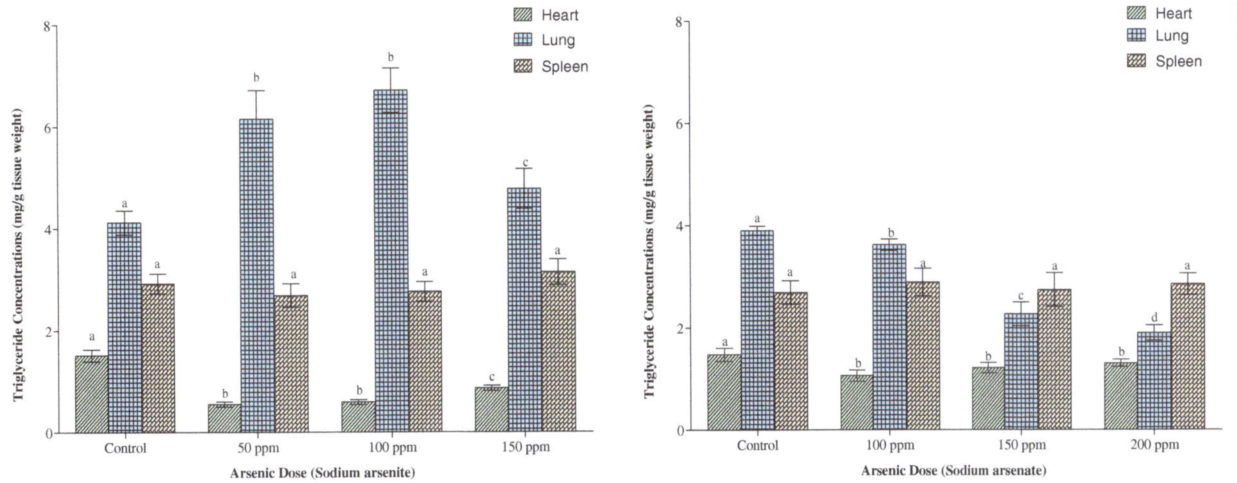

Fig. 10 Effects of arsenite and arsenate on heart, lung and spleen triglyceride concentrations. Each bar represents the mean ± S.E.M. of 7 rats. Bars with different alphabets are significantly different at $p < 0.05$

At physiological pH, trivalent arsenic compounds are neutral in charge while pentavalent arsenicals are negatively charged. Trivalent arsenic species can thus, readily transverse cell membranes than do pentavalent species [26]. Arsenite, therefore, might have been deposited in the organs at a faster rate than arsenate. Apart from blood, spleen accumulated the highest concentration of arsenic than any other tissue studied in arsenite-exposed rats. This was followed by heart and then kidney, brain, lung and liver in that order. In arsenate-exposed rats, accumulation was highest in the kidney, followed by lung, heart, brain, spleen and liver. Arsenate, in its protonated form, has similar properties and can substitute for phosphate in several biochemical reactions [27]. The high deposition in the kidney could, therefore, have resulted from the organ's physiological involvement in the reabsorption of phosphate. Arsenate and phosphate have been reported to compete for the same binding sites, with a preference for arsenate absorption [28]. Once taken up by the tissues, inorganic arsenic is methylated to MMA^{V} and DMA^{V} and excreted in the urine [24]. However, this biomethylation process may become saturated due to the different levels of methyltransferases present in each tissue, resulting in a reduced rate of clearance and hence increased deposition in the tissues [29]. Furthermore, this biomethylation process (oxidative methylation followed by reduction to trivalency) which was originally considered a detoxification process, may actually be an activation process in view of the formation of reactive intermediates like MMA^{III} and DMA^{III} [30]. In addition to these, improvement in analytical techniques has led to the discovery of new sulphur-containing

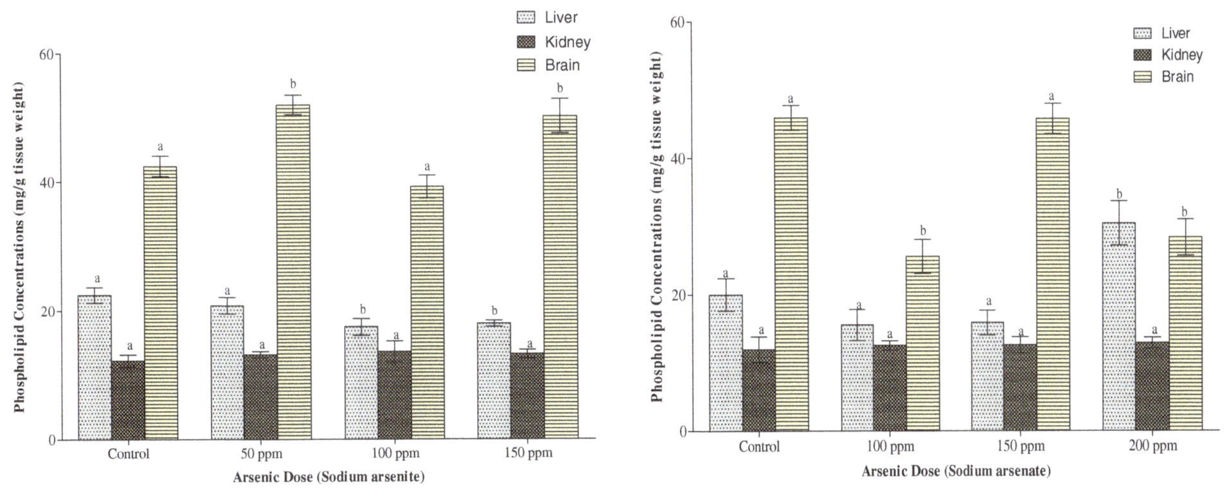

Fig. 11 Effects of arsenite and arsenate on hepatic, renal and brain phospholipid concentrations. Each bar represents the mean ± S.E.M. of 7 rats. Bars with different alphabets are significantly different at $p < 0.05$

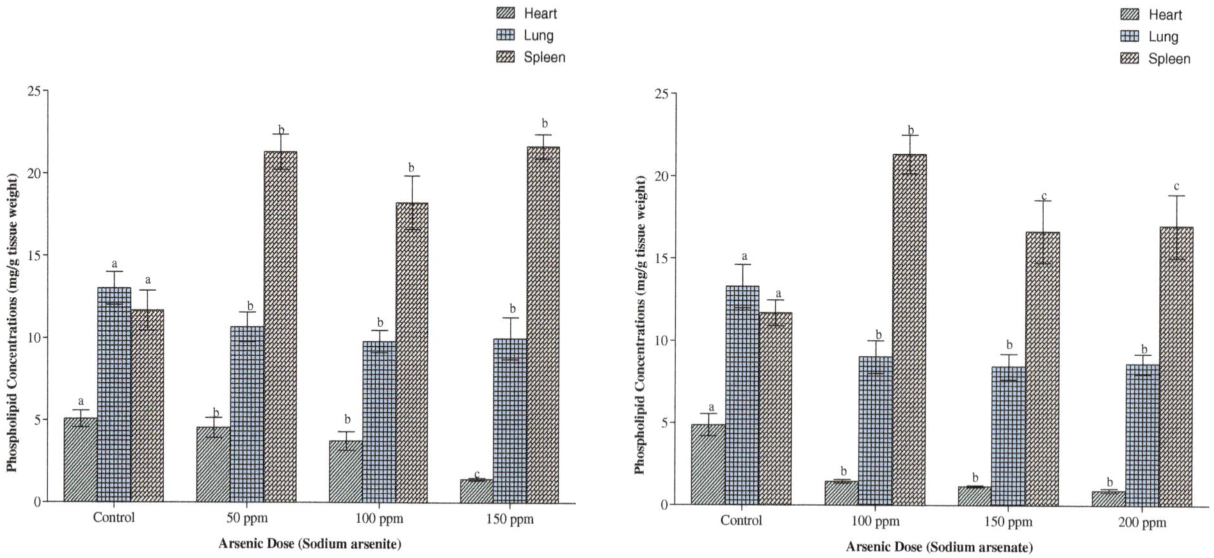

Fig. 12 Effects of arsenite and arsenate on heart, lung and spleen phospholipid concentrations. Each bar represents the mean ± S.E.M. of 7 rats. Bars with different alphabets are significantly different at $p < 0.05$

methylated arsenic metabolites, monomethylmonothioarsonic acid (MMMTA^{V}) and dimethylmonothioarsinic acid (DMMTA^{V}) in human urine [31]. To what extent this recent arsenic toxicokinetic information influences arsenic distribution/deposition in tissues on exposure to inorganic arsenic through drinking water remains to be elucidated.

The findings of this study also indicate that subchronic exposure to arsenite and arsenate through drinking water is associated with lipotoxic and non-lipotoxic perturbations in lipid homeostasis in organs, lipoproteins, plasma and erythrocytes as well as increase in HMG CoA reductase activity. Compared to control animals, lipotoxic perturbations in arsenic-exposed animals were characterised by high circulating FFA, enhanced splenic cholesterogenesis and phospholipidosis, pulmonary and hepatic cholesterogenesis as well as hypertriglyceridemia in plasma and LDL + VLDL fraction. Decrease in pulmonary and hepatic phospholipids, depletion of cardiac and brain lipids as well as depletion of erythrocyte, plasma and HDL cholesterol and phospholipids in circulation, characterised the non-lipotoxic effects of both arsenicals. An enrichment with cholesterol and depletion of phospholipids were also observed in the LDL + VLDL fraction. Since the patterns of this

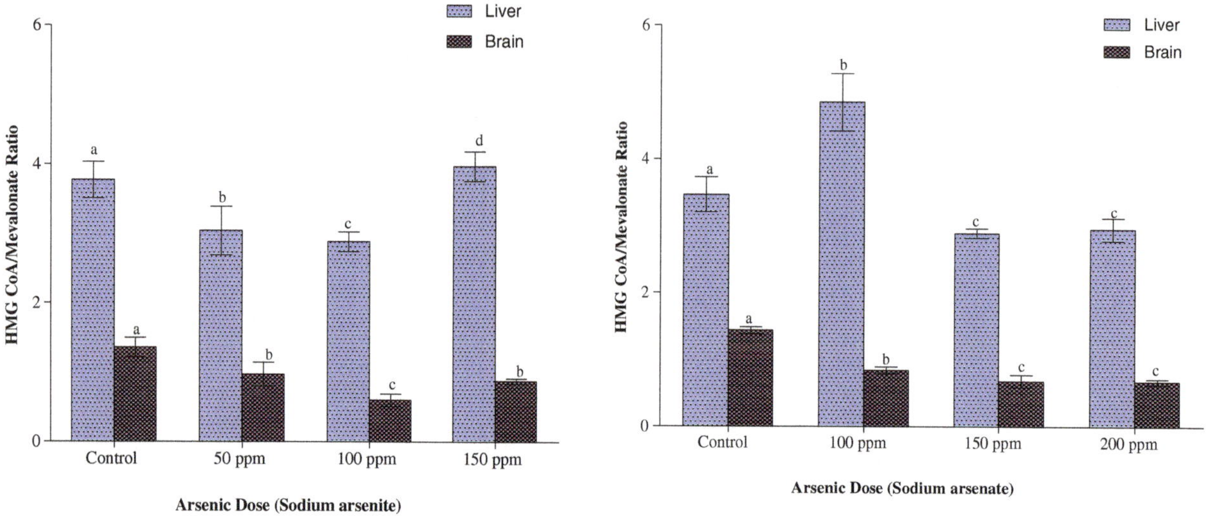

Fig. 13 Effects of arsenite and arsenate on hepatic and brain HMG CoA/ Meva-lonate ratios as an Index of HMG CoA reductase activity. Each bar represents the mean ± S.E.M. of 7 rats. Bars with different alphabets are significantly different at $p < 0.05$

Table 3 Association between tissue arsenic levels and some lipid parameters in the animals on exposure to sodium arsenite and sodium arsenate for 12 weeks through drinking water

	Plasma FFA	HDL cholesterol	Hepatic HMG CoA reductase	Brain HMG CoA reductase
Parameter	Correlation coefficient (r)	Correlation coefficient (r)	Correlation coefficient (r)	Correlation coefficient (r)
Liver arsenic	0.491[a]	−0.634[a]	NS	−0.382[a]
Kidney arsenic	0.577[a]	−0.614[a]	−0.365[a]	−0.537[a]
Brain arsenic	0.602[a]	−0.611[a]	NS	−0.556[a]
Blood arsenic	0.578[a]	−0.732[a]	NS	−0.584[a]

[a]Significant at $p < 0.05$
NS-Not Significant

homeostatic imbalance differ with each arsenic specie and dose, different mechanisms might mediate this imbalance. In addition, since exposure to the arsenic species was through the oral route, interaction between arsenic and these lipids probably did not begin at the level of the gastro-intestinal tract. Rather, lipid dynamics after absorption might be the lipotoxic target of arsenic. These observations could be discussed along several lines.

Under normal physiological conditions, all tissues avidly acquire lipids from circulating non-esterified FFA associated with albumin, esterified fatty acids bound to lipoproteins chylomicrons and very low density lipoproteins (and liberated by lipoprotein lipase-mediated lipolysis), internalization of whole lipoproteins and *de novo* synthesis [32, 33], although *de novo* synthesis might play only a minor role in some tissues [32, 34]. Excess lipid, beyond that needed for cellular structures and ATP generation is stored in lipid droplets [32, 34]. However, tissues like liver, intestine, heart and brain are able to synthesise and secrete excess lipids in lipoproteins [32, 35–38].

FFAs originating from either albumin or lipoproteins enter the organs either by passive diffusion or via a protein carrier-mediated pathway [33, 34]. While the former is a lower affinity non-saturable process operating at higher FFA concentrations, the protein carrier-mediated pathway is a low capacity but high affinity process operating at FFA/albumin ratios found in the plasma [33, 34]. Protein carriers that have been characterized include fatty acid translocase (FAT/CD 36), plasma membrane fatty-acid binding protein and fatty acid transport protein [33, 34].

Both arsenic species induced significant elevation of plasma FFA concentration. This observation implies that while arsenic exposure did not affect the absorption of dietary lipids, cellular lipid dynamics was modulated by arsenic exposure. Generally hydrolysis of triglycerides occurs in the adipose tissue and results in the production of FFA with its subsequent release into the plasma. The elevation of this lipid suggests its increased mobilization from the adipose tissue which could be induced by physiological and psychological stress [39]. With consistent report of arsenic causing oxidative stress [40–42], the elevated plasma FFA implies an arsenic-induced augmentation of triglyceride hydrolysis in the adipose tissue by triglyceride lipase, resulting in increased mobilization of the liberated FFA into the plasma. The physiological consequences of this elevated plasma FFA could be viewed from the metabolic roles of FFA. While this elevated plasma FFA should provide an immediate substrate for triglyceride synthesis as well as the source of available fuel for the tissues and also the necessary signal for tissues to oxidize them [43, 44], data in Fig. 6 indicate what while exposure to arsenic did not inhibit the uptake of FFA by the tissues, a considerable amount of the FFA was directed towards the synthesis of triglycerides in the liver, kidney and lungs as well as phospholipids in the spleen. Data in Fig. 9 also indicate that while the liver could be said to have a limited capacity for triglyceride storage, tissues like kidney and lungs accumulated the triglyceride to about 2-fold that of the liver. This further suggests that arsenic induced a dysfunction of triglyceride degradation secondary to insufficient mitochondrial ß-oxidation of FFA, thus compromising energy metabolism in these tissues. Further significant energetic and functional consequences might be expected.

The key enzyme in the distribution of circulating lipids between organs is lipoprotein lipase (LPL), an enzyme located on the walls of blood capillaries [32]. The role of LPL in lipoprotein metabolism is well known. Since majority of the circulating FFAs are present as triglycerides in lipoproteins, hydrolysis of this triglyceride by LPL is an important determinant of overall fatty acid uptake and ß-oxidation in the tissues [45, 46]. High circulating FFA (as observed in this study) is known to inhibit the activity of LPL [47]. Homeostatically, inhibition of LPL is expected to have the following consequences on lipid dynamics in the circulation:

1. Severe hypertriglyceridemia secondary to underutilisation of chylomicrons and VLDL
2. Hypocholesterolemia
3. Decrease in HDL cholesterol (otherwise known as reverse cholesterol transport) and phospholipids [48].

That arsenic exposure resulted in all these lipid metabolic derangements (Figs. 1 and 3) suggests that the inhibition of LPL might mediate these observed effects of arsenic.

Another major finding of this study was the depletion of cardiac lipids in arsenic-exposed animals. Physiologically, cardiac myocytes have regulatory pathways that regulate lipid metabolism. The myocardium has labile stores of triglyceride that serve as an endogenous source of FFAs [49, 50]. Intramyocardial triglyceride can be hydrolysed by hormone sensitive lipase and adipose triglyceride lipase [32, 33]. Insulin inhibits lipolysis, whereas catecholamines, thyroid hormone and glucagon, accelerate intramyocardial triglyceride degradation [51]. Whether arsenic-induced adrenergic stress in the animals might mediate the depletion of cardiac lipids observed in this study is not known at present. Furthermore, since the major cardiac lipids were depleted as a result of arsenic exposure, the possibility that arsenic might induce overexpression/production of cardiac apolipoprotein B (Apo B) which increased lipid secretion from the heart, cannot be ruled out [38]. Apo B expression has been found to increase in hearts of patients with coronary artery disease [52], a cardiovascular outcome that is a hallmark of arsenic exposure [53].

Due to the blood brain barrier, circulating lipoproteins cannot reach the brain except for small HDL particles [54]. Most of the lipoproteins in the brain are synthesised by the astrocytes and have been postulated to be responsible for the transfer of lipids within the brain [36, 55]. Thus, an arsenic-induced damage to the blood brain barrier might be responsible for the dyslipidemia observed in the brain of the arsenic-exposed animals [56, 57].

Enhanced cholesterogenesis observed in the spleen, lungs and liver of arsenite- and arsenate-exposed animals as well as the kidney of arsenate-exposed animals, may be attributed to an arsenic-induced activation of 3-hydroxy-3-methylglutaryl Coenzyme A (HMG CoA) reductase (the rate limiting enzyme in cholesterol synthesis) or it may be due to feedback inhibition [58, 59]. It may also be due to inhibition of the activity of cholesterol-7α-hydroxylase, a cytochrome P450 enzyme located in the endoplasmic reticulum. This could limit the biosynthesis of bile acids, which is the only significant route for elimination of cholesterol from the body [60]. Since the liver has limited capacity to store lipids, the excess cholesterol and triglycerides are packaged into VLDL particles and secreted into circulation. Consistent with this was the observation of the enrichment of LDL + VLDL fraction with cholesterol and triglycerides. Furthermore, since this fraction was depleted of phospholipids, this implies a failure occasioned by arsenic exposure in hepatic provision of phospholipids that are found in lipoproteins (Fig. 4) [61].

Compelling experimental data from animal studies have shown a positive association between high circulating FFA and pathological conditions such as diabetes mellitus, obesity, thyrotoxicosis, atherosclerosis, coronary artery disease, cardiac arrhythmia, high blood pressure and pulmonary diseases [39, 62–64]. Furthermore, elevated pulmonary cholesterol has been shown to inhibit surfactant function by disrupting the physiology and turnover of surfactant, leading to impairment of lungs mechanics [65]. Abnormalities in surfactant metabolism are the leading causes of acute respiratory distress syndrome, acute lung injury and a diverse array of other respiratory illnesses [66]. That arsenic exposure causes all these conditions have been confirmed from epidemiological studies of arsenicosis [3]. Thus, the sustained dyslipidemia observed in this study may be one of the underlying mechanisms of these arsenic-induced pathologies.

One limitation of this study was that arsenic speciation was not carried out in the tissues. Rather, arsenic in the tissues was determined as total arsenic. In view of the recent discovery of new methylsulphur derivatives of inorganic arsenic, it opens up the possibility that these organic metabolites may be more subtle and insidious in their toxic effects. Toxicological information on these newly discovered organic metabolites is scanty. However, in a recent study in our laboratory in which rats were exposed to pentavalent inorganic and organic arsenicals through drinking water, arsenic accumulation and dyslipidemia of the same magnitude were also observed. These recent data, together with the data in the present study, support a linkage between metabolism and chemical form of arsenic and lipotoxic and non-lipotoxic effects of this metalloid.

Conclusion

In conclusion, even though sub-chronic exposure to arsenite and arsenate through drinking water produced different patterns of dyslipidemia, our study identified two common denominators of dyslipidemia namely: inhibition of reverse cholesterol transport and increase in plasma FFA. These two denominators (in addition to other individual perturbations of lipid metabolism induced by each arsenical), might mediate the observed cardiovascular and other disease endpoints of inorganic arsenic exposure through drinking water.

Abbreviations

HDL: High density lipoproteins; FFAs: Free fatty acids; HMG CoA reductase: 3-hydroxy-3-methylglutaryl coenzyme A reductase; LDL: Low density lipoproteins; VLDL: Very low density lipoproteins; MMA: Monomethylarsonic acid; DMA: Dimethylarsinic acid; MMMTA: Monomethylmonothioarsonic acid; DMMTA: Dimethylmonothioarsinic acid; FAT: Fatty acid translocase; LPL: Lipoprotein lipase.

Competing interests

The authors declare that they have no competing interests

Authors' contributions

OA, EAB and OOOD (Odukoya) conceived the work. OA designed the work. OA, EAB and OOOD coordinated the study. OKA, ADW, OOOG (Ogunrinola), EOA, DOB, OAD, OBO and OA were involved in lipid and metal analyses. OKA and OA drafted the manuscript and did statistical analysis. All authors read and approved the manuscript for submission.

Acknowledgements

The technical assistance of Mr. OA. Awoyemi, Mr. OJ. Olurinde, Mrs. JO. Adebawa and Mrs. T. Osibanjo is greatly acknowledged.

Author details

[1]Department of Biochemistry, Federal University of Agriculture, Abeokuta, Nigeria. [2]Department of Chemistry, Federal University of Agriculture, Abeokuta, Nigeria. [3]Department of Biochemistry, Ladoke Akintola University of Technology, Ogbomosho, Nigeria. [4]Department of Biochemistry, Lagos State University, Ojoo, Lagos, Nigeria. [5]Department of Biochemistry, University of Ilorin, Ilorin, Nigeria. [6]Biochemistry Unit, Department of Chemical Sciences, Bells University of Technology, Ota, Nigeria.

References

1. Hughes MF, Beck BD, Chen Y, Lewis AS, Thomas DJ. Arsenic exposure and toxicology: a historical perspective. Toxicol Sci. 2011;123(2):305–32.
2. Smeester L, Rager JE, Bailey KA, Guan X, Smith N, Garcia-Vargas G, et al. Epigenetic changes in individuals with arsenicosis. Chem Res Toxicol. 2011;24:165–7.
3. Mazumder DG, Dasgupta UB. Chronic arsenic toxicity: studies in West Bengal, India. Kaohsiung J Med Sci. 2011;27:360–70.
4. States JC, Srivastava S, Chen Y, Barchowsky A. Arsenic and cardiovascular disease. Toxicol Sci. 2009;107:312–23.
5. Suwalsky M, Rivera C, Sotomayor C, Jemiola-Rzeminsky M, Strzalka K. Monomethylarsonate (MMA v) exerts stronger effects than arsenate on the structure and thermotropic properties of phospholipids bilayers. Biophys Chem. 2008;132:1–8.
6. Román DA, Pizarro I, Rivera L, Cámara C, Palacios MA, Gómez MM, et al. An approach to the arsenic status in cardiovascular tissues in patients with coronary heart disease. Human Exp Toxicol. 2011;30(9):1150–64.
7. Ademuyiwa O, Ugbaja RN, Idumebor F, Adebawo O. Plasma lipid profiles and risk of cardiovascular disease in occupational lead exposure in Abeokuta. Nigeria Lipids Health Dis. 2005;4:19.
8. Ginsberg HN. Lipoprorein metabolism and its relationship to atherosclerosis. Med Clin North Am. 1994;78:1–20.
9. Aguilar-Salinas CA, Olaiz G, Valles V, Torres JMR, Pérez FJG, Rull JA, et al. High prevalence of HDL cholesterol concentrations and mixedhyperlipidemia in a Mexican nationwide survey. J Lipid Res. 2001;42:1298–307.
10. Prozialeck WC, Edwards JR, Nebert DW, Woods JM, Barchowsky A, Atchison WD. The vascular system as a target of metal toxicity. Toxicol Sci. 2008;102(2):207–18.
11. Cheng TJ, Chuu JJ, Chang CY, Tsai WC, Chen KJ, Guo HR. Atherosclerosis induced by arsenic in drinking water in rats through altering lipid metabolism. Toxicol Appl Pharmacol. 2011;256:146–53.
12. Elsenhans B, Ademuyiwa O, Schmolke G, Scharper J, Hunder G. Arsenic-copper interactions in the kidneys of laboratory animals. In: Elsenhans B, Forth W, Schümann K, editors. Metal-metal interactions. Gütersloh, Germany: Bertelsmann Foundation Publishers; 1993. p. 110–28.
13. Hunder G, Scharper J, Ademuyiwa O, Elsenhans B. Species differences in arsenic-mediated renal copper accumulation: a comparison between rats, mice and guinea-pigs. Hum Exp Toxicol. 1999;18:699–705.
14. Xie Y, Trouba KJ, Liu J, Waalkes MP, Germolec DR. Biokinetics and subchronic toxic effects of oral arsenite, arsenate, monomethylarsonic acid, and dimethylarsinic acid in v-Ha-ras transgenic (Tg.Ac) mice. Environ Health Perspect. 2004;112(12):1255–63.
15. Yamamoto S, Konishi Y, Matsuda T, Murai T, Shibata M-A, Matsui-Yuasa I, et al. Cancer induction by an organic arsenic compound, dimethylarsinic acid (cacodylic acid), in F344/DuCrj rats after pretreatment with five carcinogens. Cancer Res. 1995;55:1271–6.
16. Ademuyiwa O, Agarwal R, Chandra R, Behari JR. Lead-induced phospholipidosis and cholesterogenesis in rat tissues. Chem Biol Interact. 2009;179:314–20.
17. Banjoko IO, Adeyanju MM, Ademuyiwa O, Adebawo OO, Olalere RA, Kolawole MO, et al. Hypolipidemic effects of lactic acid bacteria fermented cereal in rats. Lipids Health Dis. 2012;11:170.
18. Rotimi SO, Ojo DA, Talabi OA, Balogun EA, Ademuyiwa O. Tissue dyslipidemia in Salmonella-infected rats treated with amoxillin and pefloxacin. Lipids Health Dis. 2012;11:152.
19. Afolabi OK, Wusu AD, Ogunrinola OO, Abam EO, Babayemi DO, Dosumu OA, Onunkwor OB, Balogun EA, Odukoya OO, Ademuyiwa O: Paraoxonase 1 activity in subchronic low-level inorganic arsenic exposure through drinking water. Environ Toxicol 2014.
20. Folch J, Lees M, Sloane SGH. A simple method for the isolation and purification of total lipids from animal tissues. J Biol Chem. 1957;226:497–509.
21. Rose HG, Oklander M. Improved procedure for the extraction of lipids from human erythrocytes. J Lipid Res. 1965;6:428–31.
22. Rao AV, Ramakrishnan S. Indirect assessment of hydroxymethylglutaryl- CoA reductase (NADPH) activity in liver tissue. Clin Chem. 1975;21(10):1523–5.
23. Ademuyiwa O, Elsenhans B, Forth W. Arsenic-copper interaction in the kidney of the rat : influence of arsenic metabolites. Pharmacol Toxicol. 1996;78:154–60.
24. Vahter M. Biotransformation of trivalent and pentavalent inorganic arsenic in mice and rats. Environ Res. 1981;25:286–93.
25. Styblo M, Del Razo LM, LeCluyse EL, Hamilton GA, Wang C, Cullen WR, et al. Metabolism of arsenic in primary cultures of human and rat hepatocytes. Chem Res Toxicol. 1999;12:560–5.
26. Cohen SM, Arnold LL, Eldan M, Lewis AS, Beck BD. Methylated arsenicals: the implications of metabolism and carcinogenicity studies in rodents to human risk assessment. Crit Rev Toxicol. 2006;36:99–133.
27. Dixon HBF. The biochemical action of arsonic acids, especially as phosphate analogues. Adv Inorg Chem. 1997;44:191–227.
28. Gonzalez MJ, Aguilar MV, Martinez Para MC. Gastrointestinal absorption of inorganic arsenic (V): the effect of concentration and interactions with phosphate and dichromate. Vet Hum Toxicol. 1995;37:131–6.
29. Carbrey JM, Song L, Zhou Y, Yoshinaga M, Rojek A, Wang Y, Liu Y, Lujan HL, Carlo SE, Nielsen S, Rosen BP, Agre P, Mukhopadhyay R: Reduced arsenic clearance and increased toxicity in aquaglyceroporin-9-null mice. PNAS 106 (37): 15956–15960.
30. Styblo M, Drobna Z, Jaspers I, Lin S, Thomas DJ. The role of biomethylation in toxicity and carcinogenicity of arsenic. Environ Health Perspect. 2002;110 Suppl 5:767–77.
31. Naramandura H, Suzuki N, Iwata K, Hirano S, Suzuki KT. Arsenic metabolism and thioarsenicals in hamsters and rats. Chem Res Toxicol. 2007;20:616–24.
32. Goldberg IJ, Trent CM, Schulze PC. Lipid metabolism and toxicity in the heart. Cell Metab. 2012;15:805–12.
33. Lopaschuk GD, Ussher JR, Folmes CDL, Jaswal JS, Stanley WC. Myocardial fatty acid metabolism in health and disease. Physiol Rev. 2010;90:207–58.
34. Bharadwaj KG, Hiyama Y, Hu Y, Huggins LA, Ramakrishnan R, Abumrad NA, et al. Chylomicron- and VLDL-derived lipis enter the heart through different pathways: in vivo evidence for receptor- and non-receptor-mediated fatty acid uptake. J Biol Chem. 2010;285(49):37976–86.
35. Nielsen LB, Veniant M, Boren J, Raabe M, Wong JS, Tam C, et al. Genes for apoliporotein B and microsomal triglyceride transfer protein are expressed in the heart: evidence that the heart has the capacity to synthesise and secrete lipoproteins. Circul. 1998;98:13–16.
36. Postle AD. Phospholipidomics in health and disease. Eur J Lipid Sci Technol. 2009;111:2–13.
37. Walters JW, Anderson JL, Bittman R, Pack M, Farber SA. Visualisation of lipid metabolism in the zebrafish intestine reveals a relationship between NPC1L1-mediated cholesterol uptake and dietary fatty acid. Chem Biol. 2012;19:913–25.
38. Yokoyama M, Yagyu A, Hu Y, Seo T, Hirata K, Homma S, et al. Apolipoprotein B production reduces lipotoxic cardiomyopathy. Studies in heart-specific lipoprotein lipase transgenic mouse. J Biol Chem. 2004;279(6):4204–11.
39. Newsholme EA, Start C. Regulation in Metabolism. Chichester, UK: John Wiley and Sons; 1981. p. 195-246.
40. Hughes MF. Arsenic toxicity and potential mechanisms of action. Toxicol Lett. 2002;133:1–16.
41. Kitchin KT, Ahmad S. Oxidative stress as a possible mode of action for arsenic carcinogenesis. Toxicol Lett. 2003;137(1–2):3–13.
42. Pi J, Yamauchi H, Kumagai Y, Sun G, Yoshida T, Aikawa H, et al. Evidence for induction of oxidative stress caused by chronic exposure of Chinese

residents to arsenic contained in drinking water. Environ Health Perspect. 2002;110:331–6.
43. Donnelly KL, Smith CI, Schwarzenberg SJ, Jessurum J, Boldt MD, Parks EJ. Sources of fatty acid stored in liver and secreted via lipoproteins in patients with nonalcoholic fatty liver disease. J Clin Invest. 2005;115(5):1343–51.
44. Mermier P, Baker N. Flux of free fatty acids among host tissues, ascites fluid, and Ehrlich ascites carcinoma cells. J Lipid Res. 1974;15(4):339–51.
45. Lee J, Goldberg IJ. Lipoprotein lipase-derived fatty acids: physiology and dysfunction. Curr Hypertens Rep. 2007;9:462–6.
46. Pulinilkunnil T, Rodrigues B. Cardiac lipoprotein lipase: metabolic basis for diabetic heart disease. Cardiovasc Res. 2006;69:329–40.
47. Saxena U, Witte LD, Goldberg IJ. Release of endothelial cell lipoprotein lipase by plasma lipoproteins and free fatty acids. J Biol Chem. 1989;264:4349–55.
48. Rader DJ. Regulation of reverse cholesterol transport and clinical implications. Am J Cardiol. 2003;92:42J–9J.
49. Saddik M, Lopaschuk GD. Myocardial triglyceride turnover and contribution to energy substrate utilisation in isolated working rat hearts. J Biol Chem. 1991;266:8162–70.
50. Stanley WC, Recchia FA, Lopascuk GD. Myocardial substrate metabolism in the normal and failing heart. Physiol Rev. 2005;85:1093–129.
51. Swanton EM, Saggerson ED. Effects of adrenaline on triacylglycerol synthesis and turnover in ventricular myocytes from adult rats. Biochem J. 1997;328:913–22.
52. Nuotio IO, Raitakari OT, Porkka KV, Rasanen L, Moilanen T, Viikari JS. Associations between diet and the hyperapobetalipoproteinemia phenotype expression in children and young adults. The Cardiovascular Risk in Young Finns Study. Arterioscler Thromb Vasc Biol. 1997;17:820–5.
53. Li WF, Sun CW, Cheng TJ, Chang KH, Chen CJ, Wang SL. Risk of carotid atherosclerosis is associated with low serum paraoxonase (PON1) activity among arsenic exposed residents in Southwestern Taiwan. Toxicol Appl Pharmacol. 2009;236(2):246–53.
54. Kersten S. Physiological regulation of lipoprotein lipase. Biochim Biophys Acta. 2014;1841:919–33.
55. Wang H, Eckel RH. What are lipoproteins doing in the brain? Trends Endocrinol Metab. 2014;25:8–14.
56. Rosado JL, Ronquillo D, Kodas K, Rojas O, Alatorre J, Lopez P, et al. Arsenic exposure and cognitive performance in Mexican schoolchildren. Environ Health Perspect. 2007;115(9):1371–5.
57. Ross IA, Boyle T, Johnson WD, Sprando RL, O'Donnell MW, Ruggles D, Kim CS: Free fatty acids profile of the fetal brain and the plasma, liver, brain and kidneys of pregnant rats treated with sodium arsenite at mid-organogenesis. Toxicol Ind Health 2010;26(10):657–666.
58. Gesquiere L, Loreau N, Minnich A, Davignon J, Blache D. Oxidative stress leads to cholesterol accumulation in vascular smooth muscle cells. Free Radic Biol Med. 1999;27(1-2):134–45.
59. Sawada H, Takami K, Asahi S. A toxicogenomic approach to drug-induced phospholipidosis: analysis of its induction mechanism and establishment of a novel in vitro screening system. Toxicol Sci. 2005;83(2):282–92.
60. Kojima M, Masui T, Nemoto K, Degawa M. Lead nitrate induced development of hypercholesterolemia in rats: sterol independent gene regulation of hepatic enzymes responsible for cholesterol homeostasis. Toxicol Lett. 2004;154:35–44.
61. Botham KM, Mayes PA. Metabolism of acylglycerols and sphingolipids. In: Murray RK, Granner DK, Rodwell VW, editors. Harpers illustrated biochemistry 27th Edition. New York: McGraw Hill Companies Inc; 2006. p. 209–16.
62. El Hafidi M, Pérez I, Carrillo S, Cardoso G, Zamora J, Chavira R, et al. Effect of sex hormones on non-esterified fatty acids, intra-abdominal fat accumulation and hypertension induced by sucrose diet in male rats. Clin Exp Hypertens. 2006;28:669–81.
63. El Hafidi M, Valdez R, Ba˜nos G. Possible relationship between altered fatty acid composition of serum, platelets and aorta and hypertension induced by sugar feeding in rats. Clin Exp Hypertens. 2000;22:99–108.
64. Goodfreind TL, Egan BM. Nonesterified fatty acids in the pathogenesis of hypertension: theory and evidence. Prostaglandins Leukot Essent Fatty Acids. 1997;57:57–63.
65. Roszell BR, Tao J-Q, YU KJ, Gao L, Huang S, Ning Y, et al. Pulmonary abnormalities in animal models due to niemann-pick type C1 (NPC1) or C2 (NPC2) disease. Plos One. 2013;8(7), e67084.
66. Agassandian M, Mallampalli RK. Surfactant phospholipid metabolism. Biochim Biophys Acta. 2013;1831:612–25.

The pharmacokinetics and pharmacodynamics of danirixin (GSK1325756) – a selective CXCR2 antagonist – in healthy adult subjects

Bruce E. Miller[1*], Sunil Mistry[2], Kevin Smart[3,9], Paul Connolly[4], Donald C. Carpenter[5], Hiran Cooray[6,10], Jackie C. Bloomer[7], Ruth Tal-Singer[1] and Aili L. Lazaar[8]

Abstract

Background: Excessive neutrophil presence and activation is important in a number of acute and chronic inflammatory diseases. The CXCR2 chemokine receptor is important in controlling the extravasation and activation of neutrophils. Selective antagonism of the CXCR2 receptor is a potential approach to reducing neutrophil migration and activation. Danirixin, is a small molecule, CXCR2 antagonist being evaluated as a potential anti-inflammatory medicine.

Methods: (1) First time in human (FTIH) double-blind, placebo-controlled study to evaluate the safety, pharmacokinetics, and pharmacodynamics of single ascending and repeat oral doses of danirixin in healthy male subjects; (2) single-dose study of age, gender, food, and proton-pump inhibitor effects on the pharmacokinetics of danirixin in healthy adult subjects; and placebo-controlled study of the pharmacokinetics of danirixin in healthy elderly subjects.

Results: There were no serious adverse events and no adverse events considered to be of clinical relevance. There were no withdrawals due to adverse events. Systemic exposure following single doses of danirixin 10 mg, 25 mg, 50 mg, 100 mg, and 200 mg increased with increasing dose. Engagement of pharmacology was demonstrated as inhibition of ex-vivo CXCL1-induced CD11b expression on peripheral blood neutrophils when compared to placebo (approximately 50 % for 50 mg and 100 mg danirixin, and 72 % at 200 mg). There was a 37 % decrease in Cmax and a 16 % decrease in AUC (0-∞) following administration of danirixin in the presence of food. Cmax also decreased by 65 % when danirixin 100 mg was administered following omeprazole 40 mg once daily for 5 days. The AUC (0-∞) and Cmax were 50 % lower in elderly subjects compared with younger subjects.

Conclusion: The dose-dependent inhibition of agonist-induced neutrophil activation following single and repeated once daily oral administration of danirixin suggests that this CXCR2 antagonist may have benefit in neutrophil-predominant inflammatory diseases. Co-administration with food, gastric acid reducing agents, and variable exposure in the elderly have important clinical implications that need to be taken into consideration in subsequent clinical evaluations.

Trial registration: ClinicalTrials.gov identifiers: NCT01209052 and NCT01209104

Keywords: CXCR2 antagonist, Danirixin, GSK1325756, Chronic obstructive pulmonary disease, Pharmacokinetics, Pharmacodynamics, Omeprazole

* Correspondence: bruce.e.miller@gsk.com
[1]Clinical Discovery, Respiratory Therapy Area Unit, GlaxoSmithKline R&D, 709 Swedeland Road, King of Prussia, PA 19406, USA
Full list of author information is available at the end of the article

Background

Chemokines acting through specific receptors are able to recruit leukocytes to sites of inflammation, resulting in the subsequent release of a number of mediators, including neutrophil elastase and matrix metalloproteinases, which likely play an important role in disease pathophysiology [1]. For several acute and chronic pulmonary diseases, chemokines are thought to be important mediators driving the tissue destruction and airway and parenchymal remodeling associated with disease progression [2, 3].

Selective antagonism of the interaction between the CXCR2 chemokine receptor and its various ligands provides a potential targeted strategy for reducing the underlying inflammation that contributes to the deleterious effects of an excessive neutrophil response [2]. In particular, a CXCR2 antagonist may be useful in the treatment of respiratory diseases such as chronic obstructive pulmonary disease (COPD) that are associated with a high tissue burden of activated neutrophils. The potential for CXCR2 antagonism to reduce neutrophil recruitment into the lung has been demonstrated previously in experimental human models of lung inflammation (ozone challenge) [4, 5] and in initial studies in patients with severe asthma and COPD [6–8]. Transient reductions in blood neutrophils have been observed with two recent small molecule CXCR2 antagonists following short and long term oral administration leading to concerns about a potential impact on host defense and innate immunity, particularly with chronic use. It is therefore desirable to identify a CXCR2 antagonist that would have the intended efficacy in the target tissues without substantially impacting circulating neutrophil counts.

Danirixin is a small molecule, non-peptide, high affinity (IC_{50} for CXCL8 binding = 12.5 nM), selective, and reversible CXCR2 antagonist. This compound has demonstrated potent antagonism of CXCR2 activity in vitro and anti-inflammatory effects in various preclinical models. Its pharmacologic activity and duration of action following oral administration support its potential use as an oral, anti-inflammatory agent.

The results of two clinical pharmacology studies with danirixin are described in this report. The first time in human (FTIH) study was conducted to investigate the safety, tolerability, pharmacokinetics, and pharmacodynamics of single and repeat oral doses of danirixin in healthy adult male subjects. The second study explored the effects of age, gender, food (high fat meal), and a proton-pump inhibitor (omeprazole) on the pharmacokinetics of danirixin.

Methods

Danirixin formulation

The structure of danirixin free base is shown in Fig. 1. Immediate release (IR) tablets contained danirixin free base and standard excipients including mannitol, microcrystalline cellulose, HPMC, croscarmellose sodium and magnesium stearate.

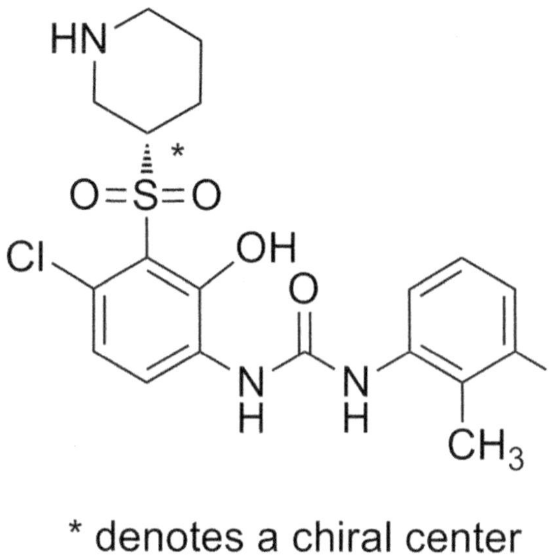

Fig. 1 Danirixin Free Base

Study designs and study subjects

Clinical studies were conducted in accordance with the Declaration of Helskini. Prior to study initiation approvals from appropriate regulatory authorities and ethics committee/institutional review boards were obtained. Written, informed consent was obtained from participating subjects prior to the performance of any study related assessments and procedures.

Study 1, FTIH (GSK Protocol CX3112483, ClinicalTrials.gov identifier NCT01209052, reviewed and approved by the Brent Medical Ethics Committee, Harrow, UK)

The first time in human study was a single-center, randomized, double-blind, placebo-controlled, adaptive design comprising five cohorts. Two cohorts of 15 healthy nonsmoking male subjects aged 18 to 65 years were randomized to receive single escalating oral doses of danirixin. Cohort 1 received doses of 10 mg, 50 mg and 200 mg; Cohort 2 received doses of 25 mg, 100 mg (as a single tablet) and 100 mg (as 2 × 50 mg tablets), as well as placebo. An interlocking design allowed a period of at least 7 days to elapse between dosing in one cohort and administration of a higher dose in the other cohort. Subjects in Cohorts 3 and 4 received repeat doses of danirixin or placebo once daily for 14 days in a parallel-group design. Fourteen subjects in each cohort were randomized 5:2 to receive danirixin 50 mg (Cohort 3) or 200 mg (Cohort 4) or placebo. Cohort 5 consisted of 15 subjects. Ten subjects were randomized to receive danirixin 400 mg and five subjects received placebo as a single dose. The schematic for the study design of the FTIH study is depicted in Fig. 2.

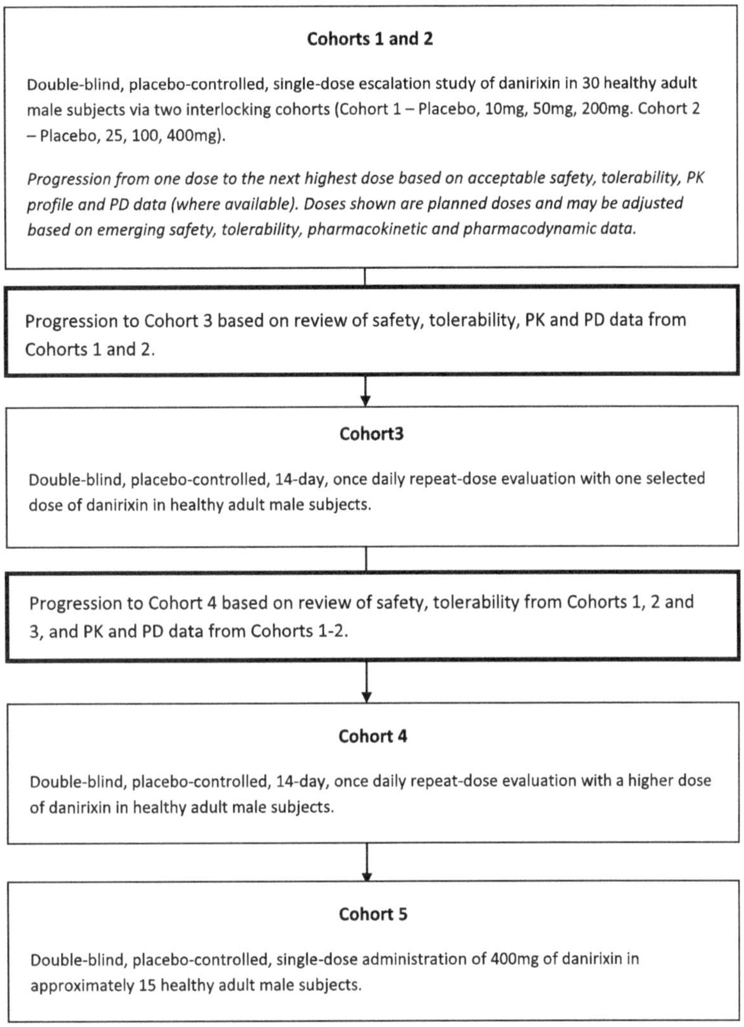

Fig. 2 Study design algorithm for Study 1 (FTIH)

Study 2, Fed versus Fasted, with Omeprazole (GSK Protocol CX3113722, ClinicalTrials.gov identifier NCT 01209104, reviewed and approved by the Western Institutional Review Board, Olympia, WA, USA)

Study 2 was conducted at a single center in two parallel parts as depicted in Fig. 3. Cohort 1 was a partially randomized, open-label, single-dose, crossover study in 16 healthy male and female adult subjects between 40 and 64 years of age. In treatment periods 1 and 2, subjects were randomized to two single dose treatment regimens in a crossover fashion, in the fed (after a high-fat meal) and fasted states. In treatment period 3, subjects were administered omeprazole once daily for 5 days. On the fifth day, all subjects received danirixin 100 mg together with the final dose of omeprazole.

Cohort 2 was a single-dose, double-blind, parallel group investigation in 16 healthy elderly individuals between 65 and 80 years of age. Subjects were randomized 3:1 to receive danirixin 100 mg or placebo in the fasting state.

Safety

For each subject, adverse events and serious adverse events were collected from the start of first dosing until the final follow-up contact. Safety was monitored by the measurement of ECGs, vital signs, clinical laboratory assessments (clinical chemistry, hematology, and urinalysis), and assessment of adverse events.

Determination of danirixin concentrations in whole blood and pharmacokinetic assessment

Whole blood concentrations of danirixin free base were determined using a validated analytical method based on extraction from a dried blood spot [9], with a 3 mm disc being punched from a 0.015 mL sample on Whatman FTA™ cards. Danirixin was extracted using methanol (0.1 mL) containing isotopically labeled [^{2}H7]-danirixin (racemic version of danirixin) at a concentration of 50 ng/mL as an internal standard. The extraction tubes were shaken for 1 h at ambient temperature, prior to the

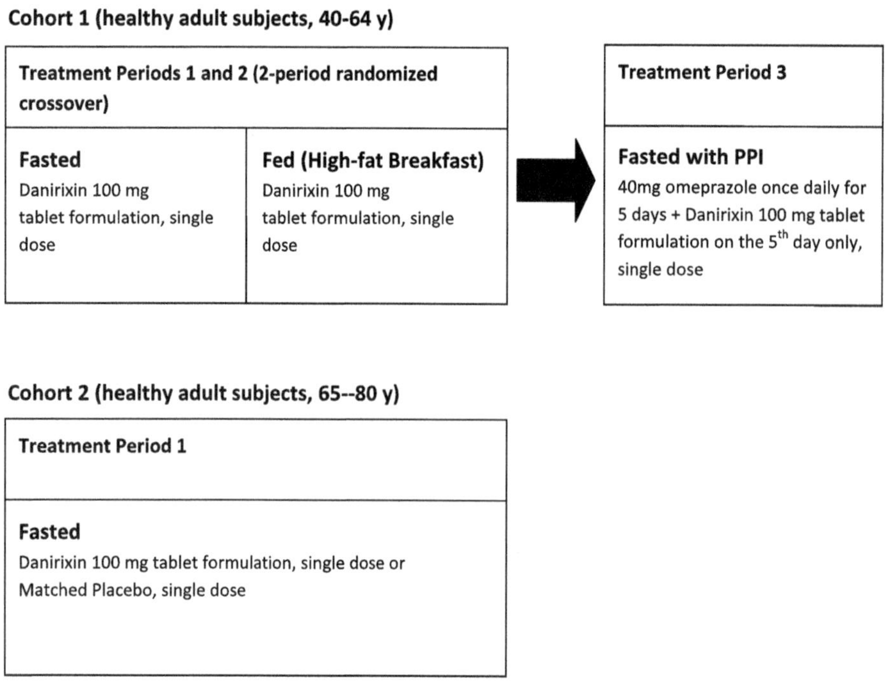

Fig. 3 Study design algorithm for Study 2 (Fed versus Fasted, Elderly, Omeprazole Interaction)

supernatant being transferred to clean tubes. The supernatant (5 μL) was injected onto a high-performance liquid chromatography system utilizing a Thermo Scientific Hypersil Gold C18 (5 μm packing 50 × 4.6 mm) column (supplied by Thermo Scientific, Hempstead, UK), eluted using an isocratic composition: 55:45 (v/v) of aqueous 10 mM ammonium formate containing 0.1 % formic acid (A) and acetonitrile (B). Danirixin free base has a retention time of approximately 1 min and was detected using tandem mass spectrometry on a Sciex 5000 (Applied Biosystems, Warrington, UK) using TurboIon Spray in positive polarity mode. Mass transitions monitored were 84 and 89 from precursor ions of 442 and 449 for danirixin and the internal standard. The assay had a linear dynamic range of 5 – 1000 ng/mL and quantification was performed using peak area ratios with $1/x^2$ weighted linear regression. Assay quality control samples were 15 ng/mL (low), 200 ng/mL (medium) and 800 ng/mL (high). The average within-run precision (%CV) was 9.9, 7.2 and 9.0 respectively, for the low, mid and high quality controls for study CX3112483 and 18.9, 5.9 and 5.2, respectively, for the low, mid and high quality controls for study CX3113722.

Pharmacokinetic parameters were determined from the blood concentration-time data for danirixin. The pharmacokinetic parameters were calculated based on actual sampling times using standard non-compartmental analysis in WinNonlin Professional, Version 5.2. The area under the blood concentration-time curve (AUC) was determined from the time of dosing to the last quantifiable concentration ($AUC_{(0\text{-}t)}$) using the lin – log trapezoidal rule. The apparent terminal elimination half-life ($t_{1/2}$) was obtained as the ratio of $\ln 2/\lambda_z$, where λ_z is the terminal phase rate constant, estimated by linear regression through the log transformed terminal data. $AUC_{(0\text{-}t)}$ was extrapolated to infinity ($AUC_{(0\text{-}\infty)}$) as the sum of $AUC_{(0\text{-}t)}$ and C_t/λ_z, where C_t is the last observed blood concentration and λ_z is the terminal phase rate constant.

Flow cytometric analysis of CD11b expression on blood neutrophils

CXCR2 ligand-induced cell surface expression of CD11b has been demonstrated to be a useful pharmacodynamic biomarker for the effects of CXCR2 antagonists [4]. To assess the pharmacodynamic effects of danirixin following oral administration, CXCL1-induced CD11b cell surface expression on blood neutrophils was determined with a whole blood assay as previously described [4, 10].

Statistical analyses

Study 1

The primary endpoint was safety and tolerability assessed by clinical monitoring of blood pressure, pulse rate, ECG, and clinical laboratory assessments as well as reporting of adverse events. Secondary endpoints included: 1) AUC (0-∞), AUC (0-t), maximum blood concentration (Cmax), time to maximum blood concentration (Tmax), and terminal half-life ($t_{1/2}$). 2) *ex vivo* CXCL1-induced CD11b cell surface expression on peripheral blood neutrophils, and 3) the relationship between the blood concentration of danirixin and *ex vivo* CXCL-1-induced CD11b cell surface expression on peripheral blood neutrophils.

In the single dose cohorts, dose proportionality was calculated on AUC (0 to ∞) and Cmax for Cohorts 1 and 2 and repeated again with Cohorts 1, 2, and 5. The power model analysis was performed on $\log_e$-transformed AUC (0 to ∞) and Cmax for danirixin. For each of these parameters, a mixed effects model was fitted with $\log_e$ (dose) as a fixed effect and individual subject intercept fitted as random effects. Estimates of the mean slope of $\log_e$ (dose) were reported along with corresponding 90 % confidence intervals.

To evaluate the accumulation ratio and time invariance of the repeat dose cohorts, a statistical analysis was performed after a log transformation of the data from all active treatment groups. A mixed effect model was fitted with treatment group, day, and treatment group by day interaction as fixed effects and subject as a random effect. Day 14 was compared with Day 1 in order to estimate the accumulation ratio and time invariance ratios for each treatment group. The ratios were calculated by back-transforming the difference between the least squares means. Using the pooled estimate of variance, 90 % confidence intervals were calculated for the difference and then back-transformed.

A mixed effects model was used to analyze the ratio to baseline fractional increase from control CD11b values over time. The model included the same effect as mentioned above except for time (hours). Subject was fitted as a random effect. In the repeat dose cohorts, a mixed effects model was used to analyze the ratio to baseline fractional increase from control CD11b values (treatment group for all pre-treatment data was set to the same dummy value, regardless of the treatment the subject went on to receive). The model included the following fixed effects (effects were fitted as categorical: time (hours) and treatment. Treatment*time and time* baseline interactions were fitted. For each day, a separate mixed model was fitted with time.

Another mixed effects model was used to analyze the weighted mean (0–9 h) ratio to baseline fractional increase from control CD11b values. The model included the following fixed effects (effects were fitted as categorical): day and treatment. Treatment*day interaction was fitted.

In the single and repeat dose cohorts, adjusted geometric means for each treatment and time point were calculated along with 95 % CIs. Point estimates of the treatment differences (each danirixin dose vs. placebo) and their associated 95 % confidence intervals were also calculated (using the pooled estimate of variance) and were back-transformed to provide point estimates and 95 % confidence intervals for the ratios. The ratios were converted into percent values to give the percent inhibition of danirixin versus placebo and 95 % confidence intervals.

A Bayesian analysis was conducted to derive the posterior probability distributions for the ratio to baseline fractional increase from control CD11b values at 24 h. The probabilities of seeing the percent inhibition of danirixin versus placebo greater than 0 %, 50 % and greater than 60 % were derived from the frequentist analysis mixed effects model. A students T cumulative distribution function was used to obtain the probabilistic statements, assuming a non-informative prior.

Study 2

The pharmacokinetic parameters AUC (0 to 24 h), AUC (0 to ∞), and Cmax were derived from the blood concentration of study drug. To assess age and gender, the exposures from Cohorts 1 and 2 (both in the fasted state) were combined. Following $\log_e$-transformation, AUC (0 to ∞) and Cmax of study drug were separately analyzed using a mixed effects model with fixed effect terms age and gender. Age-gender interaction was fitted and explored. To estimate the food effect on the primary pharmacokinetic endpoint, data from Cohort 1 were used. Following $\log_e$-transformation, AUC (0 to ∞) and Cmax of study drug were separately analyzed using a mixed effects model with fixed effect terms for regimen and period. Subject was treated as a random effect in the model. The same method of analysis, as for the food effect analysis, was applied to estimate the repeat oral doses of omeprazole on the primary pharmacokinetic endpoints, except for the exclusion of period from the model. In the single dose cohorts, a mixed effects model was used to analyse the ratio to baseline fractional increase from control CD11b values. The model included the following fixed effects (effects were fitted as categorical): period (6 levels), time (hours) and treatment. Subject baseline and period baseline were fitted as continuous covariates. Treatment*time and time*period baseline interactions were fitted. Subject was fitted as a random effect.

Results

Subject disposition

Thirty subjects were enrolled in the FTIH study and received at least one dose of study drug. One subject withdrew consent and withdrew from the study. Sixteen subjects were enrolled in Cohort 1 of Study 2; one subject was withdrawn after withdrawing consent. Sixteen subjects enrolled in Cohort 2 of Study 2; all subjects completed the study. The demographics and baseline characteristics for these subjects are shown in Tables 1 and 2.

Safety and tolerability

There were no serious adverse events and no subjects withdrawn due to adverse events. The most frequent adverse event during the FTIH study, irrespective of

Table 1 Demographics and baseline characteristics of study subjects, Study 1 (FTIH)

	Cohorts 1 and 2	Cohorts 3 and 4			Cohort 5	
		Placebo RD	danirixin 50 mg RD	danirixin 200 mg RD	Placebo SD	danirixin 400 mg SD
Age, yrs mean (SD)	35 (13)	35 (8)	29 (10)	33 (14)	27 (5)	25 (4)
n, (% male)	30 (100 %)	8 (100 %)	10 (100 %)	10 (100 %)	5 (100 %)	10 (100 %)
Race, n (%)						
White	25 (83)	6 (75)	10 (100)	9 (90)	4 (80)	7 (70)
African-American	3 (10)	2 (25)	0	0	1 (20)	1 (10)
Asian	2 (6)	0	0	1(10)	0	2 (20)
BMI (kg/m^2) mean (SD)	25 (2)	26 (3)	25 (2)	25 (3)	24 (4)	24 (2)

causality, was headache, which occurred in 14 subjects (5 subjects on placebo, 1 subject each on 10 mg and 100 mg single dose, 2 subjects each on 200 mg and 400 mg single dose, and 2 subjects on 200 mg repeat dose). Headache that was considered by the investigator to be possibly related to drug treatment occurred in 9 subjects (12 %). Somnolence occurred in five subjects (1 subject on placebo, 1 subject each on 10 mg and 200 mg single dose, and 2 subjects on 100 mg). Hot flushes occurred in four subjects (2 subjects on placebo, 1 subject on 200 mg single dose, and 1 subject on 200 mg repeat dose). Abdominal pain occurred in 4 subjects (1 subject each on 10 mg and 200 mg single dose and 1 subject each receiving 50 mg and 200 mg repeat dose).

In Study 2, 11 subjects reported 12 adverse events (34 %). Four adverse events were reported in subjects receiving danirixin 100 mg in the fasted state (headache, dizziness, nausea, and infusion site hemorrhage). Two adverse events were reported in subjects receiving danirixin 100 mg in the fed state (headache, dyspepsia). Two adverse events were reported in combination with omeprazole (nasopharyngitis, sinusitis). Three adverse events were reported in elderly subjects receiving danirixin 100 mg in the fasted state (application site rash, back pain, and dermatitis atopic) and one adverse event was reported in subjects receiving placebo (viral gastroenteritis). There were no reports of neutropenia or sustained decreases in neutrophil count. However, in the FTIH study, one subject was withdrawn from the study after the reduction in neutrophil levels met protocol stopping criteria of less than 1.5×10^9/L; the neutrophil count was fully reversed upon discontinuation of study drug. This subject was noted to have a low normal neutrophil count at screening (1.9×10^9/L).

Table 2 Demographics and baseline characteristics of study subjects, study 2 (fed vs. fasted, elderly, omeprazole interaction)

Study 2, Fed vs. Fasted Mean (range)			
	Part A	Part B	
		danirixin	Placebo
Age, years, mean (SD)	51 (8)	70 (2)	70 (6)
Sex (M/F)	8/8	6/6	2/2
Ethnicity, n (%)			
Hispanic/Latino	6 (38)	0	0
Not Hispanic/Latino	10 (63)	12 (100)	4 (100)
Race, n (%)			
African-American	1 (6)	0	0
White	15 (94)	11 (92)	4 (100)
Mixed	0	1 (8)	0
Height (cm), mean (SD)	174 (7)	172 (11)	171 (8)
Weight (kg), mean (SD)	80 (11)	80 (13)	77 (15)
BMI (kg/m^2), mean (SD)	26 (3)	27 (3)	26 (3)

Study 1: FTIH

Cohorts 1, 2, and 5 (single dose)

Systemic exposure to single daily doses of danirixin 10 mg, 25 mg, 50 mg, 100 mg (as 2×50 mg tablets), and 200 mg increased with increasing dose. The slope log versus log for the (AUC) (0 to ∞ was 1.122 (90 % CI: 0.992, 1.253) and for Cmax was 1.046 (90 % CI: 0.919, 1.172) indicating a proportional increase across the dose range. However, the 100 mg dose (2×50 mg) deviated from the dose proportionality shown by the other dose levels and had similar exposure results to 50 mg. The addition of danirixin 400 mg (Cohort 5) in the power model suggested a dose proportional increase in Cmax over the 10–400 mg dose range (1.019; 90 % CI: 0.913, 1.126) but a deviation away from dose proportionality for $AUC_{(0-\infty)}$ (1.117; 90 % CI: 1.001, 1.234).

The time at which the maximum blood concentrations were observed (Tmax) was consistent across the dose range studied (median: 1–2 h; range: 1 to 3 h). The apparent terminal half-life was approximately 6 h and was consistent across the dose range studied.

Figure 4 shows the individual and geometric means of danirixin blood dose-normalized Cmax versus dose using 10 mg as a reference dose. Subjects dosed with 100 mg had a lower Cmax than predicted and four subjects had higher Cmax values than expected (two subjects

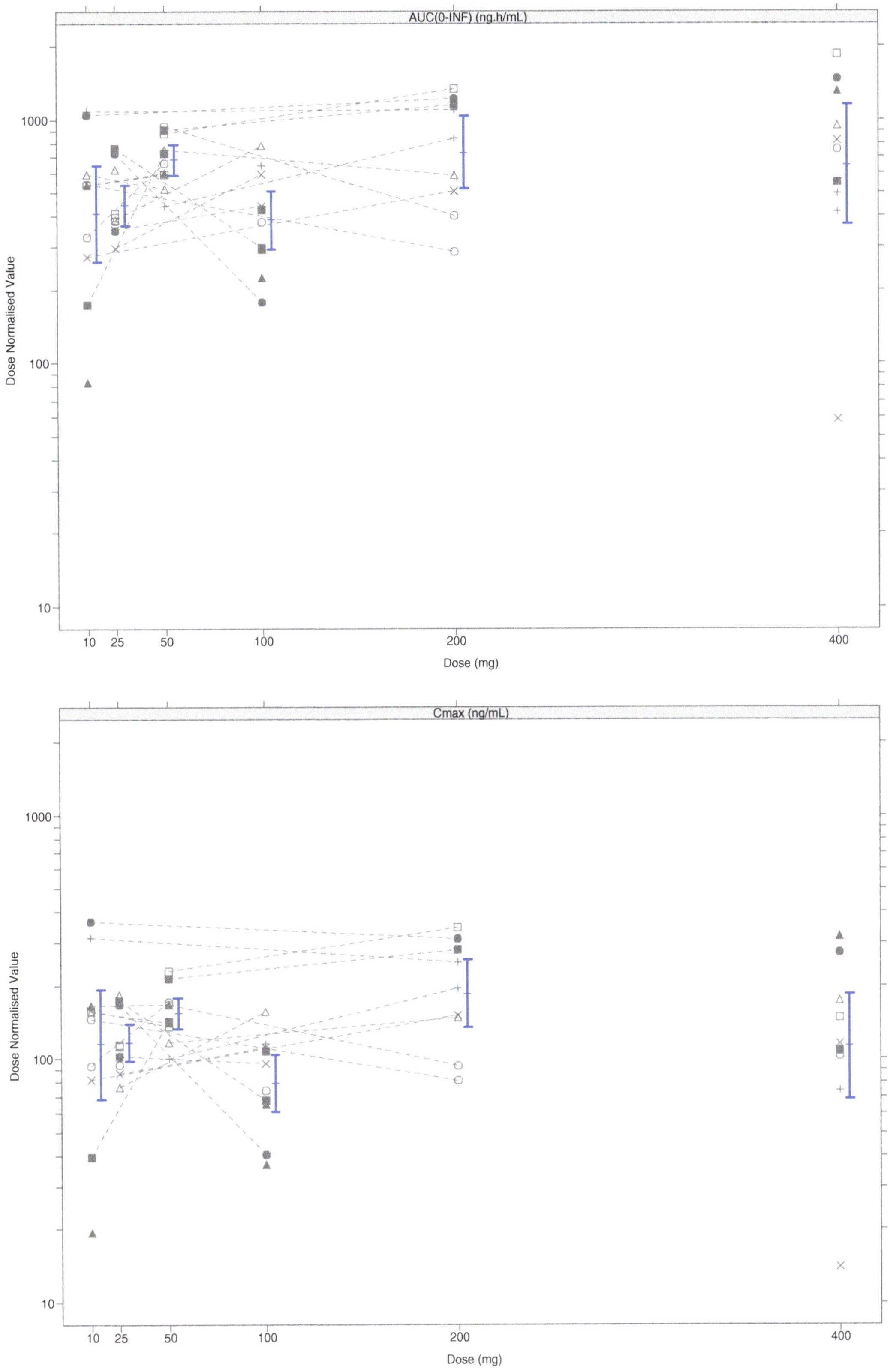

Fig. 4 Plot of individual subject danirixin blood dose-normalized AUC (A) and Cmax (B) versus dose for cohorts 1, 2, and 5 in Study 1 (FTIH). The geometric means (with 90 % confidence intervals) are also shown

randomized to 10 mg followed by 200 mg and two subjects randomized to 50 mg followed by 200 mg). These four subjects also had a comparatively high $AUC_{(0-\infty)}$. One subject had a high $AUC_{(0-\infty)}$ following dosing with danirixin 50 mg but over 2-fold lower $AUC_{(0-\infty)}$ than expected following dosing with danirixin 200 mg. Following dosing with danirixin 400 mg, two subjects had higher Cmax than expected and also had higher $AUC_{(0-\infty)}$.

Cohorts 3 and 4 (14-day repeat dose)

Repeat dosing of danirixin 50 mg and 200 mg resulted in lower exposure on Day 14 than on Day 1. The ratio of adjusted geometric means for AUC $_{(0\text{-}t)}$ was 0.846 (90 % CI: 0.553, 1.295) for danirixin 50 mg and 0.989 (90 % CI: 0.619, 1.579) for danirixin 200 mg after repeat dosing. An analysis of AUC and terminal half-life was performed to assess time invariance following repeat dosing with danirixin 50 mg and 200 mg. The AUC exposures were less, on average, on Day 14 compared with Day 1. An average decrease of 21 % (90 % CI: −48 %, 20 %) and 7 % (90 % CI: −42 %, 47 %) was observed for danirixin 50 mg and 200 mg, respectively, indicating that there was no evidence of time invariance. The t½ was greater on average by 33 % (90 % CI:-3 %, 82 %) on Day 14 compared with Day 1 for danirixin 50 mg, suggesting no evidence of time invariance based on t½. However, there was evidence to suggest an increase in t½ on Day 14 compared with Day 1 for danirixin 200 mg as t½, on average, was greater by 71 % (90 % CI: 26 %, 131 %).

CD11b surface expression on neutrophils

Approximately 50 % inhibition in weighted mean (0–9 h) CXCL1-induced CD11b expression was observed following single doses of danirixin 50 mg (ratio of active to placebo 0.445; 95 % CI: 0.257, 0.772) and 100 mg (0.502; 95 % CI: 0.299, 0.845) and 72 % inhibition (0.282; 95 % CI: 0.161, 0.493) following 200 mg compared with placebo. The ratio to baseline fractional increase from control CD11b expression at 24 h for single doses of danirixin 50 mg, 100 mg (2 × 50 mg), and 200 mg was 1.908 (95 % CI: 0.853, 4.265), 1.326 (95 % CI: 0.565, 3.110), and 0.516 (95 % CI: 0.212, 1.255), respectively. Bayesian

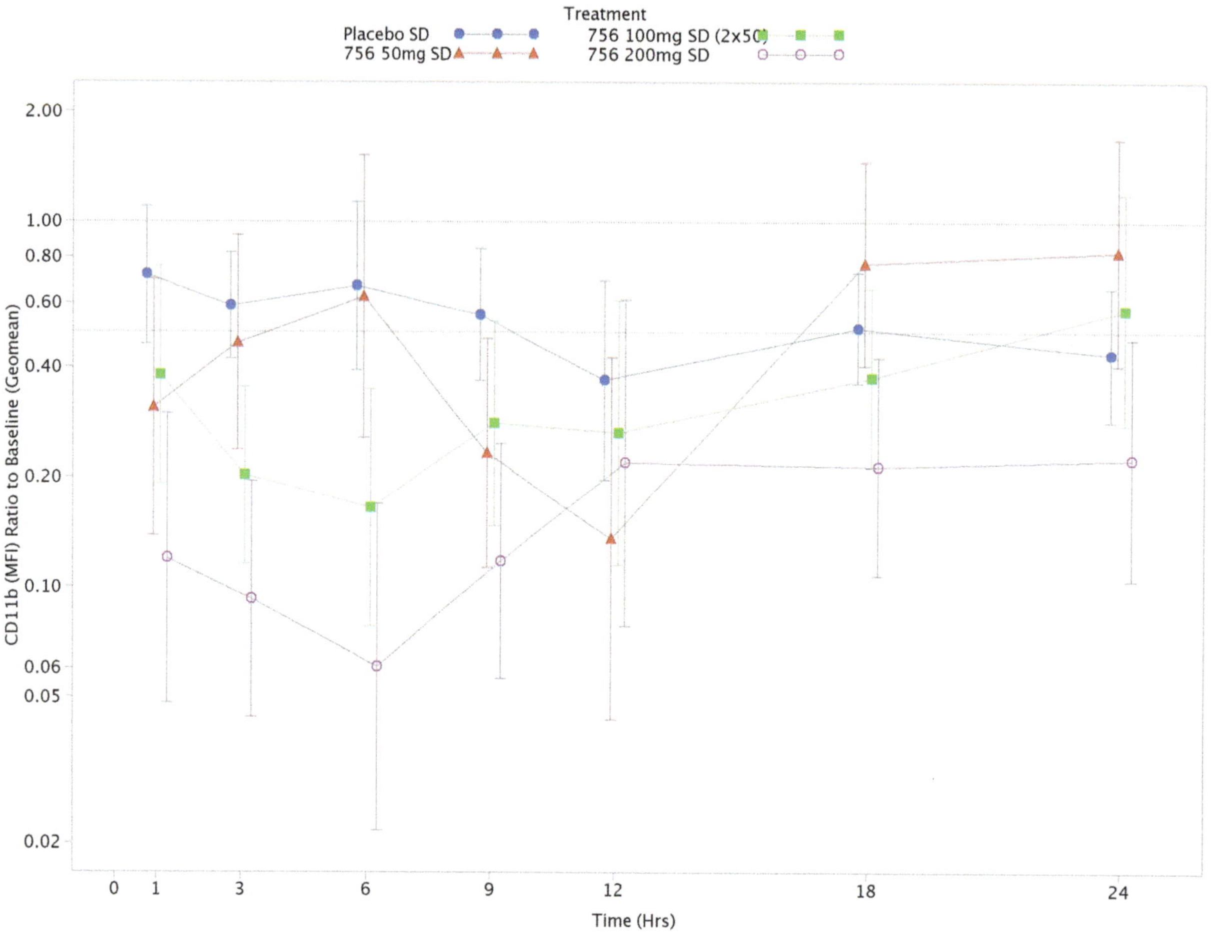

Fig. 5 Adjusted geometric means of ratio to baseline ex vivo CXCL-induced CD11b expression (0–24 h) versus time for single dose Study 1 (FTIH): fractional increase from control (CXCL1 0 nM) with 95 % CIs

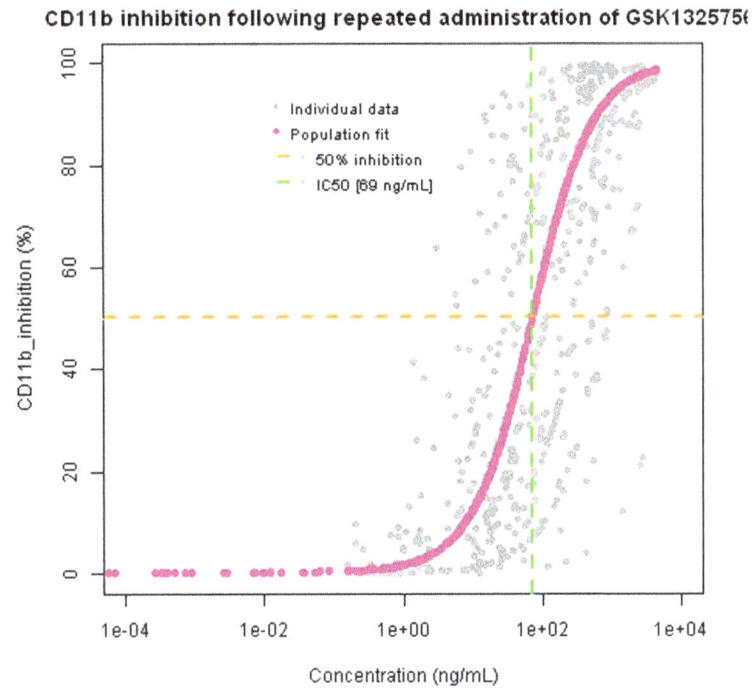

Fig. 6 Plot of inhibition of ex vivo CXCL1-induced CD11b expression versus whole blood concentration of danirixin for Study 1. The plot shows all timepoints where results are available for both danirixin whole blood concentration and ex vivo CXCL1-induced CD11b expression

analyses revealed that the probability of danirixin inhibiting CXCL1-induced CD11b expression relative to placebo at 24 h postdose at single doses of 50 mg, 100 mg, and 200 mg was 0.057, 0.26, and 0.93, respectively.

Repeat doses of danirixin 50 mg demonstrated an average of 67 % and 70 % weighted mean (0 to 9 h) CXCL1-induced CD11b inhibition on day 1 (0.335; 95 % CI: 0.227, 0.495) and day 14 (0.399; 95 % CI: 0.258, 0.617), respectively, relative to placebo. Repeat doses of danirixin 200 mg demonstrated an average of 70 % and 50 % weighted mean (0 to 9 h) CXCL1-induced CD11b inhibition on day 1 (0.301; 95 % CI: 0.209, 0.435) and day 14 (0.501; 95 % CI: 0.319, 0.788), respectively, relative to placebo. Bayesian analyses revealed that the probability of repeat doses of danirixin 200 mg inhibiting CXCL1-induced CD11b expression relative to placebo was 1.0.

In general, repeat doses of danirixin 50 mg and 200 mg demonstrated an average of 50 % inhibition in CXCL1-induced CD11b expression at various time points over the 24 h post dose on Day 1 (Fig. 5) and for most time points on Day 14, though high variability was observed across all treatments. The ratio to baseline fractional increase from control CD11b expression at 24 h for repeat doses of danirixin 50 mg on Day 1 was 0.374 (95 % CI: 0.132, 1.057) and on Day 14 was 0.403 (95 % CI: 0.226, 0.718). The ratio to baseline fractional increase from control CD11b expression at 24 h for repeat doses of danirixin 200 mg on Day 1 was 0.303 (95 % CI: 0.107, 0.861) and Day 14 was 0.348 (95 % CI: 0.192, 0.631). Fig. 6 shows the concentration-response plot for the effect of danirixin on the CXCL1-induced CD11b expression (shown in terms of percent inhibition), and clearly shows that a direct relationship exists between blood concentrations of danirixin and reduction in CXCL1-induced CD11b expression. Population PK/PD modeling of the data from the FTIH study suggests that the maximum possible inhibition of CXCL1-induced CD11b expression could be achieved and that the IC_{50} for this inhibition was 69 ng/mL (95 % CI: 17.6 to 120 ng/mL).

Study 2: Fed/fasted, omeprazole interaction and elderly pharmacokinetics

There was a statistically significant reduction in Cmax of 37 % (90 % CI: 24 % to 48 %) when danirixin 100 mg was administered following food (Table 3 and Fig. 7). The average decrease of 16 % in $AUC_{(0-\infty)}$ following administration in the presence of food was not statistically significant (90 % CI: −3.1 % to 32 %). The median Tmax was delayed in the presence of food compared with that in fasted subjects (3 h and 2 h, respectively). There was some evidence of a period effect, with lower average Cmax and less variability in Cmax in Period 2. There was also some evidence of a treatment-period interaction. Subjects randomized to fasted followed by fed had lower average Cmax and $AUC_{(0-\infty)}$ in the fed period,

Table 3 Summary of statistical analysis of fed/fasted comparison (Study 2)

	Danirixin 100 mg Fed		Danirixin 100 mg Fasted		Treatment Difference(Fed vs. Fasted)	
	n	Adjusted Geometric Mean(SE Logs)	n	Adjusted Geometric Mean(SE Logs)	Estimate	90 % CI
AUC (0-∞)(ng h/mL)	15	12,635 (0.082)	13	15,047 (0.088)	0.840	(0.684, 1.031)
Cmax(ng/mL)	16	1411 (0.076)	15	2239 (0.078)	0.630	(0.523, 0.758)

while subjects on the other treatment sequence had higher average Cmax and $AUC_{(0-\infty)}$ in the fed period. Subjects with the highest exposure in the danirixin 100 mg fasted period did not also have the highest exposure in the danirixin 100 mg fed period.

There was a reduction in exposure when danirixin was administered following dosing with omeprazole 40 mg once daily for 5 days (Fig. 5). The decreases of 56 % for $AUC_{(0-\infty)}$ (90 % CI: 41 % to 66 %) and 64 % for Cmax (90 % CI: 50 % to 73 %) were statistically significant, while the median Tmax was unchanged at 2 h for both treatments (Table 4).

In elderly subjects receiving danirixin 100 mg, the $AUC_{(0-\infty)}$ and Cmax were approximately half that observed for subjects aged 40 to 64 years ($AUC_{[0-\infty]}$, 90 % CI: 14 % to 73 %; Cmax, 90 % CI: −2.5 % to 73 %). In addition, the median Tmax for the fasted elderly cohort was earlier than that of the younger fasted cohort (1.5 h compared to 2 h).

Female subjects had approximately 1.5-fold higher average exposures compared to males ($AUC_{[0-\infty]}$, 90 % CI: 0.826 to 2.604; Cmax, 90 % CI: 0.806 to 3.064). However, due to the wide variability, these apparent differences between the sexes were not statistically significant. An exploratory analysis suggested that the absorption of danirixin was higher and that the clearance was lower in female subjects compared to male subjects. There was no evidence of an age-gender interaction; however, as the data are highly variable and the populations were

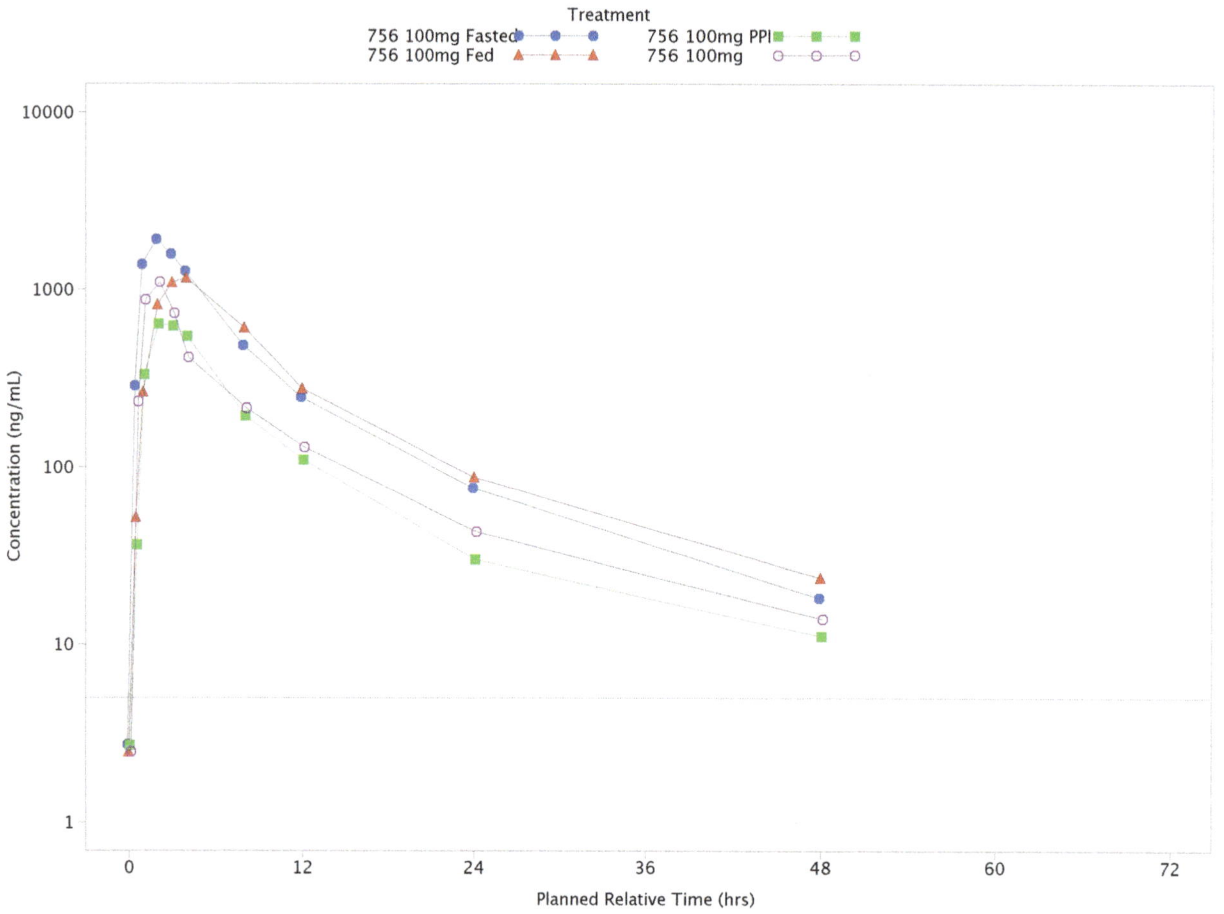

Note: LLQ = 5 ng/mL

Fig. 7 Mean pharmacokinetics concentration plot versus time for Study 2 (Fed versus Fasted, Elderly, Omeprazole Interaction)

Table 4 Summary of statistical analysis of proton pump inhibitor comparison (Study 2)

	Danirixin 100 mg Fasted + PPI		Danirixin 100 mg Fasted		Treatment Difference (Fasted + PPI vs. Fasted)	
	n	Adjusted Geometric Mean (SE Logs)	n	Adjusted Geometric Mean (SE Logs)	Estimate	90 % CI
AUC (0-∞)(ng h/mL)	12	6220 (0.1705)	13	14,020 (0.1659)	0.444	(0.337, 0.584)
Cmax (ng/mL)	15	813 (0.1646)	15	2235 (0.1646)	0.364	(0.267, 0.496)

imbalanced in terms of male and female age ranges, further work is needed to adequately define the importance of age and gender on the absorption of danirixin.

Discussion

The data presented in this report are from the first two clinical studies with danirixin in humans to assess the initial safety, tolerability, pharmacokinetics and pharmacodynamics of single and repeated doses under conditions relevant to the target patient population. Administration of danirixin was generally well-tolerated at single doses up to 400 mg and following once daily dosing for 14 days at doses of 50 mg and 200 mg. Importantly, subjects did not develop low neutrophil counts or overt neutropenia, as has been reported with other CXCR2 antagonists [6–8]. Danirixin demonstrated a dose-dependent inhibition of CXCL1-induced CD11b expression following single doses between 50 to 200 mg, which was maintained after 14 days of dosing. The optimal extent of pharmacodynamic activity needed is unknown, but it is likely that less than complete inhibition of CXCR2 activity is desirable in order to obtain a balance between clinical benefit, while minimizing the impact on innate immunity and host defense. Although the magnitude and duration of CXCR2 antagonism needed to achieve a pharmacologic and clinical effect in disease are unknown the pharmacokinetic data suggest that twice-daily dosing with danirixin may be needed to maintain blood concentrations at an appropriate level.

The prevalence of gastroesophageal reflux disease (GERD) and the use of gastric acid suppressing agents in COPD, one of the disease targets for a CXCR antagonist, is high [11–13]. Proton pump inhibitors have been reported to increase intragastric pH above 4.0 for approximately 50 % of the time over a 24 h interval [14]. Acidic conditions are required for optimal dissolution of danirixin. The formulation strategy for danirixin has thus far been focused on optimizing the disintegration and dissolution of the product in the stomach, which would then be expected to deliver a solution of the drug for absorption to the duodenal region of the small intestine. An intra-gastric pH at a steady state above 4.0 during a significant proportion of the day has potential implications for the solubility and absorption of danirixin. Statistically significant reductions in danirixin AUC and Cmax were observed in the presence of omeprazole.

The effect of omeprazole on the bioavailability of danirixin suggests an important drug interaction requiring further evaluation to determine appropriate dosing recommendations in patients using gastric acid reducing agents. Additional drug interactions that may impact danirixin have not been evaluated. However, one study has assessed the potential for metabolic drug interactions. In this study a bile sample was obtained using a non-invasive sampling technique [15]. The results demonstrated that glucuronide conjugation is likely to be the major route of metabolism for danirixin. Oxidative metabolism contributed only in a minor way indicating that cytochrome P450-mediated drug interactions are not likely to be a concern for danirixin.

In the presence of a high fat meal, the AUC and Cmax data suggest that the rate, but not the extent of absorption of danirixin was reduced, as would be expected from a molecule with this solubility profile. Furthermore, these data also suggest that in the fasted state the average exposure to danirixin in the elderly was half that of younger subjects, as reflected by lower AUC and Cmax measurements. In addition, in the fasted state, very high inter-subject variability in the exposure measurement was observed in elderly subjects. Administration of danirixin with food resulted in reduced variability in a range that is considered acceptable.

Conclusions

The data in the reported studies indicate that danirixin was well-tolerated, with a favorable pharmacokinetic and pharmacodynamic profile in healthy adult subjects, including elderly subjects. The dose-dependent inhibition of CXCL1-induced CD11b expression following single doses between 50 to 200 mg suggests the potential for clinical benefit in disease indications where an excessive neutrophil response has an important role in pathogenesis. The co-administration of daily omeprazole and use in the elderly will have to be taken into consideration when progressing to evaluation in patient populations.

Competing interests

BEM, SM, PC, DCC, JCB, RTS, and ALL are employees and shareholders of GlaxoSmithKline. KS and HC were employees of GlaxoSmithKline when the studies reported in this paper were conducted. The studies reported in this paper were funded by GlaxoSmithKline.

Authors' contributions

All listed authors meet the criteria for authorship set forth by the International Committee for Medical Journal Editors. BEM, SM, KS, PC, DCC, HC, JCB, RTS, and ALL contributed to the study design and interpretation of study results. SM and KS performed the modeling and statistical analyses. All authors participated in the preparation and editing of the manuscript. All authors approved the final version of the manuscript.

Acknowledgments

The authors wish to acknowledge Kim Poinsett-Holmes, PharmD of Poinsett Publications, Inc. for medical writing and editorial assistance.

Author details

[1]Clinical Discovery, Respiratory Therapy Area Unit, GlaxoSmithKline R&D, 709 Swedeland Road, King of Prussia, PA 19406, USA. [2]Clinical Statistics, GlaxoSmithKline R&D, Stockley Park West, Uxbridge, Middlesex UB11 1BT, UK. [3]Clinical Pharmacology Modeling and Simulation, GlaxoSmithKline, London, UK. [4]Product Development, Platform Technology and Science, GlaxoSmithKline R&D, Park Road, Ware, Hertfordshire SG 12 0DP, UK. [5]Respiratory Therapy Area Unit, GlaxoSmithKline R&D, 709 Swedeland Road, King of Prussia, PA 19406, USA. [6]Clinical Pharmacology Sciences and Study Operations, GlaxoSmithKline, London, UK. [7]Drug Metabolism and Pharmacokinetics, GlaxoSmithKline R&D, Park Road, Ware, Hertfordshire SG 12 0DP, UK. [8]Discovery Medicine, Respiratory Therapy Area Unit, GlaxoSmithKline R&D, 709 Swedeland Road, King of Prussia, PA 19406, USA. [9]Roche Pharmaceuticals, Welwyn Garden City, UK. [10]Global Development, Amgen Inc., Horsham, West Sussex, UK.

References

1. Scholten DJ, Canals M, Maussang D, Roumen L, Smit MJ, Wijtmans M, et al. Pharmacological modulation of chemokine receptor function. Br J Pharmacol. 2012;165:1617–43.
2. Chapman RW, Phillips JE, Hipkin RW, Curran AK, Lundell D, Fine JS. CXCR2 antagonists for the treatment of pulmonary disease. Pharmacol Ther. 2009;121:55–68.
3. Caramor G, Di Stefano A, Casolari P, Kirkham PA, Padovani A, Chung KF, et al. Chemokines and chemokine receptors blockers as new drugs for the treatment of chronic obstructive pulmonary disease. Curr Med Chem. 2013;20:4317–49.
4. Lazaar AL, Sweeney LE, MacDonald AJ, Alexis NE, Chen C, Tal-Singer R. SB-656933, a novel CXCR2 selective antagonist, inhibits *ex vivo* neutrophil activation and ozone-induced airway inflammation in humans. Br J Clin Pharmacol. 2011;72:282–93.
5. Holz O, Khalilieh S, Ludwig-Senqpiel A, Watz H, Stryszak P, Soni P, et al. SCH527123, a novel CXCR2 antagonist, inhibits ozone-induced neutrophilia in healthy subjects. Eur Respir J. 2010;35:564–70.
6. Todd CM, Murphy DM, Watson RM, Howie K, Strinich TX, Penk K, et al. Treatment with the CXCR2 antagonist SCH527123 reduced neutrophil levels in blood and airways but not bone marrow in mild asthmatic subjects. Am J Respir Crit Care Med. 2010;181:A4237.
7. Nair P, Gaga M, Zervas E, Alagha K, Hargreave FE, O'Byrne PM, et al. Safety and efficacy of a CXCR2 antagonist in patients with severe asthma and sputum neutrophils: a randomized, placebo-controlled clinical trial. Clin Exp Allergy. 2012;42:1097–103.
8. Magnussen H, Holz O, Watz H, Sauer M, Khanskaya I, Gann L, et al. Safety and efficacy of SCH527123, a novel CXCR2 antagonist, in patients with COPD. Eur Respir J 2010;36(Suppl 54):38S
9. Spooner N, Lad R, Barfield M. Dried blood spots as a sample collection technique for the determination of pharmacokinetics in clinical studies: considerations for the validation of a quantitative bioanalytical method. Anal Chem. 2009;81:1557–63.
10. Nicholson GC, Tennant RC, Carpenter DC, Sarau HM, Kon OM, Barnes PJ, et al. A novel flow cytometric assay of human whole blood neutrophil and monocyte CD11b levels: upregulation by chemokines is related to receptor expression, comparison with neutrophil shape change, and effects of a chemokine receptor (CXCR2) antagonist. Pulm Pharmacol Ther. 2007;20:52–9.
11. Rodriguez G, Ruigómez A, Martin-Merion E, Johannson S, Wallander MA. Relationship between gastroesophageal reflux disease and COPD in UK primary care. Chest. 2008;134:1223–30.
12. Kempainen RR, Savik K, Whelan TP, Dunitz JM, Herrington CS, Billings JL. High prevalence of proximal and distal gastroesophageal reflux disease in advanced COPD. Chest. 2007;131:1666–71.
13. Casanova C, Baudet JS, del Valle Velasco M, et al. Increased gastro-oesophageal reflux disease in patients with severe COPD. Eur Respir J. 2004;23:841–5.
14. Blum RA, Shi H, Karol MD, Greski-Rose PA, Hunt RH. The comparative effects of lansoprazole, omeprazole, and ranitidine in suppressing gastric acid secretion. Clin Ther. 1997;19:1013–23.
15. Bloomer JC, Nash M, Webb A, Miller BE, Lazaar AL, Beaumont C, et al. Assessment of potential drug interactions by characterization of human drug metabolism pathways using non-invasive bile sampling. Br J Clin Pharmacol. 2013;75:488–96.

Melatonin analgesia is associated with improvement of the descending endogenous pain-modulating system in fibromyalgia: a phase II, randomized, double-dummy, controlled trial

Simone Azevedo de Zanette[3,4], Rafael Vercelino[3,4], Gabriela Laste[3,4], Joanna Ripoll Rozisky[3,4], André Schwertner[3,4], Caroline Buzzatti Machado[1], Fernando Xavier[4], Izabel Cristina Custódio de Souza[4], Alicia Deitos[3,4], Iraci L S Torres[2,3,4] and Wolnei Caumo[1,2,3,4*]

Abstract

Background: Central disinhibition is a mechanism involved in the physiopathology of fibromyalgia. Melatonin can improve sleep quality, pain and pain threshold. We hypothesized that treatment with melatonin alone or in combination with amitriptyline would be superior to amitriptyline alone in modifying the endogenous pain-modulating system (PMS) as quantified by conditional pain modulation (CPM), and this change in CPM could be associated with serum brain-derived neurotrophic factor (BDNF). We also tested whether melatonin improves the clinical symptoms of pain, pain threshold and sleep quality.

Methods: Sixty-three females, aged 18 to 65, were randomized to receive bedtime amitriptyline (25 mg) ($n = 21$), melatonin (10 mg) ($n = 21$) or melatonin (10 mg) + amitriptyline (25 mg) ($n = 21$) for a period of six weeks. The descending PMS was assessed with the CPM-TASK. It was assessed the pain score on the Visual Analog Scale (VAS 0-100 mm), the score on Fibromyalgia Impact Questionnaire (FIQ), heat pain threshold (HPT), sleep quality and BDNF serum. Delta values (post- minus pre-treatment) were used to compare the treatment effect. The outcomes variables were collected before, one and six weeks after initiating treatment.

Results: Melatonin alone or in combination with amitriptyline reduced significantly pain on the VAS compared with amitriptyline alone ($P < 0.01$). The delta values on the VAS scores were-12.85 (19.93),-17.37 (18.69) and-20.93 (12.23) in the amitriptyline, melatonin and melatonin+amitriptyline groups, respectively. Melatonin alone and in combination increased the inhibitory PMS as assessed by the Numerical Pain Scale [$NPS_{(0\text{-}10)}$] reduction during the CPM-TASK:-2.4 (2.04) melatonin + amitriptyline,-2.65 (1.68) melatonin, and-1.04 (2.06) amitriptyline, ($P < 0.05$). Melatonin + amitriptyline treated displayed better results than melatonin and amitriptyline alone in terms of FIQ and PPT improvement ($P < 0.05$, fort both).

(Continued on next page)

* Correspondence: caumo@cpovo.net
[1]Pain and Palliative Care Service at the Hospital de Clínicas de Porto Alegre (HCPA), Universidade Federal do Rio Grande do Sul (UFRGS), Porto Alegre, Brazil
[2]Pharmacology Department, Instituto de Ciências Básicas da Saúde, UFRGS, Porto Alegre, Brazil
Full list of author information is available at the end of the article

(Continued from previous page)

Conclusion: Melatonin increased the inhibitory endogenous pain-modulating system as assessed by the reduction on $NPS_{(0-10)}$ during the CPM-TASK. Melatonin alone or associated with amitriptyline was better than amitriptyline alone in improving pain on the VAS, whereas its association with amitriptyline produced only marginal additional clinical effects on FIQ and PPT.

Trial registration: Current controlled trail is registered at clinical trials.gov upon under number NCT02041455. Registered January 16, 2014.

Keywords: Melatonin, Amitriptyline, CPM, BDNF, Clinical trial

Background

Fibromyalgia (FM) is a syndrome characterized by chronic widespread musculoskeletal pain, hyperalgesia, allodynia, stiffness of the body, fatigue, sleep disorders, circadian rhythm disturbances, anxiety, depression and, commonly, a high level of catastrophizing related to pain [1,2]. A previous study demonstrated that patients with fibromyalgia have low melatonin secretion, which could explain the lack of restorative sleep [3], which is a predisposing factor in trigger point formation [4] and dysfunction of pain modulation mechanisms [3]. Melatonin can block the cycle of impaired sleep at night, fatigue during the day [5-7], and can induce circadian rhythm synchronization [8]. In addition, melatonin administration in mice has antidepressant effects [9] and, in humans, anxiolytic properties [10].

Melatonin's effect on pain has been demonstrated in animals for inflammatory [8] and neuropathic pain [11-13], as well in acute [10,14] and chronic pain in humans [15,16]. In addition, there is some clinical evidence of melatonin's effect on FM [5,6]. However, the various study results are not consistent, possibly because the dose used has been low (3-5 mg). In regard to the melatonin dose for pain, a recent randomized clinical trial (RCT) indicated that 10 mg at bedtime produced a large size effect for chronic pelvic pain [16]. In addition, melatonin reduced the BDNF serum level in patients with chronic pelvic pain induced by endometriosis [16].

Pain is a dynamic phenomenon resulting from the activity of both endogenous pain excitatory and inhibitory systems, including inhibitory conditioned pain modulation (ICPM) [17]. The efficacy of ICPM in FM has been related to sleep quality [18]. This relationship is supported on neurobiological grounds by common neurotransmitters involved in both sleep and ICPM, including noradrenalin (NA), serotonin (5-HT) and dopamine (DA) [19-22]. Thus, it is important to investigate the therapeutic effect of drugs such as melatonin that present multifaceted mechanisms that may interfere in the peripheral and central pain mechanisms. The rationale that supports this hypothesis consists of evidence that, in long-term chronic pain situations, there is a loss of inhibitory system function, as demonstrated in FM by the pain threshold and conditioned pain modulation (CPM) [23]. Accordingly, in a recent study, we demonstrated that long-term musculoskeletal pain occurs with excessive cortical facilitation (a lack of inhibition), which is associated with lower pain threshold and higher levels of catastrophizing thinking related to pain [24]. In addition, numerous pre-clinical studies have demonstrated that ICPM depends on the recruitment of endogenous opioids in the periaqueductal gray, which trigger the release of 5-HT from neurons localized in the raphe nuclei (medulla), which, in turn, dampens nociceptive afferents at the dorsal horn of the spinal cord [25]. Noradrenergic projections from the locus coeruleus produce similar effects [25]. Together, this evidence justifies assessing the effect of melatonin in the descending modulatory pain systems, alone or combined with classic therapeutic agents such as amitriptyline, as it has been demonstrated that melatonin increases the pain threshold in healthy subjects [26], improves sleep quality [15] and modulates systems involved in pain, such as the GABAergic and opioidergic systems [12,27,28].

Taking all of this information into account, we hypothesized that melatonin treatment alone or in combination with amitriptyline is better than amitriptyline alone at modifying the endogenous pain-modulating system. Thus, to prove our hypothesis, in this study, we quantified the conditioned pain modulation (CPM)-TASK, as well BDNF serum levels in FM patients who received melatonin treatment alone or in combination with amitriptyline. We also tested whether melatonin improved clinical symptoms such as pain, pain threshold (PPT) and sleep quality related to fibromyalgia.

Methods

The Methods and Results sections are reported according to the CONSORT guidelines [29]. Figure 1 shows the flow chart of the study.

Design overview, setting, and participants

All patients provided written informed consent before participating in this randomized, double-blind, double-dummy, three-group parallel, clinical trial, which was approved by the Research Ethics Committee at the Hospital de Clínicas de Porto Alegre (HCPA) (Institutional

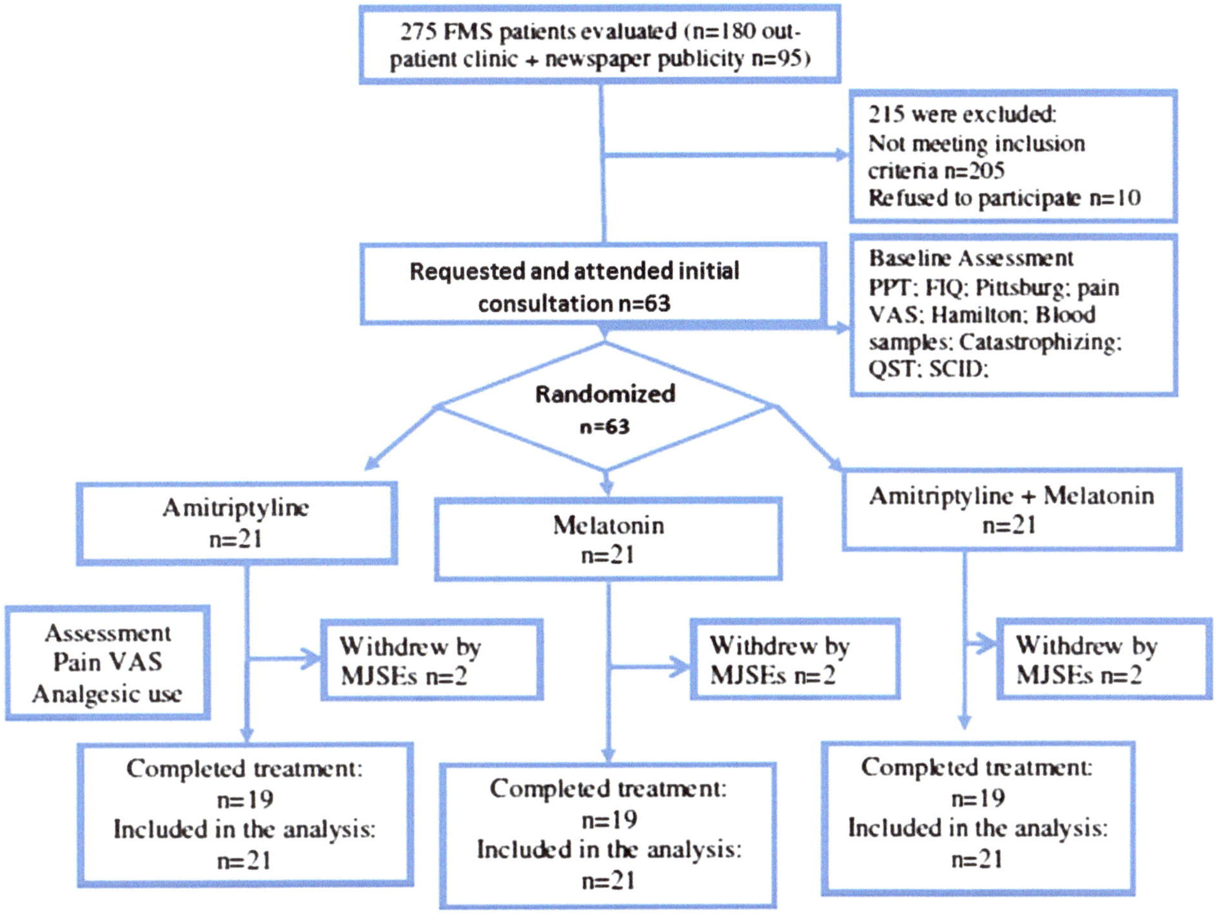

Figure 1 Flow chart showing recruitment and progress through the study. FMS: fibromyalgia syndrome; FIQ: fibromyalgia impact questionnaire; PPT: pain pressure threshold; QST: quantitative sensory testing; SCID: Structured Clinical Interview for DSM-IV; pain VAS: visual analog scale of pain; major side effects (MJSE) (severe dizziness, vivid nightmares, crippling drowsiness, severe headache, behavioral changes, and pain worsening).

Review Board IRB 0000921) in accordance with the Declaration of Helsinki (Resolution 196/96 of the National Health Council). We included 63 adult patients aged 18-years-old or older from among the pain and physiatrist clinical outpatients of the HCPA and via newspaper publicity. Patients with FM were enrolled according to American College of Rheumatology criteria [30]. To be eligible, patients had to be refractory to their current treatment. Patients were required to have a score of at least 50 mm on the 0-100 mm visual analogue scale (VAS, which 0 means "no pain" and 100 means "worst possible pain") [31] during the baseline week preceding randomization and to have completed at least four pain diaries out of seven. Patients were allowed to remain on analgesic medications, including drugs for which they were refractory, and these medications could not be adjusted during the study. At screening, all patients underwent physical examination by a pain specialist and a psychiatric interview with a psychiatrist. Patients could enroll with or without a history of major depressive disorder; however, it could not be the main reason for their functional impairment or study enrollment. Subjects were recruited solely for fibromyalgia pain. Patients were excluded if evidence was found of inflammatory rheumatic disease, autoimmune disease or other painful disorders that might confound the assessment of fibromyalgia pain or a history of substance abuse. Patients who were pregnant, breast-feeding or had a history of neurologic or oncologic disease, ischemic heart disease, kidney or hepatic insufficiency were also excluded.

Sample size justification

The number of patients in each study group was determined by previous clinical trials [32]. An *a priori* estimate indicated that a total sample size of 57 patients divided into three balanced treatment groups (n = 19) was needed to detect a 1.4-cm reduction (average standard deviation 1.2 cm) in pain intensity associated with melatonin or placebo at power and α levels of 0.8 and 0.01, respectively [33]; such a reduction would be clinically relevant and comparable to other pharmacological interventions. To account for multiple outcomes and attrition, we increased the sample size to 21 patients per group. For these calculations, we assumed that this remission was clinically relevant.

Randomization and masking

The participants were randomized into one of three groups: amitriptyline (+placebo), melatonin (+placebo), and amitriptyline + melatonin. Before the recruitment phase, envelopes containing the protocol materials were prepared. Each envelope was sealed and numbered sequentially and contained an allocated treatment. After the participant consented to participate in the trial, in the sequence, the nurse, who administered the medications, opened the envelope. During the entire protocol timeline, two investigators who were not involved in patient evaluations were responsible for the blinding and randomization procedures. Other individuals who were involved in patient care were unaware of the treatment group to which the patients belonged.

Interventions

Over a six-week period (42 days), the following oral medications were taken at bedtime by the three groups: melatonin (10 mg) tablets + placebo (Sigma Chemical, Germany, provided batch-by-batch certificates of analysis authenticating the purity of each batch), amitriptyline (25 mg) + placebo or amitriptyline (25 mg) + melatonin (10 mg) with identical characteristics. The capsules were manufactured in such a way that the placebo and active treatment had the same size, color, smell and flavor. To measure adherence to medication use, we employed the following strategies: ***i***) a researcher counted the number of tablets consumed weekly during the study period; ***ii***) the patients were asked to record a diary entry if they failed to use the medication; ***iii***) eligible patients were strongly encouraged to remain on the medication throughout the six weeks, during which time they visited the clinical center the third week after beginning the treatment. Regardless of their decision to continue or discontinue medication at this stage, the patients continued to be assessed during the study period.

Supplementary analgesic use

All of the patients were permitted to use supplementary analgesic medication (acetaminophen, ibuprofen, codeine or tramadol) to relieve their pain if necessary. Patients were allowed to take 750 mg of acetaminophen up to four times per day (QID) and 200 mg of ibuprofen at maximum QID as a rescue analgesic. If their pain persisted, patients could use Dorflex® (Sanofi Aventis, São Paulo, Brazil; 35 mg of orfenadrine citrate combined with 300 mg of dypirone and 50 mg of caffeine). If their pain persisted, patients were permitted to use 60 mg of codeine up to QID or tramadol three times per day (TID). These medications could be used a maximum of four times a day. The patients were asked to record their analgesic intake during the treatment period in their diaries, and these diaries were reviewed at the end of the treatment section. The total analgesic dose taken during the last week of treatment was considered for the analysis.

Instruments and assessments

All of the psychological tests used in this study have been validated for the Brazilian population [34,35]. Two independent medical examiners that were blind to the group assignments were trained to administer the pain scales and conduct the psychological tests. The baseline depressive symptoms of the patients were assessed using the Hamilton Depression Scale [35], and sleep quality was assessed using the Pittsburgh Sleep Quality Index [36]. Psychiatric disorders were evaluated with the Structured Clinical Interview for DSM-IV Axis I Disorders (SCID-I) [37]. To assess catastrophic thinking due to chronic pain, we used the B-PCS [38]. Demographic data and medical comorbidities were assessed using a standardized questionnaire; patients were asked about any changes that occurred during treatment, such as changes in mood, sleepiness, dizziness, headaches or allergic reactions.

Outcomes

The primary outcomes were pain score diaries on the Visual Analog Scale (VAS) [global pain in the last 24 hours] obtained during the last week of treatment and pain reduction on the Numerical Pain Scale [$NPS_{(0\text{-}10)}$] during the CPM-TASK. The secondary outcomes were the amount of analgesics used in the last week of treatment, the score on Fibromyalgia Impact Questionnaire (FIQ), Pressure Pain Thresholds (PPT), sleep quality and BDNF serum levels. The outcomes are described below.

Assessment of pain and sleep quality

a) The pain intensity was measured with a 100-mm VAS. The VAS scores ranged from no pain (zero) to worst possible pain (100 mm). The time of the worst pain during the last 24 h was recorded daily in the patients' diaries obtained at baseline during the seven days before beginning the treatment and the last week of the treatment period. They were asked to answer the following question using the pain VAS: *i*) considering your pain, how intense was your worst pain during the last 24 hours? Diary entries recorded analgesic intake (acetaminophen, non-steroidal anti-inflammatory drugs (NSAIDs) or opioids). The total analgesic dose taken during the last week of treatment was considered for analysis.

b) The quality of life of the patients in this study was evaluated using the Fibromyalgia Impact Questionnaire (FIQ), a disease-specific questionnaire initially proposed by Burckhardt et al. [39] for the evaluation of quality of life in patients with fibromyalgia. It was validated for use in the Brazilian population by Marques et al. [40]. This questionnaire is composed of 10 domains, the first consisting of 10 sub-items or questions, and the other nine of only one question each. The first domain contains questions concerning the capacity of the patient to perform certain routine activities. Responses range from 0, always able to perform the activity, to 3, never able to perform the activity. Item two refers to the number of days during that the patient felt well in the previous week, and item three refers to the number of days that the patient was unable to go to work because of the disease. Possible answers range from 0 to 7 for each item or domain. For domains 4-10, the scores range from 0 to 10 in each. These final seven items are designed to collect data on the patient's capacity to work and their perceptions of pain, fatigue, morning stiffness, mood, anxiety and depression. The data from the FIQ are arranged so that no more than 10 points can be scored for any single item. Items 2 and 3 are considered inversely proportional; therefore, the maximum possible score in this questionnaire will generally be 100.

c) Sleep quality during the study period was assessed using the Pittsburgh Sleep Quality Index [36].

Assessment of PPT and conditioned pain modulation

a) Pressure pain thresholds (PPT alone): Prior to the test trial, the patient learned to differentiate the perception of pressure versus the perception of the onset of pain. The patient was instructed to verbally report the perception of pain onset. The investigator who assessed pain threshold levels was trained, blinded to the intervention and unable to view the display of pressure intensities. An experienced rehabilitation physician (SAZ) systematically evaluated superficial and deep hyperalgesia by assessing PPT using an algometer [41]. The device had a 1-cm^2 hard-rubber probe, which was applied over eleven predefined different areas to define the PPT. These areas are among the nineteen areas corresponding to the diagnosis of FM according to the American College of Rheumatology criteria [30]. We determined the individual's PPT using the area that presented the lowest PPT. The average values of PPT in kgf/cm^2 (lb/cm^2) for three successive readings taken at intervals of 3-5 min were used as the outcomes.

b) To test CPM (the term CPM rather than diffuse noxious inhibitory control [DNIC] is chosen based on the recent recommendations of Yarnitsky et al. [17]), we used the protocol of Tousignant-Laflamme [42] and consulted the guidelines for the cold-heat task (CPM-TASK) as an experimental pain stimulus [43]. The CPM-TASK activates the diffuse noxious inhibitory control-like effect (CPM), as it is a strong nociceptive stimulus that takes place over a lengthy span of time [44] and is applied over a large body surface area [45]. Thus, the CPM-TASK allows us to modify the endogenous pain-modulating system. To quantify CPM, we evaluated the pain intensity of three heat pain (HPT) test stimuli separated by a CPM-TASK. Even if the HPT may lead to both habituation and sensitization according to the dual process theory, the cold water zero is a reliable stimulus to induce CPM [42].

c) CPM-Task: The cold-heat task was used as a conditioning stimulus to elicit a strong and prolonged pain sensation to trigger CPM. The CPM-TASK consisted of immersing the non-dominant hand cold water (zero to 1°C) for 1 minute. During the last 30 seconds of cold-water immersion, the HPT procedure was administered over the right forearm (dominant forearm). The temperature was held constant during the experiment for each subject. The mean temperature eliciting pain ratings of 0/10 on the Numerical Pain Scale [$(NPS)_{0\text{-}10}$] (HPT) was used for the HPT. After a short break, the first HPT (Pain baseline, HPT0) was applied at the extensor carpi radialis longus muscle (forearm) of the dominant forearm. Following the first HPT (HPT0), the CPM-TASK was used to trigger CPM. One minute after the CPM-TASK, we applied the second HPT (HPT1). We quantified the amount of CPM by subtracting the mean pain rating of the second HPT after the CPM-TASK (HPT1) from the first HPT before the CPM-TASK (HPT1) [46].

d) Laboratory outcomes included serum levels of BDNF. Samples of blood were collected at two time points: at baseline and at the end of treatment. The blood samples were centrifuged in plastic tubes for 10 min at 4500 × g at 4°C, and serum was stored at-80 °C for assay. Serum BDNF was determined by the Enzyme-Linked Immunosorbent Assay (ELISA) using a ChemiKine BDNF Sandwich ELISA Kit, CYT306 (Chemicon/Millipore, Billerica, MA, USA). The lower detection limit of the kit is 7.8 pg/mL of BDNF.

Statistical Analysis

The differences between the groups at baseline were examined by analysis of variance (ANOVA) for parametric variables with normal distribution or the Kruskal-Wallis test, and categorical variables were examined using chi-square or Fisher's exact tests given that our main independent outcome (intervention) was also categorical.

The results were evaluated using the absolute mean variation of pain measurements quality and BDNF were evaluating using delta values (post-treatment minus pre-treatment). Several outcomes of pain measurements (VAS, FIQ, PPT, number of tender points and PPT) did not present normal distribution. Linear mixed models were used to compare outcomes within subjects and between subjects in which the independent variable was the treatment (amitriptyline, melatonin and melatonin + amitriptyline) with Bonferroni's Multiple Comparison Test. The reduction on the $NPS_{(0-10)}$ induced by the CPM-TASK was adjusted for the baseline HPT and serum BDNF.

To identify possible predictors associated with the change on the $NPS_{(0-10)}$ during the CPM-TASK, we fitted a multiple linear regression model, using the stepwise enter method. The variables included in the model were as follows: B-PCS score, HPT0, and FIQ score obtained before treatment. In addition, the number of analgesics used in the last week of treatment was included. Finally, an exploratory analysis using the Spearman correlation coefficient (r_s) was performed to understand the reverse effect of the interaction of HPT0 and BDNF [each alone presented a negative correlation with $NPS_{(0-10)}$ during the CPM-TASK] that becomes positive. Within groups, the standardized mean difference (SMD) was computed in terms of the ratio between the mean change and the pool of baseline standard deviation (SD). The SMD was interpreted as follows: small, 0.20 to 0.4; moderate, 0.50-0.70 and large, 0.80 or higher, with respective confidence interval (CI) [47]. All of the analyses were performed assuming intention-to-treat and thus included all of the randomized subjects for whom there were observations in the study outcomes. The analyses were performed with SPSS version 18.0 (SPSS, Chicago, IL).

Results

Patient characteristics

The clinical and demographic characteristics of the patients are shown in Table 1. Twenty-one patients were allocated to the amitriptyline group, 21 were allocated to the melatonin group, and 21 patients were allocated to the melatonin + amitriptyline group. Fifty-seven patients completed the study; two patients in the melatonin + amitriptyline group and two patients in both the amitriptyline and melatonin group withdrew because of treatment side effects. Baseline characteristics are presented in Table 1. The randomization produced balance groups for most part of characteristics, but, there was observed imbalance between groups in pain on the VAS, FIQ and PPT (Table 1). Regarding the side effects, in the amitriptyline group, 38.09% (8/21) of patients presented minor side effects (MSE) (nausea, mild dizziness, weight gain, dry mouth, and mild headache) and 23.8% (5/21) of patients presented major side effects (MJSE) (severe dizziness, vivid nightmares, crippling drowsiness, severe headache, behavioral changes, and pain worsening), with two withdraw. In the melatonin group, 23.8% (5/21) of patients presented MSE and 23.8% (5/21) of MJSE, with two withdrawals. The association of melatonin + amitriptyline resulted in 14% (3/21) of patients experiencing MSE, whereas 28.57% (6/21) of patients presented MJSE with two withdrawals. The comparisons in the incidence of MSE between the amitriptyline and the melatonin + amitriptyline group was statistically significant ($P < 0.001$). However, neither the incidence of MSE nor the incidence of MJSE was significant when the groups were compared ($P > 0.05$, for all comparisons).

Analysis of the treatment effect on the main outcomes: descending modulatory system and pain on the VAS

Patients receiving melatonin alone or in combination with amitriptyline had significantly lower pain on the VAS than those receiving amitriptyline alone ($P < 0.01$) (Figure 2). A mixed model analysis revealed that the increase of one supplementary analgesic dose was associated with a 5.1% increase in the adjusted VAS pain change from baseline ($t = 5.87$; $P < 0.001$).

The change within the group was significant in all treatment groups ($P < 0.001$, for all comparisons) (Table 2). The cumulative mean (SD) on VAS one week pretreatment *vs.* the pain scores in the last week of treatment in the amitriptyline group was 62.87 (14.26) vs. 50.02 (25.60). For the melatonin group, these values were 64.90 (15.43) vs. 47.53 (21.96), respectively, and for the melatonin + amitriptyline group, the values were 69.57 (9.09) vs. 48.64 (15.38)], respectively. The effect size assessed by SDM [confidence interval (CI) 95%] within group in the amitriptyline group was 0.99 (CI 95%, 0.68-1.30), whereas in the melatonin group, it was 1.29 (CI 95%, 0.98-1.58), and in the melatonin + amitriptyline group, it was 1.47 (CI 95% 1.14-1.79) (Table 2).

The descending modulatory system function was assessed using the CPM-TASK. It was observed that in the overall treatment group, there was a reduction in pain scores during the CPM-TASK: melatonin + amitriptyline [HPT0 6.89 (1.92) vs. 4.49 (2.17) HPT1], melatonin [PPT0 7.52 (1.39) vs. 4.87 (1.97) HPT1] and amitriptyline [HPT0 6.07 (1.95) vs. 5.03 (2.17) HPT1]. The effect of treatment on CPM is presented in Figure 3. The CPM-TASK induced a reduction in pain in the melatonin group and melatonin + amitriptyline group that was significantly

Table 1 Epidemiological and clinical characteristics at baseline, according to the treatment group, values are given as the mean (SD) or frequency (n=63)

	Amitriptyline (n = 21)	Melatonin (n = 21)	Amitriptyline + melatonin (n = 21)	P value
Age (years)	49.80 ± (8.91)	47.40 ± (7.84)	49.72 ± (7.24)	0.59
Body index	27.65 ± (3.91)	27.18 ± (4.04)	27.58 ± (4.62)	0.60
Education (years)	10.95 ± (5.09)	11.30 ± (3.76)	8.22 + (5.6)	0.39
Smoking (n/%)	2 (9,5)	2 (9,5)	1 (5)	0.83
Clinical Comorbidity Yes/No	10 (47,6)	9 (42,9)	13 (65)	0.33
Hypertension (n/%)	5 (23,8)	5 (23,8)	8 (40)	
Hypothyroidism (n/%)	3 (14,3)	1 (4,8)	7 (35)	
Asthma (n/%)	1 (4,8)	1 (4,8)	2 (10)	
Other (n/%)	3 (15)	0 (0)	1 (4,8)	
Global pain on visual analogue scale[†]	62.88 ± (14.26)[a]	64.90 ± (15.44)[a]	69.57 ± (10.94)[b]	0.03
FIQ[†]	53.78 ± (12.83)[a]	64.87 ± (12.83)[b]	65.15 ± (9.94)[b]	0.005
Pain catastrophizing scale for the Brazilian population (B-PCS)[†]				
	25.90 ± (10.38)	32.90 ± (12.28)	25.90 ± (10.38)	0.07
Pittsburgh Sleep Questionnaire	19.31 ± (6.58)	22.67 ± (7.69)	24.28 ± (7.79)	0.16
Hamilton Depression Scale[†]	17.61 ± (6.37)	21.70 ± (5.88)	17.61 ± (6.33)	0.05
Pain pressure threshold[†]	2.17 ± (0.21)[a]	1.99 ± (0.16)[b]	2.05 ± (0.24)[a]	0.04
Brain-derived neurotrophic factor (BDNF)[€]				
Mean (SD)	48.28 ± (24.00)	52.54 ± (23.87)	48.28 ± (27.34)	
Median [interquartile (IQ) 25;75]	45.51 (12.8;101.51)	54.78 (20.66;97.85	37.51 (18.75;92.3)	0.79
Psychiatric disease (SCID-I)	6 (76%)	15 (71%)	13 (65)	0.45
Depression	8 (38%)	1 (62%)	11 (55%)	
Anxiety	11(52%)	12 (57%)	5 (25%)	
Analgesic used weekly in last 3 months				
Median (Q_{25-75})[€]	6 (3;28)	7 (2;26)	7 (3;29	0.91
Analgesic use: days/week in last 3 months[¥]				
(<4 = no, ≥4 = times)	20 (95%)	20 (95%)	17 (85%)	0.43
A e aminophen/Dipirone	19 (90,5%)	16 (76,2%)	15 (75%)	
NSAID	7 (33,3%)	10 (47,6%)	9 (45%)	
Opioid	1 (4,8%)	0	0	
Active use of central nervous system active medication[¥]				
Yes/No	14 (66,7%)	16 (76%)	14 (70%)	0.16
Antidepressant (n/%)	14 (66,7%)	15 (71%)	13 (65%)	
Anticonvulsant (n/%)	2 (9,5%)	2 (9,5%)	1 (5)	
Benzodiazepine (n/%)	0	5 (23,8%)	2 (10%)	

Different superscripts (a and b) indicate significant differences among treatment groups according to the Bonferroni test.
Structured Clinical Interview for DSM-IV Axis I Disorders (SCID-I).
[€]Kruskal-Wallis Test.
[¥]Chi-Square or Fisher's test.
[†]ANOVA.

higher than in the amitriptyline group. However, it was observed that there were patients in all treatment groups that reported increased pain intensity (conditioned pain modulation-CPM) between the HPT0 pain measures (test stimulus) and HPT1 after the cold pressor task (CPM-TASK, conditioning stimulus). This characterizes a summation effect, with an incidence of 15.8% (3/21) in the melatonin group, 36.8% (8/21) in melatonin + amitriptyline group and 42% (9/21) in the amitriptyline-treated group. These results reveal that

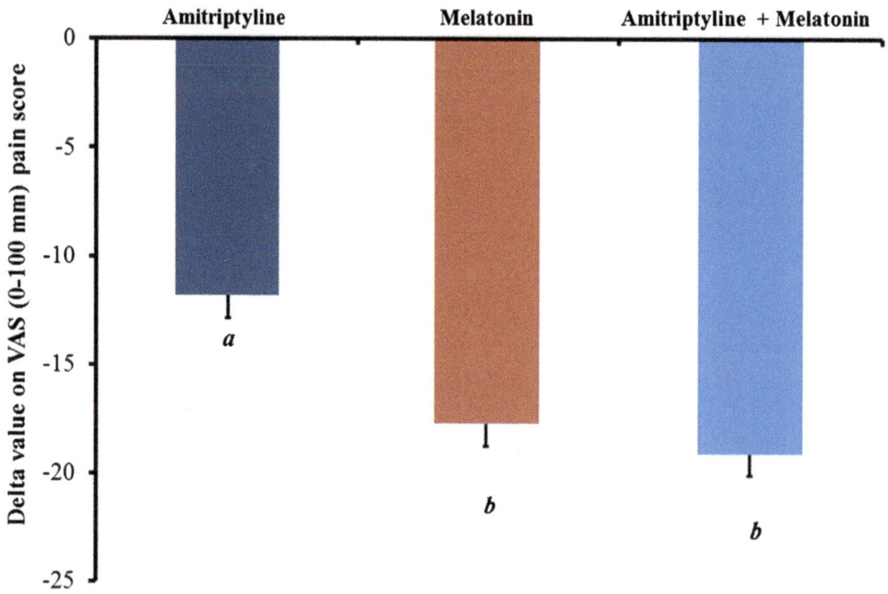

Figure 2 Mean pain levels as Delta value (scores on VAS (0-100 mm) in last week of treatment minus scores one week pretreatment) in the three experimental groups. The error bars indicate the standard error of the mean. A letter *b* indicates a significant difference between the melatonin group and melatonin + amitriptyline groups compared with the amitriptyline group (P < 0.05). All comparisons were performed using a mixed analysis of variance (ANOVA) model, followed by the Bonferroni correction for *post hoc* multiple comparisons.

the descending modulatory system lost its inhibitory function as the heterotopy stimulus induced an increase in pain, when a reduction would be expected [42].

To understand this result, we performed an exploratory analysis to identify possible factors associated with this summation effect on pain score during the CPM-TASK. To identify possible predictors, a multiple linear regression model was constructed using the stepwise method. The variables included in the model were the B-PCS score, HPT0, and FIQ score obtained before treatment. In addition, the number of analgesics used in the last week of treatment was included. Accordingly, the HPT was the only variable retained in the model, that is, associated with pain changes on NPS (0 – 10) during the CPM-TASK [(r-square =-0.21), standard β coefficient for the HPT =-5.99, $P < 0.05$)].

Thus, a mixed model was constructed to assess the effect of treatment groups and its relationship with the serum BDNF adjusted by the HPT. It was observed that the HPT and serum BDNF were inversely correlated with the change on the $NPS_{(0-10)}$ during the CPM-TASK (Table 3). However, when the interaction between HPT and BDNF was analyzed, this effect changed direction (i.e., it became positively associated with the change on the $NPS_{(0-10)}$ during the CPM-TASK) (Table 3). To understand this result, we performed a simple correlation between serum BDNF and HPT, and the Spearman coefficient (r_s) was-0.35 (P = 0.02). That is, when the HPT0 is low (higher the pain), the serum level of BDNF is high and vice versa. Thus, it is plausible to suppose that the effect of this interaction (HPT*serum BDNF) on pain score during the CPM-TASK was negatively correlated when included in the model as an isolated factor; it becomes in a factor correlated positively with the change reduction during the CPM-TASK (Table 3).

Table 2 Multivariate linear regression of the interaction between the change in NPS (0-10) during the CPM-TASK by the treatment group considering the BDNF and pain thresholds (n = 63)

Parameters	*B*	t	P	95% CI
Dependent variable: CPM-TASK				
	9.0	1.14	0.01	(4.33 to 32.35)
Treatment group				
Melatonin + Amitriptyline	-1.27	-1.72	0.09	(-2.76 to 0.21)
Melatonin	-1.75	-2.5	0.01	(-3.18 to-0.31)
Amitriptyline	0[b(reference)]			
BDNF (ng/mL)	-0.28	-2.23	0.01	(-0.53 to-0.04)
Heat pain threshold	-8.06	-2.49	0.01	(-14.56 to-1.55)
Interaction				
Serum BDNF (ng/mL) vs. PPT Pain pressure threshold (Kgf/cm^2)	0.12	2.07	0.04	(0.04 to 0.24)

[b]indicates the reference category used to do the comparisons.

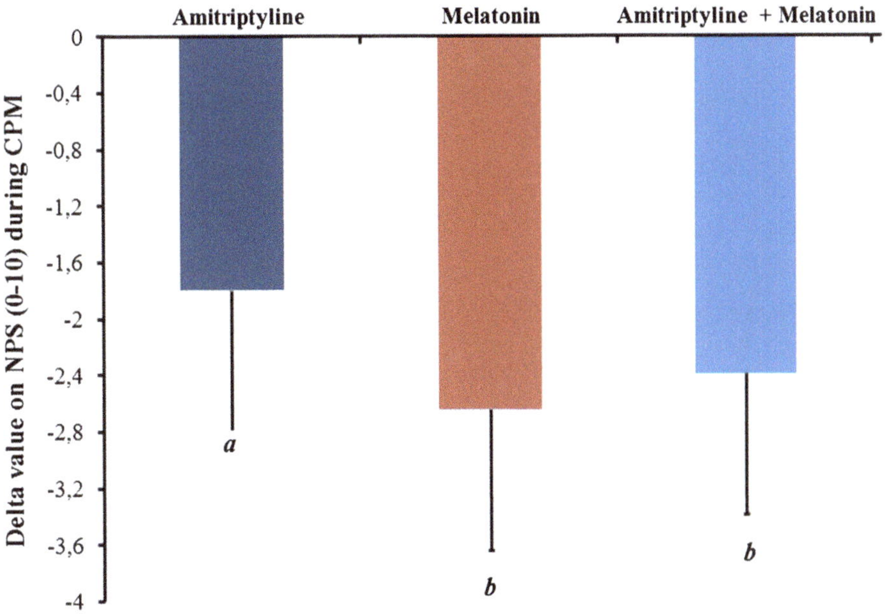

Figure 3 Delta value on the pain $NPS_{(0\text{-}10)}$ during the CPM-TASK. The error bars indicate the standard error of the mean. A letter *b* indicates a significant difference between the melatonin + and melatonin + amitriptyline compared with the amitriptyline group. All comparisons were performed using a mixed analysis of variance (ANOVA) model, followed by the Bonferroni correction for *post hoc* multiple comparisons.

Analysis of the efficacy on secondary outcomes: the Delta of pain scores for FIQ score, PPT, tender points, analgesic use, sleep quality and BDNF

The between-group changes in pain, pain threshold, analgesic consumption and sleep quality are shown in Table 3. The post hoc analysis indicated significant differences between the amitriptyline + melatonin group and the melatonin group from the amitriptyline group in terms of the FIQ score and PPT. No significant difference was observed between groups in the numbers of analgesic used in the last week of treatment, sleep quality and number of tender points. We observed a large effect size within groups considering the change pre- to post-treatment in pain measures, number of tender points and sleep quality (Table 3).

Although no significant difference between treatment groups in serum BDNF at baseline was observed, there was large variability in the serum level of this neurotrophin (Table 1). From the baseline, the mean of serum BDNF decreased 22.57% in the amitriptyline group, whereas the melatonin group and the melatonin + amitriptyline group presented a mean reduction of 36.6% and 34.49%, respectively (Figure 4). The effect size within group as assessed by SDM in the amitriptyline group was 0.43 (CI 95%, 0.05-0.83), whereas in the melatonin group, the value was 0.8 (CI 95%, 0.4-1.2), and in the melatonin + amitriptyline group, the value was 0.67 (CI 95%, 0.24-1.09) (Figure 4).

Discussion

The most clinically relevant finding of this study was melatonin's ability to improve the function of the inhibitory endogenous pain-modulating system as assessed by the reduction of the $NPS_{(0-10)}$ during the CPM-TASK. In addition, this study highlights that the HPT and BDNF serum levels at baseline were inversely correlated with the magnitude of the treatment effect on the descending modulatory system as assessed by the CPM-TASK. Furthermore, these findings revealed that in general, all treatments improved the FM symptoms (pain, sleep quality); however, the clinical effect was marginally better when the patients used melatonin alone or associated with amitriptyline.

These findings suggest that the melatonin treatment had a direct effect on pain pathways or on the levels of signaling chemicals that regulate pain. Melatonin induced a reduction that was higher than 35% on the $NPS_{(0-10)}$ during the CPM-TASK, and, as can be observed from the lower limit of the confidence interval regarding pain score on the VAS presented as SDM [1.29 (CI 95%, 0.98-1.58)], its effect was larger than that of amitriptyline alone [0.99 (CI 95%, 0.68-1.30)]. The melatonin effect on CPM is biologically plausible, and it is supported by evidence from experimental studies about its effect on GABAergic [48], opioid and glutamatergic systems [49]. In addition, this hypothesis is supported by other studies that have demonstrated a well-characterized anatomical network able to

Table 3 The mean delta score [standard deviation (SD)] (post-treatment values minus pre-treatment values) of pain measures (FIQ, PPT, analgesic consumption, tender points) and sleep quality (n = 63)

2A. Secondary outcomes					
Treatment	**Mean (SD)**	**Mean difference (SD)**	**Median of the difference (Quartile 75;25)**	**P Value†**	**SDM CI 95%**
Fibromyalgia Impact Questionnaire (FIQ) score					
Amitriptyline (n = 21)	41.16 (14.61) vs. 53.78 (12.83)	-12.19 (16.27)	-13.78 (-24.39,-4.95)**b	0.04	0.88 (0.43-1.33)
Melatonin (n = 21)	46.42 (16.18) vs. 64.87 (12.83)	-17.73 (13.0)	-16.30 (-22.29,-12.94)**b		1.28 (0.83-1.74)
Amitriptyline + melatonin (n = 21)	40.89 (10.94) vs. 65.15 (9.94)	-24.65 (12.14)	-26.41 (-32.59,-14.50)**a		1.79 (1.29-2.28)
b. Mean pressure pain threshold (PPT) in (kg/cm2/second)					
Amitriptyline (n = 21)	2.34 (0.45) vs. 2.05 (0.24)	0.29 (0.31)	0.2 (0.1, 0.5)**b	0.03	0.69 (0.34-1.04)
Melatonin (n = 21)	2.47 (0.33) vs. 1.99 (0.16)	0.47 (0.34)	0.4 (0.23, 0.55)**b		1.13 (0.79-1.47)
Amitriptyline + melatonin (n = 21)	2.70 (0.23) vs. 2.17(0.21)	0.54 (0.60)	0.6 (0.5, 0.7)**a		1.27 (0.9-1.64)
Analgesic doses (mean during the last week of treatment)†					
Amitriptyline (n = 21)	1.35 (1.2) vs. 2.07 (1.37)	-0.72 (1.40)	-0.22 (-0.82, 0.54)*	0.98	1.03 (0.33-1.67)
Melatonin (n = 21)	1.33 (1.29) vs. 2.16 (1.20)	-0.79 (1.52)	-0.14 (-1, 0.57)*		1.09 (0.51-1.66)
Amitriptyline + melatonin (n = 21)	1.04 (0.92) vs. 2.10 (1.03)	-1.1 (1.14)	-0.35 (-0.74, 0.47)*		1.33 (0.77-1.89)
Number of tender points					
Amitriptyline (n = 21)	10.62 (3.36) vs. 14.10 (2.27)	-3.45 (0.84)	- 4 (-5, 1.25)**	0.89	1.99 (1.35-2.63)
Melatonin (n = 21)	10.95 (2.94) vs. 14.71 (1.70)	- 3.75 (2.46)	- 4 (-6.5,-2.25)**		2.17 (1.53-2.80)
Amitriptyline + melatonin (n = 21)	10.29 (3.15) vs. 14.61 (2.32)	- 4.18 (1.91)	- 4 (-5,-3)**		2.41 (1.72-3.10)
Pittsburgh Sleep Questionnaire					
Amitriptyline (n = 21)	11.84 (5.82) vs. 19.31 (6.58)	-7.47 (7.34)	-7 (-11,-4)*	0.94	1.07 (0.51-1.63)
Melatonin (n = 21)	16.68 (8.38) vs. 22.67 (7.69)	-6.42 (6.53)	-5 (-11,-2)*		0.9 (0.38-1.44)
Amitriptyline + melatonin (n = 21)	16.11 (8.40) vs. 24.28 (7.79)	-7.58 (1.91)	-8 (-12,-1.5)*		1.06 (0.52-1.59)

*P < 0.01, **P < 0.0001 Comparisons using Mixed ANOVA model.

†Mixed ANOVA model. Mean difference of group. Different superscripts (a, b, and c) indicate significant differences among treatment groups according to the Bonferroni test.

Standardized mean difference (SMD) [(pre minus post)/pool baseline standard deviation] with confidence interval (CI) 95%. The size effect was interpreted as follows: small, 0.20 to 0.40; moderate, 0.50-0.70; and large, 0.80 or higher.

regulate nociceptive processing (largely within the dorsal horn) in various circumstances to produce either facilitation (pronociception) or inhibition (antinociception) [50]. Therefore, melatonin may also inhibit the descending pathways that facilitate pain transmission, which are believed to be circuits with a sustained activation that underlies chronic pain, such as in FM [51,52]. Overall, these findings suggest that melatonin increased the inhibitory descending pain system effect, which involves anatomical connections between cortical and brainstem regions in the human brain, as demonstrated by tractography [53].

The inverse correlation between CPM-TASK, BDNF and HTT0 (Table 2) corroborates the presence of central sensitization theory, which is related to a reduction in the descending inhibitory system activity [54] and to a greater activation in the brainstem [55]. Thus, the reduction of BDNF suggests that this neuromodulator is involved in central sensitization [56,57]. This neurotrophin is involved in altering the excitatory/inhibitory balance in the central nervous system (CNS) and in the amplification of pain response [58,59]. Because BDNF levels can serve as a molecular "sensor" of the global levels of neuronal activity, it has been suggested that the induction of BDNF expression in response to increases in the level of neuronal activity may dampen cortical excitability by promoting the development and/or strengthening of inhibitory synapses in local circuits [60,61]. This multifaceted mechanism of melatonin's effect on pain also results in a reduction in serum BDNF, an effect observed in this study, which corroborates the results of a previous randomized clinical trial concerning chronic pelvic pain induced by endometriosis [16].

In addition, melatonin's effect on BDNF observed in this study may be explained by its anti-inflammatory effects. This hypothesis is supported by the relation between BDNF and pro-inflammatory cytokines that has been demonstrated in FM patients [62-64]. Melatonin has marked anti-inflammatory effects on peripheral sites by inhibiting the release of pro-inflammatory cytokines [12]. Additional mechanisms involved in melatonin's effect on pain pathways include an important reduction of nitric oxide (NO) and malondialdehyde (MDA) levels,

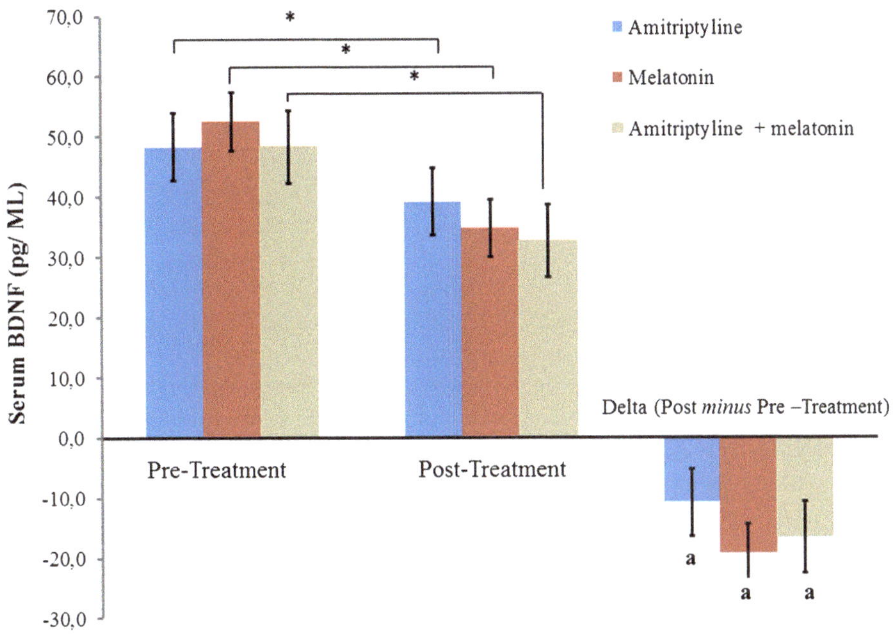

Figure 4 Mean serum BDNF (ng/mL) at baseline and the after treatment presented as the mean ± SEM. The asterisk indicates a significant within group difference according to Mixed ANOVA model with Bonferroni test. Delta values (serum BDNF before treatment minus serum BDNF after pretreatment) were performed using a Mixed ANOVA. The error bars indicate the standard error of the mean. [a]Indicates that the treatment did not induce an effect that was significantly different between treatment groups ($P > 0.05$).

two compounds that are closely related to inflammation [65]. Melatonin inhibits the inflammatory response and inducible NO synthase (iNOS) isoform expression [66], as demonstrated in FM patients by Citera et al. [5]. In addition, melatonin as an adjuvant of drugs that increase serotonin (e.g., SSRIs, tricyclic antidepressants) could be a beneficial pharmacological approach for the management of patients with FM [6]. Overall, these findings reveal that melatonin may change a response associated with a maladaptive neuroplasticity process orchestrated by neuronal, endocrinal, and immune mechanisms that can amplify sensory pain signals to the neural pain matrix.

The present study demonstrated that all treatments reduced pain, and in the melatonin-treated groups, this effect was marginally better than in the amitriptyline group. Melatonin's effect on pain was demonstrated by the VAS, FIQ and PPT. These findings corroborate evidence of experimental studies [8] and previous randomized clinical trials on acute pain [10,14] and chronic pain such as fibromyalgia [5,6], temporomandibular disorders [15], endometriosis [16] and a dose–response study with healthy subjects [26]. The highly lipid-soluble nature of melatonin allows it to easily penetrate the blood–brain barrier. The antinociceptive effect of melatonin is known to involve the activation of supraspinal sites and the inhibition of "spinal windup" [67,68].

Evidence from experimental studies suggests that the analgesic effects of melatonin are mediated by opioids [69] and by gamma-aminobutyric acid ([GABA] ergic) systems [27,28], but it is not possible to dissociate the effect of each individual neurobiological system in human experimental and clinical studies. Indeed, only the net effect can be assessed. Studies have also suggested that additional pathways play a role in the analgesic actions of melatonin, such as the nuclear signaling pathways, receptor-independent radical scavenging, and inhibition of the release of pro-inflammatory cytokines at peripheral sites.

According to previous clinical studies, the most prevalent complaints in patients with FM were sleep disturbance, fatigue, and chronic pain, and these symptoms might be a consequence of melatonin secretion disruption [70]. Moreover, serum levels of melatonin precursors (tryptophan and serotonin) have been reported to be low in patients with FM [71,72]. This could explain the lack of restorative sleep and could be a mechanism involved in dysfunctional pain modulation [3]. Thus, the restoring of melatonin could be an additional mechanism among the others not yet discussed to explain the discrepancy of its effect compared with amitriptyline. However, one can realize that, overall, the association with amitriptyline induced only a marginal increase in the clinical effect. This finding is contrary to our initial hypothesis that the combined treatment (melatonin + amitriptyline) might provide an effect with a higher clinical impact. Although the interventions were randomly allocated to balance the characteristic between arms, some baseline pain traits were higher in group that received melatonin + amitriptyline. This imbalance occurred by chance, but the random allocation ensures the groups were not systematically biased [73]. Furthermore, if any disadvantage would appear, it would be on this group (*i.e.* amitriptyline + melatonin) which had more clinical comorbidities. Accordingly, our findings highlight that melatonin alone or in combination with amitriptyline might improve the efficacy of fibromyalgia treatment in those with more severe symptoms. This finding is in accordance with a recent study that demonstrated an association between lower levels of 6-sulfatoxy-melatonin with higher severe symptoms of FM such as pain, sleep disturbances, fatigue, anxiety and depression [74]. However, to reduce the possible influence of this imbalance in the treatment effect, all analyses were fitted using the delta value of the outcomes from baseline. In addition, these results also agree with previous studies that demonstrate that antidepressant drugs (selective serotonin reuptake inhibitors, SSRIs) associated with melatonin-improved fibromyalgia symptoms [6].

The strengths of this study include the comparison of melatonin and amitriptyline association in a phase II, randomized, double-dummy factorial design, placebo-controlled trial and the use of multiple efficacy and safety measures based on previous trial experience. Although the important effects of SSRIs in FM are well known, the effects of the association of melatonin and amitriptyline in this chronic pain condition were not previously studied. We conducted this trial according to CONSORT guidelines, and given that we used the Delphi List (a list of criteria for the quality assessment of randomized controlled trials), our randomized controlled trial can be considered to be of strong quality because all 8 items in this scale can be positively scored [75]. In addition, we used the double-dummy method and shield placement to prevent the patient and team members from following the patients to control assessment bias. These findings are important because they demonstrate that the application of new therapeutics can be assessed in each particular context to determine whether they provide enough benefit over those already available [76]. The factorial design is a proposed method for examining the interactions between treatments by generating an interaction ratio. In addition, this method permits us to estimate whether the "at the margins" analyses may have overestimated or underestimated the efficacy (and adverse effects) of each agent. A potential limitation is the short treatment duration, but it would have been difficult to justify a prolonged treatment period in patients experiencing chronic pain if they had a high incidence of severe side effects. Accordingly, the incidence of MJSE in the amitriptyline group was 38.09%. This finding is in accordance with the literature reporting that the tricyclic antidepressants are effective at alleviating pain and improving sleep quality [77]; however, the complaints related to common anticholinergic side effects such as dry mouth, sedation, constipation, orthostasis and weight gain are common [78]. We emphasize that the results of this study are relevant only to the patient population investigated. Although the homogeneity of this study population is methodologically advantageous, the issue of external validity arises. Thus, additional research with a larger number of patients is needed to more widely assess the potential benefits of melatonin in several different clinical settings, and future studies are required before definitive conclusions regarding melatonin and pain treatment can be made. Finally, although several strategies were used to prevent patients and the evaluator team from unblinding, formal assessment for awareness of the allocation (either active or placebo) was not performed. However, our objective surrogates less prone to bias (i.e., serum BDNF, analgesics requirements, CPM-TASK) were consistent with pain scores, and thus, unblinding is unlikely to have influenced the direction of our conclusions.

Conclusion

In conclusion, in this 6-week, randomized, double-dummy, placebo-controlled study, melatonin alone or associated with amitriptyline was better than amitriptyline alone in improving pain on the VAS, FIQ and PPT, whereas its association with amitriptyline produced only marginal additional clinical effects. Melatonin increased the inhibitory endogenous pain-modulating system as assessed by the reduction of the $NPS_{(0-10)}$ during the CPM-TASK. In addition, this study suggests that peripheral BDNF could be used as a biomarker of central sensitization, as it is inversely correlated with pain reduction in the CPM-TASK.

Abbreviations

PMS: Pain-modulating system; BDNF: Brain-derived neurotrophic factor; HPT: Heat pain threshold; FM: Fibromyalgia; RCT: Randomized clinical trial; NA: Noradrenalin; 5- HT: Serotonin; DA: Dopamine; NO: Nitric oxide; MDA: Malondialdehyde; SSRIs: Selective serotonin reuptake inhibitors; PPT: Pressure pain thresholds; DNIC: Diffuse noxious inhibitory control; CPM: Conditional pain modulation; NPS: Numerical rating pain scale; ELISA: Enzyme-linked immunosorbent assay; NSAIDS: Non-steroidal anti-inflammatory drugs; FIQ: Fibromyalgia impact questionnaire; MSE: Minor side effects; MJSE: Major side effects; ICI: Confidence interval; B- PCS: Pain catastrophizing scale for the brazilian population; VAS: Visual analog scale.

Competing interests

The authors declare that there are no financial or other relationships that might lead to conflicts of interest involving any of the following arrangements: *financial relationship to the work, employees of a company, consultants for a company, stockholders of the company, members of a speakers bureau or any other form of financial compensation.*

Author's contribution

A participated in the sequence alignment. B participated in the design of the study and performed the statistical analysis. C conceived of the study, and participated in its design and coordination and helped to draft the manuscript. All authors read and approved the final manuscript.

Acknowledgements

This research was supported by grants and material support from the following Brazilian agencies:

Committee for the Development of Higher Education Personnel – CAPES - PNPD/CAPES (grants to Rafael Vercelino; Deitos A; I.C.C. de Souza; (G. Laste MEC/MCTI/CAPES/CNPq/FAPs No 71/2013); J.R. Rozisky International Cooperation Program – CAPES (023/11) and material support;

National Council for Scientific and Technological Development - CNPq (grants to Dr. I.L.S. Torres, Dr. W. Caumo);

Postgraduate Program in Medical Sciences at the School of Medicine of the Federal University of Rio Grande do Sul (material support);

Postgraduate Research Group at the Hospital de Clínicas de Porto Alegre (material support);

Foundation for Support of Research at Rio Grande do Sul (FAPERGS) (grant to Schwertner A).

Author details

[1]Pain and Palliative Care Service at the Hospital de Clínicas de Porto Alegre (HCPA), Universidade Federal do Rio Grande do Sul (UFRGS), Porto Alegre, Brazil. [2]Pharmacology Department, Instituto de Ciências Básicas da Saúde, UFRGS, Porto Alegre, Brazil. [3]Post Graduate Program in Medical Sciences, School of Medicine, Universidade Federal do Rio Grande do Sul (UFRGS), Porto Alegre, Brazil. [4]Laboratory of Pain & Neuromodulation, Institution: Hospital de Clínicas de Porto Alegre at UFRGS, Rua Ramiro Barcelos, 2350 - CEP 90035-003 Bairro Rio Branco, Porto Alegre, Brazil.

References

1. Mease PJ, Clauw DJ, Arnold LM, Goldenberg DL, Witter J, Williams DA, Simon LS, Strand CV, Bramson C, Martin S, Wright TM, Littman B, Wernicke JF, Gendreau RM, Crofford LJ: **Fibromyalgia syndrome.** *J Rheumatol* 2005, **32:**2270–2277.
2. Arnold LM, Hudson JI, Keck PE, Auchenbach MB, Javaras KN, Hess EV: **Comorbidity of fibromyalgia and psychiatric disorders.** *J Clin Psychiatry* 2006, **67:**1219–1225.
3. Wikner J, Hirsch U, Wetterberg L, Röjdmark S: **Fibromyalgia–a syndrome associated with decreased nocturnal melatonin secretion.** *Clin Endocrinol (Oxf)* 1998, **49:**179–183.
4. Bennett RM: **The rational management of fibromyalgia patients.** *Rheum Dis Clin North Am* 2002, **28:**181–199. v.
5. Citera G, Arias MA, Maldonado-Cocco JA, Lázaro MA, Rosemffet MG, Brusco LI, Scheines EJ, Cardinalli DP: **The effect of melatonin in patients with fibromyalgia: a pilot study.** *Clin Rheumatol* 2000, **19:**9–13.
6. Hussain SA, Al-Khalifa II, Jasim NA, Gorial FI: **Adjuvant use of melatonin for treatment of fibromyalgia.** *J Pineal Res* 2011, **50:**267–271.
7. Mahdi AA, Fatima G, Das SK, Verma NS: **Abnormality of circadian rhythm of serum melatonin and other biochemical parameters in fibromyalgia syndrome.** *Indian J Biochem Biophys* 2011, **48:**82–87.
8. Laste G, Vidor L, de Macedo IC, Rozisky JR, Medeiros L, de Souza A, Meurer L, de Souza IC, Torres IL, Caumo W: **Melatonin treatment entrains the rest-activity circadian rhythm in rats with chronic inflammation.** *Chronobiol Int* 2013, **30:**1077–1088.
9. Detanico BC, Piato AL, Freitas JJ, Lhullier FL, Hidalgo MP, Caumo W, Elisabetsky E: **Antidepressant-like effects of melatonin in the mouse chronic mild stress model.** *Eur J Pharmacol* 2009, **607:**121–125.
10. Caumo W, Levandovski R, Hidalgo MP: **Preoperative anxiolytic effect of melatonin and clonidine on postoperative pain and morphine consumption in patients undergoing abdominal hysterectomy: a double-blind, randomized, placebo-controlled study.** *J Pain* 2009, **10:**100–108.
11. Laste G, de Macedo IC, Ripoll Rozisky J, Ribeiro da Silva F, Caumo W, Torres IL: **Melatonin administration reduces inflammatory pain in rats.** *J Pain Res* 2012, **5:**359–362.
12. Ambriz-Tututi M, Granados-Soto V: **Oral and spinal melatonin reduces tactile allodynia in rats via activation of MT2 and opioid receptors.** *Pain* 2007, **132:**273–280.
13. Esposito E, Cuzzocrea S: **Antiinflammatory activity of melatonin in central nervous system.** *Curr Neuropharmacol* 2010, **8:**228–242.
14. Caumo W, Torres F, Moreira NL, Auzani JA, Monteiro CA, Londero G, Ribeiro DF, Hidalgo MP: **The clinical impact of preoperative melatonin on postoperative outcomes in patients undergoing abdominal hysterectomy.** *Anesth Analg* 2007, **105:**1263–1271. table of contents.
15. Vidor LP, Torres IL, Custódio de Souza IC IC, Fregni F, Caumo W: **Analgesic and sedative effects of melatonin in temporomandibular disorders: a double-blind, randomized, parallel-group, placebo-controlled study.** *J Pain Symptom Manage* 2013, **46:**422–432.
16. Schwertner A, Conceição Dos Santos CC, Costa GD, Deitos A, de Souza A, de Souza IC, Torres IL, da Cunha Filho JS, Caumo W: **Efficacy of melatonin in the treatment of endometriosis: a phase II, randomized, double-blind, placebo-controlled trial.** *Pain* 2013, **154:**874–881.
17. Yarnitsky D: **Conditioned pain modulation (the diffuse noxious inhibitory control-like effect): its relevance for acute and chronic pain states.** *Curr Opin Anaesthesiol* 2010, **23:**611–615.
18. Paul-Savoie E, Marchand S, Morin M, Bourgault P, Brissette N, Rattanavong V, Cloutier C, Bissonnette A, Potvin S: **Is the deficit in pain inhibition in fibromyalgia influenced by sleep impairments?** *Open Rheumatol J* 2012, **6:**296–302.
19. Houvenagel E, Forzy G, Leloire O, Gallois P, Hary S, Hautecoeur P, Convain L, Henniaux M, Vincent G, Dhondt JL: **Cerebrospinal fluid monoamines in primary fibromyalgia].** *Rev Rhum Mal Osteoartic* 1990, **57:**21–23.
20. Legangneux E, Mora JJ, Spreux-Varoquaux O, Thorin I, Herrou M, Alvado G, Gomeni C: **Cerebrospinal fluid biogenic amine metabolites, plasma-rich platelet serotonin and [3H] imipramine reuptake in the primary fibromyalgia syndrome.** *Rheumatology (Oxford)* 2001, **40:**290–296.
21. Russell IJ, Vaeroy H, Javors M, Nyberg F: **Cerebrospinal fluid biogenic amine metabolites in fibromyalgia/fibrositis syndrome and rheumatoid arthritis.** *Arthritis Rheum* 1992, **35:**550–556.
22. Wood PB, Glabus MF, Simpson R, Patterson JC: **Changes in gray matter density in fibromyalgia: correlation with dopamine metabolism.** *J Pain* 2009, **10:**609–618.
23. Potvin S, Larouche A, Normand E, de Souza JB, Gaumond I, Grignon S, Marchand S: **DRD3 Ser9Gly polymorphism is related to thermal pain perception and modulation in chronic widespread pain patients and healthy controls.** *J Pain* 2009, **10:**969–975.
24. Volz MS, Medeiros LF, Tarragô MG, Vidor LP, Dall'Agnol L, Deitos A, Brietzke A, Rozisky JR, Rispolli B, Torres IL, Fregni F, Caumo W: **The relationship between cortical excitability and pain catastrophizing in myofascial pain.** *J Pain* 2013, **14:**1140–1147.
25. Millan MJ: **Descending control of pain.** *Prog Neurobiol* 2002, **66:**355–474.
26. Stefani L, Muller S, Torres I, Razzolini B, Rozisky J, Fregni F, Markus R, Caumo W: **A Phase II, randomized, double-blind, placebo controlled, dose–response trial of the melatonin effect on the pain threshold of healthy subjects.** *PLoS One* 2013, 8(10):e74107.27.
27. Zurowski D, Nowak L, Machowska A, Wordliczek J, Thor PJ: **Exogenous melatonin abolishes mechanical allodynia but not thermal hyperalgesia in neuropathic pain. The role of the opioid system and benzodiazepine-gabaergic mechanism.** *J Physiol Pharmacol* 2012, **63:**641–647.
28. Golombek DA, Escolar E, Burin LJ, De Brito Sánchez MG, Cardinali DP: **Time-dependent melatonin analgesia in mice: inhibition by opiate or benzodiazepine antagonism.** *Eur J Pharmacol* 1991, **194:**25–30.
29. Schulz KF, Altman DG, Moher D, Group C: **CONSORT 2010 statement: updated guidelines for reporting parallel group randomised trials.** *Int J Surg* 2011, **9:**672–677.
30. Wolfe F, Clauw DJ, Fitzcharles MA, Goldenberg DL, Katz RS, Mease P, Russell AS, Russell IJ, Winfield JB, Yunus MB: **The American College of Rheumatology preliminary diagnostic criteria for fibromyalgia and measurement of symptom severity.** *Arthritis Care Res (Hoboken)* 2010, **62:**600–610.
31. Scott J, Huskisson EC: **Graphic representation of pain.** *Pain* 1976, **2:**175–184.
32. Couto C, de Souza IC, Torres IL, Fregni F, Caumo W: **Paraspinal stimulation combined with trigger point needling and needle rotation for the treatment of myofascial pain: a randomized sham-controlled clinical trial.** *Clin J Pain* 2014, **30:**214–223.
33. Dao TT, Lavigne GJ, Feine JS, Tanguay R, Lund JP: **Power and sample size calculations for clinical trials of myofascial pain of jaw muscles.** *J Dent Res* 1991, **70:**118–122.
34. Kaipper MB, Chachamovich E, Hidalgo MP, Torres IL, Caumo W: **Evaluation of the structure of Brazilian State-Trait Anxiety Inventory using a Rasch psychometric approach.** *J Psychosom Res* 2010, **68:**223–233.
35. Hamilton M: **A rating scale for depression.** *J Neurol Neurosurg Psychiatry* 1960, **23:**56–62.

36. Buysse DJ, Reynolds CF 3rd, Monk TH, Berman SR, Kupfer DJ: **The Pittsburgh Sleep Quality Index: a new instrument for psychiatric practice and research.** *Psychiatry Res* 1989, **28**:193–213.
37. Lobbestael J, Leurgans M, Arntz A: **Inter-rater reliability of the Structured Clinical Interview for DSM-IV Axis I Disorders (SCID I) and Axis II Disorders (SCID II).** *Clin Psychol Psychother* 2011, **18**:75–79.
38. Sehn F, Chachamovich E, Vidor LP, Dall-Agnol L, de Souza IC, Torres IL, Fregni F, Caumo W: **Cross-cultural adaptation and validation of the Brazilian Portuguese version of the pain catastrophizing scale.** *Pain Med* 2012, **13**:1425–1435.
39. Burckhardt CS, Clark SR, Bennett RM: **The fibromyalgia impact questionnaire: development and validation.** *J Rheumatol* 1991, **18**:728–733.
40. Marques A, Santos A, Assumpcao A, Matsutani L, Lage L, Pereira C: **Validation of a Brazilian version of the Fibromyalgia Impact Questionnaire (FIQ).** *Ann Rheum Dis* 2006, **65**:557–557.
41. Fischer AA: **Pressure algometry over normal muscles. Standard values, validity and reproducibility of pressure threshold.** *Pain* 1987, **30**:115–126.
42. Tousignant-Laflamme Y, Pagé S, Goffaux P, Marchand S: **An experimental model to measure excitatory and inhibitory pain mechanisms in humans.** *Brain Res* 2008, **1230**:73–79.
43. Magerl W, Krumova EK, Baron R, Tölle T, Treede RD, Maier C: **Reference data for quantitative sensory testing (QST): refined stratification for age and a novel method for statistical comparison of group data.** *Pain* 2010, **151**:598–605.
44. Marchand S, Arsenault P: **Spatial summation for pain perception: interaction of inhibitory and excitatory mechanisms.** *Pain* 2002, **95**:201–206.
45. Schestatsky P, Valls-Solé J, Costa J, León L, Veciana M, Chaves ML: **Skin autonomic reactivity to thermoalgesic stimuli.** *Clin Auton Res* 2007, **17**:349–355.
46. Tesarz J, Gerhardt A, Schommer K, Treede RD, Eich W: **Alterations in endogenous pain modulation in endurance athletes: an experimental study using quantitative sensory testing and the cold-pressor task.** *Pain* 2013, **154**:1022–1029.
47. Kazis LE, Anderson JJ, Meenan RF: **Effect sizes for interpreting changes in health status.** *Med Care* 1989, **27**:S178–S189.
48. Wilhelmsen M, Amirian I, Reiter RJ, Rosenberg J, Gögenur I: **Analgesic effects of melatonin: a review of current evidence from experimental and clinical studies.** *J Pineal Res* 2011, **51**:270–277.
49. Mantovani M, Kaster MP, Pertile R, Calixto JB, Rodrigues AL, Santos AR: **Mechanisms involved in the antinociception caused by melatonin in mice.** *J Pineal Res* 2006, **41**:382–389.
50. Basbaum AI, Fields HL: **Endogenous pain control systems: brainstem spinal pathways and endorphin circuitry.** *Annu Rev Neurosci* 1984, **7**:309–338.
51. Gebhart GF: **Descending modulation of pain.** *Neurosci Biobehav Rev* 2004, **27**:729–737.
52. Porreca F, Ossipov MH, Gebhart GF: **Chronic pain and medullary descending facilitation.** *Trends Neurosci* 2002, **25**:319–325.
53. Hadjipavlou G, Dunckley P, Behrens TE, Tracey I: **Determining anatomical connectivities between cortical and brainstem pain processing regions in humans: a diffusion tensor imaging study in healthy controls.** *Pain* 2006, **123**:169–178.
54. Schwenkreis P, Janssen F, Rommel O, Pleger B, Völker B, Hosbach I, Dertwinkel R, Maier C, Tegenthoff M: **Bilateral motor cortex disinhibition in complex regional pain syndrome (CRPS) type I of the hand.** *Neurology* 2003, **61**:515–519.
55. Graven-Nielsen T, Wodehouse T, Langford RM, Arendt-Nielsen L, Kidd BL: **Normalization of widespread hyperesthesia and facilitated spatial summation of deep-tissue pain in knee osteoarthritis patients after knee replacement.** *Arthritis Rheum* 2012, **64**:2907–2916.
56. Delafoy L, Gelot A, Ardid D, Eschalier A, Bertrand C, Doherty AM, Diop L: **Interactive involvement of brain derived neurotrophic factor, nerve growth factor, and calcitonin gene related peptide in colonic hypersensitivity in the rat.** *Gut* 2006, **55**:940–945.
57. Groth R, Aanonsen L: **Spinal brain-derived neurotrophic factor (BDNF) produces hyperalgesia in normal mice while antisense directed against either BDNF or trkB, prevent inflammation-induced hyperalgesia.** *Pain* 2002, **100**:171–181.
58. Sommer C, Kress M: **Recent findings on how proinflammatory cytokines cause pain: peripheral mechanisms in inflammatory and neuropathic hyperalgesia.** *Neurosci Lett* 2004, **361**:184–187.
59. Kerr BJ, Bradbury EJ, Bennett DL, Trivedi PM, Dassan P, French J, Shelton DB, McMahon SB, Thompson SW: **Brain-derived neurotrophic factor modulates nociceptive sensory inputs and NMDA-evoked responses in the rat spinal cord.** *J Neurosci* 1999, **19**:5138–5148.
60. Genoud C, Knott GW, Sakata K, Lu B, Welker E: **Altered synapse formation in the adult somatosensory cortex of brain-derived neurotrophic factor heterozygote mice.** *J Neurosci* 2004, **24**:2394–2400.
61. Rutherford LC, DeWan A, Lauer HM, Turrigiano GG: **Brain-derived neurotrophic factor mediates the activity-dependent regulation of inhibition in neocortical cultures.** *J Neurosci* 1997, **17**:4527–4535.
62. Ortega E, García JJ, Bote ME, Martín-Cordero L, Escalante Y, Saavedra JM, Northoff H, Giraldo E: **Exercise in fibromyalgia and related inflammatory disorders: known effects and unknown chances.** *Exerc Immunol Rev* 2009, **15**:42–65.
63. Bote ME, García JJ, Hinchado MD, Ortega E: **Inflammatory/stress feedback dysregulation in women with fibromyalgia.** *Neuroimmunomodulation* 2012, **19**:343–351.
64. Wallace DJ, Linker-Israeli M, Hallegua D, Silverman S, Silver D, Weisman MH: **Cytokines play an aetiopathogenetic role in fibromyalgia: a hypothesis and pilot study.** *Rheumatology (Oxford)* 2001, **40**:743–749.
65. Bilici D, Akpinar E, Kiziltunç A: **Protective effect of melatonin in carrageenan-induced acute local inflammation.** *Pharmacol Res* 2002, **46**:133–139.
66. Cuzzocrea S, Zingarelli B, Gilad E, Hake P, Salzman AL, Szabó C: **Protective effect of melatonin in carrageenan-induced models of local inflammation: relationship to its inhibitory effect on nitric oxide production and its peroxynitrite scavenging activity.** *J Pineal Res* 1997, **23**:106–116.
67. Morgan P, Barrett P, Howell H, Helliwell R: **Melatonin receptors - localization, molecular pharmacology and physiological significance.** *Neurochem Int* 1994, **24**:101–146.
68. Noseda R, Hernández A, Valladares L, Mondaca M, Laurido C, Soto-Moyano R: **Melatonin-induced inhibition of spinal cord synaptic potentiation in rats is MT2 receptor-dependent.** *Neurosci Lett* 2004, **360**:41–44.
69. Li SR, Wang T, Wang R, Dai X, Chen Q, Li RD: **Melatonin enhances antinociceptive effects of delta-, but not mu-opioid agonist in mice.** *Brain Res* 2005, **1043**:132–138.
70. Bazzichi L, Rossi A, Giacomelli C, Bombardieri S: **Exploring the abyss of fibromyalgia biomarkers.** *Clin Exp Rheumatol* 2010, **28**:S125–S130.
71. Yunus MB: **Fibromyalgia and overlapping disorders: the unifying concept of central sensitivity syndromes.** *Semin Arthritis Rheum* 2007, **36**:339–356.
72. Yunus MB: **Role of central sensitization in symptoms beyond muscle pain, and the evaluation of a patient with widespread pain.** *Best Pract Res Clin Rheumatol* 2007, **21**:481–497.
73. Fives AW, Russell D, Kearns N, Rena Lyons G, Eaton P, Canavan J, Devaney C, O'Brien A: **The role of random allocation in randomized controlled trials: distinguishing selection bias from baseline imbalance.** *J Multidisciplinary Eval* 2013, **9**:33–42.
74. Pernambuco AP, Schetino LP, Viana RS, Carvalho LS, Reis D: **The involvement of melatonin in the clinical status of patients with fibromyalgia syndrome.** *Clin Exp Rheumatol* 2014, in press. in press.
75. Verhagen AP, de Vet HC, de Bie RA, Kessels AG, Boers M, Bouter LM, Knipschild PG: **The Delphi list: a criteria list for quality assessment of randomized clinical trials for conducting systematic reviews developed by Delphi consensus.** *J Clin Epidemiol* 1998, **51**:1235–1241.
76. Cazzola M: **Application of Number Needed to Treat (NNT) as a Measure of Treatment Effect in Respiratory Medicine.** *Treat Respir Med* 2006, **5**:79–84.
77. Plesh O, Curtis D, Levine J, McCall WD: **Amitriptyline treatment of chronic pain in patients with temporomandibular disorders.** *J Oral Rehabil* 2000, **27**:834–841.
78. Bendtsen L, Jensen R: **Amitriptyline reduces myofascial tenderness in patients with chronic tension-type headache.** *Cephalalgia* 2000, **20**:603–610.

Benign elevations in serum aminotransferases and biomarkers of hepatotoxicity in healthy volunteers treated with cholestyramine

Rohit Singhal[1], Alison H Harrill[2], Francoise Menguy-Vacheron[3], Zaid Jayyosi[1], Hadj Benzerdjeb[3] and Paul B Watkins[2,4*]

Abstract

Background: There are currently no serum biomarkers capable of distinguishing elevations in serum alanine aminotransferase (ALT) that portend serious liver injury potential from benign elevations such as those occurring during cholestyramine treatment. The aim of the research was to test the hypothesis that newly proposed biomarkers of hepatotoxicity would not significantly rise in serum during elevations in serum ALT associated with cholestyramine treatment, which has never been associated with clinically relevant liver injury.

Methods: In a double-blind placebo-controlled trial, cholestyramine (8g) was administered for 11 days to healthy adult volunteers. Serum from subjects with elevations in alanine aminotransferase (ALT) exceeding three-fold the upper limit of normal (ULN) were utilized for biomarker quantification.

Results: In 11 of 67 subjects, cholestyramine treatment resulted in ALT elevation by >3x ULN (mean 6.9 fold; range 3–28 fold). In these 11 subjects, there was a 22.4-fold mean increase in serum levels of miR-122 relative to baseline, supporting a liver origin of the serum ALT. Significant elevations were noted in mean levels of necrosis biomarkers sorbitol dehydrogenase (8.1 fold), cytokeratin 18 (2.1 fold) and HMGB1 (1.7 fold). Caspase-cleaved cytokeratin 18, a biomarker of apoptosis was also significantly elevated (1.7 fold). A rise in glutamate dehydrogenase (7.3 fold) may support mitochondrial dysfunction.

Conclusion: All toxicity biomarkers measured in this study were elevated along with ALT, confirming the liver origin and reflecting both hepatocyte necrosis and apoptosis. Since cholestyramine treatment has no clinical liver safety concerns, we conclude that interpretation of the biomarkers studied may not be straightforward in the context of assessing liver safety of new drugs.

Keywords: Liver, Biomarkers, Toxicity, Hepatotoxicity

Background

Hepatotoxicity is a major reason for termination of clinical drug development programs and regulatory actions on drugs, including withdrawal from the market. The potential for a new drug candidate to cause clinically important liver injury is often difficult to ascertain in clinical trials due to deficiencies in the currently available serum tests, which have not changed in more than four decades. The most sensitive and widely employed serum test for liver injury is serum alanine aminotransferase (ALT). However, there are drugs that cause serum ALT elevations, even pronounced elevations, that do not cause clinically important liver injury [1]. To address this issue, the current FDA guidance for evaluation of drug-induced liver injury (DILI) in clinical trials recommends continuing treatment of subjects with asymptomatic ALT elevations (up to 8 × ULN) to determine whether there is subsequent loss of liver function, specifically with concurrent elevation of serum bilirubin ("Hy's Law" criteria) [2]. However, this practice may be placing clinical trial participants at risk. There exists at least one example of a patient in a clinical trial who developed fatal liver failure despite discontinuing treatment with the implicated drug prior to the occurrence of elevation in serum bilirubin [3].

* Correspondence: pwatkins@thehamner.org
[2]The Hamner-University of North Carolina Institute for Drug Safety Sciences, 6 Davis Drive, Research Triangle Park, NC 27709, USA
[4]Schools of Medicine, Pharmacy and Public Health, University of North Carolina at Chapel Hill, Chapel Hill, NC 27599, USA
Full list of author information is available at the end of the article

When ALT elevations are caused by drugs not known to cause clinically important liver injury, it has been assumed that the underlying mechanisms may not involve hepatocellular damage. Proposed mechanisms include extrahepatic sources of the ALT, leak of ALT from healthy hepatocytes, increased ALT synthesis within the liver, and/or reduced ALT clearance from blood. New serum biomarkers have been proposed to detect liver specific injury (miR-122), apoptosis (caspase cleaved cytokeratin-18 fragments), and necrosis (sorbitol dehydrogenase, full-length cytokeratin-18, glutamate dehydrogenase and HMGB1) [4-9]. It is a reasonable hypothesis that these new biomarkers may help distinguish between benign ALT elevations and those that portend potential for clinically important liver injury.

Cholestyramine, a cholesterol lowering drug, is an orally administered and non-absorbable ion-exchange resin that binds bile acids in the intestine, interrupting their enterohepatic circulation and increasing their fecal excretion [10]. Cholestyramine is also sometimes used to interrupt enterohepatic circulation of certain drugs and to accelerate their removal from the body [10,11]. To our knowledge, and in spite of the very large clinical experience with cholestyramine during decades of use, there have not been reports of clinically important hepatotoxicity associated with this treatment. Indeed, cholestyramine is commonly used in patients with advanced liver disease to relieve symptoms associated with cholestasis [12]. However, in at least two clinical studies cholestyramine treatment was reported to be associated with elevations in serum ALT [13,14].

In a clinical study involving treatment of healthy adult volunteers with cholestyramine, we observed asymptomatic elevations in serum ALT. This discrepancy between traditional interpretation of serum ALT and clinical safety experience raises the possibility that cholestyramine-associated elevations in serum ALT do not reflect true hepatocyte injury. To provide insight into mechanisms underlying these benign elevations of serum ALT, we assayed serum samples from subjects who experienced serum ALT elevations during treatment with cholestyramine for the liver specific microRNA, miR-122, and for biomarkers associated with necrosis and apoptosis. Our hypothesis was that these biomarkers would not demonstrate concomitant elevations with the serum ALT and may therefore be useful in clinical settings to distinguish benign elevations in serum ALT from those that portend potential for clinically important liver injury.

Methods

Study design

The subjects studied were a subset of a larger randomized, double blind, phase-I clinical trial conducted in healthy male and female subjects aged 18–65 years old in order to evaluate the potential for an active investigational new drug to prolong the QT interval. After a 12 day treatment phase (active drug or placebo), all subjects (including those randomized to placebo) entered a "washout" phase involving treatment with cholestyramine (8g powder, three times a day taken orally in a glass of fruit juice, milk soup or water, for 11 days, i.e., from day 13 to 23 of the clinical trial) or activated charcoal to accelerate the elimination of the investigational drug (in those that received active drug). The 67 subjects involved in the current study were all randomized to receive placebo during the treatment phase, never received the active drug, and only received cholestyramine during the washout phase. Thirty-four of these placebo treated subjects also received a single oral dose of moxifloxacin (positive control for QT prolongation), on the day before the start of cholestyramine treatment. The study protocol is shown in Figure 1. A complete description of the clinical trial has been included in CONSORT flow chart (Additional file 1) and CONSORT checklist (Additional file 2: Table S1).

Serial blood samples were obtained and serum enzymes (ALT, AST, and ALP) and total bilirubin were assayed before (baseline) and during the cholestyramine treatment period using AU 400 Olympus clinical chemistry analyzer at the Department de Biologie Clinique Centre régional de lutte contre le Cancer Eugene Marquis, Rennes Cedex, France. Samples were archived only from subjects who experienced confirmed ALT >3 times the ULN; only the baseline and the serum sample with the peak ALT value was archived from these subjects and available for biomarker analysis. The study protocol was reviewed and approved by the regional ethics committee, CPP OUEST VI, at the Centre Hospitalier Universitaire Cavale Blanche, Brest Cedex, France. The clinical trial was conducted in accordance with the International Conference of Harmonisation Guidelines for Good Clinical Practice and the Declaration of Helsinki. Written informed consent was obtained from all subjects prior to the study.

Only samples from subjects treated with cholestyramine after receiving placebo during the active treatment phase were analyzed in this study (i.e., no subjects studied received the investigational drug at any time).

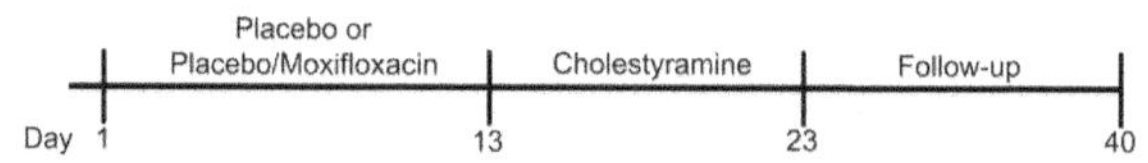

Figure 1 The study design. Subjects were administered placebo from day 1 to 12 of the study or placebo from day 1 to 12 and single dose 400 mg Moxifloxacin (Moxi) on day 12, followed by a washout phase with cholestyramine from day 13 to 23.

Investigational protein biomarker measurements

Analysis was performed on baseline serum samples and the single serum samples containing the highest value for ALT level (i.e., the only post-baseline serum sample archived and therefore available for analysis). Serum concentrations of glutamate dehydrogenase (GLDH; Randox Laboratories, Kearneysville, WV) and sorbitol dehydrogenase (SDH; Genzyme Diagnostics, Cambridge, MA) were determined using a commercial kit by quantifying the decrease in absorbance according to the manufacturer's protocol. Assay results for both GLDH and SDH were quantified using the Cobas Fara II clinical chemistry analyzer (Roche Diagnostics, Indianapolis, IN). Caspase-cleaved and total K18 were determined using the M65 and M30 (apoptosense) ELISAs, respectively, in accordance with the manufacturer's guidelines (Peviva, West Chester, OH). Total HMGB1 content was determined in serum by enzyme-linked immunosorbent assay (ELISA) per the manufacturer's protocol (IBL International, Hamburg, Germany). For all ELISA analytes, the inter- and intra-assay variability was <10%.

RNA isolation and miR-122 quantification

RNA isolation and miR-122 quantification were performed according to a protocol published previously [15], with the exception that 200μl serum was used for RNA extraction. The expression levels of miRNA hsa-miR-122 (miR-122) were quantified using the TaqMan miRNA reverse transcription kit and miRNA-specific stem-loop primers (Applied Biosystems, Foster City, CA) in a scaled-down (5μl) reverse-transcription reaction as described by Kroh *et al.* [16], using the 7900HT instrument (Applied Biosystems). MiRNA was quantified by absolute quantification via a standard curve, with quantities normalized to an exogenous spike-in control derived from *Caenorhabditis elegans*, cel-miR-39.

Statistical analysis

Clinical biochemistry parameters were expressed as fold change from upper limit of normal (ULN). Biomarker values were expressed as post-dosing fold change compared to the pre-dosing baseline. Cholestyramine-mediated changes in the concentrations of biomarkers in comparison to the pre-dosing concentrations were assessed using paired one-tailed Student's t-test. Biomarker correlation analyses were performed by calculating the Pearson correlation coefficient (σ). Descriptive statistics for liver-function tests and biomarkers included the arithmetic mean, standard error of the mean (SEM), and median. Differences in mean or correlation were deemed significant when $p < 0.05$.

Results

Clinical biochemistries

Of the 67 subjects who received placebo (and never received active study medication) and were administered cholestyramine, eleven subjects experienced asymptomatic elevations in serum ALT levels exceeding three-fold the upper limit of normal (>3× ULN). Six of these subjects had received the single oral dose of moxifloxacin the day before the start of cholestyramine treatment. The mean elevation was 255 U/L after treatment with cholestyramine compared to pre-dosing mean ALT level of 20 U/L. Four of the 11 subjects experienced peak ALT levels >5× ULN (2 men and 2 women) and one of the women experienced a 28-fold ULN increase (Figure 2). This latter subject was a 31 year old Caucasian woman with normal BMI (BMI = 25) taking oral contraceptives concomitantly. Two other young women with ALT elevation <5× ULN were also taking oral contraceptives. However, oral contraceptives were given to most of young women of child bearing potential in this trial and only one woman described above experienced an increase in ALT >5× ULN .

A rise in ALT levels was first evident three days after starting cholestyramine (study day 16), and the peak values were obtained 4 to 8 days later (between study day 20 and 24) (Figure 2). The single dose of moxifloxacin did not appear to influence the incidence or height of the serum ALT elevations observed; indeed, three subjects with the highest peak serum ALT values had not received moxifloxacin (Figure 2). The serum ALT rises were mirrored by elevations in serum AST ($\rho = 0.99$, $P < 0.0001$). The enzyme elevations were asymptomatic in each subject, returning to normal ranges

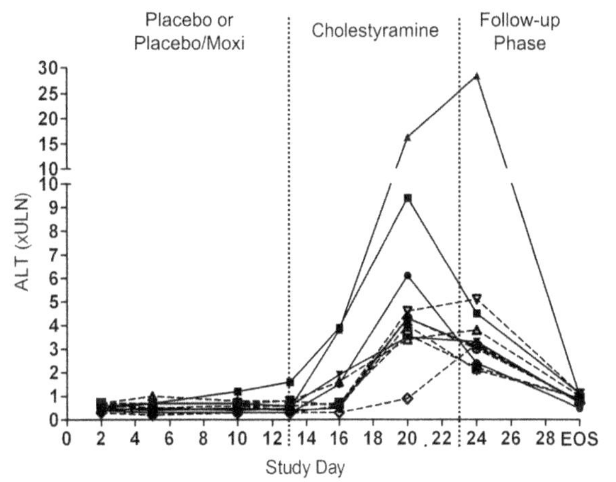

Figure 2 Alanine aminotransferase (ALT) measurement. Blood was collected before dosing on day 1 (baseline), and days 2, 5, 10, 13, 16, 20, 24, and at end of the follow-up phase. Solid and dashed lines represent placebo and moxifloxacin treatments, respectively. EOS is End of Study. Values represent fold change over upper limit of normal (ULN).

within 2 weeks. There were no consistent changes in serum ALP or total bilirubin levels (Table 1) which indicated that there was no clinical evidence of cholestasis.

Experimental biomarkers

Only the serum samples (baseline and peak) from subjects who experienced elevations in serum ALT exceeding 3 × ULN were archived and assayed for experimental biomarker analysis (Figure 3). The mean serum level of the liver-specific miRNA-122 [9] was elevated 22.4-fold over baseline ($P < 0.05$); mean levels of necrosis biomarkers SDH and HMGB1 [4,5,7,8,17] were elevated 8.1-, and 1.7 fold ($P < 0.05$), respectively over baseline. Mean serum levels of full-length cytokeratin 18 (M65) rose 2.1 fold, and its caspase-cleaved fragment (M30), a biomarker of apoptosis [5,6], also rose 1.7 fold ($P < 0.05$), Figure 3). Mean serum GLDH was elevated 7.3- fold. The single dose of moxifloxacin received by 5 of 11 subjects did not have any obvious influence on extent of elevation of any of the biomarkers measured relative to placebo. The Pearson correlation coefficient of peak ALT levels was 0.87 with SDH, 0.45 with GLDH, 0.53 with miR-122, 0.31 with cytokeratin 18, with a significant ($P < 0.05$) correlation observed between ALT and SDH, GLDH and SDH, and GLDH and full length K18 (Table 2). However, there was no correlation observed between fold elevation in serum ALT with fold elevation in caspase-cleaved K18 or HMGB1. Data obtained for each subject are listed in Additional file 3: Table S2.

Discussion

Serum alanine aminotransferase (ALT) has for more than four decades been used in clinical trials as a sensitive means to monitor liver safety of new drug candidates. However, this biomarker lacks specificity and can be elevated during treatment with drugs that are entirely safe for the liver [1]. There is urgent need for new biomarkers capable of distinguishing ALT elevations observed in a clinical trial that represent a "false positive" – *i.e.,* the drug does not cause clinically significant hepatotoxicity vs. a "true positive" – *i.e.,* the drug has potential to cause progressive and clinically important liver injury. Cholestyramine has been used for the treatment of hypercholesterolemia for more than fifty years and this treatment has never been associated with clinically important liver injury. Hence, the marked elevations in serum ALT we observed during treatment with cholestyramine represent a "false positive" safety signal for this drug. In other words, if cholestyramine were a new drug in early clinical development, the profile of serum ALT elevations observed would likely result in termination of the development program over liver safety concerns although no true safety liability exists. Our serum sample set obtained from healthy adult volunteers treated with cholestyramine therefore provided a means for investigating false positive results using additional toxicity biomarkers that have been proposed to represent advances in multiple respects over traditional liver safety biomarkers.

The eleven healthy volunteers who experienced elevations in serum ALT during cholestyramine treatment also had significant increases in serum miR-122. Circulating miR-122 is reported to be essentially liver-specific and has been established as a marker of drug-induced liver injury in humans [9]. In fact, a recent rodent study suggested a greater specificity and sensitivity of peak serum miR-122 with the extent of liver necrosis as judged histologically than that of peak serum ALT [18]. The marked rise in miR-122 we observed confirms at least a substantial contribution of liver-specific injury to the biomarker elevations we observed during cholestyramine treatment. In addition, it is doubtful that miR-122

Table 1 Classical clinical chemistry parameters following cholestyramine administration in placebo- or moxifloxacin-treated subjects

Subject#	Treatment type	ALT (U/L) baseline	ALT (U/L) peak	Peak ALT(ULN)	AST (ULN)	ALP (ULN)	Total bilirubin (ULN)
1	Placebo	16	273	6.1	1.8	1.0	0.6
2	Placebo	19	320	9.4	3.6	0.7	0.4
3	Placebo	15	967	28.4	10.9	0.9	0.6
4	Placebo	18	119	3.5	1.9	0.7	0.5
5	Placebo	16	145	4.3	2.6	0.6	0.8
6	Placebo	12	146	4.3	2.6	0.6	0.4
7	Moxifloxacin	33	164	3.6	1.8	1.1	0.3
8	Moxifloxacin	32	173	3.8	2.0	0.6	0.5
9	Moxifloxacin	30	229	5.1	2.7	1.4	0.9
10	Moxifloxacin	14	142	3.2	1.5	0.7	0.9
11	Moxifloxacin	20	136	4.0	1.9	0.8	0.4

For ALT, both absolute peak value and ULN have been included. For AST, ALP, and total Bilirubin only ULN have been included.

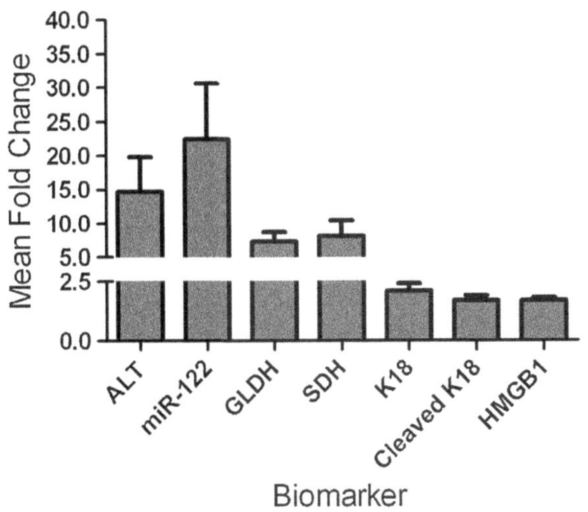

Figure 3 Fold changes in investigational new biomarkers. Values are mean ± SEM fold changes post vs pre cholestyramine administration, N = 11, represented as fold change post-dosing over pre-dosing.

and the multiple liver proteins assayed share pathways for degradation or elimination in serum, indicating that accumulation in serum due to reduced clearance is unlikely.

Cholestyramine treatment produced increases in mean serum levels of GLDH, SDH, and HMGB1 which have been proposed as specific indicators of necrosis [8,17]. SDH is located primarily in liver and kidney; activity of SDH increases rapidly in acute episodes of liver necrosis [19]. HMGB1 is a non-histone nuclear protein that is abundant in the nucleus of cells [20]. The elevations we observed in the serum levels of these biomarkers support the occurrence of hepatocellular necrosis, rather than membrane blebbing or other mechanisms that could result in cytosol leakage from viable hepatocytes.

We also observed a rise in the serum concentration of caspase-cleaved cytokeratin18 fragments (M30) which supports occurrence of hepatocellular apoptosis due to cholestyramine administration [5,6]. Because it is possible for a toxic injury to result in apoptosis when sufficient cellular ATP levels are maintained, but progress to necrosis as the injury is more severe, we examined whether the ratio of cleaved to total cytokeratin 18 differed between those subjects with highest and lowest levels of ALT or miR-122 levels. No differences were evident, (Additional file 4: Table S3) so a shift from apoptosis to necrosis with injury progression was not supported by these data. The reasons why this low-level and clinically insignificant injury never progresses toward a more serious toxicity are not clear.

The mechanisms by which cholestyramine treatment could cause mild hepatocyte necrosis/apoptosis, and why this is without any clinical consequence was not the focus of our study and remains unclear. Cholestyramine is neither metabolized nor absorbed from the GI tract so it could not have a direct effect on the liver. We speculate that the interruption of enterohepatic cycling of essential fat-soluble molecules and/or bile acids by cholestyramine may lead to alterations in membrane integrity or compensatory increase in bile acid synthesis, and this may indirectly result in transient necrosis and activation of apoptotic pathways. However, cholestyramine administration leading to increased bile acid synthesis has not been associated with significant impacts on hepatocytes, which appear to adapt to the change [21]. There is experimental evidence that cholestyramine increases activation of c-JUN N-terminal protein kinase (JNK) in the context of acetaminophen overdose in mice, but this activation is not present without the acetaminophen challenge [22]. Interestingly, cholestyramine feeding alone did not alter hepatocellular levels of glutathione, indicating that cholestyramine itself does not elicit a pro-oxidant or injurious response, even at high exposure levels comprising 2% of the diet [22]. Bertolotti *et al.* observed that *in vivo* administration of cholestyramine induced a significant dose-related increase of 7α-hydroxylation along with a decrease in the concentrations of plasma cholesterol [23]. A decrease in the concentrations of circulating bile acids trigger a disinhibition of cholesterol 7α -hydroxylase, also known as CYP7A1, resulting in enhanced production of bile acids and reduced level of cholesterol in hepatocytes. Long term cholestyramine treatment also decreased the intestinal expression of genes involved in drug transport, cholesterol metabolism, and apoprotein synthesis - MRP2,

Table 2 Pearson correlation between experimental new biomarkers and ALT

	ALT	SDH	GLDH	miR-122	K18	Cleaved K18	HMGB1
ALT		0.87*	0.45	0.53	0.31	−0.11	−0.16
SDH	0.87*		0.62*	0.39	0.44	0.22	0.08
GLDH	0.45	0.62*		0.11	0.83*	0.13	−0.25
miR-122	0.53	0.39	0.11		0.03	0.00	−0.52
K18	0.31	0.44	0.83*	0.03		0.29	−0.30
Cleaved K18	−0.11	0.22	0.13	0.00	0.29		0.17
HMGB1	−0.16	0.08	−0.25	−0.52	−0.30	0.17	

*Indicates significant correlation, P < 0.05.

ABCG5, ABCG8, SHP and SREBP-1c, and increased the hepatic expression - HMG-CoA reductase, CYP7A1, LDL receptor and LXRα genes [24,25]. How changes in the lipid, cholesterol and bile acid flux and altered hepatic metabolism by cholestyramine could rapidly translate into hepatocyte death is unclear but the rise in serum GLDH we observed may provide some insight. GLDH is a large protein localized in the mitochondrial matrix; its presence in blood reflects loss of mitochondrial integrity. Hence, it could be concluded that rises in serum GLDH during liver injury implicate mitochondrial dysfunction as a mechanisms underlying the necrosis [26]. Certain bile acids have been shown to cause mitochondrial dysfunction [27] and this could provide a mechanistic link between interruption in enterohepatic cycling, the proposed compensatory increase in bile acid synthesis, and hepatocyte death. One caveat is that our serum was not specifically prepared to eliminate mitochondria prior to freezing, and our serum samples underwent a freeze-thaw cycle which may have caused damage to intact mitochondria with leakage of detectable GLDH [26].

We have recently applied the same biomarkers used in the current study to serum samples obtained in healthy volunteers treated with various heparins [15]. Heparins, like cholestyramine, are known to cause marked elevations in serum ALT and AST, but these elevations are considered safe since heparins have not been reported to cause clinically important liver injury. In the heparin study, we also observed elevations in miR-122, serum GLDH and HMGB1 and concluded that mild and transient hepatocellular necrosis was occurring. However, despite the fact that the mean elevations of serum ALT and miR-122 are comparable in both the heparin and current cholestyramine studies, the serum HMGB1 level rose an average of 6.3-fold baseline in the heparin study but only a 1.7-fold increase was observed in the current study. Since we had only single serum samples from each subject, we could not test the hypothesis that this apparent discrepancy resulted from the kinetics of release and clearance of HMGB1. It should also be noted that in contrast to our current observations with cholestyramine, we did not find any rise in caspase-cleaved cytokeratin-18 (M-30) in the heparin study and concluded that heparins do not cause apoptosis. Because little HMGB1 is released from cells undergoing apoptosis [28], a reasonable conclusion is that the component of apoptosis caused by cholestyramine may in part explain the relatively low levels of HMGB1 we observed.

An important question is whether the magnitude of rise in the mechanistic biomarkers observed during benign ALT elevations (due to heparin or cholestyramine) is lower than would be observed during comparable ALT elevations produced by drugs capable of causing severe liver injury. If so, then there may be a threshold of concern that could be determined. Owing to the recent discovery and validation efforts for these biomarkers, standard ranges for human studies have not been established and, thus, these biomarkers may be more informative for determining tissue origin and gaining mechanistic insight. A recent publication by Antoine *et al.* investigated the same experimental liver injury biomarkers in the context of acute acetaminophen-induced liver injury in the clinic [29]. Comparison of the data from the acetaminophen study is complicated by the differences in dose, hospital presentation times, and study enrollment times of the acute injury patients. However, the values for serum ALT, GLDH, M65, and M30 measured in the present cholestyramine study were inclusive within the ranges observed for patients who developed clinically significant liver injury due to acetaminophen overdose (Additional file 5: Table S4). The observation could be partially explained by differences in sample collection and instrumentation between the two studies. However, this finding appears to support the assertion that the magnitude of elevation for GLDH, M65, and M30, does not strictly indicate a potential for overt liver injury in a given patient or study subject.

Conclusion

Our biomarker data support the conclusion that the elevation in serum aminotransferases that occurs as a result of cholestyramine treatment reflects both necrosis and apoptosis of hepatocytes. This was an unexpected finding since cholestyramine has never been reported to cause clinically important liver injury. Caution must therefore be used when interpreting elevations in these markers in the context of assessing liver safety of new drug candidates in clinical trials. We believe that the application of these and other new biomarkers will have a future role in monitoring liver safety in clinical trials but additional validation studies with DILI negative and DILI positive compounds in both nonclinical and clinical settings are needed.

Additional files

Additional file 1: CONSORT 2010 Flow Diagram.

Additional file 2: CONSORT 2010 checklists.

Additional file 3: Pre and post-dosing values for investigational protein biomarkers.

Additional file 4: Ratio of cleaved to total cytokeratin 18 in individuals with largest and smallest elevation in ALTs.

Additional file 5: A comparison of Cholestyramine vs. Acetaminophen-induced elevation in biomarkers of liver safety.

Abbreviations

ALT: Alanine aminotransferase; AT: Aminotransferase; M65: Cytokeratin-18 full length; M30: Cytokeratin cleaved; DILI: Drug-induced liver injury; GLDH: Glutamate dehydrogenase; HMGB1: High-mobility group box- 1; MiR-122: MicroRNA-122; SDH: Sorbitol dehydrogenase; ULN: Upper limit of normal.

Competing interests

Authors: A.H. had no support from any organization for the submitted work; no financial relationships with any organizations that might have an interest in the submitted work in the previous 3 years. R.S., F.M-V, Z.J., and H.B. are currently employed and have had support from Sanofi in the previous 3 years. P.W. serves as a scientific advisor to Sanofi. There are no other relationships or activities that could appear to have influenced the submitted work.

Authors' contributions

RS, AH, and PW analyzed the biomarker data. FM-V, ZJ, and HB designed the clinical protocol and helped analyze the biomarker data. All authors contributed to the writing of the manuscript.

Acknowledgements

We thank James Morelli for helping us with the figures.

Author details

[1]Sanofi, Disposition, Safety and Animal Research, Framingham, MA 01701, USA. [2]The Hamner-University of North Carolina Institute for Drug Safety Sciences, 6 Davis Drive, Research Triangle Park, NC 27709, USA. [3]Sanofi, 1 Ave Pierre Brossolette - 91385 Chilly-Mazarin Cedex, Paris, France. [4]Schools of Medicine, Pharmacy and Public Health, University of North Carolina at Chapel Hill, Chapel Hill, NC 27599, USA.

References

1. Senior JR: **Alanine aminotransferase: a clinical and regulatory tool for detecting liver injury-past, present, and future.** *Clin Pharmacol Ther* 2012, **92**:332–339.
2. *Guidance for Industry: Drug-Induced Liver Injury: Premarketing Clinical Evaluation.* [http://www.fda.gov/downloads/Drugs/GuidanceCompliance RegulatoryInformation/Guidance/UCM174090.pdf]
3. Watkins PB: **Drug safety sciences and the bottleneck in drug development.** *Clin Pharmacol Ther* 2011, **89**:788–790.
4. Antoine DJ, Jenkins RE, Dear JW, Williams DP, McGill MR, Sharpe MR, Craig DG, Simpson KJ, Jaeschke H, Park BK: **Molecular forms of HMGB1 and keratin-18 as mechanistic biomarkers for mode of cell death and prognosis during clinical acetaminophen hepatotoxicity.** *J Hepatol* 2012, **56**:1070–1079.
5. Antoine DJ, Williams DP, Kipar A, Jenkins RE, Regan SL, Sathish JG, Kitteringham NR, Park BK: **High-mobility group box-1 protein and keratin-18, circulating serum proteins informative of acetaminophen-induced necrosis and apoptosis in vivo.** *Toxicol Sci: Off J Soc Toxicol* 2009, **112**:521–531.
6. Guicciardi ME, Gores GJ: **Apoptosis: a mechanism of acute and chronic liver injury.** *Gut* 2005, **54**:1024–1033.
7. Rovere-Querini P, Capobianco A, Scaffidi P, Valentinis B, Catalanotti F, Giazzon M, Dumitriu IE, Muller S, Iannacone M, Traversari C, Bianchi ME, Manfredi AA: **HMGB1 is an endogenous immune adjuvant released by necrotic cells.** *EMBO Rep* 2004, **5**:825–830.
8. Schmidt ES, Schmidt FW: **Glutamate dehydrogenase: biochemical and clinical aspects of an interesting enzyme.** *Clin Chim Acta* 1988, **173**:43–55.
9. Starkey Lewis PJ, Dear J, Platt V, Simpson KJ, Craig DG, Antoine DJ, French NS, Dhaun N, Webb DJ, Costello EM, Neoptolemos JP, Moggs J, Goldring CE, Park BK: **Circulating microRNAs as potential markers of human drug-induced liver injury.** *Hepatology* 2011, **54**:1767–1776.
10. Ast M, Frishman WH: **Bile acid sequestrants.** *J Clin Pharmacol* 1990, **30**:99–106.
11. Jahnchen E, Meinertz T, Gilfrich HJ, Kersting F, Groth U: **Enhanced elimination of warfarin during treatment with cholestyramine.** *Br J Clin Pharmacol* 1978, **5**:437–440.
12. Mela M, Mancuso A, Burroughs AK: **Review article: pruritus in cholestatic and other liver diseases.** *Aliment Pharmacol Ther* 2003, **17**:857–870.
13. **A multicenter comparison of lovastatin and cholestyramine therapy for severe primary hypercholesterolemia. The Lovastatin Study Group III.** *JAMA* 1988, **260**:359–366.
14. **Comparative efficacy and safety of pravastatin and cholestyramine alone and combined in patients with hypercholesterolemia. Pravastatin Multicenter Study Group II.** *Arch Intern Med* 1993, **153**:1321–1329.
15. Harrill AH, Roach J, Fier I, Eaddy JS, Kurtz CL, Antoine DJ, Spencer DM, Kishimoto TK, Pisetsky DS, Park BK, Watkins PB: **The effects of heparins on the liver: application of mechanistic serum biomarkers in a randomized study in healthy volunteers.** *Clin Pharmacol Ther* 2012, **92**:214–220.
16. Kroh EM, Parkin RK, Mitchell PS, Tewari M: **Analysis of circulating microRNA biomarkers in plasma and serum using quantitative reverse transcription-PCR (qRT-PCR).** *Methods* 2010, **50**:298–301.
17. O'Brien PJ, Slaughter MR, Polley SR, Kramer K: **Advantages of glutamate dehydrogenase as a blood biomarker of acute hepatic injury in rats.** *Lab Anim* 2002, **36**:313–321.
18. Laterza OF, Lim L, Garrett-Engele PW, Vlasakova K, Muniappa N, Tanaka WK, Johnson JM, Sina JF, Fare TL, Sistare FD, Glaab WE: **Plasma MicroRNAs as sensitive and specific biomarkers of tissue injury.** *Clin Chem* 2009, **55**:1977–1983.
19. Dooley JF: **The role of clinical chemistry in chemical and drug safety evaluation by use of laboratory animals.** *Clin Chem* 1979, **25**:345–347.
20. Harris HE, Andersson U, Pisetsky DS: **HMGB1: a multifunctional alarmin driving autoimmune and inflammatory disease.** *Nat Rev Rheumatol* 2012, **8**:195–202.
21. Jolley CD, Dietschy JM, Turley SD: **Induction of bile acid synthesis by cholesterol and cholestyramine feeding is unimpaired in mice deficient in apolipoprotein AI.** *Hepatology* 2000, **32**:1309–1316.
22. Bhushan B, Borude P, Edwards G, Walesky C, Cleveland J, Li F, Ma X, Apte U: **Role of bile acids in liver injury and regeneration following acetaminophen overdose.** *Am J Pathol* 2013, **183**:1518–1526.
23. Bertolotti M, Abate N, Loria P, Concari M, Guicciardi ME, Dilengite MA, Bozzoli M, Carubbi F, Carulli N: **Regulation of bile acid synthesis in humans: studies on cholesterol 7 alpha-hydroxylation in vivo.** *Ital J Gastroenterol* 1995, **27**:446–449.
24. Kamisako T, Ogawa H, Yamamoto K: **Effect of cholesterol, cholic acid and cholestyramine administration on the intestinal mRNA expressions related to cholesterol and bile acid metabolism in the rat.** *J Gastroenterol Hepatol* 2007, **22**:1832–1837.
25. Felgines C, Mazur A, Rayssiguier Y: **Effect of the interruption of enterohepatic circulation of bile acids by cholestyramine on apolipoprotein gene expression in the rat.** *Life Sci* 1994, **55**:1053–1060.
26. Jaeschke H, McGill MR: **Serum glutamate dehydrogenase–biomarker for liver cell death or mitochondrial dysfunction?** *Toxicol Sci: Off J Soc Toxicol* 2013, **134**:221–222.
27. Schulz S, Schmitt S, Wimmer R, Aichler M, Eisenhofer S, Lichtmannegger J, Eberhagen C, Artmann R, Tookos F, Walch A, Krappmann D, Brenner C, Rust C, Zischka H: **Progressive stages of mitochondrial destruction caused by cell toxic bile salts.** *Biochimica Biophysica Acta* 1828, **2013**:2121–2133.
28. Scaffidi P, Misteli T, Bianchi ME: **Release of chromatin protein HMGB1 by necrotic cells triggers inflammation.** *Nature* 2002, **418**:191–195.
29. Antoine DJ, Dear JW, Lewis PS, Platt V, Coyle J, Masson M, Thanacoody RH, Gray AJ, Webb DJ, Moggs JG, Bateman DN, Goldring CE, Park BK: **Mechanistic biomarkers provide early and sensitive detection of acetaminophen-induced acute liver injury at first presentation to hospital.** *Hepatology* 2013, **58**:777–787.

Permissions

All chapters in this book were first published in BMCPT, by BioMed Central; hereby published with permission under the Creative Commons Attribution License or equivalent. Every chapter published in this book has been scrutinized by our experts. Their significance has been extensively debated. The topics covered herein carry significant findings which will fuel the growth of the discipline. They may even be implemented as practical applications or may be referred to as a beginning point for another development.

The contributors of this book come from diverse backgrounds, making this book a truly international effort. This book will bring forth new frontiers with its revolutionizing research information and detailed analysis of the nascent developments around the world.

We would like to thank all the contributing authors for lending their expertise to make the book truly unique. They have played a crucial role in the development of this book. Without their invaluable contributions this book wouldn't have been possible. They have made vital efforts to compile up to date information on the varied aspects of this subject to make this book a valuable addition to the collection of many professionals and students.

This book was conceptualized with the vision of imparting up-to-date information and advanced data in this field. To ensure the same, a matchless editorial board was set up. Every individual on the board went through rigorous rounds of assessment to prove their worth. After which they invested a large part of their time researching and compiling the most relevant data for our readers.

The editorial board has been involved in producing this book since its inception. They have spent rigorous hours researching and exploring the diverse topics which have resulted in the successful publishing of this book. They have passed on their knowledge of decades through this book. To expedite this challenging task, the publisher supported the team at every step. A small team of assistant editors was also appointed to further simplify the editing procedure and attain best results for the readers.

Apart from the editorial board, the designing team has also invested a significant amount of their time in understanding the subject and creating the most relevant covers. They scrutinized every image to scout for the most suitable representation of the subject and create an appropriate cover for the book.

The publishing team has been an ardent support to the editorial, designing and production team. Their endless efforts to recruit the best for this project, has resulted in the accomplishment of this book. They are a veteran in the field of academics and their pool of knowledge is as vast as their experience in printing. Their expertise and guidance has proved useful at every step. Their uncompromising quality standards have made this book an exceptional effort. Their encouragement from time to time has been an inspiration for everyone.

The publisher and the editorial board hope that this book will prove to be a valuable piece of knowledge for researchers, students, practitioners and scholars across the globe.

List of Contributors

Marina N Fogaça
Psychobiology Department, Federal University of São Paulo, Edifício de Ciências Biomédicas, Rua Botucatu 862 - 1° Andar, São Paulo, Brasil

Ruth F Santos-Galduróz
Laboratory of Physical Activity and Aging of Rio Claro Biosciences Institute - Universidade Paulista Júlio de Mesquita Filho, Rio Claro, São Paulo, Brasil and Centro de Matemática, Computação e Cognição da UFABC, Santo Andrá, São Paulo, Brasil

Jaqueline K Eserian
Psychobiology Department, Federal University of São Paulo, Edifício de Ciências Biomédicas, Rua Botucatu 862 - 1° Andar, São Paulo, Brasil

José Carlos F Galduróz
Psychobiology Department, Federal University of São Paulo, Edifício de Ciências Biomédicas, Rua Botucatu 862 - 1° Andar, São Paulo, Brasil

Kathryn A Ramsey
Division of Clinical Sciences, Telethon Institute for Child Health Research, 100 Roberts Road, Subiaco, WA 6008, Australia
Centre for Child Health Research, University of Western Australia, 100 Roberts Road, Subiaco, WA 6008, Australia

Alexander N Larcombe
Division of Clinical Sciences, Telethon Institute for Child Health Research, 100 Roberts Road, Subiaco, WA 6008, Australia
Centre for Child Health Research, University of Western Australia, 100 Roberts Road, Subiaco, WA 6008, Australia

Peter D Sly
Queensland Children's Medical Research Institute, University of Queensland, Level 4, Foundation Building, Herston Road, Herston, QLD 4029, Australia

Graeme R Zosky
Division of Clinical Sciences, Telethon Institute for Child Health Research, 100 Roberts Road, Subiaco, WA 6008, Australia
Centre for Child Health Research, University of Western Australia, 100 Roberts Road, Subiaco, WA 6008, Australia

Ian F Burgess
Medical Entomology Centre, Insect Research & Development Limited, Cambridge, UK

Nazma A Burgess
Medical Entomology Centre, Insect Research & Development Limited, Cambridge, UK

Elizabeth R Brunton
Medical Entomology Centre, Insect Research & Development Limited, Cambridge, UK

Oluseyi C Ayinde
Department of Biochemistry, College of Medicine, University of Lagos, Idi-Araba, Lagos, Nigeria

Sunday Ogunnowo
Department of Biochemistry, College of Medicine, University of Lagos, Idi-Araba, Lagos, Nigeria

Rita A Ogedegbe
Department of Biochemistry, College of Medicine, University of Lagos, Idi-Araba, Lagos, Nigeria

Angela Peichen Sun
Division of Applied Health Sciences, University of Aberdeen, King's College, Aberdeen AB24 3FX, UK

Bradley Kirby
Division of Applied Health Sciences, University of Aberdeen, King's College, Aberdeen AB24 3FX, UK

Corri Black
Division of Applied Health Sciences, University of Aberdeen, King's College, Aberdeen AB24 3FX, UK

Peter John Helms
Division of Applied Health Sciences, University of Aberdeen, King's College, Aberdeen AB24 3FX, UK

Marion Bennie
National Medicines Utilisation Unit, Information Services Division, NHS National Services Scotland, Edinburgh, Scotland

James Stuart McLay
Division of Applied Health Sciences, University of Aberdeen, King's College, Aberdeen AB24 3FX, UK
Department of Child Health, Royal Aberdeen Children's Hospital, Westburn Road, Aberdeen, Scotland AB25 2ZG, UK

Davide Crobu
Bio-Ker S.r.l.-Multimedica Group, Sardinia Scientific and Technological Park, Building 3, I-09010 Pula Cagliari, Italy

Gaia Spinetti
IRCCS MultiMedica, Laboratory of Diabetological Research, Milan, Italy

Rodolfo Schrepfer
Bio-Ker S.r.l.-Multimedica Group, Sardinia Scientific and Technological Park, Building 3, I-09010 Pula Cagliari, Italy

Giancarlo Tonon
Bio-Ker S.r.l.-Multimedica Group, Sardinia Scientific and Technological Park, Building 3, I-09010 Pula Cagliari, Italy

Gloria Saccani Jotti
Department of Biomedical, Biotechnological and Traslational Science (S.Bi.Bi.T.), University of Parma, via Volturno 39, 43121 Parma, Italy

Pierluigi Onali
Department of Biomedical Sciences, Laboratory of Cellular and Molecular Pharmacology, University of Cagliari, 09042 Monserrato Cagliari, Italy

Simona Dedoni
Department of Biomedical Sciences, Laboratory of Cellular and Molecular Pharmacology, University of Cagliari, 09042 Monserrato Cagliari, Italy

Gaetano Orsini
Bio-Ker S.r.l.-Multimedica Group, Sardinia Scientific and Technological Park, Building 3, I-09010 Pula Cagliari, Italy

Andrea Di Stefano
CROSS Research S.A, Phase I Unit, via F. A. Giorgioli 14, CH-6864 Arzo, Switzerland

Ann-Sofie Albrekt
Department of Immunotechnology, Lund University, Medicon Village building 406, 223 81 Lund, Sweden

Henrik Johansson
Department of Immunotechnology, Lund University, Medicon Village building 406, 223 81 Lund, Sweden

Anna Börje
Department of Chemistry and Molecular Biology, Dermatochemistry and Skin Allergy, University of Gothenburg, SE-412 96 Gothenburg, Sweden

Carl Borrebaeck
Department of Immunotechnology, Lund University, Medicon Village building 406, 223 81 Lund, Sweden

Malin Lindstedt
Department of Immunotechnology, Lund University, Medicon Village building 406, 223 81 Lund, Sweden

Hatem Sallam
Experimental Cancer Medicine (ECM), Laboratory Medicine, Karolinska Institutet, 141 86, Stockholm, Sweden

Ibrahim El-Serafi
Experimental Cancer Medicine (ECM), Laboratory Medicine, Karolinska Institutet, 141 86, Stockholm, Sweden

Laurent Meijer
C.N.R.S., 'Protein Phosphorylation and Human Disease' Group, C.N.R.S., Station Biologique, B.P. 74, 29682Roscoff cedex, Bretagne, France

Moustapha Hassan
Experimental Cancer Medicine (ECM), Laboratory Medicine, Karolinska Institutet, 141 86, Stockholm, Sweden
Experimental Cancer Medicine (ECM), Clinical Research Center, Novum, Karolinska University Hospital-Huddinge, 141 86, Stockholm, Sweden
ECM, KFC, Karolinska University Hospital, 141 86, Stockholm, Sweden

Sagita Dewi
Centre for Epidemiology and Biostatistics, Faculty of Veterinary Medicine and Biosciences, Norwegian University of Life Sciences, P.O. Box 5003, 1432 Ås, Norway

Tore Aune
Department of Food Safety and Infection Biology, Faculty of Veterinary Medicine and Biosciences, Norwegian University of Life Sciences, P.O. Box 5003, 1432 Ås, Norway

John A Aasen Bunæs
Department of Food Safety and Infection Biology, Faculty of Veterinary Medicine and Biosciences, Norwegian University of Life Sciences, P.O. Box 5003, 1432 Ås, Norway

Adrian J Smith
Norecopa, c/o Norwegian Veterinary Institute, P.O. Box 750, Sentrum 0106 Oslo, Norway

Stig Larsen
Centre for Epidemiology and Biostatistics, Faculty of Veterinary Medicine and Biosciences, Norwegian University of Life Sciences, P.O. Box 5003, 1432 Ås, Norway

José Antonio Vázquez
Grupo de Reciclado e Valorización de Residuos (REVAL), Instituto de Investigacións Mariñas (IIM-CSIC), C/ Eduardo Cabello 6, CP36208 Vigo, Spain

Therese Bredholt
Department of Clinical Science, University of Bergen, Bergen, Norway

Elisabeth Ersvær
Department of Clinical Science, University of Bergen, Bergen, Norway
Institute of Biomedical Laboratory Sciences, Bergen University College, Bergen, Norway

Bjarte Skoe Erikstein
Department of Clinical Science, University of Bergen, Bergen, Norway

André Sulen
Department of Clinical Science, University of Bergen, Bergen, Norway

Håkon Reikvam
Department of Clinical Science, University of Bergen, Bergen, Norway
Department of Internal Medicine, Haukeland University Hospital, Bergen, Norway

Hans Jørgen Aarstad
Department of Head and Neck Surgery, Haukeland University Hospital, Bergen, Norway
Department of Clinical Medicine, University of Bergen, Bergen, Norway

Anne Christine Johannessen
Department of Clinical Medicine, University of Bergen, Bergen, Norway
Department of Pathology, Haukeland University Hospital, Bergen, Norway

Olav Karsten Vintermyr
Department of Clinical Medicine, University of Bergen, Bergen, Norway
Department of Pathology, Haukeland University Hospital, Bergen, Norway

Øystein Bruserud
Department of Clinical Science, University of Bergen, Bergen, Norway
Department of Internal Medicine, Haukeland University Hospital, Bergen, Norway

Bjørn Tore Gjertsen
Department of Clinical Science, University of Bergen, Bergen, Norway
Department of Internal Medicine, Haukeland University Hospital, Bergen, Norway

Sergio Parra
Department of Pharmacology, University of Michigan, Ann Arbor, Michigan 48109, USA

Xinyan Huang
Department of Pharmacology, University of Michigan, Ann Arbor, Michigan 48109, USA

Raelene A Charbeneau
Department of Pharmacology, University of Michigan, Ann Arbor, Michigan 48109, USA

Susan M Wade
Department of Pharmacology, University of Michigan, Ann Arbor, Michigan 48109, USA

Kuljeet Kaur
Department of Pharmacology, University of Michigan, Ann Arbor, Michigan 48109, USA

Boyd R Rorabaugh
Department of Pharmaceutical and Biomedical Sciences, Ohio Northern University College of Pharmacy, Ada, OH 45810, USA

Richard R Neubig
Department of Pharmacology and Toxicology, B440 Life Sciences, Michigan State University, 1355 Bogue St, East Lansing, MI 48824, USA

Qing Wang
Department of Molecular Medicine and Surgery, Karolinska Institutet, SE-171 76 Stockholm, Sweden

Rickard Ljung
Department of Molecular Medicine and Surgery, Karolinska Institutet, SE-171 76 Stockholm, Sweden
Unit of Epidemiology, Institute of Environmental Medicine, Karolinska Institutet, Stockholm, Sweden

Jesper Lagergren
Department of Molecular Medicine and Surgery, Karolinska Institutet, SE-171 76 Stockholm, Sweden
Division of Cancer Studies, King's College London, London, United Kingdom

Yunxia Lu
Department of Molecular Medicine and Surgery, Karolinska Institutet, SE-171 76 Stockholm, Sweden
Department of Epidemiology and Biostatistics, Imperial College London, London, United Kingdom

Venkategowda Sunil
Connexios Life Sciences Pvt Ltd, #49, "SHILPA VIDYA" 1st Main, 3rd Phase, JP Nagar, Bangalore 560078, India

Mahesh Kumar Verma
Connexios Life Sciences Pvt Ltd, #49, "SHILPA VIDYA" 1st Main, 3rd Phase, JP Nagar, Bangalore 560078, India

Anup M Oommen
Connexios Life Sciences Pvt Ltd, #49, "SHILPA VIDYA" 1st Main, 3rd Phase, JP Nagar, Bangalore 560078, India

Manojkumar Sadasivuni
Connexios Life Sciences Pvt Ltd, #49, "SHILPA VIDYA" 1st Main, 3rd Phase, JP Nagar, Bangalore 560078, India

Jaideep Singh
Connexios Life Sciences Pvt Ltd, #49, "SHILPA VIDYA" 1st Main, 3rd Phase, JP Nagar, Bangalore 560078, India

Dasarahalli N Vijayraghav
Connexios Life Sciences Pvt Ltd, #49, "SHILPA VIDYA" 1st Main, 3rd Phase, JP Nagar, Bangalore 560078, India

Bhawna Chandravanshi
Connexios Life Sciences Pvt Ltd, #49, "SHILPA VIDYA" 1st Main, 3rd Phase, JP Nagar, Bangalore 560078, India

Jayalaxmi Shetty
Connexios Life Sciences Pvt Ltd, #49, "SHILPA VIDYA" 1st Main, 3rd Phase, JP Nagar, Bangalore 560078, India

Sanghamitra Biswas
Connexios Life Sciences Pvt Ltd, #49, "SHILPA VIDYA" 1st Main, 3rd Phase, JP Nagar, Bangalore 560078, India

Anilkumar Dandu
Connexios Life Sciences Pvt Ltd, #49, "SHILPA VIDYA" 1st Main, 3rd Phase, JP Nagar, Bangalore 560078, India

Yoganand Moolemath
Connexios Life Sciences Pvt Ltd, #49, "SHILPA VIDYA" 1st Main, 3rd Phase, JP Nagar, Bangalore 560078, India

Marikunte V Venkataranganna
Connexios Life Sciences Pvt Ltd, #49, "SHILPA VIDYA" 1st Main, 3rd Phase, JP Nagar, Bangalore 560078, India

Baggavalli P Somesh
Connexios Life Sciences Pvt Ltd, #49, "SHILPA VIDYA" 1st Main, 3rd Phase, JP Nagar, Bangalore 560078, India

Madanahalli R Jagannath
Connexios Life Sciences Pvt Ltd, #49, "SHILPA VIDYA" 1st Main, 3rd Phase, JP Nagar, Bangalore 560078, India

Lisa Drange Hole
Section of Clinical Pharmacology, Laboratory of Clinical Biochemistry, Haukeland University Hospital, 5021 Bergen, Norway

Terje Hjalmar Larsen
Institute of Biomedicine, University of Bergen, 5021 Bergen, Norway
Department of Heart Disease, Haukeland University Hospital, 5021 Bergen, Norway

Kjell Ove Fossan
Section of Clinical Pharmacology, Laboratory of Clinical Biochemistry, Haukeland University Hospital, 5021 Bergen, Norway

Fredrik Limé
Section of Clinical Pharmacology, Laboratory of Clinical Biochemistry, Haukeland University Hospital, 5021 Bergen, Norway

Jan Schjøtt
Section of Clinical Pharmacology, Laboratory of Clinical Biochemistry, Haukeland University Hospital, 5021 Bergen, Norway
Institute of Clinical Science, Faculty of Medicine and Dentistry, University of Bergen, 5021 Bergen, Norway

Robert Eggertsen
Department of Medicine/Primary Health Care, University of Gothenburg, Mölnlycke vårdcentral, Ekdalavägen 2, S 435 30, Mölnlycke, Sweden

Åke Andreasson
Landvetter vårdcentral, Centrumhuset, S 438 32, Landvetter, Sweden

Lennart Andrén
Department of Clinical Pharmacology, University of Gothenburg, Sahlgrenska University Hospital, S 413 45, Göteborg, Sweden

Ali S Alfazari
Department of Internal Medicine, United Arab Emirates University, Al Ain, Abu Dhabi, United Arab Emirates

Bayan Al-Dabbagh
Department of Internal Medicine, United Arab Emirates University, Al Ain, Abu Dhabi, United Arab Emirates

Saeeda Almarzooqi
Department of Pathology, United Arab Emirates University, Al Ain, Abu Dhabi, United Arab Emirates

Alia Albawardi
Department of Pathology, United Arab Emirates University, Al Ain, Abu Dhabi, United Arab Emirates

Abdul-Kader Souid
Department of Pediatrics, United Arab Emirates University, Al Ain, Abu Dhabi, United Arab Emirates

Nagesh Gowda
Connexios Life Sciences Pvt Ltd, #49, "SHILPA VIDYA" 1st Main, 3rd Phase, JP Nagar, Bangalore 560078, India

Anilkumar Dandu
Connexios Life Sciences Pvt Ltd, #49, "SHILPA VIDYA" 1st Main, 3rd Phase, JP Nagar, Bangalore 560078, India

Jaideep Singh
Connexios Life Sciences Pvt Ltd, #49, "SHILPA VIDYA" 1st Main, 3rd Phase, JP Nagar, Bangalore 560078, India

Sanghamitra Biswas
Connexios Life Sciences Pvt Ltd, #49, "SHILPA VIDYA" 1st Main, 3rd Phase, JP Nagar, Bangalore 560078, India

Vijaya Raghav
Connexios Life Sciences Pvt Ltd, #49, "SHILPA VIDYA" 1st Main, 3rd Phase, JP Nagar, Bangalore 560078, India

Mudigere N Lakshmi
Connexios Life Sciences Pvt Ltd, #49, "SHILPA VIDYA" 1st Main, 3rd Phase, JP Nagar, Bangalore 560078, India

Pavagada C Shilpa
Connexios Life Sciences Pvt Ltd, #49, "SHILPA VIDYA" 1st Main, 3rd Phase, JP Nagar, Bangalore 560078, India

Venkategowda Sunil
Connexios Life Sciences Pvt Ltd, #49, "SHILPA VIDYA" 1st Main, 3rd Phase, JP Nagar, Bangalore 560078, India

Ashokkumar Reddy
Connexios Life Sciences Pvt Ltd, #49, "SHILPA VIDYA" 1st Main, 3rd Phase, JP Nagar, Bangalore 560078, India

Manojkumar Sadasivuni
Connexios Life Sciences Pvt Ltd, #49, "SHILPA VIDYA" 1st Main, 3rd Phase, JP Nagar, Bangalore 560078, India

Kumaraswamy Aparna
Connexios Life Sciences Pvt Ltd, #49, "SHILPA VIDYA" 1st Main, 3rd Phase, JP Nagar, Bangalore 560078, India

Mahesh Kumar Verma
Connexios Life Sciences Pvt Ltd, #49, "SHILPA VIDYA" 1st Main, 3rd Phase, JP Nagar, Bangalore 560078, India

Yoganand Moolemath
Connexios Life Sciences Pvt Ltd, #49, "SHILPA VIDYA" 1st Main, 3rd Phase, JP Nagar, Bangalore 560078, India

Mammen O Anup
Connexios Life Sciences Pvt Ltd, #49, "SHILPA VIDYA" 1st Main, 3rd Phase, JP Nagar, Bangalore 560078, India

Marikunte V Venkataranganna
Connexios Life Sciences Pvt Ltd, #49, "SHILPA VIDYA" 1st Main, 3rd Phase, JP Nagar, Bangalore 560078, India

Baggavalli P Somesh
Connexios Life Sciences Pvt Ltd, #49, "SHILPA VIDYA" 1st Main, 3rd Phase, JP Nagar, Bangalore 560078, India

Madanahalli R Jagannath
Connexios Life Sciences Pvt Ltd, #49, "SHILPA VIDYA" 1st Main, 3rd Phase, JP Nagar, Bangalore 560078, India

Lisa Drange Hole, Kjell Ove Fossan and Fredrik Limé
Section of Clinical Pharmacology, Laboratory of Clinical Biochemistry, Haukeland University Hospital, 5021 Bergen, Norway

Terje Hjalmar Larsen
Institute of Biomedicine, University of Bergen, 5021 Bergen, Norway
Department of Heart Disease, Haukeland University Hospital, 5021 Bergen, Norway

Jan Schjøtt
Section of Clinical Pharmacology, Laboratory of Clinical Biochemistry, Haukeland University Hospital, 5021 Bergen, Norway
Institute of Clinical Science, Faculty of Medicine and Dentistry, University of Bergen, 5021 Bergen, Norway

Robert Eggertsen
Department of Medicine/Primary Health Care, University of Gothenburg, Mölnlycke vårdcentral, Ekdalavägen 2, S 435 30, Mölnlycke, Sweden

Åke Andreasson
Landvetter vårdcentral, Centrumhuset, S 438 32, Landvetter, Sweden

Lennart Andrén
Department of Clinical Pharmacology, University of Gothenburg, Sahlgrenska University Hospital, S 413 45, Göteborg, Sweden

Ali S Alfazari and Bayan Al-Dabbagh
Department of Internal Medicine, United Arab Emirates University, Al Ain, Abu Dhabi, United Arab Emirates

Saeeda Almarzooqi and Alia Albawardi
Department of Pathology, United Arab Emirates University, Al Ain, Abu Dhabi, United Arab Emirates

Abdul-Kader Souid
Department of Pediatrics, United Arab Emirates University, Al Ain, Abu Dhabi, United Arab Emirates

Nagesh Gowda, Anilkumar Dandu, Jaideep Singh, Sanghamitra Biswas, Vijaya Raghav, Mudigere N Lakshmi, Pavagada C Shilpa, Venkategowda Sunil, Ashokkumar Reddy, Manojkumar Sadasivuni, Kumaraswamy Aparna, Mahesh Kumar Verma, Yoganand Moolemath, Mammen O Anup, Marikunte V Venkataranganna, Baggavalli P Somesh and Madanahalli R Jagannath
Connexios Life Sciences Pvt Ltd, #49, "SHILPA VIDYA" 1st Main, 3rd Phase, JP Nagar, Bangalore 560078, India

Kennon Heard and Richard C Dart
Rocky Mountain Poison and Drug Center, Denver Health, Denver, CO, USA
University of Colorado Department of Emergency Medicine, Aurora, CO, USA

Jody L Green
Rocky Mountain Poison and Drug Center, Denver Health, Denver, CO, USA
Vanderbilt School of Nursing, Nashville, TN, USA

Victoria Anderson
Rocky Mountain Poison and Drug Center, Denver Health, Denver, CO, USA

Becki Bucher-Bartelson
Rocky Mountain Poison and Drug Center, Denver Health, Denver, CO, USA
Colorado School of Public Health, Aurora, CO, USA

Justin Mandala
FHI 360, 1825 Connecticut Ave, Suite 800, NW, Washington, DC 20009, USA

Kavita Nanda, Meng Wang, Jennifer Deese, and Douglas Taylor
FHI 360, Durham, NC, USA

Irith De Baetselier
Institute of Tropical Medicine, Antwerp, Belgium

Johan Lombaard
JOSHA Research, Bloemfontein, South Africa

Fredrick Owino
Impact Research and Development Organization, Kisumu, Kenya

Mookho Malahleha
Setshaba Research Centre, Soshanguve, Pretoria, South Africa

Rachel Manongi
Kilimanjaro Christian Medical Center, Kilimanjaro region, Tanzania

Lut Van Damme
FHI 360, 1825 Connecticut Ave, Suite 800, NW, Washington, DC 20009, USA
The Bill & Melinda Gates Foundation, Seattle, WA, USA

Sung Min Park, Sook Jin Seong, Mi-Ri Gwon, and Young-Ran Yoon
Clinical Trial Center, Kyungpook National University Hospital, Daegu, South Korea
Department of Biomedical Science, Kyungpook National University Graduate School, Daegu, South Korea
BK21 Plus KNU Bio-Medical Convergence Program for Creative Talent, Kyungpook National University Graduate School, 680 Gukchaebosang-ro, Jung-gu, Daegu 700-842, South Korea

Joomi Lee
Clinical Trial Center, Kyungpook National University Hospital, Daegu, South
Department of Biomedical Science, Kyungpook National University Graduate Korea School, Daegu, South Korea

Jong Gwang Park
Clinical Trial Center, Kyungpook National University Hospital, Daegu, South Korea

Mi-sun Lim
College of Pharmacy, Yeungnam University, Daegu, South Korea

Hae Won Lee
Clinical Trial Center, Kyungpook National University Hospital, Daegu, South Korea

Dong Heon Yang
Department of Internal Medicine, Division of Cardiology, Kyungpook National University School of Medicine, Daegu, South Korea

Kwang-Il Kwon
College of Pharmacy, Chungnam National University, Daejeon, South Korea

Seunghoon Han
Department of Pharmacology, College of Medicine, The Catholic University of Korea, Seoul, South Korea
PIPET (Pharmacometrics Institute for Practical Education and Training), Seoul, South Korea

Simon P Ramseier
Cantonal Hospital Aarau, Aarau, Switzerland

Serge Roth
Clinique de Carouge SA, Carouge, Switzerland

Adam Czaplinski
Neurocentre Bellevue, Theaterstrasse 8, Zurich CH-8001, Switzerland

Andrea C Tricco, Charlene Soobiah, Wing Hui, Jesmin Antony and Vladi Struchkov
Li Ka Shing Knowledge Institute, St. Michael's Hospital, 209 Victoria Street, East Building, Toronto, Ontario M5B 1 W8, Canada

Brian Hutton and David Moher
Clinical Epidemiology Program, Centre for Practice-Changing Research, Ottawa Hospital Research Institute, 725 Parkdale Ave., Ottawa, Ontario K1Y 4E9, Canada

Brenda Hemmelgarn
Departments of Medicine and Community Health Sciences, University of Calgary, TRW Building, 3rd Floor, 3280 Hospital Drive NW, Calgary, Alberta T2N 4Z6, Canada

Sharon E Straus
Li Ka Shing Knowledge Institute, St. Michael's Hospital, 209 Victoria Street, East Building, Toronto, Ontario M5B 1 W8, Canada
Department of Geriatric Medicine, Faculty of Medicine, University of Toronto, 27 Kings College Circle, Toronto, Ontario M5S 1A1, Canada

Olusegun K. Afolabi
Department of Biochemistry, Federal University of Agriculture, Abeokuta, Nigeria
Department of Biochemistry, Ladoke Akintola University of Technology, Ogbomosho, Nigeria

Adedoja D. Wusu and Olabisi O. Ogunrinola
Department of Biochemistry, Federal University of Agriculture, Abeokuta, Nigeria
Department of Biochemistry, Lagos State University, Ojoo, Lagos, Nigeria

Esther O. Abam
Department of Biochemistry, Federal University of Agriculture, Abeokuta, Nigeria
Biochemistry Unit, Department of Chemical Sciences, Bells University of Technology, Ota, Nigeria

David O. Babayemi, Oluwatosin. A. Dosumu, Okechukwu. B. Onunkwor and Oladipo Ademuyiwa
Department of Biochemistry, Federal University of Agriculture, Abeokuta, Nigeria

Elizabeth. A. Balogun
Department of Biochemistry, Federal University of Agriculture, Abeokuta, Nigeria
Department of Biochemistry, University of Ilorin, Ilorin, Nigeria

Olusegun O. Odukoya
Department of Chemistry, Federal University of Agriculture, Abeokuta, Nigeria

Bruce E. Miller and Ruth Tal-Singer
Clinical Discovery, Respiratory Therapy Area Unit, GlaxoSmithKline R&D, 709 Swedeland Road, King of Prussia, PA 19406, USA

Sunil Mistry
Clinical Statistics, GlaxoSmithKline R&D, Stockley Park West, Uxbridge, Middlesex UB11 1BT, UK

Kevin Smart
Clinical Pharmacology Modeling and Simulation, GlaxoSmithKline, London, UK
Roche Pharmaceuticals, Welwyn Garden City, UK

Paul Connolly
Product Development, Platform Technology and Science, GlaxoSmithKline R&D, Park Road, Ware, Hertfordshire SG 12 0DP, UK

Donald C. Carpenter
Respiratory Therapy Area Unit, GlaxoSmithKline R&D, 709 Swedeland Road, King of Prussia, PA 19406, USA

Hiran Cooray
Clinical Pharmacology Sciences and Study Operations, GlaxoSmithKline, London, UK
Global Development, Amgen Inc., Horsham, West Sussex, UK

Jackie C. Bloomer
Drug Metabolism and Pharmacokinetics, GlaxoSmithKline R&D, Park Road, Ware, Hertfordshire SG 12 0DP, UK

Aili L. Lazaar
Discovery Medicine, Respiratory Therapy Area Unit, GlaxoSmithKline R&D, 709 Swedeland Road, King of Prussia, PA 19406, USA

Simone Azevedo de Zanette, Rafael Vercelino, Gabriela Laste, Joanna Ripoll Rozisky, André Schwertner and Alicia Deitos
Post Graduate Program in Medical Sciences, School of Medicine, Universidade Federal do Rio Grande do Sul (UFRGS), Porto Alegre, Brazil
Laboratory of Pain & Neuromodulation, Institution: Hospital de Clínicas de Porto Alegre at UFRGS, Rua Ramiro Barcelos, 2350 - CEP 90035-003 Bairro Rio Branco, Porto Alegre, Brazil

Caroline Buzzatti Machado
Pain and Palliative Care Service at the Hospital de Clínicas de Porto Alegre (HCPA), Universidade Federal do Rio Grande do Sul (UFRGS), Porto Alegre, Brazil

Fernando Xavier and Izabel Cristina Custódio de Souza
Laboratory of Pain & Neuromodulation, Institution: Hospital de Clínicas de Porto Alegre at UFRGS, Rua Ramiro Barcelos, 2350 - CEP 90035-003 Bairro Rio Branco, Porto Alegre, Brazil

Iraci L S Torres
Pharmacology Department, Instituto de Ciências Básicas da Saúde, UFRGS, Porto Alegre, Brazil
Post Graduate Program in Medical Sciences, School of Medicine, Universidade Federal do Rio Grande do Sul (UFRGS), Porto Alegre, Brazil

Laboratory of Pain & Neuromodulation, Institution: Hospital de Clínicas de Porto Alegre at UFRGS, Rua Ramiro Barcelos, 2350 - CEP 90035-003 Bairro Rio Branco, Porto Alegre, Brazil

Wolnei Caumo
Pain and Palliative Care Service at the Hospital de Clínicas de Porto Alegre (HCPA), Universidade Federal do Rio Grande do Sul (UFRGS), Porto Alegre, Brazil
Pharmacology Department, Instituto de Ciências Básicas da Saúde, UFRGS, Porto Alegre, Brazil
Post Graduate Program in Medical Sciences, School of Medicine, Universidade Federal do Rio Grande do Sul (UFRGS), Porto Alegre, Brazil
Laboratory of Pain & Neuromodulation, Institution: Hospital de Clínicas de Porto Alegre at UFRGS, Rua Ramiro Barcelos, 2350 - CEP 90035-003 Bairro Rio Branco, Porto Alegre, Brazil

Rohit Singhal and Zaid Jayyosi
Sanofi, Disposition, Safety and Animal Research, Framingham, MA 01701, USA

Alison H Harrill
The Hamner-University of North Carolina Institute for Drug Safety Sciences, 6 Davis Drive, Research Triangle Park, NC 27709, USA

Francoise Menguy-Vacheron and Hadj Benzerdjeb
Sanofi, 1 Ave Pierre Brossolette - 91385 Chilly-Mazarin Cedex, Paris, France

Paul B Watkins
The Hamner-University of North Carolina Institute for Drug Safety Sciences, 6 Davis Drive, Research Triangle Park, NC 27709, USA
Schools of Medicine, Pharmacy and Public Health, University of North Carolina at Chapel Hill, Chapel Hill, NC 27599, USA